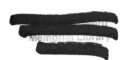

SONOGRAPHY

**Introduction to Normal Structure
and Function**

SONOGRAPHY

Introduction to Normal Structure and Function

REVA ARNEZ CURRY, PhD, RT(R), RDMS, FSDMS
Vice-President of Student Services
Salem Community College
Carney's Point, New Jersey

BETTY BATES TEMPKIN, BA, RT(R), RDMS
Ultrasound Consultant
Formerly, Clinical Director
Diagnostic Medical Sonography Program
Hillsborough Community College
Tampa, Florida

SECOND EDITION

with 1200 illustrations

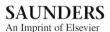

SAUNDERS
An Imprint of Elsevier

SAUNDERS
An Imprint of Elsevier

11830 Westline Industrial Drive
St. Louis, Missouri 63146

Previous edition copyrighted 1995

ISBN-13: 978-0-7216-9780-2
ISBN-10: 0-7216-9780-1

Publisher: Andrew Allen
Acquisitions Editor: Jeanne Wilke
Senior Developmental Editor: Linda Woodard
Publishing Services Manager: Pat Joiner
Project Manager: David Stein
Design Manager: Gail Morey Hudson

Printed in the United States of America

Last digit is the print number: 9 8 7 6 5

My efforts with this textbook would not have been possible
without the love, encouragement, and support from my husband, **Dwight,**
and growing adult family: **Tiana, Serena, Omar,** and **Jeremy.**
Thank you, **Dr. Raymond M. Gordon,** for your guidance and support.
I'd like to extend a special thank you to **Dr. Jerome Cunningham,**
my first teacher in ultrasound, who taught me to appreciate
sonography and what I could contribute to the profession,
and to my mentor, **Dr. Barry B. Goldberg,** who has been unfailing in his
support for sonographers, and a teacher, guide, and role model for me.

R.A.C.

Gratefully dedicated to M.M.T. and D.L.T. for the time this edition
required and for always sharing the best of themselves with me.

B.B.T.

Reviewers

GINA M. AUGUSTINE, MLS, RT(R)
Director, School of Radiography and Specialty Programs
Jameson Health System
New Castle, Pennsylvania

JAN D. BRYANT, MS, RDMS
Program Director
El Centro College
Dallas, Texas

ADELIA THAL BULLINS, RDMS, RVT, BS, AAS, CNMT, RT(N)
Clinical Coordinator
Forsyth Technical Community College
Winston Salem, North Carolina

JOAN M. CLASBY, BvE, RDMS, RT, RDCS
Professor, Diagnostic Medical Sonography
Program Director, Orange Coast College
Costa Mesa, California

CAROLYN T. COFFIN, MPH, RT, RDMS, RVT, RDCS
Educational Coordinator
University of Colorado Hospital
University of Colorado Health Science Center
Denver, Colorado

STEPHANIE J. ELLINGSON, BA, RDMS, RDCS, RVT, RTR
Program Director
University of Iowa Hospitals and Clinics
Iowa City, Iowa

SUSANNA OVEL, RDMS, RVT
Senior Sonographer / Trainer
Radiological Associates of Sacramento
Sacramento, California

REGINA SWEARENGIN, BS, RDMS (AB, ON, NE)
Sonography Department Chair
Austin Community College
Austin, Texas

THOMAS F. WALSH, MA, RDMS
Program Director
Middlesex Community College
Bedford, Massachusetts

Contributors

PEGGY MALZI BIZJAK, BBA, RDMS, RT(R)(M)
Imaging Chief/Manager
Department of Radiology, Ultrasound Division
University of Virginia Health System
Charlottesville, Virginia
The Female Pelvis, First Trimester Obstetrics, Second and Third Trimester Obstetrics, High-Risk Obstetric Sonography

REVA ARNEZ CURRY, PhD, RT(R), RDMS, FSDMS
Dean of Student Services
Salem Community College
Carney's Point, New Jersey
The Pancreas, The Urinary System, The Neonatal Brain, Three-Dimensional Ultrasound

MARILYN DICKERSON, MEd, MPH, RDMS
Vascular Technologist
Department of Radiology
Crawford Long Hospital of Emory Hospital
Atlanta, Georgia
The Liver, The Gastrointestinal System

KATHRYN A. GILL, MS, RT, RDMS
Program Director
Institute of Ultrasound Diagnostics
Daphne, Alabama
Introduction to Ultrasound of Human Disease, Appendices I and V

CANDYCE JAMES, BS, RDMS
Sonographer
The Imaging Center of Aiken
Aiken, Georgia
The Abdominal Aorta, The Inferior Vena Cava, The Portal Venous System, The Biliary System, The Pancreas, The Urinary System, The Spleen

MICHAEL J. KAMMERMEIER, BSRT, RDMS, RVT
Clinical Specialist
GE Ultrasound, Inc.
Milwaukee, Wisconsin
The Male Pelvis, Three-Dimensional Ultrasound

ALEXANDER LANE, PhD
Coordinator of Anatomy and Physiology
Triton College
River Grove, Illinois
Anatomy Layering and Sectional Anatomy

WAYNE C. LEONHARDT, BA, RT, RDMS, RVT, APS
Lead Sonographer,
Technical Director and Continuing Education Coordinator
Alta Bates Summit Medical Center
Summit Campus Ultrasound Section
Oakland, California
Clinical Instructor, Foothill College School of Ultrasound
Los Altos, California
The Thyroid and Parathyroid Glands

VIVIE MILLER, BA, BS, RDMS, RDCS
Clinical Specialist
Hephizabah, Georgia
The Abdominal Aorta, The Inferior Vena Cava, The Portal Venous System, The Biliary System, The Pancreas, The Urinary System, The Spleen, Pediatric Echocardiography

MARSHA M. NEUMYER, BS, RVT
Director, Vascular Diagnostic Educational Services
A Division of Inside/Outside, L.L.C.
Harrisburg, Pennsylvania
Abdominal Vasculature, Vascular Technology

M. NATHAN PINKNEY, BS, RDMS
Medical Physicist, Sonicor, Inc.
West Point, Pennsylvania
Physics, Instrumentation

J. CHARLES POPE III, PAC, RDCS, RVS
Assistant Clinical Professor
Director, Echocardiography Laboratory
Cardiovascular Associates of Augusta
Augusta, Georgia
Adult Echocardiography

LISA STROHL, BS, RT(R), RDMS, RVT
Marketing Manager
Jefferson City Imaging
Philadelphia, Pennsylvania
Breast Sonography, Appendices I, II, III, and IV

BETTY BATES TEMPKIN, BA, RT(R), RDMS
Ultrasound Consultant, Formerly, Clinical Director
Diagnostic Medical Sonography Program
Hillsborough Community College
Tampa, Florida
Body Systems, Anatomy Layering and Sectional Anatomy, The Pancreas, The Urinary System, The Female Pelvis, First Trimester Obstetrics, Second and Third Trimester Obstetrics, High-Risk Obstetric Sonography, The Neonatal Brain, Introduction to Ultrasound of Human Disease, Interventional and Intraoperative Ultrasound, Appendix I

Preface

Many of you have told us how much you enjoyed the first edition of this textbook and workbook. Thank you for your support and encouragement over the years. As you will see in the following pages, we have pulled out all the stops for the second edition!

Several years in the making, we feel that we have improved on what was already a good product—a thorough overview of normal ultrasound anatomy and physiology delivered in a student-friendly manner, with easy to understand text, images, charts, tables, and study questions.

We have incorporated the comments and suggestions from many of our colleagues, ultrasound educators, supervisors, staff sonographers, and ultrasound students into the second edition. This new edition includes the following changes:

- New images and illustrations throughout the text
- Multiple examples of how to describe ultrasound findings
- Expanded information on how to image pathology
- Additional study questions added to each chapter of the workbook
- Addition of an appendix on Universal Precautions
- Expanded liver, gastrointestinal, vascular technology, and adult echocardiography chapters
- Substantially rewritten chapters including First Trimester Obstetrics, Second and Third Trimester Obstetrics, High-Risk Obstetric Sonography, The Female Pelvis, Introduction to Ultrasound of Human Disease, and Appendix I: Ultrasound Documents Related to Patient Examination
- New chapters, including Interventional and Intraoperative Ultrasound, Abdominal Vasculature, Three-Dimensional Ultrasound, and Your First Scanning Experience (moved from the previous edition's workbook to the textbook)
- Chapters reorganized as you requested: the abdominal vascular chapters now precede the abdominal organ chapters.

Our philosophy toward ultrasound education is simple: the more comfortable the new sonographer is with normal anatomy and physiology and normal ultrasound appearance, the easier it will be to recognize pathophysiology and differentiate abnormal ultrasound appearances. Hence, we spend a lot of time presenting many normal images with correlative gray scale illustrations to help the student understand sectional anatomy and its sonographic presentation.

Our learning strategy is a two-part repetition approach: first, repetition *within* each chapter through key words, multiple images, and detailed illustrations. Second, repetition *between* the textbook and the workbook—students are given another chance to study and work with images, this time without labeling. We feel this dual repetition approach is an effective method to help students process what they have learned from short-term into long-term memory. The end result, we hope, is improved didactic and clinical student performance from having studied and worked with our textbook and workbook.

Finally, we want to extend a special "thank you" to our contributors. Without you, this edition would not have been possible.

We hope you are as excited as we are about the second edition textbook and workbook. Please let us know what you think.

With Warm Regards and Best Wishes for Your Ultrasound Career.

Reva Arnez Curry
Betty Bates Tempkin

FOR INSTRUCTORS
Evolve—Online Course Management

Evolve is an interactive learning environment designed to work in coordination with *Sonography: Introduction to Normal Structure and Function.* Instructors may use Evolve to provide an Internet-based course component that reinforces and expands on the concepts delivered in class. Evolve may be used to publish the class syllabus, outlines, and lecture notes; set up "virtual office hours" and email communication; share important dates and information through the online class Calendar; and encourage student participation through Chat Rooms and Discussion Boards. Evolve allows instructors to post exams and manage their grade book online. For more information, visit http://www.evolve.elsevier.com or contact an Elsevier sales representative.

Contents

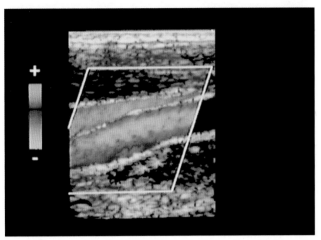

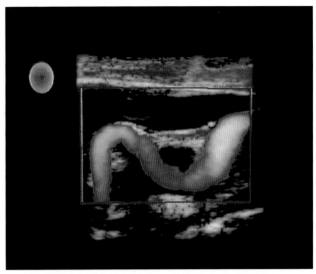

Plate 1   Color flow Doppler image (see Fig. 2-33).

Plate 2   Power Doppler image (see Fig. 2-34).

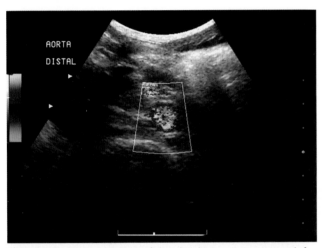

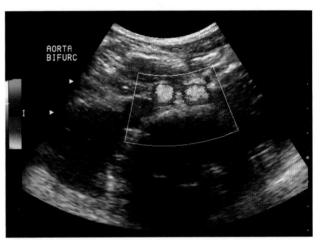

Plate 3   Transverse section of the distal aorta just prior to bifurcation into the common iliac arteries (see Fig. 5-13, *B*).

Plate 4   Color Doppler sonogram demonstrating the common iliac arteries (see Fig. 5-19).

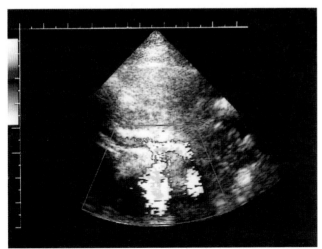

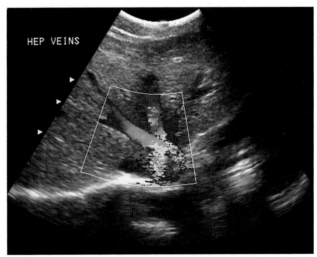

Plate 5   Color Doppler sonogram demonstrating flow within the aorta, celiac artery, splenic artery, and common hepatic artery (see Fig. 5-20).

Plate 6   Color image showing hepatic veins emptying into the inferior vena cava (see Fig. 6-7, *B*).

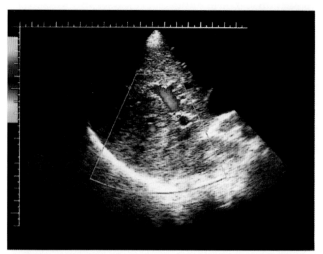

Plate 7 Longitudinal section of the right lobe of the liver demonstrating normal color flow Doppler. Note that flow toward the transducer is indicated in red. Thus the flow is toward the transducer (into the liver) in this case (see Fig. 7-12).

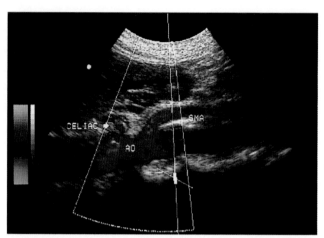

Plate 8 Longitudinal Doppler color flow image of the abdominal wall of the aorta (see Fig. 8-2).

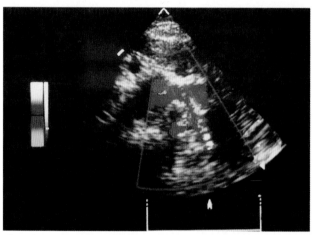

Plate 9 Transverse color flow image of the abdominal aorta showing the origin of the left renal artery (see Fig. 8-3).

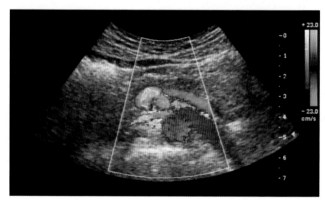

Plate 10 Transverse color flow image of the abdominal aorta (see Fig. 8-10).

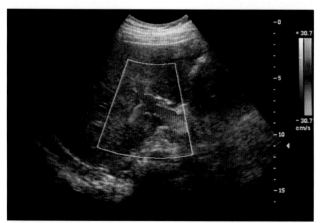

Plate 11 Oblique, longitudinal, intercostal color flow image of the main, right, and left portal veins (see Fig. 8-11).

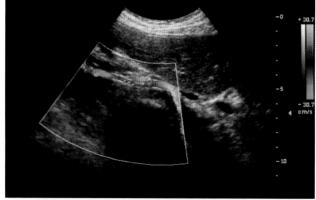

Plate 12 Color flow image of the hepatic artery at its origin from the celiac artery bifurcation (see Fig. 8-12, A).

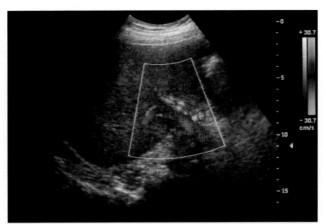

Plate 13 Color flow image of hepatic artery as it courses with portal vein in the portal hepatic (see Fig. 8-12, *B*).

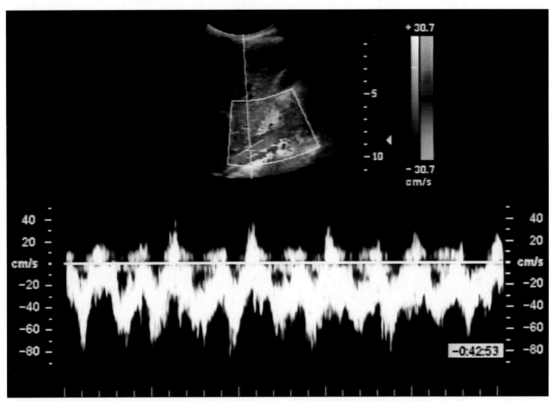

Plate 14 Doppler spectral waveform from the distal inferior vena cava (see Fig. 8-13, *A*).

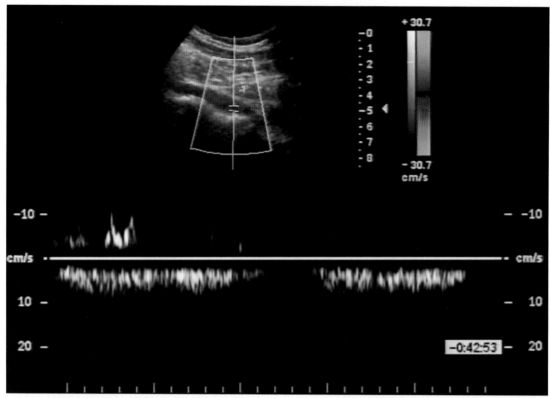

Plate 15 Doppler spectral waveform from the proximal inferior vena cava (see Fig. 8-13, *B*).

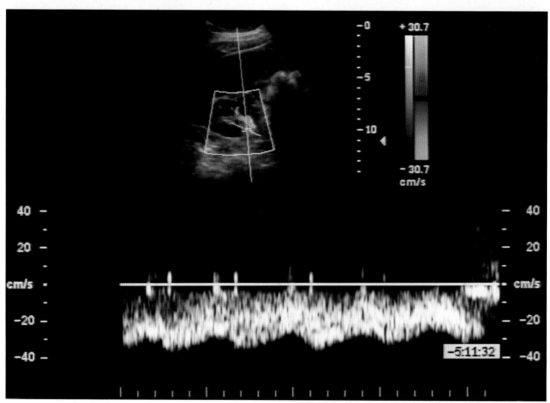

Plate 16 Doppler spectral waveform from the right renal vein (see Fig. 8-14).

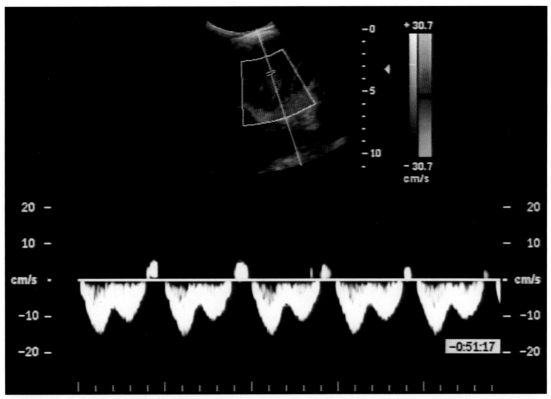

Plate 17 Doppler spectral waveform from the right renal vein (see Fig. 8-15).

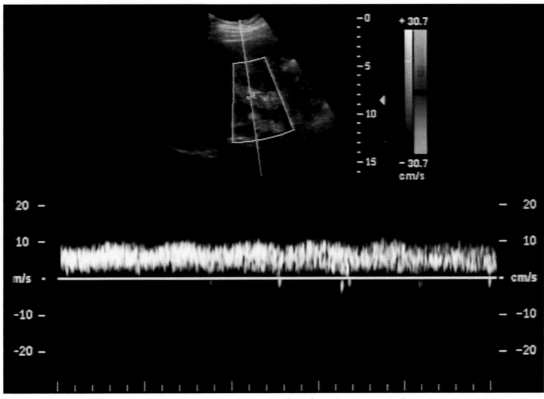

Plate 18 Minimally phasic Doppler spectral waveform from the main portal vein (see Fig. 8-16).

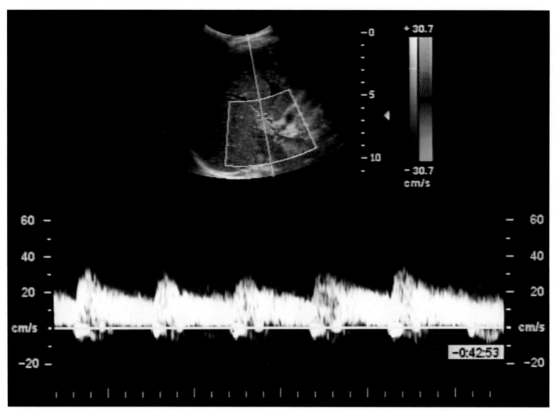

Plate 19 Low resistance Doppler spectral waveform pattern from the hepatic artery (see Fig. 8-17).

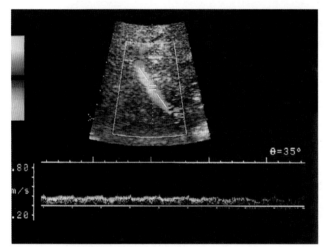

Plate 20 Color Doppler image showing the characteristic waveform of a normal portal vein. Note that the blood flow is in the direction of the liver toward the transducer (see Fig. 9-23).

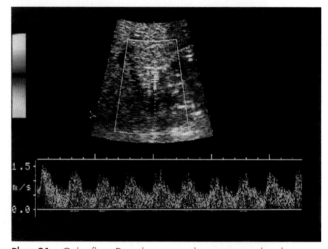

Plate 21 Color flow Doppler image demonstrating the characteristic arterial waveform of the normal hepatic artery (see Fig. 9-24).

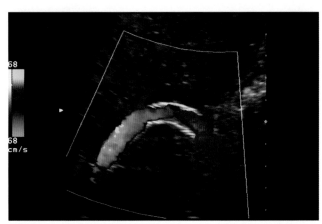

Plate 22 Color Doppler evaluation of a TIPS shunt connecting the hepatic vein to the intrahepatic portal vein. Note that the color blue represents flow away from the transducer (portal vein) (see Fig. 9-26).

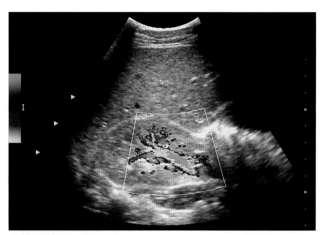

Plate 23 Color Doppler image of the right renal hilum. Transverse section of the right kidney shows the rounded pole. The liver is anterior. Note the hilar area, where the renal artery and vein are located (see Fig. 12-16).

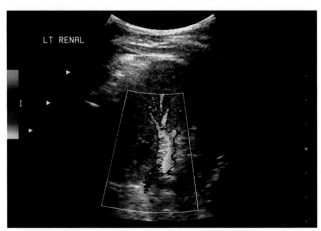

Plate 24 Transverse scan with color Doppler of the renal hilum of the left kidney (see Fig. 12-24).

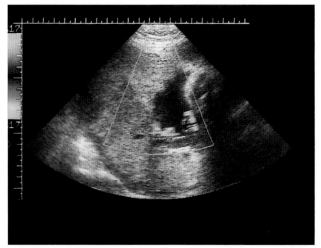

Plate 25 Color flow demonstration of the placental cord insertion site (see Fig. 17-24).

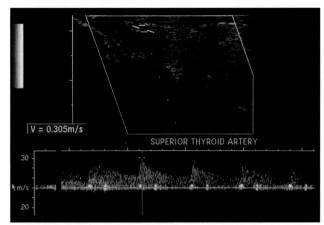

Plate 26 Color Doppler longitudinal section of the thyroid gland and superior thyroid artery demonstrating arterial flow with a peak systolic velocity of 0.305 m/s (see Fig. 20-3, *B*).

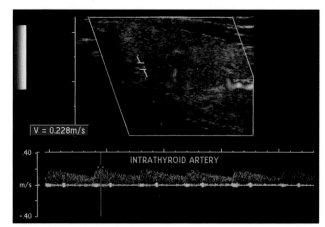

Plate 27 Color Doppler imaging of an intrathyroidal artery demonstrating a peak systolic velocity of 0.228 m/s (see Fig. 20-3, *C*).

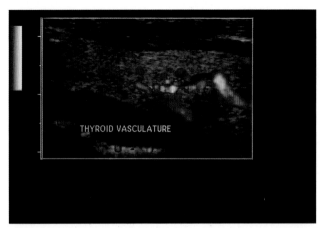

Plate 28 Color imaging longitudinal section of the thyroid gland demonstrating intrathyroid and extrathyroid vasculature (see Fig. 20-3, *D*).

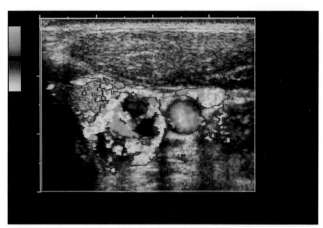

Plate 29 Color Doppler transverse image of a mid left parathyroid adenoma. Note the hypervascularization of the adenoma. Areas without color represent cystic areas. Note the relationship of the adenoma to the thyroid gland, common carotid artery, and jugular vein (see Fig. 20-17).

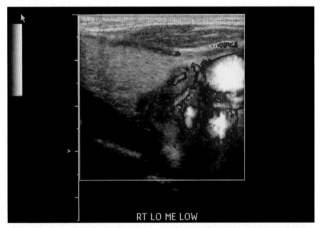

Plate 30 Color Doppler image of an inferior parathyroid adenoma. Note the feeder inferior thyroid artery supplying the adenoma (see Fig. 20-19).

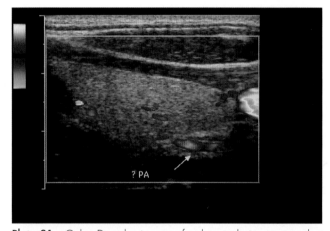

Plate 31 Color Doppler image of a hypoechoic structure that fills with color, indicating a vascular structure and not a parathyroid adenoma (see Fig. 20-20, *B*).

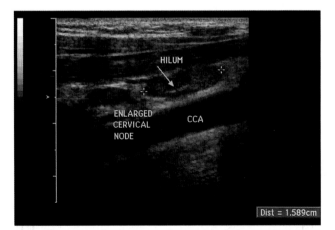

Plate 32 Longitudinal section of an enlarged hypoechoic cervical lymph node with echogenic hilum *(arrow)* adjacent to the common carotid artery. Note the position of calipers (see Fig. 20-21).

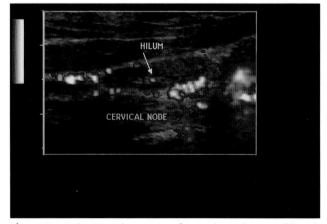

Plate 33 Color Doppler image of an enlarged cervical lymph node. Note the vascular flow within the hilum (see Fig. 20-22).

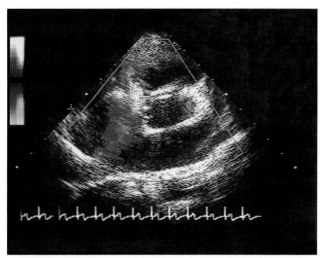

Plate 34 Parasternal short axis view showing color flow through the tricuspid valve. Note the blue color as the flow turns to move away from the transducer (see Fig. 23-21, *C*).

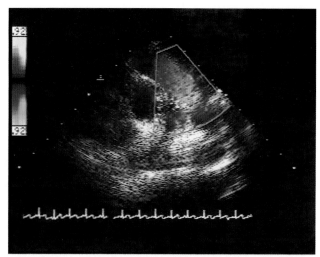

Plate 35 As flow continues from Plate 34, it is going away from the transducer through the pulmonary valve and into the right and left pulmonary branches (see Fig. 23-21, *D*).

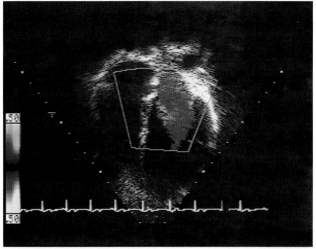

Plate 36 Color flow Doppler of the mitral valve. Echocardiographic image of inflow from the left atrium through the mitral valve into the left ventricle. The flow is red because it is moving toward the transducer positioned at the apex. Note the laminar flow (no turbulence) (see Fig. 23-25, *B*).

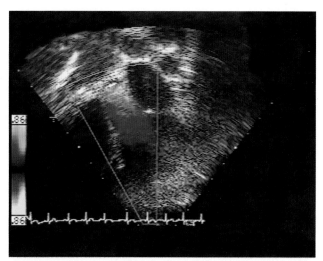

Plate 37 Apical long axis view showing color flow in the left ventricular outflow tract, through the aortic valve and a limited section of the ascending aorta. The transducer is at the apex of the heart with the flow moving away from it. Therefore the blood flow is shown in blue (see Fig. 23-26, *B*).

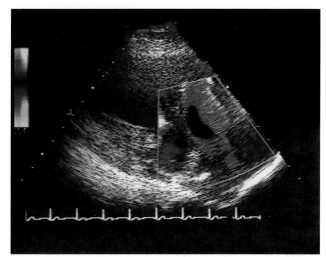

Plate 38 Color flow Doppler of the right ventricular inflow tract. The flow is toward the transducer from the right atrium through the tricuspid valve into the right ventricle (see Fig. 23-32, *C*).

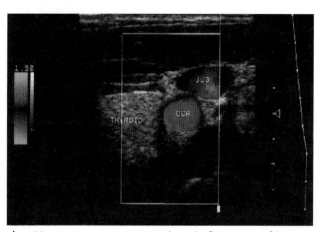

Plate 39 Transverse section, Doppler color flow image of the common carotid artery, jugular vein, and thyroid gland (see Fig. 25-3).

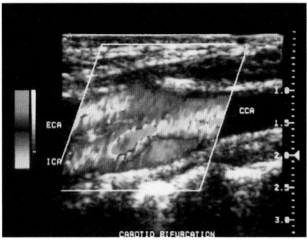

Plate 40 Long axis section, Doppler color flow image of the carotid bifurcation demonstrates the common, external and internal carotid arteries. Note the zone of retrograde flow in the carotid bulb caused by boundary layer separation (see Fig. 25-4).

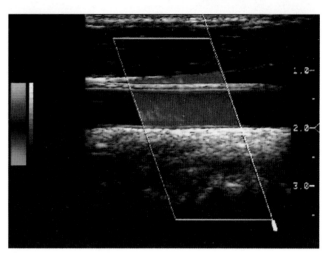

Plate 41 Long axis section of the common carotid artery. Arterial wall definition reveals linear reflectivity resulting from the echogenicity of collagen found in the intima and media (see Fig. 25-5).

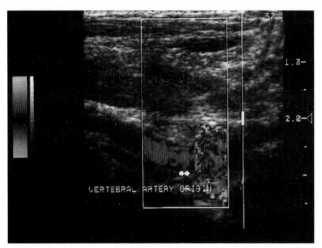

Plate 42 Doppler color flow image of the vertebral artery origin. The subclavian artery is seen in the transverse plane just distal to the origin of the right common carotid artery (see Fig. 25-6).

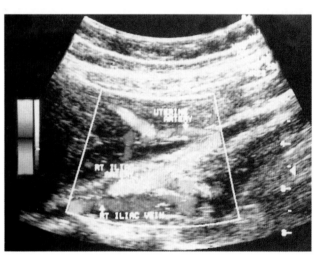

Plate 43 Doppler color flow image of the aortic bifurcation (see Fig. 25-13). (Courtesy Advanced Technology Labs.)

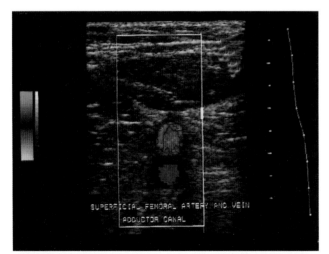

Plate 44 Transverse section, Doppler color flow image of the superficial femoral artery and vein in Hunter's canal (see Fig. 25-14).

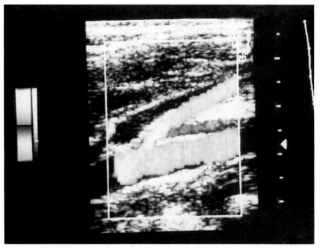

Plate 45 Long axis color flow image of the popliteal artery (see Fig. 25-15).

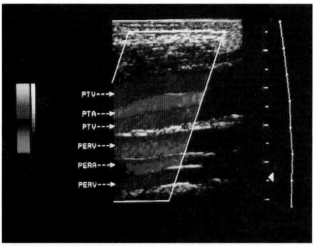

Plate 46 Long axis section, Doppler color flow image of the posterior tibial and peroneal arteries surrounded by their companion tibial veins of the same name (see Fig. 25-16).

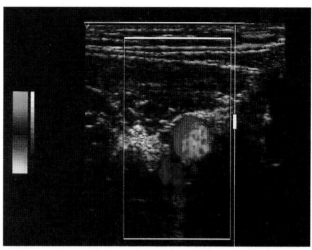

Plate 47 Transverse section, Doppler color flow image of the superficial femoral artery and vein (see Fig. 25-20, *B*).

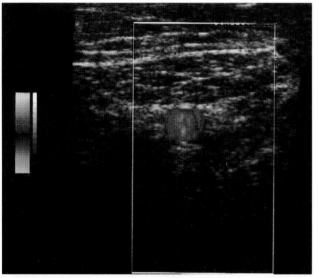

Plate 48 Transverse section, Doppler color flow image of the superficial femoral artery and vein demonstrating coaptation of the venous walls that occurs with gentle transducer pressure (see Fig. 25-20, *C*).

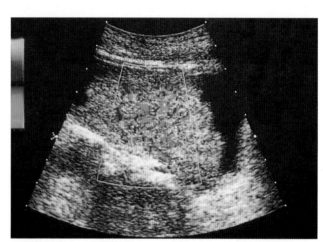

Plate 49 A bladder mass with irregular borders (see Fig. 26-21). (Courtesy Acuson Corp, Mountain View, Calif.)

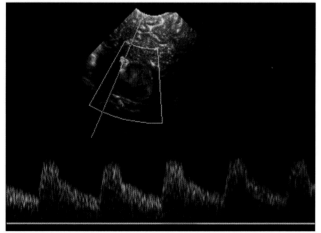

Plate 50 Intraoperative image of a brain aneurysm (see Fig. 28-4).

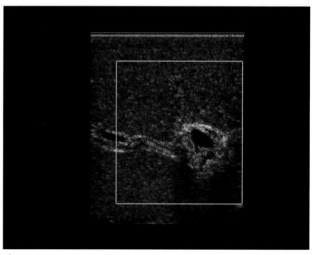

Plate 51 Intraoperative, color Doppler image of the hepatic artery (see Fig. 28-5, *J*).

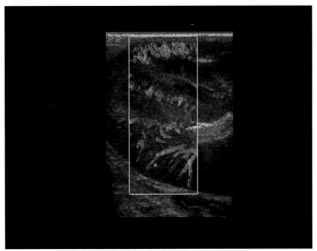

Plate 52 Color Doppler of intraoperative transverse section of the kidney (see Fig. 28-6, *B*).

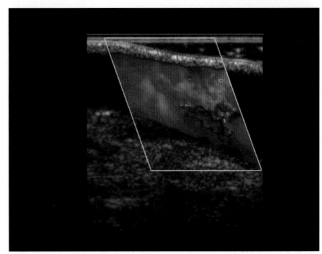

Plate 53 Intraoperative color Doppler image of the internal carotid artery (see Fig. 28-7, *C*).

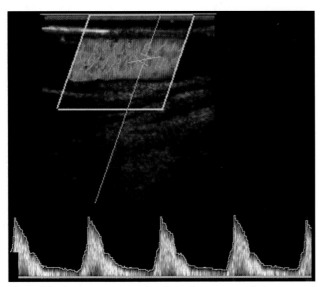

Plate 54 Intraoperative color Doppler image of the internal carotid artery (see Fig. 28-7, *D*).

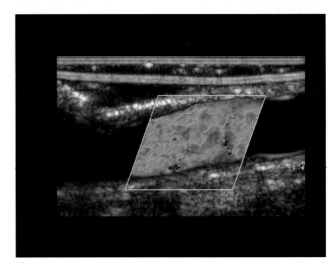

Plate 55 Intraoperative color Doppler image of an arterial graft (see Fig. 28-7, *G*).

INTRODUCTION

Your First Scanning Experience

BETTY BATES TEMPKIN

The primary role of a sonographer is to provide interpretable images for diagnosis by a physician. This goal is totally dependent on the skill of the operator. Becoming an accomplished sonographer happens with practice and the development of good scanning techniques. Informing yourself with established scanning criteria should take the struggle out of scanning while ensuring accuracy, standardization, and quality. To master this skill is to directly contribute to an integral part of patient evaluation.

Before you scan for the first time, review the eight orientation guidelines for learning sectional anatomy in Chapter 4.

Whether you are in a classroom or clinical setting, certain professional and clinical standards should be followed. First, you must be able to properly handle the ultrasound equipment. Practice attaching and detaching transducers from the machine. Be comfortable operating the image documenting system. Experiment with the machine controls to be familiar with their results (see Chapters 1 and 2: "Physics" and "Instrumentation," and "Knobology" in the appendix.)

Second, be sure you have the right patient. Check patient identification bracelets and the chart. Introduce yourself and briefly explain the ultrasound examination. Assist the patient in every possible way; always practice safety and be courteous and respectful. Keep conversations professional and never give a patient your opinion of the study or a diagnosis.

Your first scan will be of the abdominal aorta because it is easy to recognize sonographically. It is important at this stage to review the location, gross anatomy, and sonographic appearance of the aorta in Chapter 5. Also, a valuable exercise is to duplicate with Playdough the abdominal layers that include the aorta. Use the layering illustrations from Chapter 4 as a guide. Choose one color for arteries, another for veins, and so on. This exercise helps differentiate the intricate relationship of adjacent structures and reinforces the layering concept.

Use a scanning protocol—it is essential for comparable studies and ensures that you will be methodical and organized while scanning. Following a scanning protocol is like following a recipe. You take certain steps to achieve a specific goal. The following is a suggested scanning protocol for the abdominal aorta.

A. Patient preparation: The patient should fast for at least 8 hours prior to the examination. This is supposed to reduce the amount of gas in the overlying bowel that can obscure visualization of posterior structures. Even if the patient has recently eaten, you still attempt the examination on the chance that you can evaluate the area of interest.

B. Patient position: The best position is determined by what will produce the optimal view. In this case a supine position is the best approach for evaluating the aorta. Alternatively, the aorta can also be seen from a right or left lateral decubitus, from a right or left posterior oblique, or with the patient sitting semierect to erect. (See Figure 1 for different patient positions.) This should alert you to the fact and advantage that multiple approaches are available for solving imaging needs. Simply put, if it does not work in one position, try another.

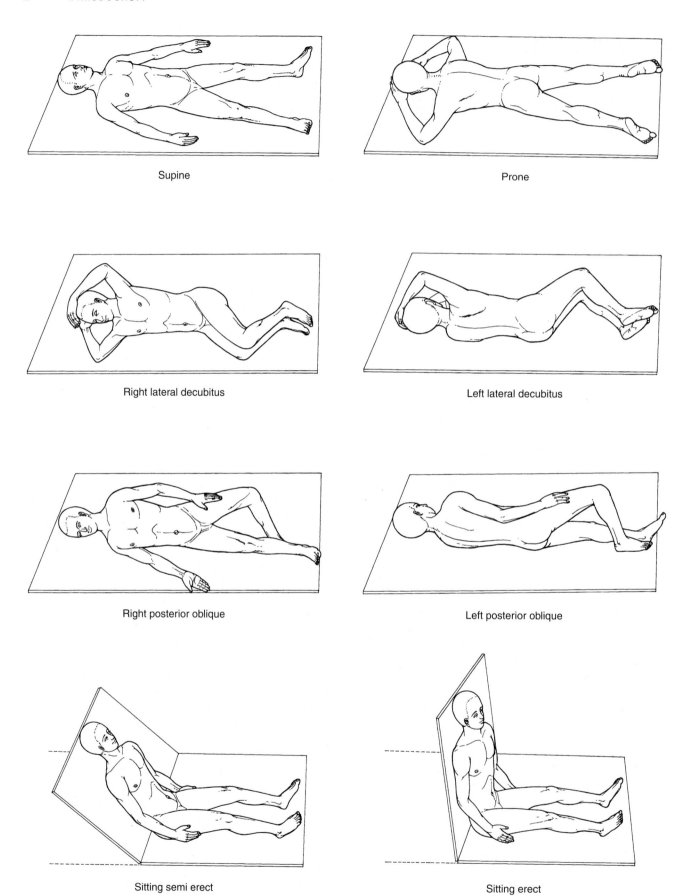

Supine

Prone

Right lateral decubitus

Left lateral decubitus

Right posterior oblique

Left posterior oblique

Sitting semi erect

Sitting erect

Figure 1 Standard patient positions.

C. Choosing a transducer: You will learn in Chapter 2 of the text that the higher number megahertz transducers are best for imaging superficial structures, and the lower number megahertz transducers are best for evaluating deep structures. Because the aorta is retroperitoneal and one of the deepest structures of the body, the transducer of choice is usually a 3.0 MHz or 3.5 MHz. Try a 5.0 MHz transducer if the patient is very thin. If you are not achieving the desired results with one transducer, switch to another.

D. Breathing technique: Respiration causes body structures to move. Deep inspiration forces the diaphragm and everything below it in the abdomen to move down. Deep exhalation causes abdominal structure to move up. You will have to experiment with different breathing techniques to achieve optimal visualization of body structures. The suggested breathing technique for imaging the aorta is normal respiration. If you find that a patient's normal respiration causes too much movement for taking clear images, have the patient momentarily stop breathing without inhaling or exhaling.

E. The survey: A survey is a detailed comprehensive observation. All ultrasound examinations should begin with a survey of the area of interest and adjacent structures in at least two scanning planes. In most cases, abdominal and pelvic structure studies include evaluation of the entire cavity. However, some clinical circumstances warrant a limited study, confined to the structure or area of interest only. For our purpose of a first scan, the study will be limited to the aorta.

No images are taken during the survey. This is the time to investigate the areas of interest, adjust technique, and rule out any normal variants or abnormalities.

The longitudinal survey of the abdominal aorta is generally performed first. This is usually from an anterior approach in the sagittal plane (see Chapter 4, Figure 4-6). Alternatively, the aorta may also be visualized from a left lateral approach in the coronal plane. The steps of the *longitudinal survey* from an *anterior approach in the sagittal plane* are as follows:

■ Begin with the transducer perpendicular, at the midline of the body, just inferior to the xiphoid process of the sternum. (See Figure 2 for transducer positions and Figure 3 for surface landmarks.) Always use a scanning couplant, such as scanning gel, to reduce air between the transducer and surface of the skin.

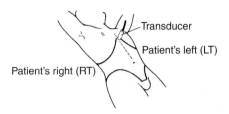

■ It is preferable to start the study by differentiating the inferior vena cava from the aorta because they are similar in size and sonographic appearance. Slightly move or angle the transducer to the patient's right and identify the distal portion of the inferior vena cava posterior to the liver. You can identify the inferior vena cava by its long, tubular, anechoic appearance and echogenic walls.

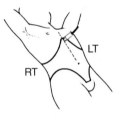

■ Slightly move or angle the transducer to the patient's left and identify the proximal portion of the aorta posterior to the liver. The aorta can be recognized as a long, tubular, anechoic structure with echogenic walls and anterior branches.

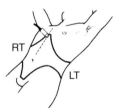

■ While viewing this proximal portion of the aorta, slowly move the transducer inferiorly, using a rock-and-slide motion (Figure 4). Slightly rock the transducer from side to side, scanning through each side of the aorta, while slowly sliding the transducer inferiorly. It may be necessary to rotate the transducer at varying degrees to oblique the scanning plane according to the lie (or position) of the aorta (Figure 5). You should be able to view the long axis (full length) of this proximal portion of the aorta and its anterior branches: the celiac axis and superior mesenteric artery.

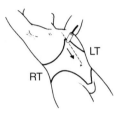

■ Continue rocking and sliding the transducer inferiorly through the mid and distal portions of the aorta to the bifurcation (usually at or just beyond the level of the umbilicus).

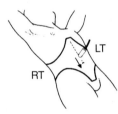

■ From the lateral aspects of the most distal portion of the aorta, angle the transducer back toward the aorta and slightly move inferiorly until the bifurcation and common iliac arteries are seen.

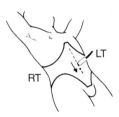

NOTE: As mentioned, the bifurcation may be easier to visualize from a *left lateral approach* in the coronal plane:

■ Begin with the transducer perpendicular, midcoronal plane, just superior to the iliac crest. Use the inferior pole of the left kidney as a landmark and look for the aortic bifurcation medial, as you slowly move along inferiorly. Again, it may be necessary to rotate the transducer varying degrees to visualize the long axis of the bifurcation and the common iliac arteries.

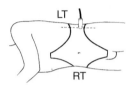

The next step is the transverse survey of the aorta. This is usually performed from an anterior approach in the transverse plane. Alternatively, like the longitudinal views of the aorta, the transverse views may also be obtained from a left lateral approach in the transverse plane. The steps of the **transverse survey** from an *anterior approach in the transverse plane* are as follows:

■ Begin with the transducer perpendicular, at the midline of the body, just inferior to the xiphoid process of the sternum (see Figures 2 and 3).

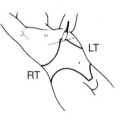

■ Angle the transducer superiorly until the heart is seen, then slowly straighten the transducer back to a perpendicular position and look for the aorta just to the left of midline in the posterior portion of the image. The aorta will appear round or oval and anechoic with bright, echogenic walls.

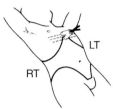

NOTE: Alternatively, locating the transverse section of the proximal aorta may be easier by starting with a longitudinal view of the proximal aorta in the sagittal plane. Simply rotate the transducer 90 degrees into the transverse plane, visualizing the aorta the entire time.

■ While viewing the traversed section of proximal aorta, slightly rock the transducer superiorly to inferiorly while slowly sliding inferiorly; this way you should never lose sight of the aorta. As you move inferiorly, note and evaluate the aorta's anterior branches: the celiac axis and superior mesenteric artery.

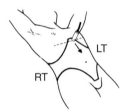

■ Continue rocking and slowly sliding the transducer inferiorly through the mid and distal portions of the aorta to the bifurcation. As you move inferiorly through the mid portion of the aorta, note and evaluate the lateral branches: the renal arteries.

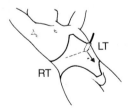

■ At the level of the bifurcation, evaluate the proximal portion of the common iliac arteries by scanning through them inferiorly until you lose sight of them. The sonographic appearance of the distal aorta to the common iliac arteries is from a single large round anechoic vessel to two small round anechoic vessels.

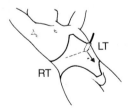

F. Required images: Ultrasound images reflect isolated sections of structures or samples of the whole. These image sections must clearly represent examples of what was determined during the survey. Just as surveys are done in at least two scanning planes, images must be documented in at least two scanning planes. This gives a more dimensional and therefore accurate representation. Generally, the scanning planes used during the survey should be the same scanning planes used to document the images.

For legal purposes and clinical standardization, images should be labeled to include the patient's name, any identification number, the date, the scanning site, and the initials of the sonographer scanning. Additionally, the area of interest, the scanning plane, and the transducer megahertz must also be included. When endocavital studies are performed, another health professional should witness the procedure and his or her initials should be recorded as well.

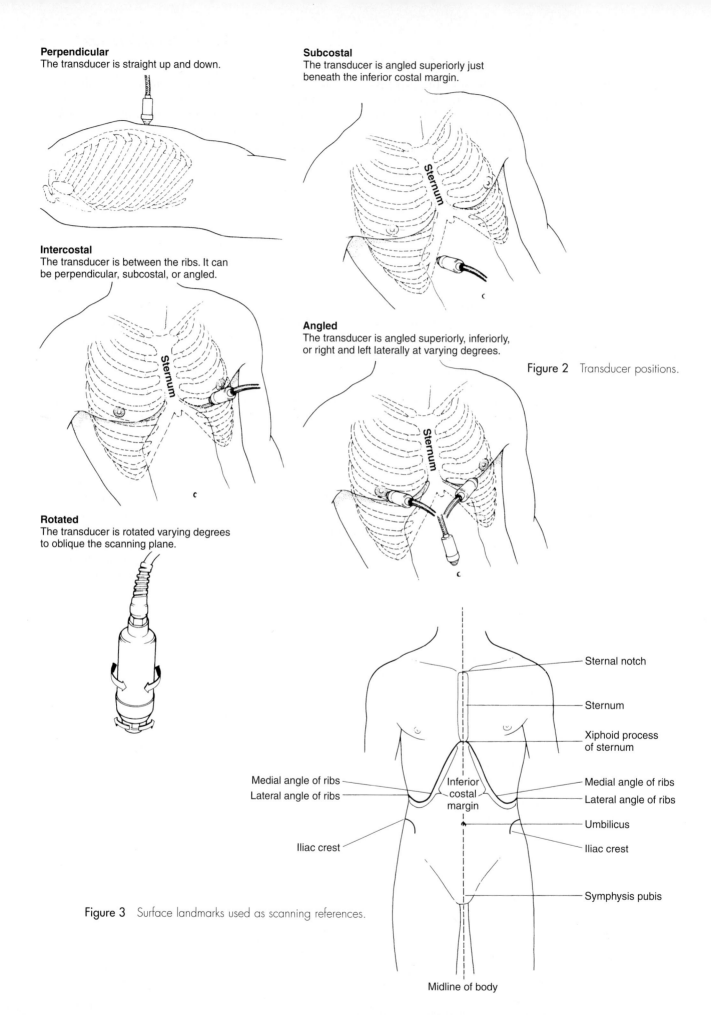

Perpendicular
The transducer is straight up and down.

Intercostal
The transducer is between the ribs. It can be perpendicular, subcostal, or angled.

Rotated
The transducer is rotated varying degrees to oblique the scanning plane.

Subcostal
The transducer is angled superiorly just beneath the inferior costal margin.

Angled
The transducer is angled superiorly, inferiorly, or right and left laterally at varying degrees.

Figure 2 Transducer positions.

Sternal notch

Sternum

Xiphoid process of sternum

Medial angle of ribs
Lateral angle of ribs

Inferior costal margin

Medial angle of ribs
Lateral angle of ribs

Umbilicus

Iliac crest

Iliac crest

Symphysis pubis

Midline of body

Figure 3 Surface landmarks used as scanning references.

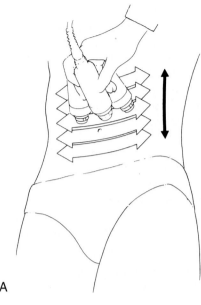

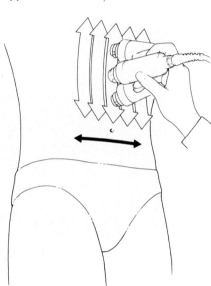

Figure 4 Rock and slide scanning method. **A,** When scanning in a sagittal plane, slightly rock the transducer right and left while slowly sliding the transducer superiorly or inferiorly. **B,** When scanning in a transverse plane, slightly rock the transducer superiorly or inferiorly while slowly sliding the transducer laterally.

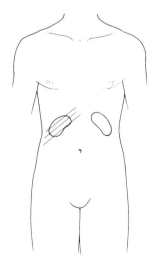

Figure 5 Scan according to the lie (or position) of a structure. In this example, slightly rotating the transducer obliques the sagittal planes used to visualize the lie or longitudinal views of the kidney.

Remember that the images you take for the physician should be the best representation for diagnostic interpretation. Also keep in mind that you survey the entire abdominal aorta from its proximal portion to its bifurcation, but you take only one representative longitudinal and transverse image of each major section. Therefore those images have to embody the overall condition of the aorta.

It is standard practice to take certain views that give the physician the most information. In some institutions additional views may be included. For instance, some physicians prefer that the longitudinal image of the proximal aorta be at the level of and demonstrate the celiac and superior mesenteric branches, and the transverse image of the mid aorta must include the renal arteries. Although there may be slight variations in the scanning protocol according to the interpreting physician, the basic comprehensive images (including those with measurements) should always be the same.

It is important to note that whenever an image is taken with measurement calipers or any type of labeling directly on the image, that very same image must be taken again without the calipers or labels. This is done for the interpreting physician in case the measurement(s) or label(s) happens to cover some area of interest.

Since the survey of the aorta was done in the sagittal and transverse planes from an anterior approach, the required pictures should be taken in the same manner. The following are the standard longitudinal and transverse images of the abdominal aorta and how they should be labeled:

Longitudinal Images/Sagittal Plane/Anterior Approach

    1. Longitudinal image of the proximal aorta:

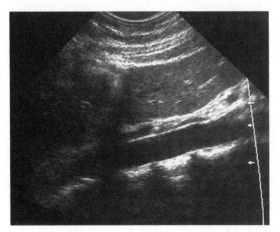
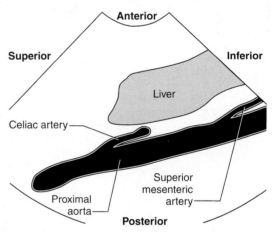

Labeled: **AORTA SAG PROX**

2. Longitudinal image of the mid aorta:

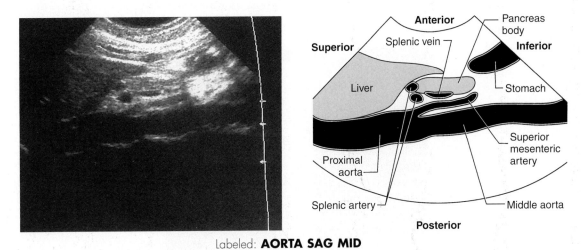

Labeled: **AORTA SAG MID**

3. Longitudinal image of the distal aorta:

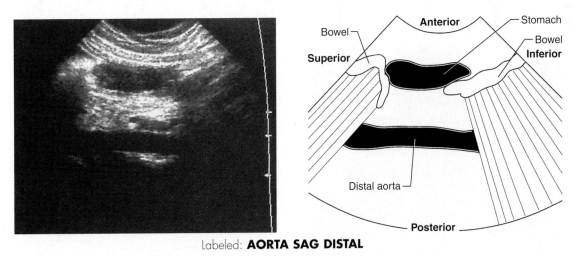

Labeled: **AORTA SAG DISTAL**

4. Longitudinal image of the aorta bifurcation (common iliac arteries):

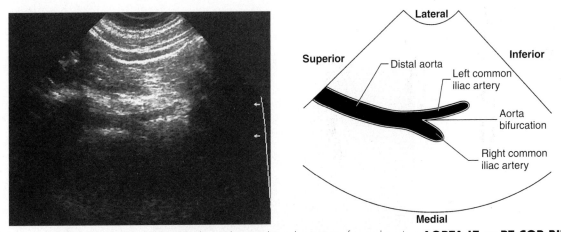

Labeled: **AORTA SAG BIF RT or LT** (depending on lateral position of transducer) or **AORTA LT or RT COR BIF**

Transverse Images/Transverse Plane/Anterior Approach

5. Transverse image of the proximal aorta with anterior to posterior measurement (calipers placed on outside wall to outside wall):

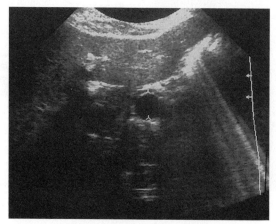

Labeled: **AORTA TRV PROX**

6. The same image as number 5 without the measurement calipers:

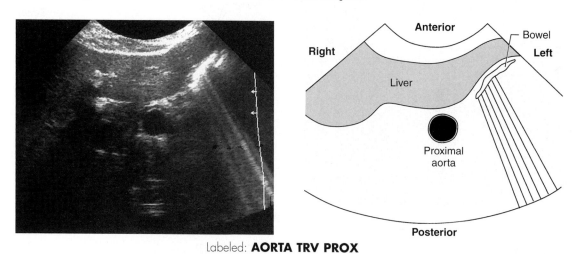

Labeled: **AORTA TRV PROX**

7. Transverse image of the mid aorta with anterior to posterior measurement (calipers placed on outside wall to outside wall):

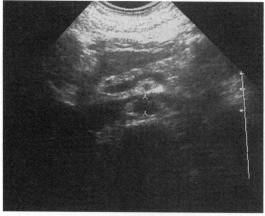

Labeled: **AORTA TRV MID**

8. The same image as number 7 without the measurement calipers:

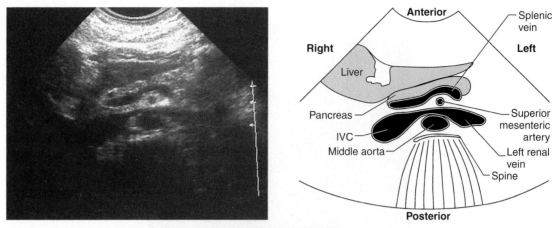

Labeled: **AORTA TRV MID**

NOTE: If the renal arteries are not represented on the previous images, an additional image(s) of the renal arteries should be taken here and labeled accordingly.

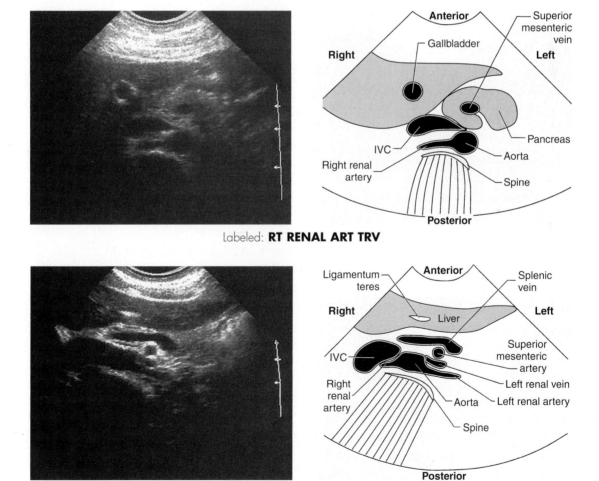

Labeled: **RT RENAL ART TRV**

Labeled: **LT RENAL ART TRV**

9. Transverse image of the distal aorta with anterior to posterior measurement (calipers placed on outside wall to outside wall):

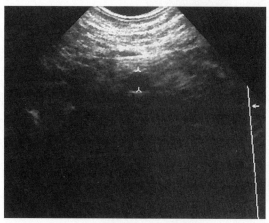

Labeled: **AORTA TRV DISTAL**

10. The same image as number 9 without the measurement calipers:

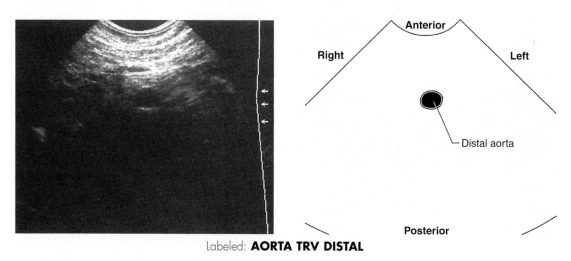

Labeled: **AORTA TRV DISTAL**

11. Transverse image of the aorta bifurcation (common iliac arteries):

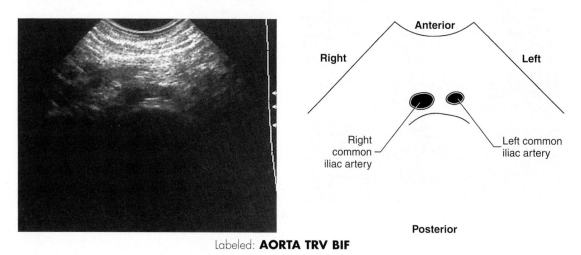

Labeled: **AORTA TRV BIF**

This sample protocol addresses the basic comprehensive images that should be taken when the abdominal aorta is the area of interest or examination ordered.

Keep in mind that if you see something abnormal about the aorta during the survey you must be prepared to document it. Basically, all abnormalities or pathologies can be evaluated and documented the same way. First, during the survey determine which organ(s) or structure(s) is primarily involved, which of the adjacent structures, if any, are involved, and the composition of the abnormality, such as solid, cystic, complex, septated, or dissected. (See Chapter 26, "Introduction to Ultrasound of Human Disease.") The pathology images should come after the standard protocol images and document the clearest representation of the aforementioned, including measurement images in two scanning planes at the greatest dimensions (excluding gallstones, renal stones, hydronephrosis, thrombosis, pleural effusion, or ascites).

The clinical portion of a sonographer's expertise is the most direct and important contribution that a sonographer makes to a patient's ultrasound evaluation. Since this clinical competence is not directly evaluated by registry or licensing, it takes personal initiative and discipline to master scanning skills. Match the quality of your images with other established protocol images and use feedback from your instructors and/or physicians to monitor your personal progress.

BIBLIOGRAPHY

Tempkin BB: *Ultrasound scanning: principles and protocols,* Philadelphia, 1993, WB Saunders.

Physics

CHAPTER 1

Physics

M. NATHAN PINKNEY

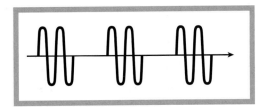

BASIC PRINCIPLES OF ULTRASOUND

Ultrasound is sound whose frequency is above the range of human hearing. Ultrasound is widely used in medical imaging for the evaluation of a patient's internal organs. Ultrasound energy is transmitted into the patient; then, because the various internal structures reflect and scatter sound differently, returning echoes can be used to form an image of a structure.

Sound Energy

Sound waves consist of mechanical variations containing **condensations** and **rarefactions** that are transmitted through a medium. Unlike x-rays, sound is not electromagnetic. **Matter** must be present for sound to travel, which explains why sound cannot propagate through a vacuum. **Propagation** of sound is the transfer of energy—not matter—from one place to another.

Categories of Sound

Sound is categorized according to its frequency. Frequency describes the number of mechanical variations or vibrations that occur per unit time. **Infrasound** is subsonic sound with a frequency less than 20 hertz, where each **hertz** (Hz) represents one cycle per second. **Audible sounds** have frequencies that range from 20 to 20,000 Hz. Sounds that have frequencies greater than 20,000 Hz (20 kHz) are ultrasonic. When ultrasound is used for medical diagnostic applications, operating frequencies greater than 1 million hertz (1 megahertz [MHz]) are used.

Propagation Speed

Sound waves propagate through matter by causing molecules to vibrate successively along the sound path. **Stiffness, elasticity,** and **density** properties of a material determine the **velocity** of sound propagation. Normally, the velocity of sound is significantly higher in materials that are very stiff (Table 1-1).

■ ■ ■ **Table 1-1**   Sound Velocities

Material	Meters Per Second (m/sec)
Air	330
Pure water	1430
Metal	5000
Fat	1450
Soft tissue	*1540*
Liver	1550
Blood	1570
Muscle	1585
Bone	4080

From Pinkney N: *A review of concepts of ultrasound physics and instrumentation*, 4th ed, Philadelphia, 1992, Sonicor.

Piezoelectric Effect

High-frequency **transducers** are used to generate the ultrasonic energy. The major component of an ultrasound transducer is the piezoelectric element. Piezoelectric materials are capable of converting one form of energy into another (Figure 1-1).

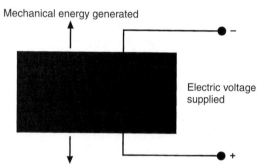

Figure 1-1   Piezoelectric effect: Electrical energy into mechanical energy.

A voltage supplied to a piezoelectric element initiates vibrations at the element's resonant (operating) frequency. The **resonant frequency** is related to the element's thickness. The thinner the element, the higher the resonant frequency of the transducer.

Another function of the piezoelectric element is to receive echoes that return from the object being studied. When the mechanical energy is received, the piezoelectric element converts it into an electrical voltage, which forms a visual image of the studied structure (Figure 1-2). Although a single piezoelectric element is capable of either transmitting or receiving, it cannot be used to perform both functions simultaneously.

Medical diagnostic ultrasound transducers use ceramic materials for piezoelectric elements. To make a ceramic material piezoelectric, it is necessary to heat it above a certain temperature, called the **Curie point.** It is at this temperature that a material's **dipoles** move freely and will align themselves with an electric field. An elec-

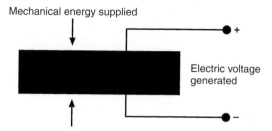

Figure 1-2   Piezoelectric effect: Mechanical energy into electrical energy.

trical potential is applied, and the material is then cooled to room temperature while the voltage remains. This **polarization** of the ceramic material remains as long as the temperature of the material is kept below the Curie point. Ceramic materials typically used are **lead zirconate titanate** and **barium titanate.**

There are two basic modes of transducer operation that are used in medical diagnostic applications: continuous and pulsed (Figure 1-3).

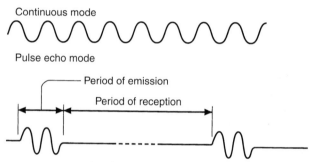

Figure 1-3   Graphs of continuous mode and pulse-echo mode in ultrasound.

The continuous mode or **continuous wave** (CW) is used in some Doppler ultrasound systems. Separate elements are required for continuous sending and receiving. **Doppler** is used to detect blood flow through vessels. The Doppler technique detects not only the presence of blood flow but also the direction of flow by measuring the difference in the frequency of the reflected sound compared with the transmitted sound.

Pulsed transducers can use the same piezoelectric elements for sending and receiving because separate time intervals are provided for emission and reception.

Pulse-Echo Ultrasound

Pulse-echo ultrasound transducers operate by periodically sending short bursts of sound energy into the area being studied. Echoes are produced when changes in the characteristic of the material are encountered. When these echoes return to the transducer, they are converted into electrical signals. After processing, the information received forms an image of the studied area. The ultrasound system measures the time that it takes to receive the echoes after each transmitted pulse. By keeping track of the time between transmitted pulses and the returning echoes, the ultrasound system can determine the distances to the various reflectors. Most diagnostic ultrasound systems are calibrated for a velocity of 1540 m/sec (1.54 mm/μsec), which is the average velocity of sound through human soft tissue. Large propagation speed errors will result in improper positioning of echoes on a display.

Shock excitation is used to generate sound energy in pulse-echo ultrasound systems (Figure 1-4). The excitation is normally several hundred volts. The frequency of the excitation, which is the **pulse repetition frequency** (PRF), is normally greater than 1000 pulses/sec (1 kHz). The **pulse repetition period,** which is the reciprocal of the PRF, decreases as the PRF is increased. Shorter pulse repetition periods may be used only when structures that are not very deep are examined. This is because an ultrasound transducer should not be permitted to send out a pulse until sufficient time has been allowed to receive all returning echoes that are the result of the previous pulse.

Shock excitation is used to generate sound energy in pulse-echo systems

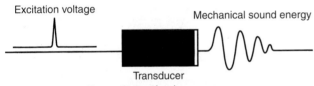

Figure 1-4 Shock excitation.

Backing materials are present in pulse-echo transducers to provide **damping** of the piezoelectric element so that each transmitted sound pulse consists of only a few cycles to ensure a very short period of emission compared with a longer period of reception (Figure 1-5).

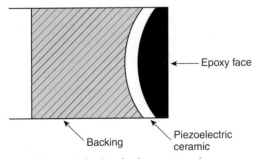

Figure 1-5 Single-element transducer.

The relationship between the period of emission and the period of reception is called the **duty factor,** or duty cycle.

The duty factor of pulse-echo ultrasound instruments is very small, usually less than 1%. CW Doppler systems operate with duty factors of 100% because they are capable of sending and receiving at the same time (Figure 1-6).

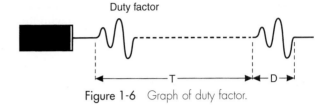

Figure 1-6 Graph of duty factor.

Ultrasound Beam Generation

Any sound source creates waves from individual **point sources. Huygen's principle** demonstrates how these multiple single-point sources produce spherical secondary wavelets. Successive wave fronts will be present in areas of tangency to the secondary wavelets (Figure 1-7).

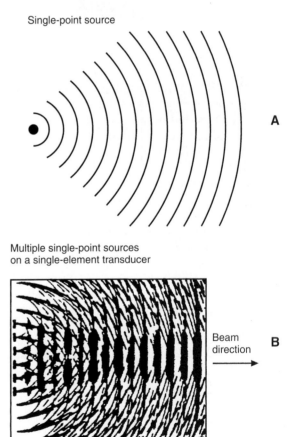

Figure 1-7 **A,** Single-point source. **B,** Beam formation resulting from Huygen's principle.

Normally, the waves emanating from a piezoelectric element follow a defined beam path, but occasionally undesirable extraneous energy components are produced. These energy components, which are not in the primary direction of the ultrasound beam, are called **sidelobes.**

Each cycle from an expanding and contracting piezo-electric element results in condensation and rarefaction. The condensations and rarefactions of the molecules produce longitudinal sound waves (Figure 1-8). **Longitudinal sound waves** have particle motion that is back and forth along the direction of propagation. Longitudinal waves are very useful in medical diagnostic ultrasound.

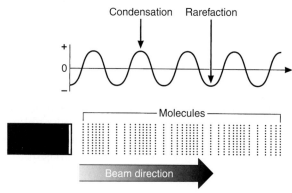

Figure 1-8 Graph representing longitudinal waves.

A graph of ultrasound waves may represent a scale of time. The time required to produce each cycle depends on the operating frequency of the transducer. This time interval is the **period** of the wave. The period of a diagnostic ultrasound cycle is typically less than 1 microsecond (Table 1-2). The total time of each sound pulse is the period multiplied by the number of cycles in each pulse. This time interval, which is the **pulse duration,** decreases along with the period when higher-frequency transducers are used. It is the pulse duration divided by the pulse repetition period that gives the duty factor. Figure 1-9 is a representation of period and pulse duration.

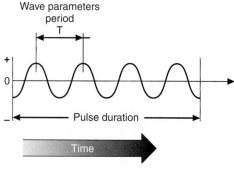

Figure 1-9 Graph of period and pulse duration.

A graph of ultrasound waves may also represent a scale of distance. The distance occupied by each cycle depends on the operating frequency of the transducer and the velocity of the sound. This distance interval is the **wavelength** of the cycle. The wavelength of a diagnostic ultrasound cycle is typically less than 1 millimeter (Table 1-3).

■ ▨ ▨ **Table 1-2** Frequency vs. Period
Examples
Period of a 1 MHz wave is 1 microsecond
Period of a 2 MHz wave is 0.5 microsecond
Period of a 3 MHz wave is 0.33 microsecond
Period of a 5 MHz wave is 0.2 microsecond

■ ▨ ▨ **Table 1-3** Frequency vs. Wavelength
Examples For a Velocity of 1540 m/sec
Wavelength for 1 MHz is 1.54 mm
Wavelength for 2 MHz is 0.77 mm
Wavelength for 3 MHz is 0.51 mm

From Pinkney N: *A review of concepts of ultrasound physics and instrumentation,* 4th ed, Philadelphia, 1992, Sonicor.

The total distance occupied by a sound pulse is the wavelength multiplied by the number of cycles in the pulse. This distance, which is the **spatial pulse length,** decreases along with the wavelength when higher-frequency transducers are used (Figure 1-10).

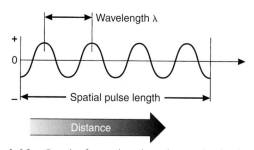

Figure 1-10 Graph of wavelength and spatial pulse length.

Sound Reflection

Sound reflection occurs at an acoustic interface, which is the boundary between two media of different acoustic impedance. The **acoustic impedance** (measured in rayls) of a material is the product of the material's density and the velocity of sound in the material (Table 1-4).

■ ▨ ▨ **Table 1-4** Typical Acoustic Impedance Values	
Material	**Z**
Air	400
Fat	1,380,000
Water	1,430,000
Tissue	1,630,000
Muscle	1,700,000
Bone	7,800,000

From Pinkney N: *A review of concepts of ultrasound physics and instrumentation,* 4th ed, Philadelphia, 1992, Sonicor.

The difference in the acoustic impedance of the two materials determines the amount of sound energy transmitted and reflected at a boundary. The greater the difference in the acoustic impedance, the higher the reflection and the lower the transmission through the interface. As a general rule, medical diagnostic ultrasound energy will not travel through air (Table 1-5). This is why acoustic couplants (water, oil, or gel) are needed. Acoustic couplants are used to provide a good sound path between the transducer and the skin.

■ ▩ ▩ **Table 1-5** Typical Reflection Percentages (Approximate)

Interface	% Reflection
Fat-muscle	1
Fat-bone	50
Tissue-air	100

From Pinkney N: *A review of concepts of ultrasound physics and instrumentation*, 4th ed, Philadelphia, 1992, Sonicor.

Reflections most frequently received are those that occur at normal (perpendicular) incidence. The angle of reflection is usually equal to the angle of incidence. This is true at most **specular interfaces,** where the boundary of the interface is smooth and where the dimensions of the interface are larger than the wavelength (Figure 1-11). Examples of specular interfaces include the diaphragm, the walls of vessels and anechoic structures, and the boundaries of many organs.

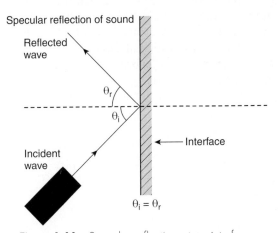

Figure 1-11   Specular reflection at an interface.

Sound that is not reflected is transmitted through the interface. Refraction can occur if the incident angle is not zero and if the velocities of sound in the two materials forming the boundary are not equal. **Refraction** is a change in direction of sound as it passes through a boundary. The **transmitted angle** will be larger or smaller than the angle of incidence in proportion to an increase or decrease in the respective velocity. Refraction can result in improper placement of displayed echoes (Figure 1-12).

Interfaces that are either smaller than the wavelength or not smooth are nonspecular. Scattering of the sound

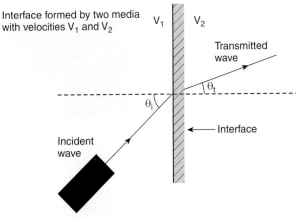

Figure 1-12   Refraction.

occurs at **nonspecular interfaces** (Figure 1-13). Examples of nonspecular interfaces include red blood cells, liver parenchyma, and other materials representing the tissue characteristics of an organ.

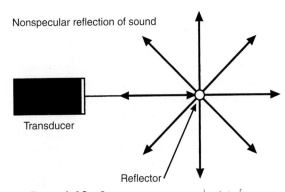

Figure 1-13   Scatter at a nonspecular interface.

Resolution

Resolution is the minimum reflector separation required to produce separate reflections in a pulse-echo system. **Axial resolution** is the minimum reflector separation along the sound path required to produce separate echoes.

The axial resolution, which does not vary with depth, is improved by using short spatial pulse lengths. High-frequency, highly damped transducers produce shorter spatial pulse lengths. Figure 1-14 depicts good and poor axial resolution. **Lateral resolution** is the minimum reflector separation perpendicular to the sound path required to produce separate echoes. Lateral resolution, which is the **beam width,** can change with depth. Lateral resolution is affected by the diameter of the piezoelectric element and transducer focusing. **Focusing** creates a beam pattern with a smaller cross-sectional area. Lateral resolution is also improved when high-frequency transducers are used. Figure 1-15 illustrates good and poor lateral resolution.

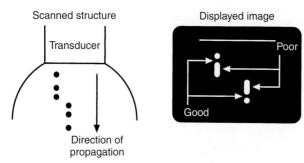

Figure 1-14 Good and poor axial resolution.

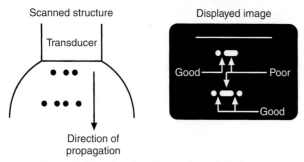

Figure 1-15 Good and poor lateral resolution.

Attenuation

Although higher-frequency transducers provide improved axial and lateral resolution, there is increased attenuation. Increased attenuation results in less penetration through the medium. **Attenuation** is the decrease in energy as a wave travels through a medium. Attenuation is caused by absorption, reflection, beam divergence, and scattering. Scattering increases with an increase in frequency. In human soft tissue, sound is attenuated at the rate of 0.5 **decibel**/cm/MHz. In bone, attenuation is greater and more frequency dependent, but in water, it is very low. (NOTE: The decibel [dB] is a relative measure and is used to compare the relative intensities of two ultrasound beams. The dB is a function of the logarithm of the ratio of the two intensities [Tables 1-6 and 1-7].)

■ ■ ■ Table 1-6   Intensity Ratio vs. Decibel Value

Intensity Ratio	dB
1	0
2	3
4	6
8	9
1,000,000	60
0.50	−3
0.25	−6

From Pinkney N: *A review of concepts of ultrasound physics and instrumentation,* 4th ed, Philadelphia, 1992, Sonicor.

■ ■ ■ Table 1-7   Typical Transducer Frequencies

1.9 MHz	2.25 MHz
3.0 MHz	3.5 MHz

5.0 MHz   7.5 MHz   10.0 MHz

The lower frequencies are used for large patients or for any study that requires imaging at great depths.

Transducers in the 3.0 or 3.5 MHz range are used for general-purpose imaging.

For studies of thin patients or small parts, higher frequencies may be used.

From Pinkney N: *A review of concepts of ultrasound physics and instrumentation,* 4th ed, Philadelphia, 1992, Sonicor.

BIOEFFECTS

Bioeffects (biological effects) are the effects of ultrasound on tissue. The categories of bioeffects are (1) heat, (2) cavitation, and (3) other. Heat is the effect created by the motion of the vibrating molecules. Any heating is negligible when pulse ultrasound is used for diagnostic purposes. **Cavitation** results in the production of gas bubbles. Cavitation is possible when pulsed ultrasound with very high intensity is used. Cavitation can eventually result in damage to cell walls. The "other" category includes various minor mechanical effects that are not related to heat or cavitation.

Bioeffects have not been confirmed for pulsed ultrasound intensities less than 100 mW/cm², SPTA. (NOTE: SPTA refers to a method often used to measure ultrasound intensities, in which SP [spatial peak] is intensity measured at the center of a beam. TA [temporal average] indicates that the intensity is the average value during the periods of emission and reception.)

CHAPTER 2

Instrumentation

M. NATHAN PINKNEY

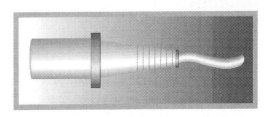

OBJECTIVES ■

Describe the basic pulse-echo display modes.
Compare linear and sector scanning formats.
Describe transducer configurations for real-time imaging.
Describe the digital scan converter functions.
Describe Doppler principles and instrumentation.
Describe the various image-recording techniques.
Define the key words.

KEY WORDS ■

A mode	Focusing
A scan	Frame rate
Acoustic line	Frequency shift
Aliasing	Gain
Amplification	Gated Doppler
Analog	Gray scale
B mode	Hard-copy recording
B scan	Harmonic
Bit	Linear
Cathode ray tube	Linear array
Cine-loop	M mode
Color flow Doppler	Magnetic recording
Compression	Magnification
Continuous wave	Mechanically steered
Convex array	Multiimage camera
Curved linear array	Nyquist limit
Depth ambiguity	Phased array
Digital to analog	Pixel
Digital memory	Postprocessing
Doppler shift	Preprocessing
Duplex ultrasound	Pulse-echo ultrasound
Dynamic range	Pulse repetition frequency
Electronic beam	Pulsed wave Doppler

Pulser	Spectral Doppler
Real-time imaging	Spectrum analyzer
Read-magnification	Swept gain
Receiver	Television monitor
Scan converter	TGC curve
Sector	Time gain compensation
Sector scanning format	Transducer
Sequenced array	Write-magnification

BASIC PULSE-ECHO INSTRUMENTATION

A basic **pulse-echo ultrasound** system (Figure 2-1) contains a **transducer** that, depending on its configuration, can contain one or more piezoelectric elements. The energy within a pulse-echo system is electrical, but the energy in the patient's body is sound, which is mechanical. The function of the transducer is to convert electrical energy into mechanical energy during transmission and to convert mechanical energy back into electrical energy during reception.

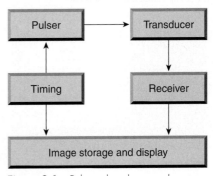

Figure 2-1   Pulse-echo ultrasound system.

The **pulser** section of a pulse-echo system provides the shock excitation to the transducer. The excitation voltage from the pulser can be varied in some ultrasound systems. Varying the transducer's excitation voltage affects the amount of energy leaving the transducer. Typical controls that affect the pulser's voltage could be labeled:

TRANSMITTER
TRANSMIT POWER
OUTPUT
ACOUSTIC POWER
PULSER POWER
ENERGY OUTPUT

The rate of recurrence of the pulser's excitation to the transducer is the **pulse repetition frequency** (PRF), which is determined by the timing section. The timing section also provides synchronization to the rest of the system so that the returning echoes will be processed and displayed according to their proper axial positions.

A **receiver** is used to provide the initial processing of the received echo information. **Time gain compensation** (TGC), or **swept gain,** is a receiver function used to equalize differences in received echo amplitudes caused by reflector depth. TGC provides gradually increasing amplification with depth. **Amplification** is the increasing of smaller voltages to larger ones. The TGC control is just one of the receiver-associated controls that affect the amplification of echoes. The actual names of the various controls will vary with each manufacturer. Typical controls that affect the amplification of echoes could be labeled:

NEAR GAIN
TGC DELAY
SLOPE (TGC)
FAR GAIN
GAIN OR OVERALL GAIN

Many manufacturers incorporate a group of sliding potentiometers to control the amplification of received echoes (Figure 2-2). Each potentiometer in the group is programmed to affect echoes returning from a specific depth. Some ultrasound displays include a **TGC curve,** which is a graphic display of the settings of the receiver's gain controls. Figure 2-3 shows image examples of abnormal and normal TGC settings. Notice how the TGC is too low in A, making it impossible to evaluate that portion of the liver. TGC settings and manipulation are essential for accurate ultrasound evaluation. (See Appendix II for further discussion.)

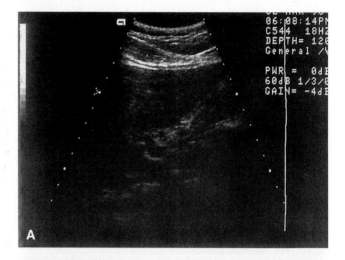

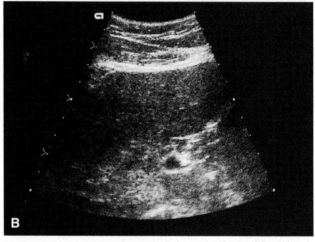

Figure 2-3 Images with abnormal and normal TGC settings. A, Without TGC. B, With TGC.

Another receiver function is **dynamic range,** which is the ratio of the largest signal to the smallest signal that a system can handle. A wider dynamic range, which is often expressed in decibels (dB), ensures a wider range of displayed gray levels. **Compression** is a related function that decreases the difference between small and large amplitude signals. Compression effectively reduces the dynamic range of the receiver. Figure 2-4 is an image that shows narrow and wide dynamic range settings. Controls that permit the operator of an ultrasound system to vary the dynamic range could include:

DYNAMIC RANGE
COMPRESSION
LOG COMPRESSION
COMPRESS

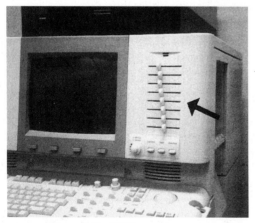

Figure 2-2 TGC potentiometers.

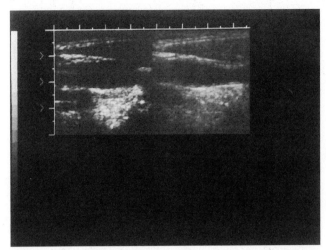

Figure 2-4 Images with narrow (left) and wide (right) dynamic ranges.

Some ultrasound equipment manufacturers have incorporated harmonic detection capabilities into their receivers. A **harmonic** is a wave whose frequency is a whole-number multiple of that of some fundamental frequency. The fundamental frequency is the frequency that is produced by the transducer. Harmonic echoes are often created when tissue or some contrast agents interact with ultrasound energy. Some harmonics are "native" to specific types and characteristics of tissue or contrast agents. The receiver in a system with harmonic capabilities is designed to filter echoes returning at the fundamental frequency while detecting only the harmonics. Detecting these harmonics permits enhancement of selected areas of an image and often reduces unwanted artifacts caused by interaction with low-frequency sound waves.

DISPLAY MODES

There are two basic display modes for returning echo information: A mode and B mode (Figure 2-5).

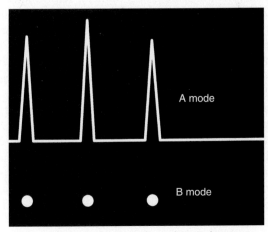

A mode

B mode

Figure 2-5 A mode and B mode.

A mode (A scan) provides an amplitude-modulated display. The escalation of the displayed spikes is a relative indication of the strength of returning echoes. The distance from the reference spike ("main bang") to other spikes along the baseline is an indication of the relative distances to the various reflectors. Although some ultrasound systems have A-mode display capabilities, its current use is limited.

B mode provides a brightness-modulated display in which there is a change in spot brightness for each echo received by the transducer. In a B-mode ultrasound imaging system, the returning echoes are eventually displayed on a **television monitor** as shades of gray, which are discrete brightness levels. Typically, the brighter gray shades represent echoes with greater intensity levels.

M mode (TM mode) is a graphic B-mode display that is a single-dimension time display that represents the motion of structures along a single line penetrated by a single ultrasound beam. M mode, which is commonly used during echocardiographic studies, is often provided as an option on general-purpose ultrasound systems. Figure 2-6 shows examples of A mode, B mode, and M mode.

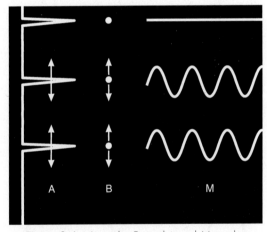

A   B   M

Figure 2-6 A mode, B mode, and M mode.

B scans are B-mode displays that provide cross-sections of objects through scanning planes. The term *B scan* applies to the older static and the newer **real-time imaging** systems. See Figure 2-7 for an image example of B scan, A mode, and M mode.

CROSS-SECTIONAL IMAGE DISPLAY PATTERNS

The two basic real-time scanning formats for cross-sectional imaging are **linear** and **sector** (Figure 2-8).

The linear format provides a rectangular field of view. The sector format displays wedge-shaped sections that are termed pie-shaped, blunted-pie, or trapezoidal. The linear format displays a large field of view for structures close to the transducer. The linear format is created by sequentially transmitting a series of **acoustic lines,** each

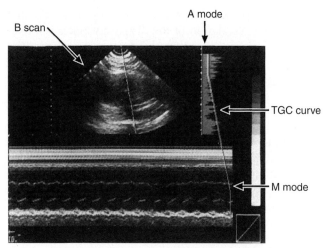

Figure 2-7 Image of A mode and M mode with real-time sector B scanning.

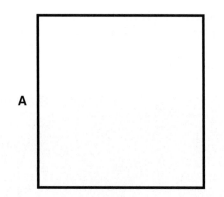

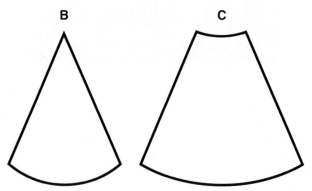

Figure 2-8 **A,** Linear scanning pattern. **B** and **C,** Sector scanning patterns.

in a direction that is parallel to the previous acoustic line. The linear format also provides greater accuracy when horizontal digital caliper measurements are made. However, the parallel acoustic beam format of the linear pattern often makes it difficult to obtain im-

ages of structures located beneath other anatomic areas. Moreover, it is often difficult to maintain complete skin contact with the large scanning surface of a linear transducer. Ultrasound scanners that produce sector images have overcome this primary disadvantage of the large linear transducer. The sector format is created by transmitting a series of acoustic lines, each at an angle that is different from that of the previous acoustic line.

TRANSDUCER CONFIGURATIONS

A transducer typically used to provide a linear (rectangular) scanning pattern is a **linear array** transducer. The term *linear array* normally refers to a flat **sequenced array,** which contains a number of linearly arranged piezoelectric elements that are pulsed sequentially in groups. Figure 2-9 gives examples of flat linear array transducers.

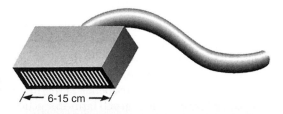

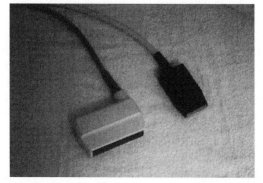

Figure 2-9 Flat linear array transducers.

Each group of elements, when pulsed, generates an acoustic line; the same group waits for returning echoes before the next group is pulsed. The acoustic line from each group of elements of a flat sequenced array is parallel to the other acoustic lines produced. See Figure 2-10 for a drawing of the cross-sectional slice produced by a flat sequenced linear array, and Figure 2-11 for an image produced with flat sequenced array.

Another sequenced array transducer is the **curved linear array,** which is often termed **convex array.** Figure 2-12 depicts examples of curved linear array transducers.

Similar to the flat sequenced array, a curved linear array also contains a number of piezoelectric elements that are pulsed sequentially in groups. The curved scanning surface of this transducer produces a blunted-pie sector cross-sectional image (Figure 2-13).

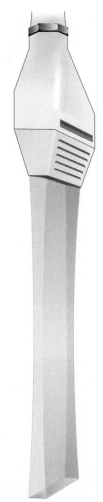

Figure 2-10 Cross-sectional slice produced by a flat sequenced linear array.

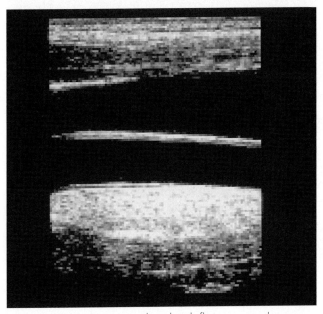

Figure 2-11 Image produced with flat sequenced array.

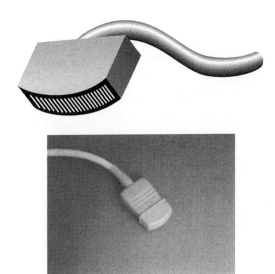

Figure 2-12 Curved linear array transducers.

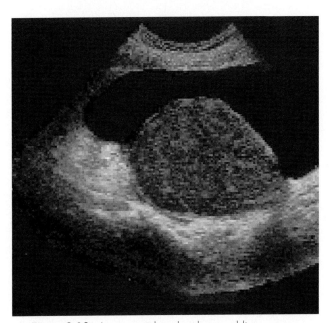

Figure 2-13 Image produced with curved linear array.

A **phased array** transducer contains a number of piezoelectric elements along a small scanning surface. Figure 2-14 gives examples of phased array transducers. Each acoustic line from a phased array transducer is steered by pulsing all of the elements as one group but with small time (phase) differences between them (Figure 2-15).

The phased array transducer produces a sector image; however, compared with the curved linear array, the skin contact area is much smaller, and the pie-shaped sector image produced has a limited field of view of structures located near the skin surface. Figure 2-16 shows an image produced with a phased array transducer. Some manufacturers have combined sequenced

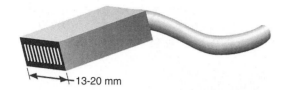

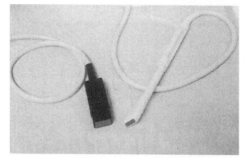

13-20 mm

Figure 2-14 Phased array transducers.

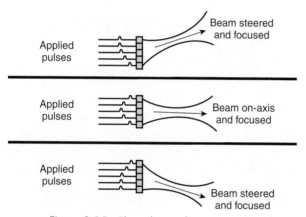

Applied pulses — Beam steered and focused

Applied pulses — Beam on-axis and focused

Applied pulses — Beam steered and focused

Figure 2-15 Phased array beam steering.

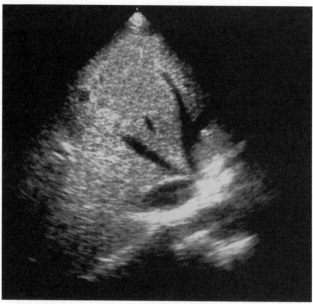

Figure 2-16 Image produced with phased array transducer.

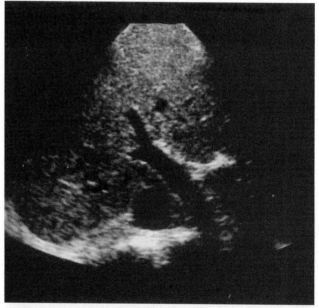

Figure 2-17 Image produced with a trapezoidal (vector) array transducer.

array and phased array techniques to produce a trapezoidal (often termed vector) imaging format. This is accomplished by adding sector field of view to both sides of a rectangular linear image (Figure 2-17).

Unlike earlier **mechanically steered** (motorized) transducers, flat linear array, curved linear array, phased array, and trapezoidal array transducers have no moving parts. The electronics in the systems using these transducers can rapidly switch between different modes of operation to provide simultaneous display modes. The simultaneous display modes could include real time, M mode, or Doppler. Additionally, transducers containing arrays have **electronic beam focusing** capability. Electronic beam focusing is accomplished by varying the delays of the excitation voltages applied to an array's individual piezoelectric elements. This allows control of the width of each acoustic line to provide an improvement in the lateral resolution of the image.

REAL-TIME FRAME RATES
A real-time ultrasound image is updated every fraction of a second to produce a live display. The **frame rate** rep-

resents how often the updating occurs. Generally, higher frame rates are useful for imaging rapidly moving structures, whereas lower frame rates improve image quality by increasing the number of acoustic lines that make up the image. Higher PRFs can also increase the number of acoustic lines, but high PRFs can limit the maximum depth that can be accurately imaged. Depending on the system, frame rates can be fixed or operator selectable or can vary automatically. Frame rates that vary automatically often depend on the transducer frequency or the field of view size chosen by the operator.

IMAGE STORAGE AND DISPLAY

The heart of the image storage component is the digital scan converter. A **scan converter** is used to convert the echo-amplitude information from its original format into a signal format that can be fed to a standard television monitor (Figure 2-18).

IMAGE STORAGE
(Digital scan converter)

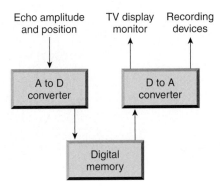

Figure 2-18   Block diagram of digital scan converter.

During the conversion process, the information is temporarily stored in the scan converter's digital memory. The **digital memory** is an electronic device that stores discrete signals. A typical digital memory is configured with an image-matrix memory size of 512 × 512, which represents the number of rows and columns of digital picture elements, or **pixels** (Figure 2-19). Each pixel in a 512 × 512 matrix represents one of 262,144

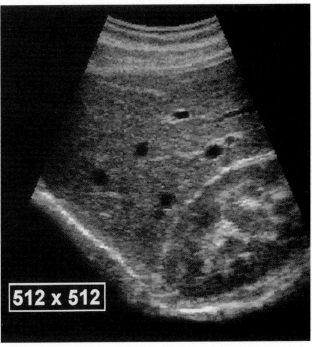

Figure 2-19   Image produced with a typical pixel (picture element) matrix of 512 × 512.

discrete horizontal-vertical echo locations, each displayed as a specific shade of gray. Using multiple digital memories permits **cine-loop,** which is the real-time recording and playback of multiple image frames.

The echo amplitude and position information is normally **analog,** which means that it does not represent discrete values. Before being fed to the scan converter's digital memory, it must first enter the digital scan converter's analog-to-digital (A to D) converter. One function of the A to D converter is to assign discrete shades of gray to the incoming echo amplitudes. This process is called **preprocessing.** Figure 2-20 shows preprocessing assignments.

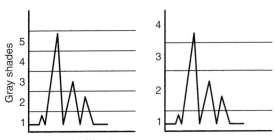

Figure 2-20   Preprocessing assignments.

Selectable preprocessing permits the operator to vary the texture of the displayed image. Because preprocessing occurs before the digital memory, changing the selection will not affect any image information once it is stored.

The maximum number of possible **gray scale** levels depends on the number of **bits** (binary digits) of information that can be stored in the digital memory for each horizontal-vertical location. Typical bit values are 4, 5, 6, 7, 8, 9, and 10 to provide 16, 32, 64, 128, 256, 512, or 1024 gray scale levels, respectively. See Figure 2-21 for an example of a 4-bit (16 gray shade) image and Figure 2-22 for an example of an 8-bit (256 gray shade) image.

Because a television monitor is designed to display analog information, the information that is stored in the scan converter's digital memory must be fed to a **digital-to-analog** (D to A) converter. One function of the D to A converter is to determine the brightness level that will be displayed for each gray scale level. This function is called **postprocessing.** Selectable postprocessing permits the operator to vary the emphasis that is given to various gray scale ranges. Because postprocessing occurs after the digital memory, it can affect stored and live images. Most ultrasound systems use some form of selectable postprocessing. See Figure 2-23 for image examples of different postprocessing selections.

Another image processing function that occurs before the digital memory is **write-magnification.** Selectable write-magnification permits the operator to electronically change the size of the displayed image before storage in the digital memory. With write-magnification,

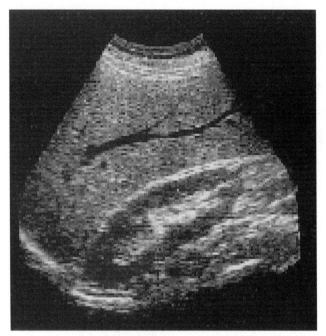

Figure 2-21 Four-bit (16 gray shade) image.

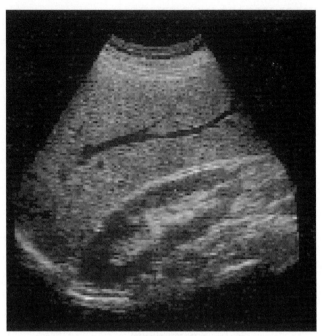

Figure 2-22 Eight-bit (256 gray shade) image.

there is no reduction in the number of displayed pixels. All ultrasound systems use some form of write-magnification. Controls often associated with write-magnification include:

SCALE
SIZE
FIELD OF VIEW
DEPTH
RES

Figure 2-24 shows write-magnification of a selected area.

Read-magnification is an image-size function in some ultrasound systems that occurs after the digital memory. Selectable read-magnification permits an operator to enlarge a selected area of the display by enlarging each pixel. By enlarging each pixel, fewer pixels are present on the display. Images magnified in this manner are coarse when compared with images that are

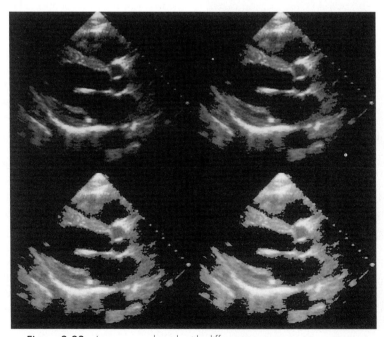

Figure 2-23 Images produced with different postprocessing settings.

IMAGE STORAGE AND DISPLAY

The heart of the image storage component is the digital scan converter. A **scan converter** is used to convert the echo-amplitude information from its original format into a signal format that can be fed to a standard television monitor (Figure 2-18).

IMAGE STORAGE
(Digital scan converter)

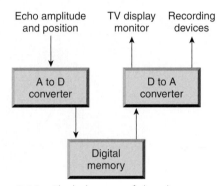

Figure 2-18 Block diagram of digital scan converter.

During the conversion process, the information is temporarily stored in the scan converter's digital memory. The **digital memory** is an electronic device that stores discrete signals. A typical digital memory is configured with an image-matrix memory size of 512 × 512, which represents the number of rows and columns of digital picture elements, or **pixels** (Figure 2-19). Each pixel in a 512 × 512 matrix represents one of 262,144

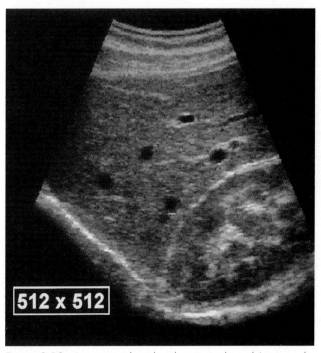

Figure 2-19 Image produced with a typical pixel (picture element) matrix of 512 x 512.

discrete horizontal-vertical echo locations, each displayed as a specific shade of gray. Using multiple digital memories permits **cine-loop,** which is the real-time recording and playback of multiple image frames.

The echo amplitude and position information is normally **analog,** which means that it does not represent discrete values. Before being fed to the scan converter's digital memory, it must first enter the digital scan converter's analog-to-digital (A to D) converter. One function of the A to D converter is to assign discrete shades of gray to the incoming echo amplitudes. This process is called **preprocessing.** Figure 2-20 shows preprocessing assignments.

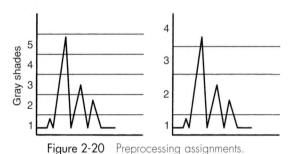

Figure 2-20 Preprocessing assignments.

Selectable preprocessing permits the operator to vary the texture of the displayed image. Because preprocessing occurs before the digital memory, changing the selection will not affect any image information once it is stored.

The maximum number of possible **gray scale** levels depends on the number of **bits** (binary digits) of information that can be stored in the digital memory for each horizontal-vertical location. Typical bit values are 4, 5, 6, 7, 8, 9, and 10 to provide 16, 32, 64, 128, 256, 512, or 1024 gray scale levels, respectively. See Figure 2-21 for an example of a 4-bit (16 gray shade) image and Figure 2-22 for an example of an 8-bit (256 gray shade) image.

Because a television monitor is designed to display analog information, the information that is stored in the scan converter's digital memory must be fed to a **digital-to-analog** (D to A) converter. One function of the D to A converter is to determine the brightness level that will be displayed for each gray scale level. This function is called **postprocessing.** Selectable postprocessing permits the operator to vary the emphasis that is given to various gray scale ranges. Because postprocessing occurs after the digital memory, it can affect stored and live images. Most ultrasound systems use some form of selectable postprocessing. See Figure 2-23 for image examples of different postprocessing selections.

Another image processing function that occurs before the digital memory is **write-magnification.** Selectable write-magnification permits the operator to electronically change the size of the displayed image before storage in the digital memory. With write-magnification,

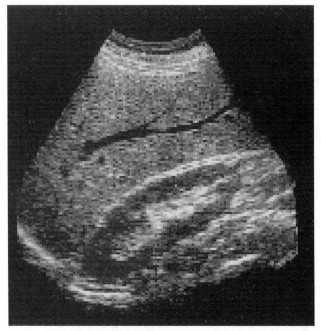

Figure 2-21 Four-bit (16 gray shade) image.

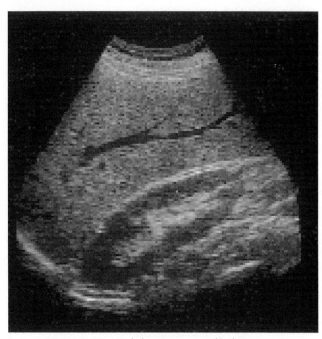

Figure 2-22 Eight-bit (256 gray shade) image.

there is no reduction in the number of displayed pixels. All ultrasound systems use some form of write-magnification. Controls often associated with write-magnification include:

    SCALE
    SIZE
    FIELD OF VIEW
    DEPTH
    RES

Figure 2-24 shows write-magnification of a selected area.

Read-magnification is an image-size function in some ultrasound systems that occurs after the digital memory. Selectable read-magnification permits an operator to enlarge a selected area of the display by enlarging each pixel. By enlarging each pixel, fewer pixels are present on the display. Images magnified in this manner are coarse when compared with images that are

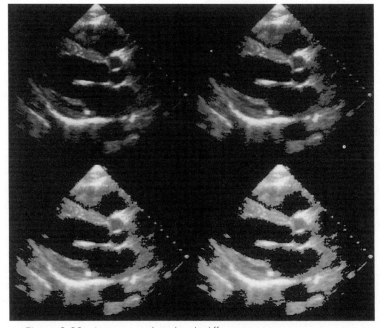

Figure 2-23 Images produced with different postprocessing settings.

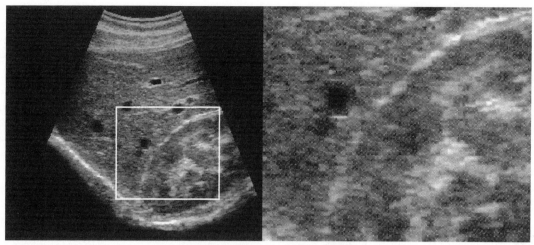

Figure 2-24   Write-magnification.

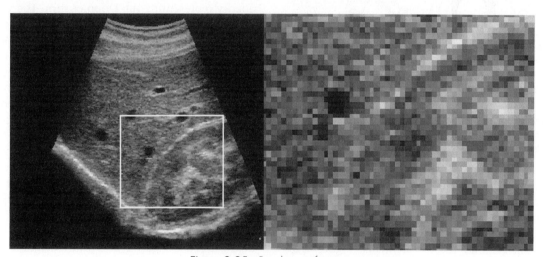

Figure 2-25   Read-magnification.

magnified using write-magnification techniques. Controls often associated with read magnification include:

ZOOM
MAG
SIZE

Figure 2-25 shows read-magnification of a selected area.

Most displays used in diagnostic ultrasound systems are television monitors designed to operate according to National Television Standards Committee (NTSC) specifications. Complete television pictures, or frames, are displayed 30 times every second ($^1/_{30}$ second for each frame). Each frame contains 525 horizontal scan lines with brightness variations produced as a result of an electron beam scanning the phosphor of the television monitor's cathode ray tube.* The frame's odd-numbered scan lines are produced first by starting at the top of the television monitor's cathode ray tube and moving from left to right, dropping down to the next

odd-line position at the left, moving again from left to right. This process repeats at every odd-line position for $^1/_{60}$ second until the line at the bottom is produced. This first pass, or television field, results in $262^1/_2$ lines. The process is then repeated during another $^1/_{60}$-second interval, producing a second (even) television field of $262^1/_2$ lines. The lines in the odd field are interlaced with the lines in the even field to produce the 525-line television frame.

---

*A **cathode ray tube** (CRT) is constructed of glass and encloses a vacuum. An electron gun at the rear of the CRT produces a narrow beam of electrons that travels through the CRT until it strikes the tube's face, which has a phosphor coating. When the electrons strike the phosphor, light is produced. Before reaching the phosphor, the electron beam passes through a changing magnetic field and is deflected to illuminate various areas of the phosphor. The beam's intensity is varied as it is being deflected to produce the various gray shades that are displayed.

DOPPLER INSTRUMENTATION

The **Doppler shift,** or **frequency shift,** is a change in frequency of a reflected wave caused by relative motion between the reflector and the transducer's beam. The change in frequency is proportional to the velocity of the moving reflector. The higher the original (transmitted) frequency, the greater the shift in frequency for a given reflector velocity. The returning frequency increases if the reflector is moving toward the transducer and decreases if the reflector is moving away from the transducer. The Doppler effect produces the shift that is the reflected frequency minus the transmitted frequency (Figure 2-26).

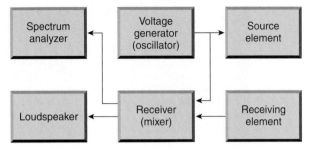

Figure 2-27 Block diagram of continuous wave Doppler system.

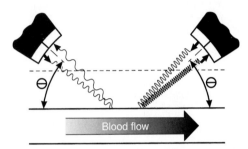

Figure 2-26 Doppler shifts from blood vessel. *Left,* away from the beam causes a shift to a lower frequency. *Right,* toward the beam causes a shift to a higher frequency.

A Doppler shift can only occur if the angle between the transducer's beam and the direction of movement of the reflector (red blood cells) is not 90 degrees. The maximum Doppler shift occurs if the angle is zero. **Continuous wave** (CW) Doppler transducers that are designed to be used without B-mode imaging contain separate transmit and receive elements. Figure 2-27 shows a diagram of a CW Doppler system.

A voltage generator that oscillates at the transducer's resonant frequency energizes the sending or source element. When the reflected sound returns to the receiving

element, it is converted into an electrical voltage, which is fed to a receiver. The receiver also receives a voltage with a frequency that was supplied to the source element. The receiver electronically "mixes" the two voltages and produces, at its output, a voltage having a frequency representing the Doppler shift. The voltage can be fed to a loudspeaker to produce an audible sound or to a **spectrum analyzer** to provide a visual representation of the shift frequencies. CW Doppler is capable of detecting a wide range of shift frequencies that are caused by high blood flow velocities. A disadvantage of CW Doppler is that it detects all movement in the path of the beam and cannot selectively detect Doppler shifts from specific depths.

When CW Doppler is used in conjunction with B-mode imaging, to assist in proper transducer positioning, a single line cursor is positioned on the two-dimensional (2D) image to guide the Doppler ultrasound beam (Figure 2-28).

A **pulsed wave** (PW) or **gated Doppler** system is depth selective. Figure 2-29 shows a diagram of a pulsed Doppler system.

The gate section of the system controls the timing of the oscillation voltage that is periodically supplied to the transducer. Another function of the gate is to syn-

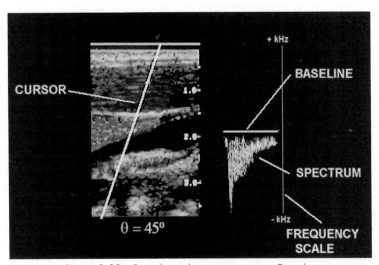

Figure 2-28 B-mode and continuous wave Doppler.

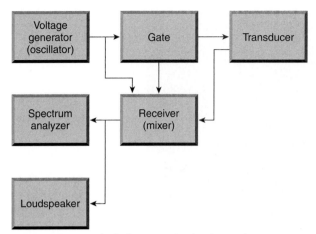

Figure 2-29 Block diagram of pulsed Doppler system.

PRF of a PW Doppler system represents intervals of transducer excitation controlled by the gate's timing function. Increasing the PRF raises the Nyquist limit, which increases the possibility of detecting greater velocities without aliasing. A high PRF may also result in **depth ambiguity.** Depth ambiguity reduces the maximum depth from which the location of a Doppler shift can be accurately detected. Other methods that can reduce the chances for aliasing include using a lower-frequency transducer or a steeper Doppler angle.

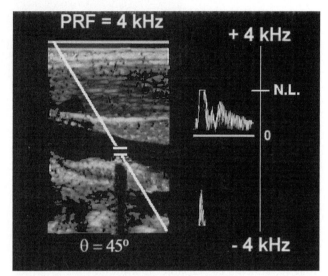

Figure 2-31 Pulsed wave Doppler with aliasing, a result of exceeding the Nyquist limit (NL).

chronize the receiver of the PW Doppler system. This synchronization results in information from the loudspeaker or spectrum analyzer that represents only the Doppler shifts from selected depths. A cursor can be superimposed over a cross-sectional B-mode image to select the direction from which Doppler shift frequencies are to be sampled. For PW Doppler operation, the cursor's gate is positioned to select the desired depth for Doppler frequency shift detection (Figure 2-30).

A drawback of pulsed Doppler is the possibility of **aliasing,** which occurs when high blood flow velocities are present. Aliasing, which does not occur with CW Doppler, results in the display of incorrect Doppler shift information. It occurs when the Doppler shift exceeds the Nyquist limit (Figure 2-31). The **Nyquist limit,** which represents the maximum accurately detectable Doppler shift, is equal to one half the Doppler PRF. The

Doppler ultrasound systems are designed only to measure frequency shifts. Most systems also provide indications of blood flow velocity. Blood flow velocity is

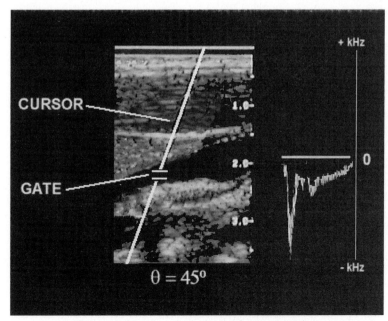

Figure 2-30 B-mode and pulsed wave Doppler.

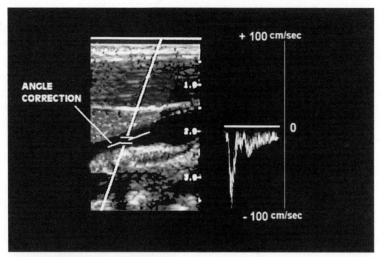

Figure 2-32 Pulsed wave Doppler with angle correction.

not measured but calculated. The operator must position an "angle-correction" cursor parallel with the walls of the vessel to ensure an accurate velocity calculation (Figure 2-32).

A **duplex ultrasound** system makes imaging and Doppler possible with the same transducer. A "true" duplex system is capable of providing "simultaneous" Doppler and real-time imaging from a single probe. Most linear array and electronically steered phased array imaging systems are capable of simultaneous Doppler and real-time imaging. In these systems, the same piezoelectric elements can be rapidly switched to permit their nearly simultaneous use for both functions.

Unlike **spectral Doppler** (CW or PW), which detects Doppler shifts along a single line, **color flow Doppler** permits instantaneous global detection of the Doppler shift frequencies by superimposing colors over the normal white and black cross-sectional image. The displayed colors, with hues that normally range from red to blue, are used to indicate the direction of blood flow relative to the selected angle of Doppler detection. See Figure 2-33 for an image with color flow Doppler.

All forms of ultrasound imaging of red blood cells are derived from the reflections that are received from them in response to the transmitted sound. The main characteristics of the reflections are frequency and amplitude. Whereas the velocity of the red blood cells determines the reflected frequency, the density (or concentration) of the moving blood cells producing the Doppler shifts determines their amplitude. The density of cells is controlled by the dynamics of blood flow within the vessel. With power Doppler, blood flow is detected using normal Doppler techniques to establish a threshold for discrimination of tissue motion. Signals with velocities below the threshold are assumed to originate from tissue, whereas signals with velocities above the threshold are

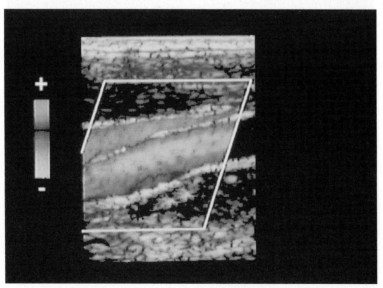

Figure 2-33 Color flow Doppler image (see Color Plate 1).

associated with blood flow. After discrimination of tissue motion, the remaining frequency shift information is ignored so that the display is free of normal Doppler characteristics such as angle and direction dependence and aliasing. Whereas normal color flow Doppler assigns color hues dependent on the direction and velocity of moving blood cells, power Doppler assigns a narrow range of hues dependent on the concentration of the moving blood cells (Figure 2-34).

Power Doppler is inherently more sensitive than normal color flow Doppler. This enables power Doppler to demonstrate very low velocity blood flow. Additionally, power Doppler is able to show smaller vessels at greater depths. The increased sensitivity, however, makes power Doppler more susceptible to tissue-motion artifacts.

Various terms that are used by different manufacturers to describe the power Doppler technique include:
POWER DOPPLER
POWERFLOW DOPPLER
DOPPLER ENERGY
COLOR ENERGY
COLOR AMPLITUDE
COLOR ANGIO
ULTRASOUND ANGIO
COLOR POWER ANGIO

IMAGE-RECORDING DEVICES
Ultrasound images may be recorded using various methods.

Photographic methods are routinely used to provide permanent **hard copies** by capturing images directly from television monitors supplied with video signals from ultrasound system scan converters.

Multiimage cameras are self-contained photographic devices with built-in television monitors that can record multiple images on single sheets of film or photographic paper. The multiple recording positions are produced using moving lenses, multiple lenses, moving film cassettes, or combinations of techniques. The exposed film or paper is normally developed in an x-ray film processor to provide transparent or opaque hardcopy images.

Laser imagers also produce multiple images on single sheets of film using nonphotographic techniques. Laser imagers operate by capturing video frames in digital memories. The stored digital information is then used to control the intensity of a laser beam that exposes the film using a sequential scanning technique.

Other nonphotographic hard-copy devices use thermal recording techniques. Black-and-white thermal printers use heat-sensitive paper as a recording medium. The image recorded on the paper is the result of the paper's passing over a multielement thermal head. The temperatures of the various elements are controlled by the television signal information fed to the printer from the ultrasound system. A color thermal printer produces a hard-copy color image by using a thermal head to melt portions of a multicolored ribbon onto a sheet of paper.

Video tape recorders and disk recorders store television image information using a magnetic medium. A video tape recorder can store live or frozen images. Disk recorders are designed to record frozen images. Some disk recorders use optical recording, rather than **magnetic recording,** methods. Because playback equipment is required for viewing the recorded information, the recordings themselves are not considered to be hard copies.

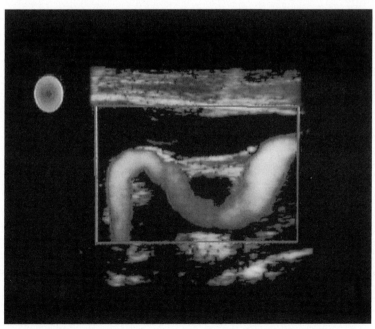

Figure 2-34 Power Doppler image (see Color Plate 2).

SECTION II

Sonographic Approach to Understanding Anatomy

■ CHAPTER 3

Body Systems

BETTY BATES TEMPKIN

OBJECTIVES ■

Describe the function of the musculoskeletal system.
Explain the motor, storage, and support capabilities provided by the musculoskeletal system.
Describe the function of the circulatory system.
Describe an artery and a vein, noting their differences.
Describe the function of the urinary system.
Trace the production of urine from the kidney to the urethra.
Describe the function of the digestive system.
Explain the digestive process from oral cavity to anus.
Describe the function of the respiratory system.
List the organs used in breathing.
Describe the function of the reproductive system.
Explain the normal menstrual cycle.
Describe male and female gamete production.
Describe the function of the endocrine system.
Explain the interrelationship of the various hormone-producing organs.
Describe the function of the central nervous system.
Explain how nerve impulses are transmitted.
Define the key words.

KEY WORDS ■

Abdominopelvic cavity	Diastolic
Alveoli	Dorsal cavity
Anastomose	Endocrine
Apex	Estrogen
Arteries	Follicle stimulating hormone
Autonomic system	Gametes
Base	Homeostasis
Bone marrow	Hormone
Collaterals	Human chorionic go-
Compact bone	nadotropin
Corpus luteum cyst	Involuntary muscles
Cranial cavity	Kidneys
Diaphragm	Large intestine

Ligaments	Spinal cavity
Luteinizing hormone	Spermatozoa
Lymph	Spongy bone
Metabolism	Suprarenal glands
Nephron	Sweat glands
Neurons	Systolic
Ovum	Tendons
Peripheral system	Thoracic cavity
Peritoneal	Trachea
Phagocytes	Tunica media
Pleura	Ureter
Renal pelvis	Urinary bladder
Retroperitoneal	Veins
Rugae	Ventral cavity
Sequelae	Voluntary muscles
Small intestine	

Although the importance of having a thorough understanding of the individual anatomic organs and areas within the body will be stressed throughout this textbook, a general knowledge of body systems and their relationship(s) to one another is significantly important. A general comprehension not only enables the sonographer to determine underlying events but also may be the determining factor leading to further investigation of related body systems during a sonographic examination.

An important concept for sonographers to master is how body systems function interdependently with each other. Although each body system has a unique, primary function(s), the function(s) may also relate in kind to another body system with the exact same function(s), or the function(s) may act as an accessory function to another body system. Body systems rely on each other to maintain homeostasis, and systems that share the same function can replace each other if one system's performance fails. With this understanding, it becomes obvious how pathologic conditions can affect more than one body system at a time. For a sonographer, this knowledge helps differentiate main or primary sites of disease processes from their potential secondary site(s) and consequently provides the interpreting physician with precise image representations from which to make an accurate diagnosis.

HUMAN DEVELOPMENT

During embryo-fetal development, molecules from specific specialized cells are determined by deoxyribonucleic acid (DNA). These cells unite to develop organs that work together to form a system (e.g., several anatomic organs make up the digestive system). Each organ has a specialized function, or possibly multiple functions, that it must carry out (e.g., ovaries are both endocrine and exocrine organs) based on the type of tissue cells that were formed as a group. There are a multitude of cell and tissue types that have specific functions (e.g., nephrons within the kidneys, neurons within the brain). Body systems work together to control the body's **metabolism** (buildup and breakdown of various chemicals) to maintain **homeostasis** (equilibrium).

BODY CAVITIES

As seen in Figure 3-1, the body has several natural "vaults" composed of cavities and spaces that contain organs within a specific region. A brief list is presented below; further details will be provided in upcoming chapters.

- **Ventral cavity:**
  - **Abdominopelvic cavity:** Cavity whose boundaries are the pubic bone inferiorly and the diaphragm superiorly.
    - **Thoracic cavity:** Enclosed area that basically corresponds to the rib cage. It is separated from the abdominal cavity by the diaphragm.
    - **Peritoneal space:** Anterior area of the abdominopelvic cavity within the peritoneal lining.
    - **Retroperitoneal space:** Posterior area of the abdominopelvic cavity, located posterior to the peritoneal lining.
- **Dorsal cavity:**
  - **Cranial cavity** (calvarium): Contains the brain.
  - **Spinal cavity:** Contains the spinal cord.

MUSCULOSKELETAL SYSTEM
Function

The musculoskeletal system (Figure 3-2) is a support system best compared to a high-rise building. Similar to the framework of a building, the bones enable other systems to attach and provide a means to counteract gravity.

This system has several functions. **Ligaments** attach bones to one another; **tendons** attach muscle to bone, allowing for *movement*. The bony skeleton and the muscles themselves unite to perform movement. The bones provide areas for muscle attachment via the tendons; with articulation areas, movement is now possible through contraction and relaxation. Various joint types (e.g., ball and socket, hinge) allow movement.

As seen in Figure 3-3, each bone is composed of a hard outer shell termed **compact bone** and a softer inner core, the **bone marrow.** Between the hard outer core and the soft marrow is a honeycomb type of bone structure termed **spongy bone.** This is similar to aircraft wings, which are made of a hard outer shell and a hon-

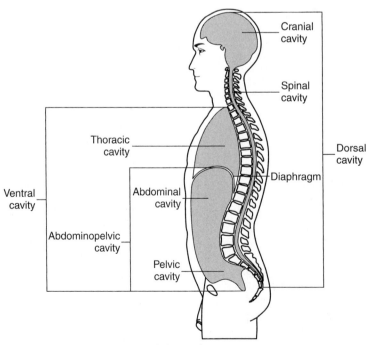

Figure 3-1 Body cavities.

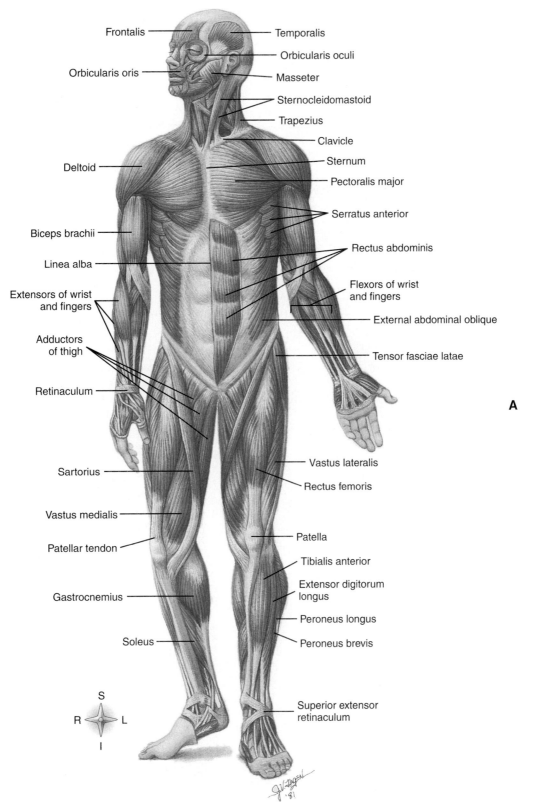

Frontalis

Temporalis

Orbicularis oculi

Orbicularis oris

Masseter

Sternocleidomastoid

Trapezius

Clavicle

Deltoid

Sternum

Pectoralis major

Serratus anterior

Biceps brachii

Rectus abdominis

Linea alba

Flexors of wrist
and fingers

Extensors of wrist
and fingers

External abdominal oblique

Adductors
of thigh

Tensor fasciae latae

Retinaculum

Sartorius

Vastus lateralis

Rectus femoris

Vastus medialis

Patella

Patellar tendon

Tibialis anterior

Extensor digitorum
longus

Gastrocnemius

Peroneus longus

Peroneus brevis

Soleus

S

R — L

I

Superior extensor
retinaculum

A

Figure 3-2   A, Skeletal muscles.

continued

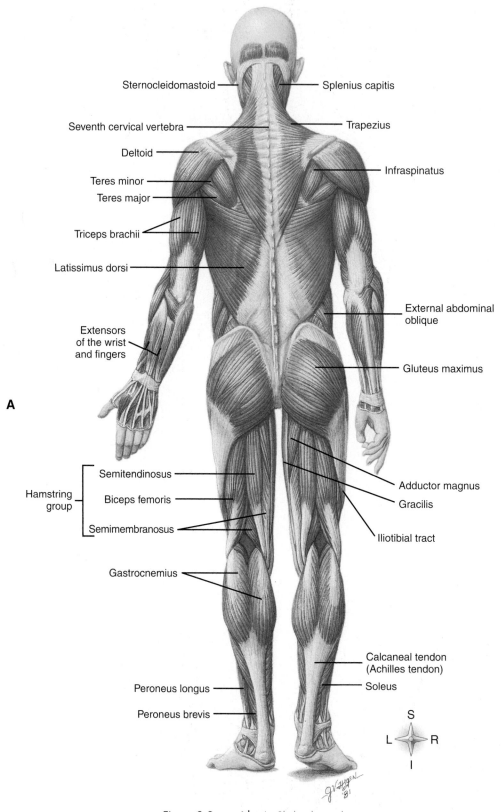

A

Figure 3-2, cont'd A, Skeletal muscles.

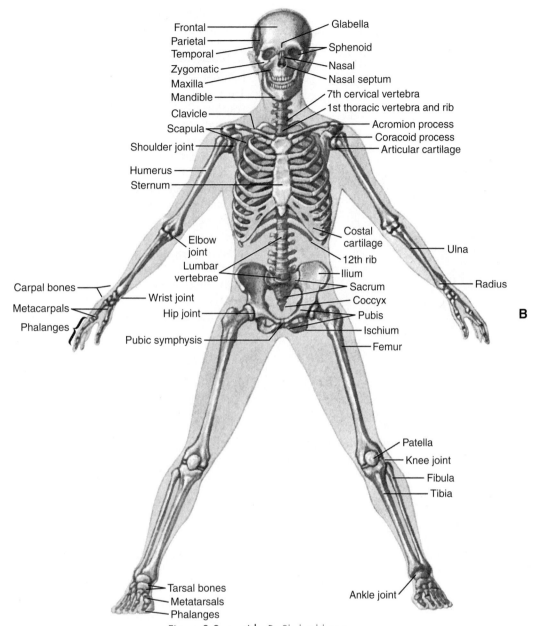

Frontal — Glabella
Parietal — Sphenoid
Temporal
Zygomatic — Nasal
Maxilla — Nasal septum
Mandible — 7th cervical vertebra
Clavicle — 1st thoracic vertebra and rib
Scapula — Acromion process
Shoulder joint — Coracoid process
— Articular cartilage
Humerus
Sternum
Elbow joint — Costal cartilage
— Ulna
Lumbar vertebrae — 12th rib
Carpal bones — Ilium
Metacarpals — Wrist joint — Sacrum
Phalanges — Hip joint — Coccyx
Pubic symphysis — Pubis
— Ischium
— Femur
Radius

B

Patella
Knee joint
Fibula
Tibia

Tarsal bones
Metatarsals — Ankle joint
Phalanges

Figure 3-2, cont'd B, Skeletal bones.

eycomb inner carbon material. This construction permits moderate flexing without causing stress fractures.

Bone and muscle provide *protection* from external forces. Although there are many other protective mechanisms within the body, as described elsewhere in this book, bone and muscle combine to form a protective covering for the vital organs. The brain and heart are excellent examples. The brain is encased in the bony protective calvarium, and the heart and lungs are surrounded by the bony rib cage.

Blood cell production occurs within the bone marrow and plays a vital role. Blood cells usually function for only 120 days before wearing out, at which time they

break down into amino acids and other proteins. Should the marrow cease to function appropriately as in cases such as leukemia or severe radiation damage, death is certain because of the inability of the marrow to replace the dying blood cells. In these instances, the urinary system provides an accessory function to the musculoskeletal system by assisting with the production of red blood cells (RBCs). In addition to their urinary system functions, the kidneys secrete the hormone erythropoietin, which stimulates bone marrow stem cells to manufacture RBCs (erythrocytes). Clearly, this demonstrates how independent yet interrelating body systems support one another. Other following examples

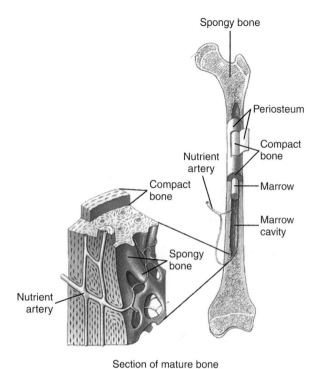

Section of mature bone

Figure 3-3 Bone composition.

show how the circulatory system and nervous system closely relate to the musculoskeletal system.

Muscle *contractions* function to move blood up through the veins against the effects of gravity. Normal muscle contraction and relaxation occur when one walks. As the blood moves up, valves located within the veins prevent the blood from returning downward after each contraction.

The bones *provide minerals* to any part of the body as needed. This is accomplished via the release of specific hormones and chemicals that break down bone to pass calcium, sodium, and potassium into the blood stream, which transports the minerals to the necessary site(s).

Muscle Types

The ability to move depends on the musculoskeletal system and its interdependent relationships with the nervous system and circulatory system.

The three different types of muscle tissue, skeletal, smooth, and cardiac, fall into two categories: voluntary and involuntary. **Voluntary muscles** are skeletal muscles that stabilize the skeleton and move it in response to commands from the brain. **Involuntary muscles** include smooth and cardiac muscles, which are controlled by the autonomic nervous system. Smooth muscle is found in the walls of blood vessels and the walls of digestive organs. It involves involuntary contractions that move venous blood from the lower limbs as previously discussed and moves digestive contents through the digestive tract. Cardiac muscle is unique to the heart and provides the

involuntary stimulus that results in the contraction and relaxation of the muscle that becomes the heart beat.

CIRCULATORY SYSTEM
Function

The circulatory system is a network of tubes and tubules responsible for providing blood, oxygen, and nutrients throughout the body and removing toxins. These provisions are primarily dependent on the pumping action of the heart.

Composition of Arteries and Veins

The circulatory system is composed of arteries, arterioles, veins, venules, and capillary beds. There are differences in structure, mainly related to the thickness of the musculature area (the **tunica media**) within an artery or vein (Figure 3-4). The difference in structure is directly related to the pressures that are maintained within those vessels. Arteries must withstand higher pressures than veins; thus their muscular layers are proportionately thicker.

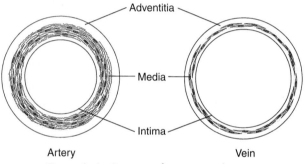

Figure 3-4 Structure of arteries and veins.

The difference in structure is an asset during renal dialysis procedures. An artery is connected to a vein in the forearm, forcing the vein to expand; a tube inserted within the vein sustains this distended state. As a result, the patient can undergo dialysis several times per week with much less likelihood of rupture of the vein.

Blood Flow Throughout the Body

The left side of the heart and the arterial system are under high pressure **(systolic),** whereas the right side of the heart and venous vessels are under low pressure **(diastolic).** Generally, the **arteries** (Figure 3-5) carry oxygenated blood, and the **veins** (Figure 3-6) transport deoxygenated blood. There are two exceptions: during fetal circulation, the umbilical vein carries oxygenated blood; the umbilical arteries carry deoxygenated blood. Also, the pulmonary artery and pulmonary veins are functionally reversed: the artery carries deoxygenated blood, and the veins carry oxygenated blood.

As previously described, blood in the legs would stagnate were it not for the presence of valves within the

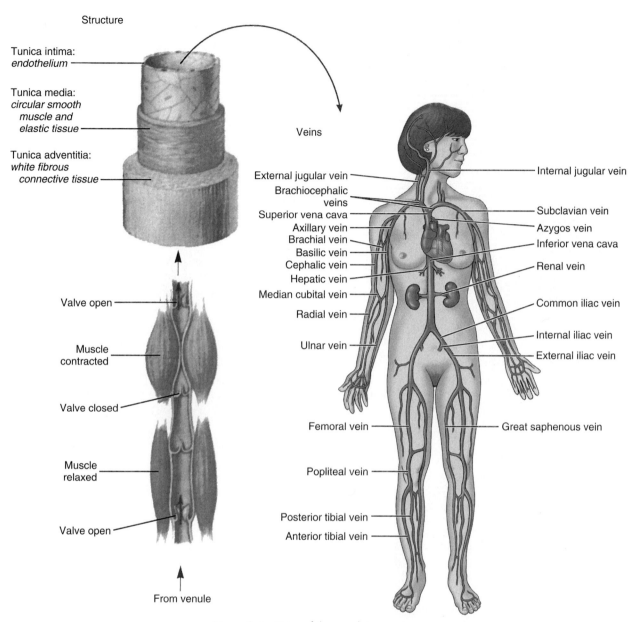

Figure 3-5 Veins of the circulatory system.

veins, along with muscular contraction provided by the musculoskeletal system. Arteries do not contain valves, the exception being the pulmonic and aortic valves. The thick muscular wall in the arteries squeezes the blood forward (see Figure 3-4).

Special Situations

There are two body areas in which the blood flow is unique—the liver and the kidney. In most organs, blood flow is as follows:

Artery → Arteriole → Capillary → Venule → Vein

Blood enters the liver via the hepatic artery. In the liver, the hepatic artery conveys blood to the liver cells to provide nourishment and energy. The unusual circumstance is that there is simultaneously free mixing of portal venous and hepatic arterial blood (deoxygenated with oxygenated). Blood is carried away from the liver via the hepatic veins, which drain into the inferior vena cava.*

Also, the kidney contains two sets of capillary beds rather than a single set (as is the case in all other areas). This additional set enables the kidney to maintain a state of blood pressure equilibrium, a safety feature that maintains blood pressure even when systemic pressure changes occur (Figure 3-7). This is a good example of

---

*Mixing of oxygenated and deoxygenated blood within the liver is possible because of the close proximity of the heart.

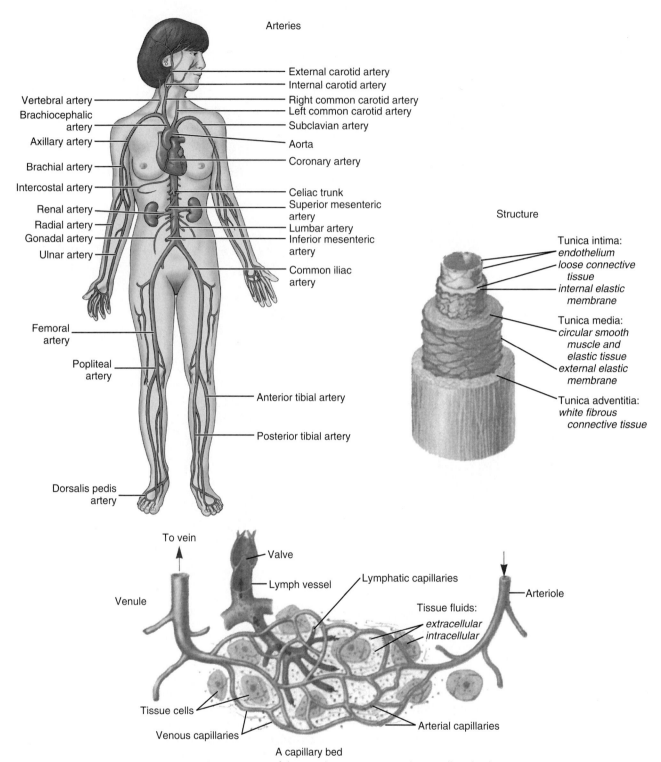

Figure 3-6   Arteries of the circulatory system, and a capillary bed.

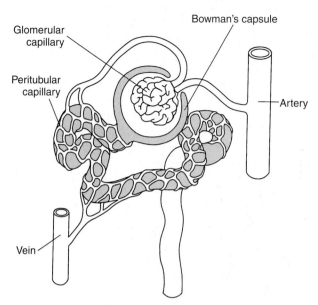

Figure 3-7 The two capillary beds of the kidney.

how interdependent body systems share functions and provide protective back up assistance if the primary system's function fails.

Conditions Resulting From Prolonged Venous Hypertension

Veins under constant pressure begin to expand. The result is an increase in the size of a vein or organ (e.g., hepatomegaly, splenomegaly). As a result, **collateral** veins, forming detours, may develop. The vessel under pressure seeks assistance from nearby vessels and **anastomoses** or connects to those vessels.

Lymphatic System

The lymphatic system has two major functions, the first being to transport excess fluid from tissue back into the bloodstream, and the second being to attack harmful bacteria and foreign substances through **phagocytes** within the lymph nodes. (The special function of phagocytes is to destroy foreign substances.) Without this transport capability, excess fluid in the tissues would develop (called edema).

When harmful bacteria are destroyed, an immune response may occur in which a foreign substance is recognized as hostile and is destroyed by white blood cells (WBC). In patients with an infection, macrophages (large phagocytes) are created in such large numbers within the lymph nodes that the lymph node increases in size.

Unlike blood flow, lymph travels in one direction only (Figure 3-8). Lymphatic flow is identical to and parallels venous flow via muscle contraction. During blood exchange in the capillary beds, some fluid **(lymph)** remains within the tissues and must be eliminated. The excess fluid is transported via the lymphatic vessels and is

filtered through the lymph nodes as the lymph courses toward the thorax. Lymph nodes are located along the lymphatic tract (e.g., groin, axilla, neck, and periaortic area [see Figure 3-8]) and act as "filtering stations" that the lymph must pass through. Once in the chest, lymph reenters the bloodstream, which is essential to maintain correct fluid levels within the blood. The spleen is part of the lymphatic system; its function is to eliminate worn-out blood cells from the circulatory system.

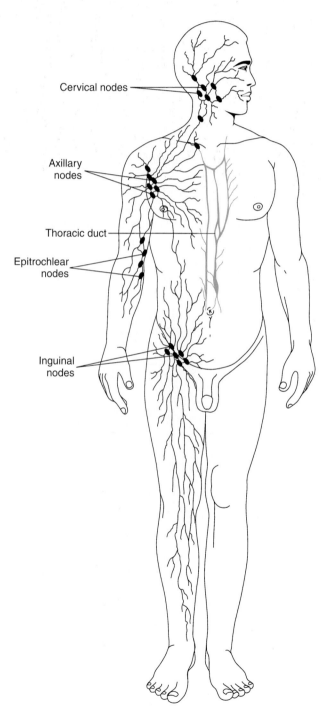

Figure 3-8 The lymphatic system.

URINARY SYSTEM

Function

The basic function of the urinary system is to filter waste products such as urea, uric acid, and creatinine, while maintaining a state of equilibrium within the body. When blood is filtered in the **kidneys** (bean-shaped organs situated in the posterior part of the abdomen at approximately the height of the elbows), wastes are removed, but much of the water and other substances required by the body is reabsorbed and becomes part of the general circulation. As previously mentioned, kidney function also includes the production of substances that influence blood pressure, the production of erythrocytes, and the maintenance of serum levels of phosphate and calcium.

Anatomy

The urinary system is composed of paired kidneys and **ureters** (one on each side of the body) and a bladder and urethra. On the superior medial surface of each kidney is an adrenal gland (also called **suprarenal glands**), which is discussed in the endocrine system section of this chapter (Figure 3-9). The **renal pelvis** is a funnel-shaped reservoir that collects urine from all parts of the kidney.

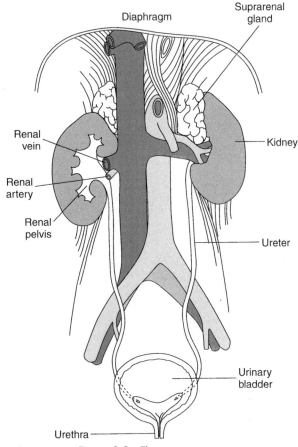

Figure 3-9   The urinary system.

Each kidney has its own artery, vein, and ureter emanating from the renal hilum. As noted earlier, there is a slight variation in the circulation of blood within the kidney related to the existence of an additional capillary bed not commonly found in other areas (blood pressure regulators).

The functional structure of the kidney is the **nephron.** There are more than 1 million microscopic nephrons in each kidney. A nephron is shown in Figure 3-10; its major components are a glomerulus and tubules. Each glomerulus is a cluster of capillaries derived from the afferent arteriole.

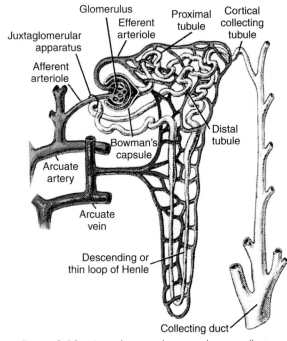

Figure 3-10   A nephron and surrounding capillaries.

Filtration

Within the renal cortex, the glomeruli inside Bowman's capsule act to filter the blood passing through (see Figure 3-10). This action is similar to that of a washing machine: cells within Bowman's capsule have "slits" that allow smaller molecules to pass through and keep out larger molecules, while in a washing machine, waste products are removed by size in much the same way. Laundry is spun, allowing water to run through the small holes (waste) yet keeping the clothes (blood cells) where they belong. Damage to the kidneys would be the equivalent of increasing the hole size and letting unwanted substances such as blood cells pass through (i.e., gross hematuria).

Urine Flow

Using gravity, urine leaves the renal pyramids toward the renal pelvis via the major and minor calyces, one drop at a time. Urine leaves the renal pelvis, descends the ureter, and enters the **urinary bladder** in streams

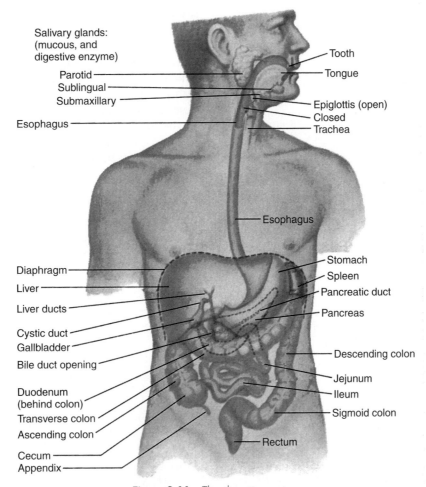

Salivary glands:
(mucous, and
digestive enzyme)

Parotid

Sublingual

Submaxillary

Esophagus

Tooth

Tongue

Epiglottis (open)

Closed

Trachea

Esophagus

Diaphragm

Liver

Liver ducts

Cystic duct

Gallbladder

Bile duct opening

Duodenum
(behind colon)

Transverse colon

Ascending colon

Cecum

Appendix

Stomach

Spleen

Pancreatic duct

Pancreas

Descending colon

Jejunum

Ileum

Sigmoid colon

Rectum

Figure 3-11   The digestive system.

termed "jets" that are commonly seen on ultrasound. The bladder temporarily stores the urine until it is excreted from the body via the urethra.

DIGESTIVE SYSTEM

Function

The function of the digestive system is to convert ingested food into substances the body uses to maintain metabolism. The mouth, esophagus, stomach, small intestine, colon, liver, and pancreas work together in the breakdown and absorption process. The biliary system plays an accessory role by storing and releasing bile (produced in the liver) into the small intestine when fatty chyme (semidigested material) is detected.

Anatomy

From the oral cavity to the anus, the digestive canal is one long unbroken "tube" (Figure 3-11). The stomach consists of folds called **rugae** that allow expansion and contraction. Between the rugae are glands that secrete acid and mucus that breakdown or digest solid food products into a liquid called chyme.

The **small intestine** consists of villi, which are finger-like projections that add to the overall surface volume of the intestine and function to absorb substances such as nutrients and minerals from chyme (Figure 3-12). In addition to producing enzymes capable of digesting lipids (fats), carbohydrates, and proteins, the small intestine receives accessory enzymes from bile, as previously mentioned, via the common bile duct and from the pancreas via the pancreatic duct to aid in digestion.

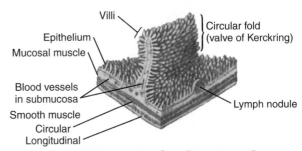

Villi

Epithelium

Mucosal muscle

Blood vessels
in submucosa

Smooth muscle

Circular

Longitudinal

Circular fold
(valve of Kerckring)

Lymph nodule

Figure 3-12   Section of small intestine wall.

The **large intestine** transports unabsorbed material to the sigmoid colon and anus to be expelled. Occasionally, the vermiform appendix, a small appendage of the intestinal cecum, becomes full and inflamed by the unabsorbed material. In some cases this is demonstrable on ultrasound.

RESPIRATORY SYSTEM
Function
The respiratory system provides a means of supplying oxygen to the body while eliminating carbon dioxide, a natural byproduct of cellular activity (Figure 3-13).

Anatomy
Air enters the body via the **trachea,** which subdivides into bronchi, bronchioles, alveolar ducts, and alveoli. The **alveoli** are small sacs with a very thin tissue lining, which facilitates the exchange of gases (i.e., oxygen and carbon dioxide). The lungs receive their blood supply from the descending aorta.

The lungs, contained within the thoracic cavity, are somewhat triangular in shape, with their **apex** superior and **base** inferior. They are separated from the abdomi-

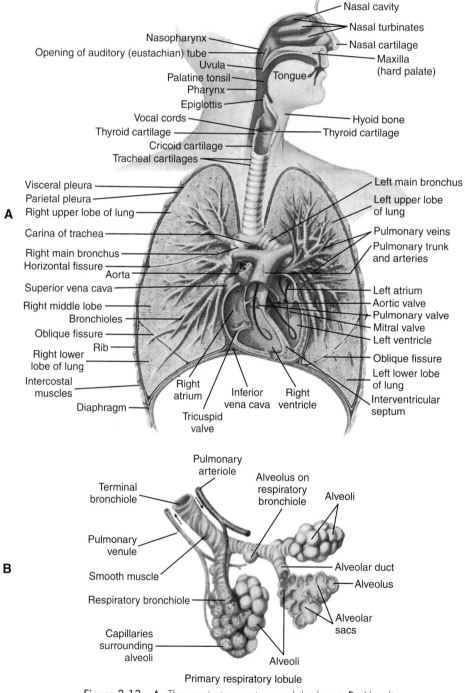

Figure 3-13   **A,** The respiratory system and the heart. **B,** Alveoli.

nal cavity by the muscular **diaphragm** located at their base. For descriptive purposes, the lungs are divided into lobes, with the right lung having three lobes and the left having two. A double-walled sac called the **pleura** (visceral and parietal pleura) surrounds the lungs. These two sacs, with pleural fluid between them, enable the lung to expand and contract without adhering to the chest walls. Diaphragmatic movement enables inhalation and exhalation.

Pressure within the lungs is below atmospheric pressure, which causes the lungs to remain partially inflated at all times. In the fetus, the pressure within the lungs is above atmospheric pressure, which causes the fetal lungs to stay collapsed until birth.

REPRODUCTIVE SYSTEM

Function

The reproductive system provides a means to perpetuate the species. The male and female reproductive systems differ from the previously described body systems because they do nothing directly to contribute to the survival of the human body such as breathing, blood flow, and digestion (Figures 3-14 and 3-15).

In a process called fertilization, **gametes** or germ cells (male **sperm cell,** female **egg cell**) fuse to form a zygote and ultimately perpetuate the species.

Male Gamete Production

Spermatozoa are produced in the testes and mature in the epididymis. The vas deferens transports the spermatozoa from the epididymis and is joined by the seminal vesicle before becoming the ejaculatory duct. The ejaculatory duct courses through the prostate, joining the prostatic urethra, and exits the penis via the urethra. The scrotum is capable of protraction and retraction, which aids spermatozoa production and maintenance. The scrotum actually moves away from the body if the temperature is too high and closer to the body if the temperature is too low.

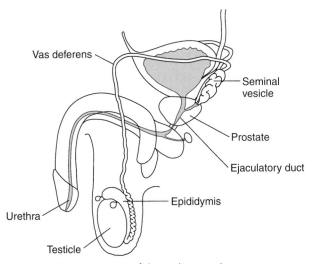

Figure 3-14 Organs of the male reproductive system.

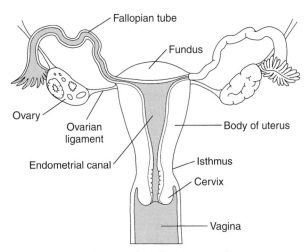

Figure 3-15 Organs of the female reproductive system.

Female Gamete Production and Fertilization

Following is the process involved in ovulation and attempted fertilization, beginning with the female menstrual cycle:

1. **Follicle stimulating hormone** (FSH) is released by the pituitary gland, which stimulates the ovaries to produce follicles.
2. **Estrogen** is released by ovarian tissue during the FSH release to prepare the endometrial lining of the uterus for potential zygote implantation.
3. **Luteinizing hormone** (LH) is released on approximately the fourteenth day of the menstrual cycle and stimulates the follicle to burst and release its ovum. The empty follicle becomes a corpus luteum cyst, which is maintained by LH release. The ovum enters the fallopian tube, moving toward the endometrial canal of the uterus.
4. The **corpus luteum cyst** releases estrogen and progesterone.
5. The detection of progesterone released by the corpus luteum cyst causes LH to stop being released. This disrupts maintenance of the corpus luteum cyst and subsequent menstruation (sloughing off of the endometrial lining).

If pregnancy occurs, the corpus luteum cyst is maintained. No other follicles are stimulated during the remaining months of the pregnancy. Below are the differences that occur in the presence of fertilization:

1. The blastocyst (embryonic cell) releases an enzyme before implantation that "loosens" the implantation site, enabling it to bury itself deep into the endometrial lining of the uterus.
2. A second release from the blastocyst prevents the endometrium from being shed and maintains the corpus luteum, thus suppressing menstruation. The hormone BhCG or **human chorionic gonadotropin** can now be detected via blood or urine for pregnancy testing.

Zygote formation usually occurs within the fallopian tube. The cells undergo multiple cell divisions, forming a tiny blastocyst containing hundreds of cells before implantation within the uterus. Following implantation, the cells organize to form the embryo. Over several weeks the embryonic cells multiply and undergo the beginnings of structural development. By the eighth week, organs are formed and limb buds begin to enlarge to form the fetus. Development of body systems continues along with growth. The respiratory system continues to develop through the eighth month, just prior to birth.

Twins develop after either the fertilization of two separate ova or division of the embryo before implantation (see Chapter 19 for diamniotic and dichorionic definitions). Embryonic division beyond the twelfth day after fertilization results in the development of conjoined twins.

ENDOCRINE SYSTEM
Function
The endocrine or neuroendocrine system regulates specific functions performed by other body systems. It is regulated by the hypothalamus of the brain, which communicates with the endocrine system's pituitary gland (also located in the brain) to regulate the hormonal activity of the other seven endocrine glands located throughout the body (Figure 3-16).

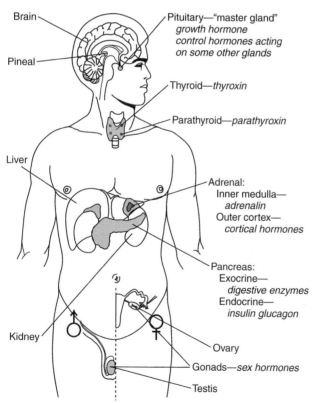

Figure 3-16 Location of the eight glands of the endocrine system.

Between the hypothalamus and pituitary gland, **hormones** or "chemical messengers" are released to regulate body functions such as growth, metabolism, blood sugar levels, production of adrenalin, maturation of ova and sperm, ovulation, lactation, and others. Target areas or receptors within the hypothalamus monitor the levels of many chemicals within the body. These receptors are said to control whether a releasing or inhibiting hormone is released, which acts directly on the pituitary gland.

The double-lobed, pea-size pituitary or "master" gland is influenced by the hormones released from the hypothalamus and, in response, produces its own hormones that stimulate the other endocrine glands to produce their own hormones that control specific functions to help maintain the body's chemical equilibrium and homeostasis. The effect of each hormone on the body varies. The term hormone is a general classification. For example, the hormone insulin has a different function from the reproductive or thyroid hormones.

The term **endocrine** means ductless; the endocrine glands release the hormones directly into the blood stream.

Glands of the Endocrine System
Table 3-1 lists the endocrine glands, the hormones they produce, and their endocrine function.

CENTRAL NERVOUS SYSTEM
Function
The central nervous system is the body's "computer." It is responsible for processing input data from all areas of the body. **Neurons** (nerve cells} transmit messages to and from the brain, controlling everything from pain sensation to coordination, from high-level cognitive processing to the endocrine-regulating hypothalamus.

Anatomy
The brain and spinal cord are the main components of the central nervous system. They are well protected by bone, the cranial vault, and the spinal column, which surround these structures like protective armor.

The central nervous system is classified into peripheral and autonomic nervous systems, also referred to as voluntary and involuntary control. The **peripheral system** is responsible for voluntary actions such as walking. The **autonomic system** controls involuntary actions of the heart, endocrine glands, and other internal organs.

The brain receives blood via two carotid arteries and two vertebral arteries. Although relatively small, these vessels receive approximately 20% of the total blood flow. Blood exits the cranium via the jugular veins. Because of its blood supply requirements, the brain is susceptible to severe perfusion **sequelae** (conditions associated with changes in blood flow).

■ ■ ■ **Table 3-1** Hormones of the Endocrine Glands and Their Function

Gland	Function
Pituitary Gland	
Follicle stimulating hormone (FSH)	Assists in ovarian follicle development in females and sperm maturation in males.
Luteinizing hormone (LH)	
Thyrotropin (TSH)	Thyroid-stimulating hormone.
Adrenocorticotropin (ACTH)	Adrenal stimulating hormone.
Growth hormone (GH)	Stimulates growth in general.
Prolactin	Initiates and maintains milk secretion in females.
Thyroid Gland	
Thyroxine (T_4)	Responsible for assisting in metabolism of lipids, proteins, and carbohydrates. Their presence can increase the body's need for oxygen. This leads to increased heat production (body temperature elevation) that will influence most tissues.
Triiodothyronine (T_3)	
Note: The number in parentheses indicates the number of attached iodine cells (e.g., thyroxine + 4 iodine cells)	
Calcitonin	Responsible for removing calcium via absorption. This causes calcium to be removed from the blood and sent to the bones for storage.
Parathyroid Glands	
Parathyroid hormone (PTH)	Basic antagonist for calcitonin. PTH sends a signal causing bone reabsorption. If the body is low in calcium, it will take what it needs from the bones, adding calcium to the bloodstream.
Adrenal Glands	
Epinephrine	Causes blood glucose levels to elevate. The heart races and major vessels dilate. It also causes ACTH to be released from the pituitary.
Norepinephrine	Causes diastolic and systolic blood pressure to increase. It is also a vasoconstrictor, and causes peripheral vessels to constrict. It makes sense to keep the blood flow where needed in the heart, lungs, and voluntary muscles—for running.
Mineralocorticoids	Control sodium and potassium levels.
Glucocorticoids	Control glucose use by conserving consumption (ACTH controlled).
Pancreas	
Insulin	Controls the uptake/use of glucose to prevent glycogen breakdown within the liver; it is responsible for decreasing the blood sugar level. Glucagon antagonist to glucocorticoids; it increases the blood sugar level.
Ovaries	
Estrogen	Responsible for female secondary sex characteristics. Released during the menstrual cycle to prepare the uterus for possible implantation.
Progesterone	Released during the menstrual cycle to prepare the uterus for possible implantation.
Testes	
Testosterone	Responsible for male sex characteristics.

Neuron

A neuron is a nerve cell, responsible for transmitting impulses much the same way that a wire carries an electric charge. Most nerve cells are covered by a myelin sheath, which is analogous to the plastic covering or insulation of a wire or cord. When neurons are damaged, other neurons often attempt to compensate by assuming additional tasks.

Special Sensory Organs: The Ear and the Eye (Figure 3-17)

The ear is composed of three parts: outer, middle, and inner. The outer ear (i.e., the pinna or auricle) focuses sound toward the middle ear. The middle ear consists of the tympanic membrane and the three smallest bones of the body—malleus, incus, and stapes. Their function is to conduct sound to the inner ear, which is composed of the cochlea and semilunar canals. The inner ear is responsible for balance and conversion of physical sound waves to electrical impulses that the brain can recognize. This is similar to a reverse piezoelectric effect (see Chapter 1).

The eye functions like a camera. Light is focused toward the back of the eye to be recorded or converted into a signal recognizable by the brain. The eye focuses on thousands of objects every day. It is estimated that 12 video cameras would be required to match the recording capabilities that the eye performs in a single day.

The cornea of the eye serves to refract (bend) light through the iris and lens toward the retina at the back for processing. Problems with the lens or cornea cause light to be refracted to the back of the eye but not toward the retina. In this case, glasses are needed to correct the refraction problem.

The eyelids shield the eye from debris and impact. They also clean the surface of the eyes similarly to the action of windshield wipers.

SUMMARY

The body has many specialized cells and tissues with highly specific functions. These cells and tissues allow the body to maintain a state of equilibrium (balance) by performing their individual duties and working together. Body compartments (cavities) separate many of these systems from one another.

Muscles and bones afford physical protection and work together in movement. Bones are a reservoir for calcium and produce blood cells within the marrow. Muscles are divided into those that the person controls (voluntary) and those that the person does not control (involuntary).

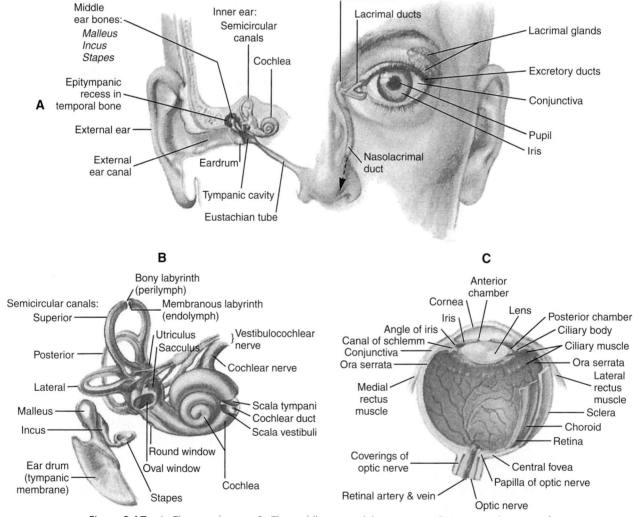

Figure 3-17 **A,** The ear; the eye. **B,** The middle ear and the inner ear. **C,** Horizontal section of the eye.

The circulatory system (blood and lymph) carries vital nutrients to the tissues and removes excess fluid. Lymph in the capillaries is filtered as it passes through the lymph nodes to remove foreign bodies. The circulatory system and the lymphatic system depend on muscle contraction for transport.

The urinary system filters waste from the blood and helps maintain the body's equilibrium. Blood is filtered through the nephrons of the kidney, which also serve to reabsorb water and other substances that the body can use. The kidneys also influence blood pressure, the production of RBCs, and serum levels of phosphate and calcium.

The digestive system metabolizes ingested food. Starting at the oral cavity, mastication (chewing) and saliva begin the initial breakdown of food. The stomach is the organ in which gastric acids begin to further break down the food so that it may enter the small intestine. At the duodenum, pancreatic enzymes and hepatic bile aid in breaking down lipids and proteins, illuminating the importance of the pancreas and liver as accessory organs to the digestive system. The small intestine also absorbs essential nutrients and then passes the chyme on to the large intestine for expulsion.

Oxygen and carbon dioxide are exchanged across a thin alveolar membrane during inhalation and exhalation assisted by the diaphragm. Although the lungs are not routinely evaluated by ultrasound, excess fluid in the pleural sac (pleural effusion) and infectious pus pockets (empyema) may be demonstrated.

Reproduction of the species is very intricate as demonstrated by the number of hormones required to prepare for and maintain a pregnancy. Equally important is the capability of protraction and retraction of the scrotum to aid spermatozoa maintenance.

The endocrine system enables the body to regulate a multitude of functions by detecting changes in blood chemistry. Release of hormones directly into the bloodstream ensures immediate response to the hypothalamus's signal regulating blood pressure, blood sugar, calcium levels, and other body functions.

The brain controls all actions within the body via voluntary and involuntary muscle signaling. Additional functions of the brain include control of sensory areas (sight, hearing, smelling, and touch) and regulatory areas (hypothalamus and pituitary control of the endocrine system).

General comprehension of body systems and how they interrelate is necessary for accurate ultrasound evaluation of the body. Later chapters describe details of individual organs and vessels to facilitate sonographic assessment. However, it is essential to keep in mind the interdependency of specific organs and vessels. Knowledge of this interaction not only enables the sonographer to determine underlying events but also may be the determining factor leading to further investigation of other areas or body systems during a sonographic examination.

BIBLIOGRAPHY

Larson D: *Mayo Clinic family healthbook,* ed 2, New York, 1996, William Morrison.

Rothenberg D: *The new Lexicon illustrated medical encyclopedia and guide to family health,* New York, 1988, Lexicon Publishing.

Spence A: *Basic human anatomy,* ed 3, Massachusetts, 1990, Addison-Wesley/Cummings.

CHAPTER 4

Anatomy Layering and Sectional Anatomy

ALEXANDER LANE AND BETTY BATES TEMPKIN

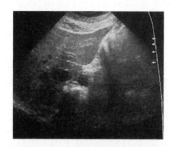

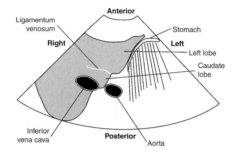

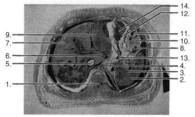

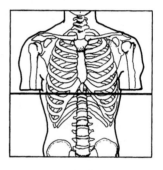

1. Spinal cord
2. Spleen
3. Hilum of spleen
4. Descending abdominal aorta
5. Inferior vena cava
6. Caudate lobe
7. Right lobe of the liver
8. Descending colon
9. Left lobe of the iver
10. Splenic flexure (left colic flexure)
11. Transverse colon
12. Greater curvature of stomach
13. Lesser curvature of stomach
14. Lumen of stomach

Cadaver section and ultrasound image section. See Figure 4-14 for more details.

OBJECTIVES ■

Define the directional terminology used in sonography.
Describe how the body is divided.
Classify body layers (anatomic tissue layers) into four classes and describe each briefly.
Describe the visceral layers (including muscles and blood vessels) of the abdomen and pelvis.
Describe body planes and sonographic scanning planes and their interpretation.
Describe the positional orientation of body structures.
Define the significance of describing the relationship of adjacent body structures.
Describe the similarities and differences among body structures as they appear in cadaver sections and ultrasound image sections.
Describe the sonographic appearance of body structures.
Define the key words.

KEY WORDS ■

Abdominal cavity	Lateral
Anechoic	Lesser sac
Anterior	Medial
Coronal plane	Mesentery
Crura of the diaphragm	Omentum
Diaphragm	Parietal peritoneum
Distal	Pelvic cavity
Dorsal cavity	Pelvic inlet
Echogenicity	Peritoneal cavity
Extravisceral layers	Peritoneal membrane
False pelvis	Posterior
Foramen of Winslow	Proximal
Greater sac	Retroperitoneal
Homogeneous	Sagittal plane
Hyperechoic	Somatic layers
Hypoechoic	Superficial
Inferior	Superior
Intraperitoneal	Thoracic cavity
Intravisceral luminal layers	Transverse plane
Intravisceral nonluminal layers	True pelvis
Isosonic	Ventral cavity
	Visceral peritoneum

This chapter relates to the methodology for learning sectional anatomy. Advances and expansions in the field of radiologic diagnostic medicine demanded an update in the teaching of human anatomy. Therefore a new methodology guided by computer imaging modalities was formulated. Each computer imaging modality, including ultrasound, depicts the body in sections in various views, layer by layer. Thus an analysis of body sections is essential to the interpretive process.

The guidelines for the sonographic study of sectional anatomy can be standardized and are outlined below. These guidelines use a systematic search pattern for the accurate identification and description of layered anatomy, sectional anatomy, cadaver sections, and clinical images. These eight orientation guidelines for sectional anatomy follow:

1. *Directional terminology.* Understanding the directional terminology that sonographers use is the key to accurate description and communication. Table 4-1 defines those terms, and Figure 4-1 demonstrates them.
2. *Divisions of the body.* It is important that sonographers are able to differentiate the natural cavities and spaces of the body, not only because of the bulk of structures they contain but also because of the potential abnormalities that can invade them. A brief list of all the body cavities is covered in Chapter 3. The peritoneal cavity is the primary focus of this section.

The human body consists of two main cavities, **ventral** and **dorsal**, with one situated on the **ante-**rior (ventral) area and the other on the **posterior** (dorsal) area. Each of these cavities, in turn, is divided into smaller cavities. The **diaphragm** (a muscular partition that assists inspiration) separates the ventral cavity into the **thoracic cavity** and the **peritoneal cavity.** The peritoneal cavity is the largest body cavity, encompassing the abdomen and pelvis.

The **peritoneal membrane,** a thin sheet of tissue that secretes serous fluid, lines the peritoneal cavity; the fluid acts as a lubricant and facilitates free movement between organs. The peritoneum is classified as **parietal,** the portion of peritoneum lining the cavity, and **visceral,** the portion of peritoneum covering the organs. The parietal peritoneum forms a closed sac, except in females, in whom a portion of the fallopian tubes opens into it. The enclosed, or **intraperitoneal,** structures include the liver (except for a bare area posterior to the dome), gallbladder, spleen (except for its hilum), stomach, the majority of the intestines, and the ovaries. The intraperitoneal abdominal organs are connected to the cavity wall by the **mesentery,** a double fold of peritoneum.

Retroperitoneal structures are located posterior to the sac and are covered anteriorly with peritoneum. This applies to the kidneys, ureters, adrenal glands, pancreas, aorta, inferior vena cava, urinary bladder, uterus, and prostate gland. The ascending colon, descending colon, and most of the duodenum are also situated in the retroperitoneum, as are the abdominal lymph nodes and somatic nerves.

■ ▥ ▥ **Table 4-1**   Directional Terminology

Term	Definition	Examples
Anterior (ventral)	Situated at or directed toward the front. A structure in front of another structure.	The liver is situated anteriorly in the body. The head of the pancreas is anterior to the inferior vena cava.
Posterior (dorsal)	Situated at or directed toward the back. A structure behind another structure.	The kidneys are situated posteriorly in the body. The inferior vena cava is posterior to the head of the pancreas.
Superior (cranial)	Situated above or directed upward. Toward the head. A structure higher than another structure.	The lungs are situated superiorly in the body. The diaphragm is superior to the liver.
Inferior (caudal)	Situated below or directed downward. Toward the feet. A structure lower than another structure.	The uterus is situated inferiorly in the body. The superior mesenteric artery is inferior to the celiac axis.
Medial	Situated at, on, or toward the middle or midline of the body.	The spine is situated medially in the body. The aorta is medial to the left kidney.
Lateral	Situated at, on, or toward the side. To the right or left of the middle or the midline of the body.	The spleen is situated left laterally in the body. The carotid arteries are lateral to the thyroid.
Ipsilateral	Situated on or affecting the same side.	The spleen and left kidney are ipsilateral.
Contralateral	Situated on or affecting the opposite side.	The ovaries are contralateral.
Proximal	Situated closest to the point of origin or attachment.	The common hepatic duct is proximal to the common bile duct.
Distal	Situated farthest from the point of origin or attachment.	The abdominal aorta is distal to the thoracic aorta.
Superficial	Situated on or toward the surface. External.	The testicles are superficial structures.
Deep	Situated away from the surface. Internal.	The pancreas is a deep structure.

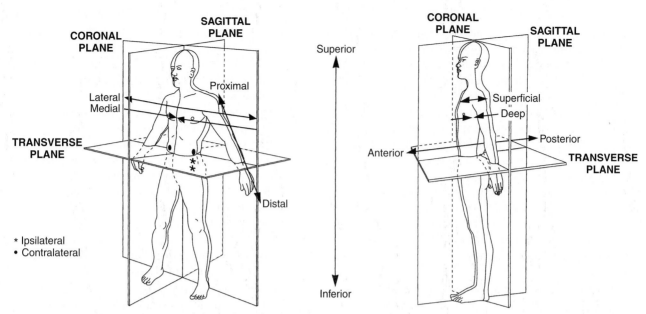

Figure 4-1 View of the body in the anatomic position (standing erect, arms at the sides, face and palms directed forward) with body planes (sagittal, coronal, transverse) and directional terms.

The abdominal portion of the peritoneal cavity can be divided further into two peritoneal compartments: the greater sac and the lesser sac. The **greater sac** extends from the diaphragm to the pelvis and covers the width of the abdomen. The **lesser sac,** or omental bursa, is a diverticulum of the greater sac located posterior to the stomach. The neck, or area of communication between the sacs, is termed epiploic foramen or **foramen of Winslow.** Table 4-2 summarizes several additional peritoneal cavity spaces created by the complex arrangement of the peritoneum. These spaces are particularly appreciated sonographically when filled with free fluid.

The **omentum** is a double layer of peritoneum that extends from the stomach to adjacent abdominal organs. It is classified into the greater omentum, which attaches to the anterior surface of the transverse colon, and the lesser omentum, which joins the lesser curvature of the stomach and the first part of the duodenum to the porta hepatis (area of the liver where the hepatic artery and main portal vein enter the liver and the biliary ducts leave). In some instances, there are folds of peritoneum running from one organ to another, called ligaments. The names of the ligaments are directly related to the organs to which they are attached.

The abdominal portion of the peritoneal cavity, or **abdominal cavity,** excluding the retroperitoneum and the pelvis, is bounded superiorly by the diaphragm, anteriorly by the abdominal wall muscles, and posteriorly by the vertebral column, ribs, and iliac fossa. It is continuous with the pelvic cavity inferiorly through the pelvic in-

let. The abdominal contents include the liver, gallbladder and biliary tract, pancreas, adrenal glands, kidneys, ureters, spleen, stomach, intestines, and lymph nodes. Also included are the abdominal aorta and its branches, which supply blood to these structures, and the inferior vena cava and the main portal vein, which receive and remove blood from them. The left and right **crura of the diaphragm** (muscular bands that arise from the lumbar vertebrae and insert into the diaphragm) are also within the abdominal cavity.

The peritoneal cavity is routinely described as nine regions and four quadrants. Sonographers use these divisions to accurately describe the location of abdominal structures. Figure 4-2 demonstrates those divisions and also the surface landmarks used to describe the abdominal wall.

The pelvic portion of the peritoneal cavity, or **pelvic cavity,** is bounded anteriorly and laterally by the hipbones and posteriorly by the sacrum and coccyx. It extends superiorly from the iliac crests to the pelvic diaphragm inferiorly. Deep to this bony framework lie the muscles that line the pelvic cavity. The pelvic contents include the distal portion of the ureters, urinary bladder, urethra, distal portion of the ileum, cecum, appendix, sigmoid colon, rectum, lymph nodes, and iliac vessels. Additionally, the female pelvis includes the uterus, fallopian tubes, and ovaries, and the male pelvis contains the prostate gland and seminal vesicles.

The pelvis is divided into the false and the true pelves by an oblique plane circumscribing the

■ ■ ■ **Table 4-2** Peritoneal Cavity Spaces

Space	Location
Supracolic compartment (supramesocolic space)	The area above the transverse colon constitutes the supracolic compartment, which includes the right subhepatic space, left subhepatic space, right subphrenic space, and left subphrenic space.
Subhepatic spaces	Classified as right and left because they are respectively located posterior to the right and left lobes of the liver. The right subhepatic space includes Morison's pouch, which lies between the superior pole of the right kidney and the posterior aspect of the right lobe of the liver. The left subhepatic space includes the lesser sac.
Subphrenic spaces	Classified as right and left because they are respectively located on each side of the falciform ligament. The spaces lie between the diaphragm and the anterior portion of the right and left lobes of the liver.
Infracolic compartment (inframesocolic space)	The area inferior to the transverse colon constitutes the infracolic compartment, which includes the right paracolic gutter, left paracolic gutter, the gutter to the right of the mesentery, and the gutter to the left of the mesentery.
Paracolic gutters	The right paracolic gutter is located between the right lateral abdominal wall and the ascending colon. The left paracolic gutter is between the left lateral abdominal wall and the descending colon. The gutter to the right of the mesentery is a space between the mesentery and the ascending colon. The gutter to the left of the mesentery is a space between the mesentery and the descending colon.
Perirenal space	An area located around the kidney, adrenal gland, and fat, surrounded by fascia (Gerota's fascia).
Pararenal space	Classified as anterior and posterior. The anterior pararenal space is located between the anterior surface of the renal fascia (Gerota's fascia) and the posterior portion of the peritoneum. The posterior pararenal space is located between the posterior surface of the renal fascia and the transversalis fascia.
Posterior cul-de-sac (pouch of Douglas or rectouterine pouch)	The most posterior and dependent portion of the peritoneal sac. A space located between the urinary bladder and rectum in the male and the rectouterine pouch in the female.
Anterior cul-de-sac (vesicouterine pouch)	A shallow space located between the anterior wall of the uterus and the urinary bladder. This space all but disappears as the urinary bladder fills with urine. This space does not exist in the male.

sacral promontorium, ala of the sacrum, arcuate line of the ilium, pectineal line of the pubis, pubic crest, and upper edge of the pubic symphysis. The circumference of this plane is the **pelvic inlet.** The **false pelvis (greater pelvis or pelvis major)** forms the walls of the most superior portion of the pelvic cavity. It is situated superior to the pelvic inlet. The **true pelvis (lesser pelvis or pelvis minor)** is shorter than the false pelvis, with considerably greater depth on its posterior wall than on its anterior wall. It is situated inferior to the pelvic inlet and contains the bladder, distal portion of the ileum, cecum, appendix, sigmoid, rectum, and some of the reproductive organs.

The pelvic portion of the peritoneal cavity is described as three regions: right iliac, hypogastric, and left iliac. These regions are subdivisions of the hypogastrium (see Figure 4-2, *top left*). Sonographers use these regions to accurately describe the location of the pelvic viscera. For example, the right iliac region includes the cecum and appendix. The hypogastric region contains structures such as the distal end of the ileum, urinary bladder, uterus (nonpregnant), and prostate. The sigmoid colon, distal end of the left ureter, and left ovary are found in the left iliac region.

3. *Tissue layers.* Tissue layers (anatomic layers) are classified based on location into four classes: (1) *somatic,* (2) *extravisceral (visceral),* (3) *intravisceral luminal,* and (4) *intravisceral nonluminal.* The **somatic layers** include the multilayers found on each body region from skin to cavity. In a region where no cavity exists, the somatic tissue layers consist of the entire region from peripheral to deep. The **extravisceral layers** (visceral layers) indicate the serial sequence of viscera (internal organs), blood vessels, and spaces between each organ within each cavity. **Intravisceral luminal layers** are found within the walls of organs with a lumen, such as the stomach. **Intravisceral nonluminal layers** involve organs without a prominent lumen. An excellent example of an intravisceral nonluminal organ would be the adrenal glands.

The extravisceral layers (visceral layers) of the abdomen and pelvis are outlined and discussed, going from deep to superficial. Each visceral layer (organ layers including muscles and blood vessels) from posterior to anterior is named and discussed. For example, the stomach is anterior to the pancreas. This layering approach is the best method for clarifying the intricate relationships of adjacent body

Regional Divisions of the Abdomen

Quadrant Divisions of the Abdomen

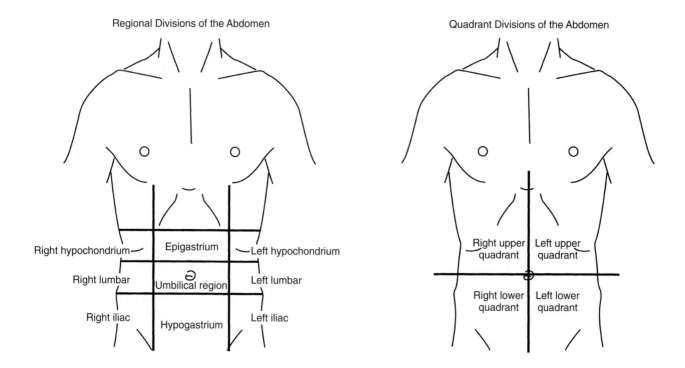

Surface Landmarks of the Abdominal Wall

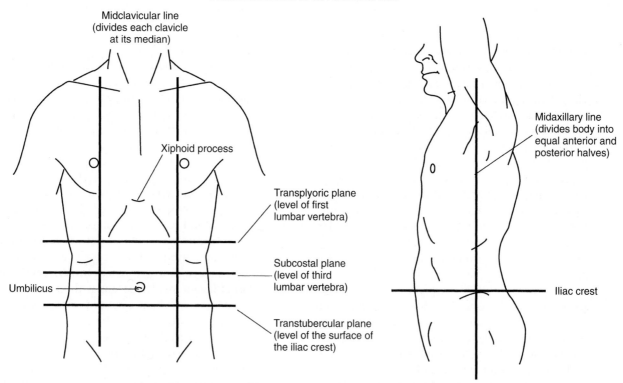

Figure 4-2 Divisions of the peritoneal cavity and surface landmarks.

plane. For further information on the layering concept and visceral unit layers of the abdominal and pelvic regions see Figures 4-3 and 4-4.

4. *Classification of structures.* Classification of the structures in cadaver and ultrasound sections into four anatomic units follows mastery of the anatomic layers. The four units are the musculoskeletal, vascular, visceral, and enclosing units. In the musculoskeletal unit, the skeletal muscles in the body wall are specified. In the vascular unit, origin and distribution of the vessels are noted. In the visceral unit, the location and course are discussed. The structures of the enclosing unit include membranes, fossae, spaces, depressions, and recesses. See Figures 4-3 and 4-4 for assistance in classifying structures.

5. *Positional orientation of body structures.* Note, in the layering illustrations, that some structures lie in a vertical position (inferior vena cava), and some are vertical oblique (portal vein, kidneys). Other body structures lie transversely (renal arteries and veins) or transverse oblique (pancreas), and some vary in position (gallbladder). Figure 4-5 illustrates these examples. Knowledge of the specific position of body structures makes their identification more recognizable on cadaver and ultrasound sections.

6. *Sectional planes.* The classic anatomic planes are the transverse, sagittal, and coronal (see Figure 4-1). The **transverse plane** divides the body into unequal superior and inferior sections perpendicular to the long axis of the body. The **sagittal plane** divides the body into unequal right and left sections parallel to the long axis of the body. Equal right and left sections are described as being from the midsagittal plane. The **coronal plane** divides the body into unequal anterior and posterior sections perpendicular to the sagittal planes and parallel to the long axis of the body. Equal anterior and posterior body sections at the midaxillary line are described as being from the midcoronal plane. The scanning planes used in sonography are the same as anatomic body planes, whereas their interpretations depend on the location of the transducer and the sound wave approach. Positional orientation of the transducer and its location on the body determine the scanning plane viewed. Generally, the manufacturer of the transducer sets the positional orientation. Sagittal plane orientation, for example, is usually indicated when a notch or raised portion of the transducer appears on the top surface. Rotating the transducer 90 degrees changes the scanning plane. Figures 4-6 and 4-7 demonstrate standard scanning plane interpretations. The endovaginal and endorectal scanning plane interpretations are shown in Figure 4-8. Figure 4-9 demonstrates how to interpret neurosonography (sonography of the brain) scanning planes.

7. *Relationship of adjacent body structures.* Describing the relationship of adjacent body structures is the best way to accurately classify specific anatomy. Currently, most ultrasound is performed with real-time sector scanners. This results in ultrasound images of isolated sections of the body that may contain major body structures such as the spine for locational reference. For this reason, the specific area of the body being imaged, patient position (scanning approach), and scanning plane must be clarified on the image for accurate interpretation. With clarification of the aforementioned specifics and determination of the relationship of adjacent structures, the anatomy in an image section can be classified. This is a critical discipline for the sonographer to adopt because errors can occur when structures are identified solely based on their expected standard location and sonographic appearance. Too many normal variants exist to rely strictly on memorization as to where a structure "ought" to be or what its sonographic appearance "should" be. Consideration must also be given to disease processes that can affect the standard location of body structures and most certainly their sonographic appearance. Because of these variables and the fact that ultrasound images are isolated sections, classifying anatomy according to the relationship of adjacent structures is the most accurate form of interpretation. For example, in a sagittal section, the target organ or area of interest is related to a structure immediately anterior to it, posterior to it, superior to it, and inferior to it (Figure 4-10). In a coronal section, the target organ or area of interest is related to a structure immediately **lateral** (right or left) to it, **medial** (toward the midline) to it, **superior** (above) to it, and **inferior** (below) to it (Figure 4-11). In a transverse section taken from either an anterior or a posterior approach (transducer position), the target organ or area of interest is related to a structure immediately anterior to it, posterior to it, right lateral to it, and left lateral to it (Figure 4-12). In a transverse section taken from either a right or left lateral approach, the target organ or area of interest is related to a structure immediately lateral (right or left) to it, medial to it, anterior to it, and posterior to it (Figure 4-13).

Figure 4-3 The anatomic layers of the abdomen. The layering approach is the best method for clarifying the intricate relationships of adjacent body structures regardless of body plane or scanning plane.

A, The posterior muscle layer is the most dorsal layer of the abdomen, which includes the lumbar spine, psoas major muscle, and quadratus lumborum muscle. The psoas major muscle is a somewhat triangular, bilateral muscle that originates from the lower thoracic and the lumbar vertebrae. It courses slightly anterior and slightly lateral as it descends through the lower abdomen immediately lateral to the spine. Near the fifth lumbar vertebra, the psoas major separates from the spine and courses more laterally on its descent to the iliac crests. This separation creates a space between the vertebral column and psoas major through which the iliac vessels run. The quadratus lumborum muscle is also a bilateral muscle tissue that extends from the iliolumbar ligament, the adjacent portion of the iliac crest, and the transverse processes of the lower lumbar vertebrae. The muscle courses upward, lateral to the psoas major muscle, until it reaches the twelfth rib.

B, This layer includes the kidneys and adrenal glands. The kidneys are retroperitoneal organs that lie on each side of the spine in the area between the twelfth thoracic and fourth lumbar vertebrae. The adrenals are located superior, anterior, and slightly medial to each kidney. The kidneys and adrenal glands lie just anterior to the quadratus lumborum and psoas major muscles; however, the largest portion of the psoas muscle is located more medially.

C, The inferior vena cava originates at the junction of the two common iliac veins anterior to the body of the fifth lumbar vertebrae. It ascends the retroperitoneum anterior to the spine and psoas major muscle and passes through the diaphragm to enter the right atrium of the heart. Note the location and transverse lie of the renal vein tributaries. Also note the location of the hepatic vein tributaries.

D, The aorta originates at the left ventricle of the heart and then descends (thoracic aorta) posterior to the diaphragm into the retroperitoneum of the abdominal cavity (abdominal aorta). The aorta continues to descend, anterior to the spine and psoas major muscle, and then bifurcates into the common iliac arteries at the level of the fourth lumbar vertebra. Note the anterior branches of the abdominal aorta: the celiac axis and the superior mesenteric artery. The celiac axis has three branches: the splenic artery, which courses left laterally toward the spleen; the hepatic artery, which courses right laterally toward the liver; and the left gastric artery, which travels superiorly and then left laterally toward the stomach and esophagus. Note the gastroduodenal artery, a branch of the hepatic artery that travels inferiorly toward the head of the pancreas. The superior mesenteric artery runs anterior and parallel to the aorta. Note the layers and the left renal vein passing right between the aorta and superior mesenteric artery as it traverses the body from the left kidney to the inferior vena cava. Note that both renal arteries lie just posterior to the renal veins. Also, the right renal artery runs just posterior to the inferior vena cava on its course to the right kidney.

E, This layer includes the portal venous system, which supplies blood to the liver for metabolic processes. This blood originates from the stomach, small intestine, large intestine, and spleen. The splenic vein courses laterally to medially, adjacent and inferior to the splenic artery. Note that it passes just anterior to the superior mesenteric artery. The splenic vein terminates posterior to the neck of the pancreas as it unites with the superior mesenteric vein to form the portal vein. Note that the superior mesenteric vein and inferior mesenteric vein tributaries course from inferior to superior. Also note the proximity of the superior mesenteric vein and superior mesenteric artery. Note that after the main portal vein forms, it courses superiorly approximately 5 to 6 cm and then bifurcates into right and left branches. Note that the hepatic artery is anterior to the portal vein.

The Layers of the Abdomen

A. POSTERIOR MUSCLES

Right   Left

Diaphragm

Quadratus lumborum

Quadratus lumborum

Lumbar vertebra

Psoas major

B. KIDNEYS AND ADRENAL GLANDS

Right   Left

Diaphragm

Right adrenal gland

Left adrenal gland

Right kidney

Left kidney

Quadratus lumborum muscle

Quadratus lumborum muscle

Ureter

Lumbar vertebra

Psoas major

C. VENA CAVA

Right   Diaphragm   Left

Hepatic veins

Left adrenal gland

Right adrenal gland

Left kidney

Right renal vein

Left renal vein

Right kidney

Quadratus lumborum muscle

Lumbar vertebra

Inferior vena cava

Psoas major muscle

Common iliac veins

D. AORTA

Right   Diaphragm   **Aorta**   Left

Hepatic veins   **Left gastric artery**

Hepatic artery   **Celiac axis**

Right renal artery   **Splenic artery**

Right renal vein   **Left renal artery**

Left renal vein

Gastroduodenal artery

Superior mesenteric artery

Inferior vena cava

Psoas major muscle

Common iliac veins   **Common iliac arteries**

E. PORTAL VENOUS SYSTEM

Right   Left gastric artery   Left

Diaphragm   Aorta

Hepatic veins   Celiac axis

Hepatic arteries   Spleen

                            Splenic artery

Portal vein   **Splenic vein**

Right renal vein   Left renal vein

Gastroduodenal artery   **Inferior mesenteric vein**

Inferior vena cava   Superior mesenteric artery

Psoas major muscle   **Superior mesenteric vein**

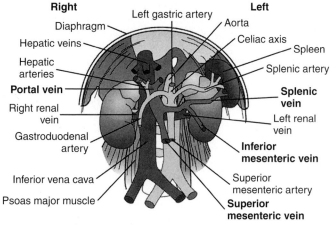

Figure 4-3 A to E   *continued*

Figure 4-3, cont'd

F, The pancreas is a retroperitoneal organ that traverses the body from the hilum of the spleen to the duodenum. The head of the pancreas lies to the right of the superior mesenteric vein and immediately anterior to the inferior vena cava. Note that the head lies slightly inferior to the body and tail. Also note the gastroduodenal artery that lies on the anterolateral surface of the head. The uncinate process is a medial projection of the head that lies just posterior to the superior mesenteric vein. Because it varies in size, it may extend to lie between the superior mesenteric artery and the aorta. The pancreatic neck is immediately anterior to the superior mesenteric vein, and slightly superior to that level, it lies anterior to the formation of the portal vein. The body of the pancreas lies to the left of the pancreatic neck, immediately anterior to the splenic vein. Note the layers, as the splenic vein is then anterior to the superior mesenteric artery, which branches anteriorly from the aorta. The pancreatic body extends left laterally to the tail of the pancreas. The tail, like the body, lies just anterior to the splenic vein. The tail of the pancreas extends left lateral to the hilum of the spleen. Note that the body and tail of the pancreas are inferior to the splenic artery.

G, This layer includes the intraperitoneal gallbladder and the biliary tract. The position of the gallbladder is variable, but it is common to see the fundus anterior to the superior pole of the right kidney or the head of the pancreas. The gallbladder neck is fixed in its position. Note that the cystic duct is immediately superior to the gallbladder neck. The common hepatic duct courses inferomedially and meets the cystic duct to form the common bile duct. Note that the common hepatic duct is anterior to the portal vein. The common bile duct also courses inferomedially, running behind the duodenum on its way to the head of the pancreas. Note the layers, as the common bile duct is anterior to the portal vein and hepatic artery at certain levels. Also note that at other levels, the common bile duct is right lateral to the hepatic artery.

H, In this layer, the gastrointestinal (GI) tract consists of the stomach and duodenum. Note the anterior lay of this portion of the GI tract and the numerous structures it covers. The anterior surface of the stomach is in contact with the diaphragm; the thoracic wall formed on the left by the seventh, eighth, and ninth ribs; the left lobe of the liver; and the anterior abdominal wall. The posterior surface of the stomach is related to the diaphragm, spleen, left adrenal gland, superior pole of the left kidney, anterior surface of the pancreas, and splenic flexure of the colon. The course of the duodenum presents a remarkable curve, somewhat in the shape of an imperfect circle, so that its termination is not far removed from its starting point. The first portion of the duodenum begins at the pylorus of the stomach and ends at the neck of the gallbladder. This portion is usually posterior to the gallbladder and anterior to the gastroduodenal artery, head of the pancreas, common bile duct, common hepatic artery, and portal vein (note the layers). It then takes a sharp curve and descends along the right margin of the head of the pancreas for a variable distance, usually to the level of the superior edge of the fourth lumbar vertebra. Now it curves again, passing from right to left with a slight inclination upward, anterior to the inferior vena cava, aorta, and vertebral column. The duodenum ends opposite the second lumbar vertebra at the jejunum.

I, The liver is the most anterior visceral organ of the peritoneal cavity and is intraperitoneal except for a bare area that is posterior to its dome. It occupies the right upper quadrant and often extends past the midline into the left upper quadrant. The superior and lateral surfaces of the liver border the diaphragm. The left lobe is just anterior to the stomach and body of the pancreas. The right lobe is immediately anterior to the gallbladder, right kidney (primarily the superior pole), right adrenal gland, and head of the pancreas.

J, The most anterior layer of the abdomen is the abdominal wall, which extends from the xiphoid process of the sternum to the pelvic bones. It consists of subcutaneous tissue and muscles. The subcutaneous tissue contains fat, fibrous tissue, fascia, small vessels, and nerves. The rectus abdominis muscle is an anterior, bilateral muscle immediately lateral to the linea alba (a white line of connective tissue in the median of the abdomen). This muscle originates at the pubis and then ascends to insert at the xiphoid process and costal cartilages of the fifth, sixth, and seventh ribs. The rectus sheath encloses the rectus abdominis muscle. The external oblique muscle is a bilateral muscle tissue that originates from the outer surface of the lower eight ribs and then fans out to insert into the xiphoid process, linea alba, pubic bones, and anterior iliac crest. The internal oblique muscle is also a bilateral muscle immediately deep to the external oblique muscle. Its muscle fibers run at right angles to those of the external oblique.

F. PANCREAS

Right   **Left**

Left gastric artery

Aorta

Diaphragm

Celiac axis

Hepatic veins

Spleen

Hepatic artery

Splenic artery

Portal vein

Pancreas

Body

Tail

Neck

Right renal
vein

Left renal
vein

Head

Gastroduodenal
artery

Inferior
mesenteric vein

Psoas major
muscle

Superior
mesenteric artery

Inferior vena cava

Superior
mesenteric vein

G. GALLBLADDER AND BILIARY TRACT

Right   **Left**

Portal vein

Diaphragm

**Common
hepatic duct**

Hepatic veins

Splenic artery

Hepatic artery

Main
pancreatic duct

Cystic duct

Right kidney

Pancreas

Gallbladder

Inferior
mesenteric vein

Gastroduodenal
artery

Superior
mesenteric artery

**Common bile
duct**

Psoas major muscle

Aorta

Superior
mesenteric vein

Inferior vena cava

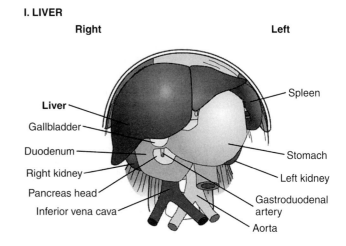

H. GASTROINTESTINAL TRACT

Right   Common hepatic duct   **Left**

Diaphragm

Portal vein

Hepatic veins

Celiac axis

Spleen

Hepatic artery

Splenic
artery

Gallbladder

Right kidney

Gastroduodenal
artery

Stomach

Duodenum

Left kidney

Pancreas head

Aorta

Inferior vena cava

I. LIVER

Right   **Left**

Liver

Spleen

Gallbladder

Duodenum

Right kidney

Stomach

Left kidney

Pancreas head

Gastroduodenal
artery

Inferior vena cava

Aorta

J. ANTERIOR MUSCLES

Right   **Left**

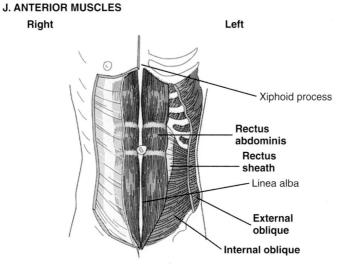

Xiphoid process

**Rectus
abdominis**

**Rectus
sheath**

Linea alba

**External
oblique**

Internal oblique

Figure 4-3 cont'd   F to J

Figure 4-4 The anatomic layers of the pelvis. The layering approach is the best method for clarifying the intricate relationship of adjacent body structures regardless of body plane or scanning plane.

A, The true pelvis muscle layer is the deepest layer of the pelvis. The muscles of this layer include the obturator internus, piriformis, coccygeus, iliococcygeus, and pubococcygeus. The obturator internus muscle is a triangular, bilateral muscle tissue that originates at the pelvic brim. It courses parallel and adjacent to the lateral pelvic wall, narrowing inferiorly to pass through the lesser sciatic foramen to the greater trochanter of the femur. It is lateral to the pelvic viscera. The piriformis muscle is also a triangular, bilateral muscle that originates from the sacrum. It extends laterally, narrowing to pass through the greater sciatic foramen to the greater trochanter of the femur. The pubococcygeus, iliococcygeus, and coccygeus muscles are a group referred to as the pelvic diaphragm. This muscle group lines the floor of the true pelvis. The pubococcygeus, puborectalis, and iliococcygeus muscles form the hammocklike portion of the pelvic floor, and together are termed the levator ani muscles. The pubococcygeus muscles course from the pubic bone to the coccyx. There is a separation in a section of the muscle termed the genital hiatus, which allows the passage of the urethra, vagina, and rectum (as demonstrated here). A section of the puborectalis muscle embraces the sides of the prostate. This portion is called the levator prostate and the pubovaginalis in women. The most medial and anterior muscles of the pelvic diaphragm are the pubococcygeus muscle pair. The iliococcygeus muscles extend from the ischial spine to the coccyx. They lie just lateral to the pubococcygeus muscles. The coccygeus muscles also course from the ischial spine to the coccyx. They are the most posterior muscle pair of the pelvic diaphragm.

B, Muscles of the posterior body wall and false pelvis include the quadratus lumborum, psoas major, iliacus, and iliopsoas. The quadratus lumborum muscle is a bilateral muscle tissue that extends from the iliolumbar ligament, the adjacent portion of the iliac crest, and the transverse processes of the lower lumbar vertebrae. It courses upward, lateral to the psoas major muscle, until it reaches the twelfth rib. The psoas major muscle is a somewhat triangular, bilateral muscle that originates from the lower thoracic and lumbar vertebrae. It courses slightly anteriorly and slightly laterally as it descends through the lower abdomen immediately lateral to the spine. Near the fifth lumbar vertebra, the psoas major separates from the spine and courses more laterally on its descent to the iliac crests. This separation creates a space between the vertebral column and the psoas major through which the iliac vessels run. At the level of the iliac crests, the psoas major muscles join the iliacus muscles to form the iliopsoas muscles. The iliacus muscles originate from the iliac fossa and the base of the sacrum and extend to meet the psoas major. The iliopsoas muscles continue a lateral descent, passing over the pelvic inlet to insert into the lesser trochanter of the femur.

C, This layer includes the rectum and a portion of the colon. The descending colon passes downward through the abdominal cavity along the lateral border of the left kidney. It curves medially at the inferior pole of the kidney toward the lateral border of the psoas major muscle and then descends in the angle between the psoas major and quadratus lumborum muscle to the iliac crest. The distal portion (iliac colon) begins at the iliac crest and runs just anterior to the psoas major and iliacus muscle to the sigmoid portion of the colon. The sigmoid colon is continuous with the descending colon and passes transversely, anterior to the sacrum to the right side of the pelvis. It then curves toward the left to reach the midline of the pelvis, where it bends downward and ends at the rectum. The sigmoid colon is anterior to the external iliac vessels and the left piriformis muscle. The rectum is continuous with the sigmoid colon above and ends in the anal canal below. It courses inferiorly, anterior to the coccyx, where it bends back sharply into the anal canal. This inferior portion lies directly anterior on the sacrum and coccyx, and levator ani muscle.

D, The anatomy of the female pelvis and the urinary bladder are appreciated at this layer. Note that a large portion of the bladder has not been drawn to facilitate the location of the organs just adjacent to it. The organs of the female pelvis include the uterus, vagina, fallopian tubes, and ovaries. The nonpregnant uterus is located in the true pelvis, anterior to the rectum and posterior to the bladder. There are spaces posterior and anterior to the uterus not demonstrated here that are referred to as the posterior cul-de-sac (pouch of Douglas or rectouterine pouch) and anterior cul-de-sac formed by the peritoneum. The fundus is the superior, anteriorly tilted part of the uterus. The body is the vertical, oblique portion between the fundus and the cervix. The cervix is inferior to the body of the uterus and adjacent to the vagina. The vagina is a vertically elongated structure located just anterior to the rectum and posterior to the bladder (trigone) and urethra. Note that the distal portion of the ureters is lateral to the vagina. The fallopian tubes lie in the superior part of the broad ligament and extend laterally toward the ovaries. The broad ligament is actually a double fold of peritoneum covering the anterior surface of all of the pelvic viscera except for the ovaries, which are located on the posterior portion of the broad ligament and entirely inside the peritoneal sac. For this reason, the ovaries are not demonstrated here because, although "attached" laterally to the uterus by the fallopian tubes and broad ligament, they are posterior to both structures. The ovary is also immediately anterior to a portion of the ureter and internal iliac vessels. The urinary bladder is situated in a vertical and oblique position in the anterior pelvis. The superior portion is anterior to the inferior part.

E, The organs of the male pelvis appreciated at this layer are the prostate gland, seminal vesicles, and urinary bladder. The prostate gland is retroperitoneal. The prostate is anterior to the rectum and inferior to the bladder. The lateral surfaces are in close proximity to the levator prostate muscles, which are separated from the gland by a plexus of veins. Not demonstrated here but important to note is that the prostate is perforated by the urethra and ejaculatory duct. The seminal vesicles lie superior to the prostate and posterior to the bladder. The urinary bladder is situated in a vertical and oblique position in the anterior pelvis. The superior portion is anterior to the inferior part. It is immediately anterior to the rectum.

F, The most anterior muscle of the pelvis is the rectus abdominis muscle, a bilateral muscle tissue immediately lateral to the linea alba (a white line of connective tissue in the median of the abdomen). It originates at the pubis and then ascends to insert at the xiphoid process and costal cartilages of the fifth, sixth, and seventh ribs.

The Layers of the Pelvis

A. POSTERIOR MUSCLES/TRUE PELVIS

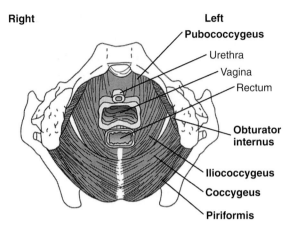

Right

Left
Pubococcygeus
Urethra
Vagina
Rectum
Obturator internus
Iliococcygeus
Coccygeus
Piriformis

B. POSTERIOR MUSCLES/FALSE PELVIS

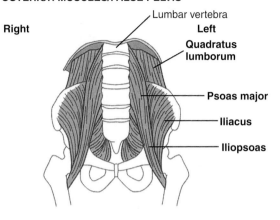

Right
Lumbar vertebra

Left
Quadratus lumborum
Psoas major
Iliacus
Iliopsoas

C. RECTUM/COLON

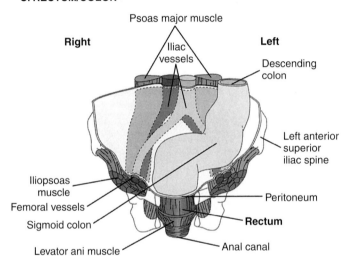

Psoas major muscle
Iliac vessels

Right

Left
Descending colon
Left anterior superior iliac spine
Peritoneum
Rectum
Anal canal

Iliopsoas muscle
Femoral vessels
Sigmoid colon
Levator ani muscle

D. UTERUS/BLADDER

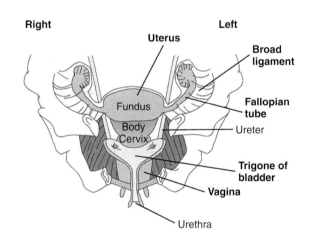

Right

Left
Uterus
Broad ligament
Fallopian tube
Fundus
Ureter
Body
Cervix
Trigone of bladder
Vagina
Urethra

E. PROSTATE GLAND/BLADDER

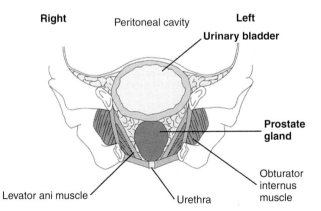

Right
Peritoneal cavity

Left
Urinary bladder
Prostate gland
Obturator internus muscle
Levator ani muscle
Urethra

F. ANTERIOR MUSCLE

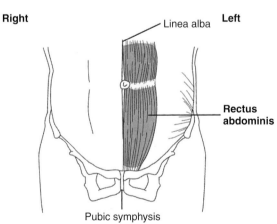

Right
Linea alba
Left
Rectus abdominis
Pubic symphysis

Figure 4-4   A to F

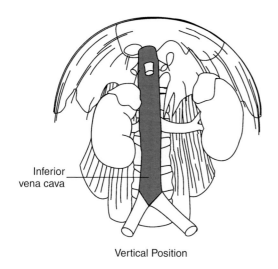

Inferior
vena cava

Vertical Position

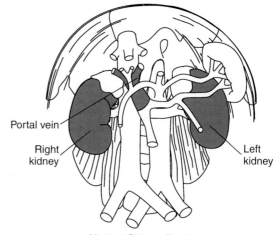

Portal vein

Right
kidney

Left
kidney

Vertical Oblique Position
(the superior pole of the kidneys is medial to the inferior pole—
the portal vein's inferior portion is medial to its superior portion)

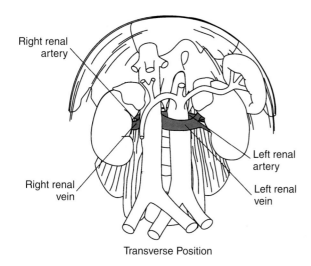

Right renal
artery

Left renal
artery

Right renal
vein

Left renal
vein

Transverse Position

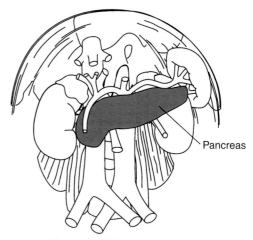

Pancreas

Transverse Oblique Position
(the lateral end of the pancreas is slightly more
superior than the medial end)

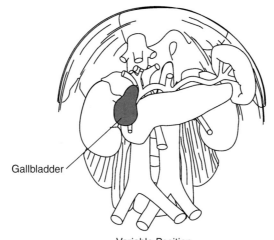

Gallbladder

Variable Position
(the variable position of the gallbladder is dependent on the amount of bile
it contains and/or the length of its mesenteric attachment)

Figure 4-5 Positional orientations of structures within the body.

A. ANTERIOR APPROACH/SAGITTAL PLANE

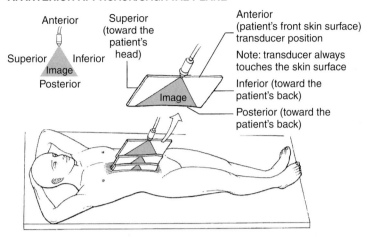

B. POSTERIOR APPROACH/SAGITTAL PLANE

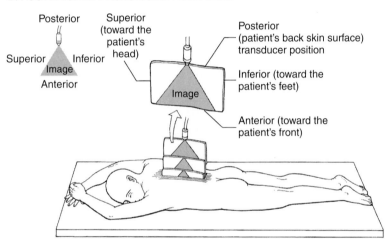

C. ANTERIOR APPROACH/TRANSVERSE PLANE

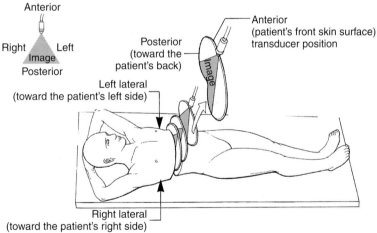

Figure 4-6 **A** and **B,** A sagittal plane image is obtained from either an anterior or a posterior scanning surface approach. From either approach, the interpretation includes the following specific anatomic areas as seen on the ultrasound image: anterior, posterior, superior, and inferior.

C to **E,** A transverse plane image is obtained from an anterior, posterior, or lateral scanning surface approach.

C and **D,** From the anterior or posterior approach, the interpretation includes the following anatomic areas: anterior, posterior, right, and left.

continued

D. POSTERIOR APPROACH/TRANSVERSE PLANE

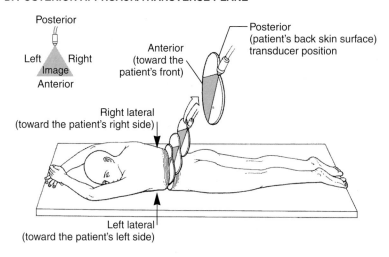

E. LATERAL APPROACH/TRANSVERSE PLANE

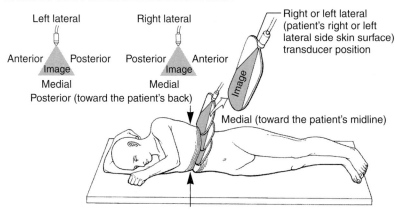

F. LATERAL APPROACH/CORONAL PLANE

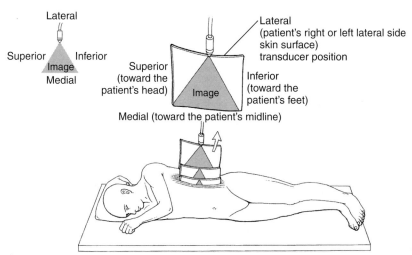

Figure 4-6, cont'd   E, From the right or left lateral approach, the interpretation includes the following anatomic areas: lateral (right or left), medial, anterior, and posterior.

F, A coronal plane image is obtained from either a right or a left lateral scanning surface approach. From either approach, the interpretation includes the following anatomic areas: lateral (right or left), medial, superior, and inferior.

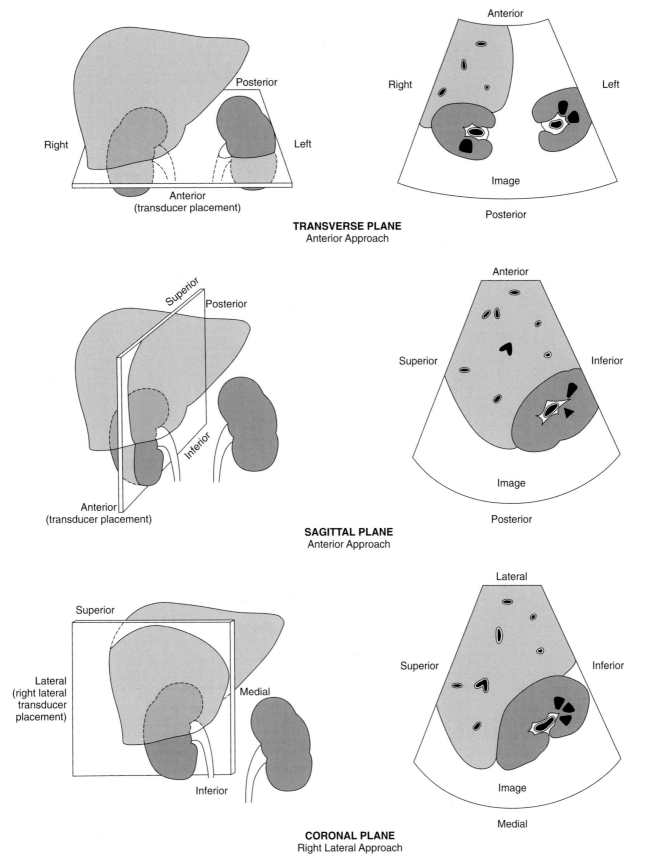

TRANSVERSE PLANE
Anterior Approach

SAGITTAL PLANE
Anterior Approach

CORONAL PLANE
Right Lateral Approach

Figure 4-7 Transverse, sagittal, and coronal planes through the liver and kidneys.

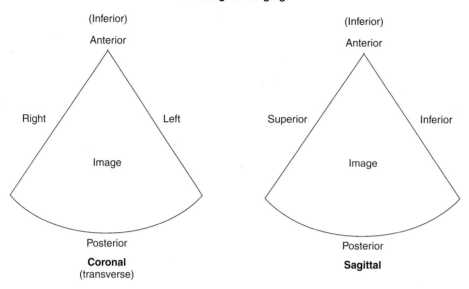

Endovaginal Imaging

Coronal
(transverse)

Sagittal

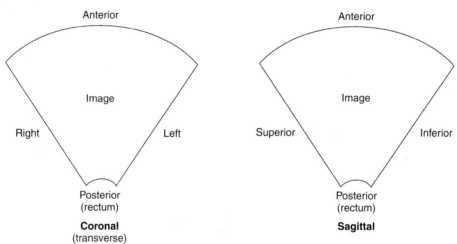

Endorectal Imaging

Coronal
(transverse)

Sagittal

Figure 4-8 Endovaginal imaging and endorectal imaging are obtained from an inferior endocavital approach, which is technically organ oriented. Image orientation still varies among authors and textbooks; however, many institutions are currently using the scanning plane interpretations shown here.

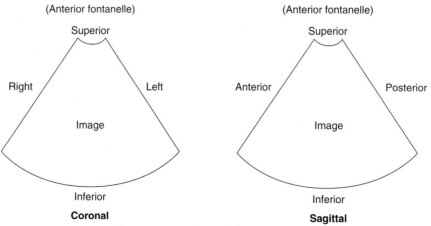

Neurosonography Imaging
(Brain Imaging)

Coronal

Sagittal

Figure 4-9 Neurosonography imaging is obtained from a superior scanning surface approach in which the transducer is placed on the head. Coronal and sagittal views are standard.

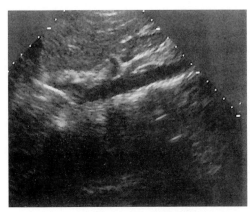
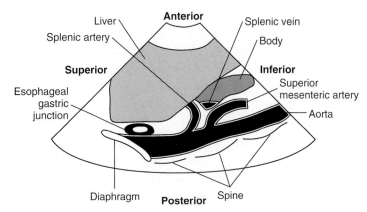

Figure 4-10 In this sagittal section, the area of interest is the body of the pancreas. Note that the liver is just anterior to the pancreas, and the splenic vein and superior mesenteric artery are posterior to it. Also note that the pancreatic body lies just inferior to the splenic artery.

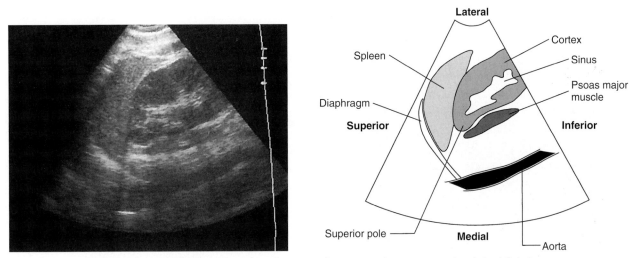

Figure 4-11 In this coronal section, the area of interest is the superior pole of the left kidney. Note the spleen just lateral and superior to the left kidney. Also note the psoas muscle and aorta medial to the kidney.

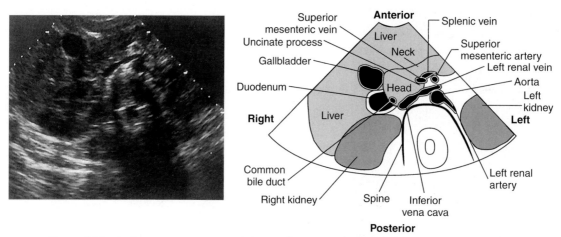

Figure 4-12 In this transverse section, the area of interest is the head of the pancreas. Note the liver just anterior to the pancreas head and the inferior vena cava immediately posterior to it. Also note the duodenum and gallbladder right lateral to the pancreas and the superior mesenteric vein left lateral.

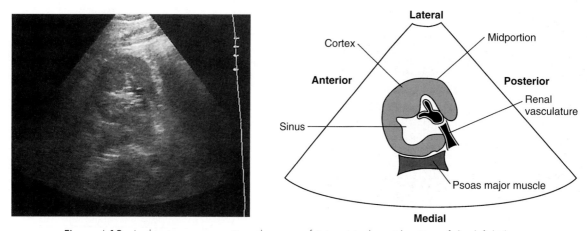

Figure 4-13 In this transverse section, the area of interest is the midportion of the left kidney. Note the psoas major muscle and vasculature just medial to the kidney.

8. *Comparison of cadaver sections and ultrasound image sections.* It is immediately apparent that the size, shape, and relationship of adjacent structures, positional orientation, and location of body structures do not change in regard to cadaver sections and ultrasound images (Figure 4-14). The one difference is the sonographic appearance of the structures. It is important to note that the standard sonographic appearance of body structures does not depend on the scanning plane from

which they are imaged. An understanding of the normal appearance provides the baseline against which to recognize variations and abnormalities. Each structural characteristic varies in sonographic appearance as follows.

Organ parenchyma, muscles, placenta, and abdominopelvic wall tissues are described in terms of echo textures. The normal echo texture of organ parenchymas, muscles, and tissues is described as **homogeneous** (uniform composition or structure throughout) with ranges in **echogenicity** (echoes produced or reflections of the sound beam). For example, the liver may be described as homogeneous and moderately echogenic (Figure 4-15). In the same respect, the echogenic textures of organs are commonly compared with one another. For instance, the liver can be **isosonic** (the same relative echodensity) or slightly more echogenic compared with renal parenchyma (Figure 4-16). The liver is generally isosonic or slightly less echogenic compared with the pancreas (Figure 4-17). Another example of the sonographic appearance of organ parenchyma is the myometrium of the uterus. It may be described as homogeneous with low to moderate echogenicity (Figure 4-18). Other considerations in describing organ parenchyma depend on an organ's density, vascular components, and normal variations, and the presence of disease processes.

Muscle echo texture appears homogeneous with low echogenicity (Figure 4-19). Muscles are usually less echogenic than the organ(s) they are adjacent to. Normal variations and the presence of disease processes are other factors to consider when describing muscle texture.

The echo texture of the placenta varies throughout a pregnancy and can be described as homogeneous with moderate to high echogenicity (Figure 4-20). The otherwise homogeneous texture may be interrupted by vascular components termed venous pools or lakes. Comparatively, the placenta is more echogenic than the adjacent myometrium of the uterus. Other considerations in describing the placenta would depend on any disease or abnormal processes that may be present.

Tissue echo texture, specifically the distinguishable abdominopelvic subcutaneous tissue layers anterior to the muscles, appears homogeneous with moderate echogenicity and strongly reflective borders (Figure 4-21). Description would also depend on any disease or abnormal processes present.

Any fluid-filled structure, such as blood vessels, ducts, umbilical cord, amniotic sac, ventricles of the heart and brain, ovarian follicles, urine-filled medullary pyramids and urinary bladder, and bile-filled gallbladder, are described as having **anechoic** (echo-free) lumens and highly echogenic walls (Figure 4-22). Sound waves readily pass through these fluid-filled structures into surrounding tissues. The sonographic appearance of this through transmission or acoustic enhancement of the surrounding structures is an increase in echogenicity (Figure 4-23). Other considerations in description depend on normal variations and the existence of disease processes.

The gastrointestinal (GI) tract is described as having generally **hypoechoic** (echoes not as bright as surrounding tissues) thin walls, though they may appear **hyperechoic** (echoes brighter than surrounding tissues) depending on the amount of fat surrounding them. The sonographic appearance of the GI tract lumen depends on its contents. Therefore the appearance of the lumen varies from anechoic (fluid), to highly echogenic (gas, air, or collapsed lumen), to a mixed pattern (fluid, gas, air, digested food, or feces) (Figure 4-24). The GI lumen containing gas or air may cast a shadow because gas and air reflect the sound beam, preventing through transmission. When the bowel is empty and collapsed, it is described as having a bull's-eye appearance because of the highly echogenic collapsed lumen and hypoechoic walls. Other considerations in description depend on normal variations and disease processes that may be present.

Bone, fat, air, fissures, ligaments, and the diaphragm are described as echogenic. The degree of echogenicity depends on the density of the structure, its distance from the sound beam, and the angle at which the beam strikes the structure. In most cases, these structures are hyperechoic to adjacent tissues (Figure 4-25). Bone, for example, is so dense that it absorbs or attenuates the sound beam, preventing through transmission. This attenuation means that the surface of the bone is generally all that is seen. It appears highly echogenic, with a shadow cast behind it (Figure 4-26). Other considerations in description depend on normal variations and any existing disease processes.

Structures not routinely imaged using sonography include normal lymph nodes, nerves, normal fallopian tubes, normal ureters, and second-order vascular branches. However, with the advancement of ultrasound technology, it may become possible to sonographically evaluate these structures.

A

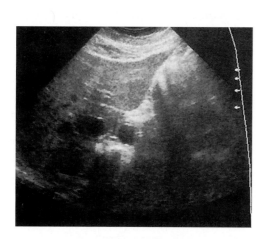

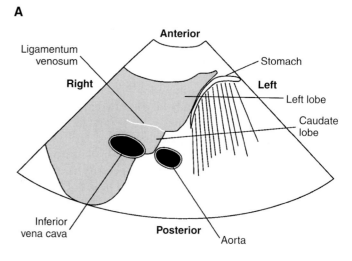

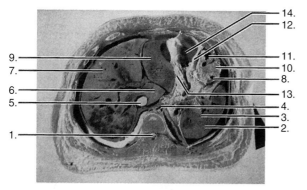

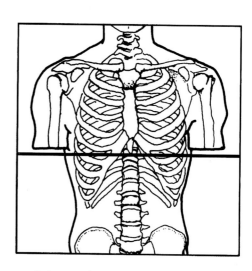

1. Spinal cord
2. Spleen
3. Hilum of spleen
4. Descending abdominal aorta
5. Inferior vena cava
6. Caudate lobe
7. Right lobe of the liver
8. Descending colon
9. Left lobe of the liver
10. Splenic flexure (left colic flexure)
11. Transverse colon
12. Greater curvature of stomach
13. Lesser curvature of stomach
14. Lumen of stomach

Figure 4-14 Comparison of structures of cadaver sections and ultrasound image sections.

A, In this comparison of cadaver section and ultrasound image at the level of the tenth thoracic vertebra, it is apparent that the size, shape, positional orientation, and location of the left lobe and caudate lobe of the liver are the same. Note the location and adjacent relationships of the inferior vena cava, aorta, and stomach.

B

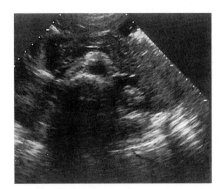

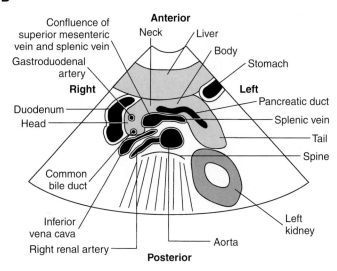

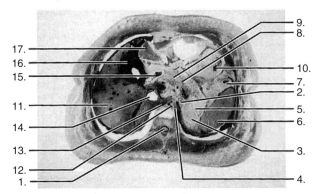

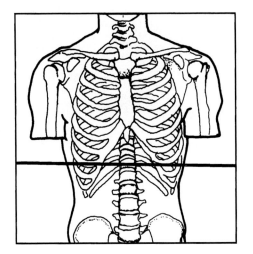

1. Spinal cord
2. Left suprarenal gland (adrenal gland)
3. Left kidney
4. Left crus of diaphragm
5. Tail of pancreas
6. Spleen
7. Colon
8. Body of pancreas
9. Head of pancreas
10. Colon
11. Right lobe of liver
12. Descending abdominal aorta
13. Right crus of the diaphragm
14. Inferior vena cava
15. Descending duodenum (second segment of duodenum)
16. Gallbladder
17. Stomach

Figure 4-14 cont'd

B, Comparing this cadaver section and ultrasound image at the level of the twelfth thoracic vertebra, it is apparent that the size, shape, positional orientation, and location of the pancreas and adjacent structures are the same. Note that the head of the pancreas rests against the duodenum and sits immediately anterior to the inferior vena cava. Also note the location and adjacent relationships of the aorta, tail of the pancreas, and left kidney.

continued

C

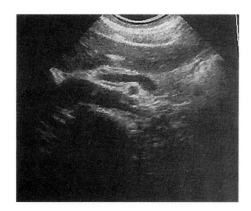

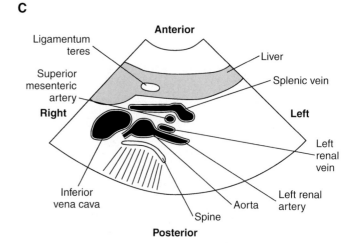

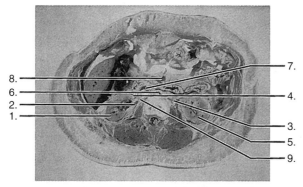

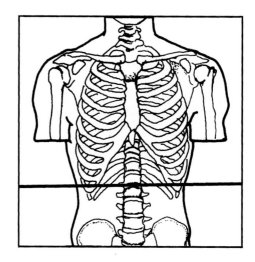

1. Right kidney
2. Right renal artery
3. Left sympathetic nerve trunk
   (sympathetic chain)
4. Right renal vein
5. Left kidney
6. Descending abdominal aorta
7. Inferior vena cava
8. Superior mesenteric artery
9. Right sympathetic nerve trunk
   (sympathetic chain)

Figure 4-14 cont'd

C, This cadaver and ultrasound section is at the level of the second lumbar vertebra. Compare the identical size, location, and positional orientation of the superior mesenteric artery and aorta. Note the comparable relationship of the right renal artery and inferior vena cava. Note the adjacent relationship of the kidneys on the cadaver section.

D

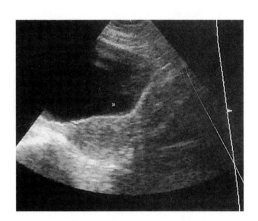

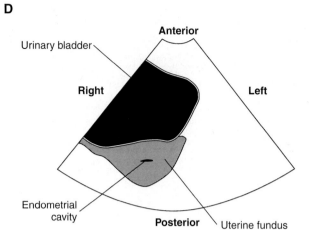

Urinary bladder

Anterior

Right

Left

Endometrial
cavity

Posterior   Uterine fundus

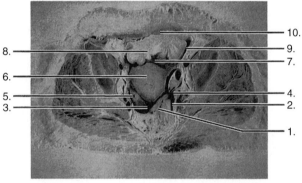

8.
6.
5.
3.

10.
9.
7.

4.
2.

1.

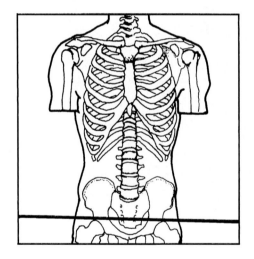

1. Rectum
2. Pararectal fossa
3. Rectouterine pouch
   (posterior cul-de-sac)
4. Ureter
5. Ovary
6. Uterus (Womb)

7. Uterovesical (vesicouterine)
   pouch (anterior cul-de-sac)
8. Urinary bladder
9. Paravesical fossa
10. Retropubic space

Figure 4-14 cont'd

D, In this comparison of cadaver section and ultrasound image at the level of the fifth vertebra of the sacrum, it is obvious that the size, shape, and positional orientation of the uterus are the same on both sections. Note the comparable locations of the urinary bladder. Also note the location and adjacent relationships of the rectum, rectouterine pouch (posterior cul-de-sac), and ovary as indicated on the cadaver section.

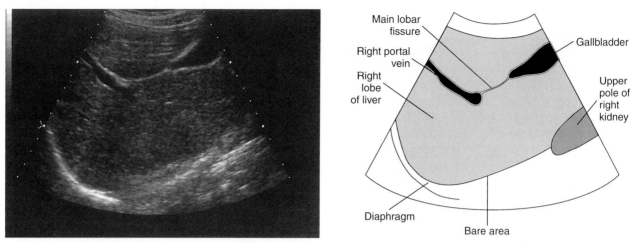

Figure 4-15 The sonographic appearance of the liver is normally homogeneous and moderately echogenic.

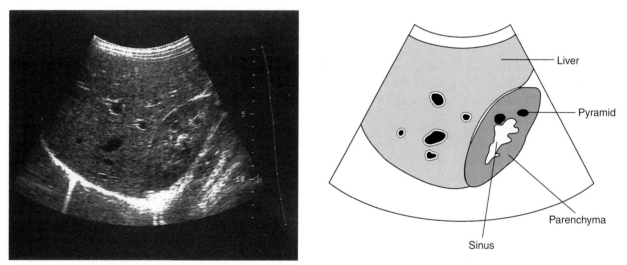

Figure 4-16 In this comparison of the sonographic appearance of liver and renal parenchyma, the liver may be described as being more echogenic than the kidney.

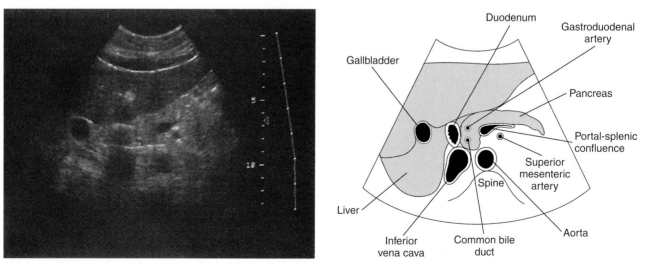

Figure 4-17 In this comparison of the sonographic appearance of liver and pancreatic parenchyma, the liver may be described as being less echogenic than the pancreas.

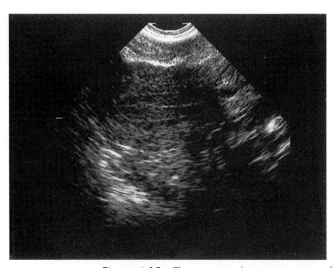
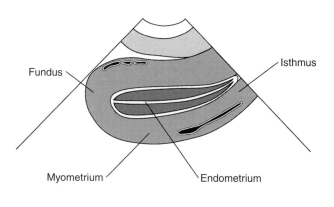

Figure 4-18 The sonographic appearance of the myometrium of the uterus is normally homogeneous, with low to moderate echogenicity.

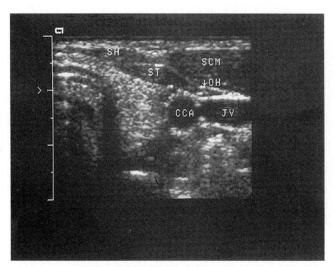
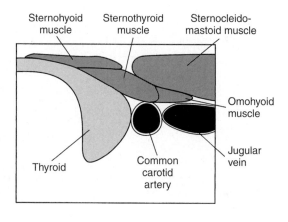

Figure 4-19 The sonographic appearance of muscles is normally homogeneous, with low echogenicity. Note that the muscles are less echogenic than the thyroid.

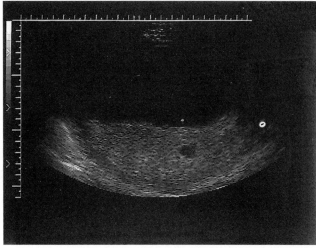
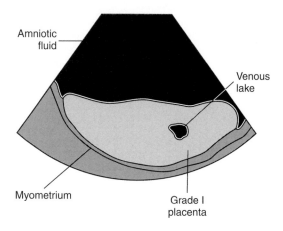

Figure 4-20 The sonographic appearance of the placenta is normally homogeneous, with moderate to high echogenicity. Note that the placenta is more echogenic than the myometrium.

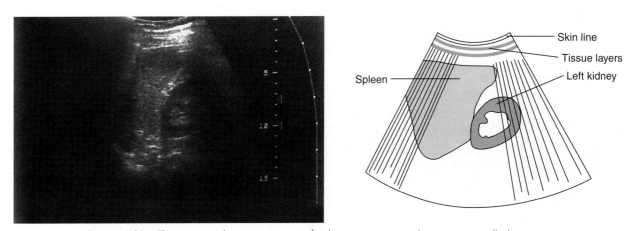

Figure 4-21 The sonographic appearance of subcutaneous tissue layers is normally homogeneous with moderate echogenicity. Note the highly reflective borders.

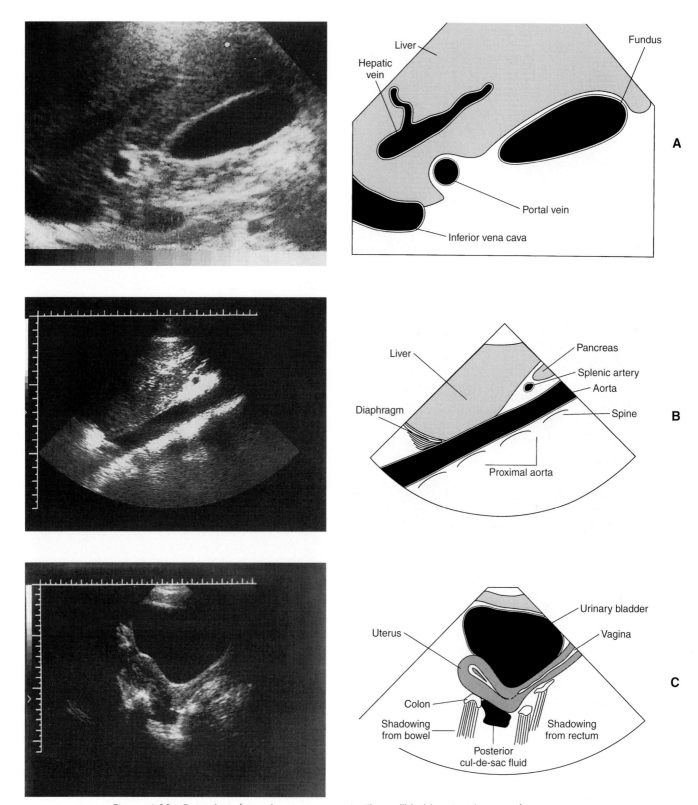

Figure 4-22 Examples of anechoic structures. **A,** The gallbladder, portal vein, inferior vena cava, and hepatic vein. **B,** The aorta and splenic artery. **C,** The urinary bladder. Note the anechoic free fluid in the posterior cul-de-sac.

continued

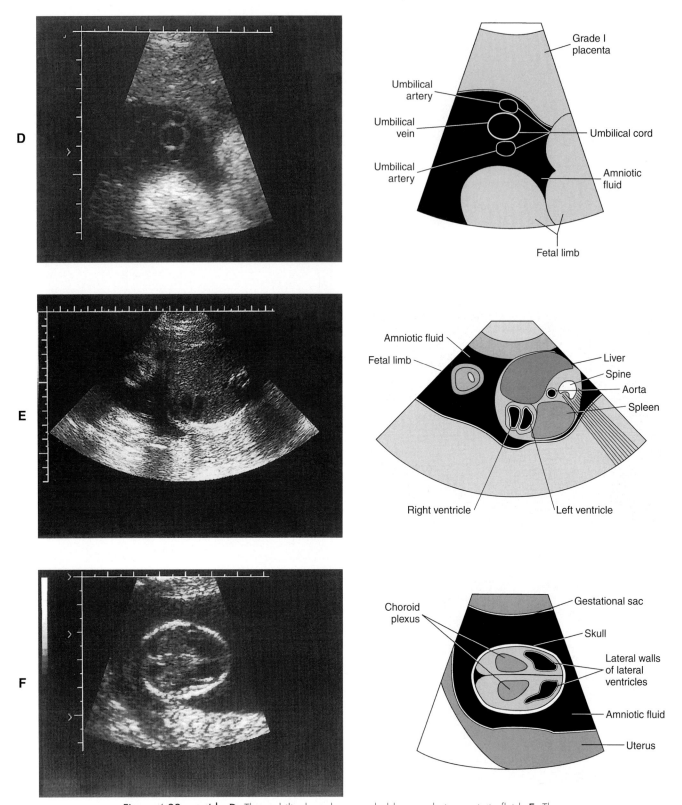

Figure 4-22, cont'd **D,** The umbilical cord surrounded by anechoic amniotic fluid. **E,** The ventricles of the fetal heart, the fetal aorta. Note the surrounding anechoic amniotic fluid. **F,** The ventricles of the fetal brain. Note the surrounding anechoic amniotic fluid.

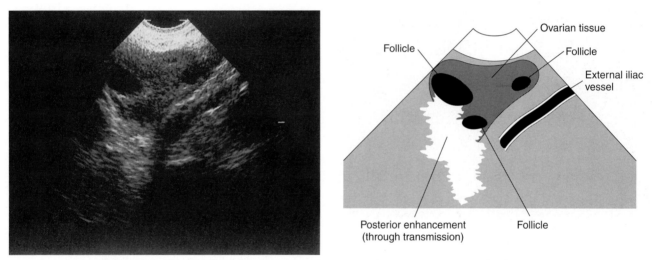

Figure 4-23 The sonographic appearance of acoustic enhancement is increased echogenicity.

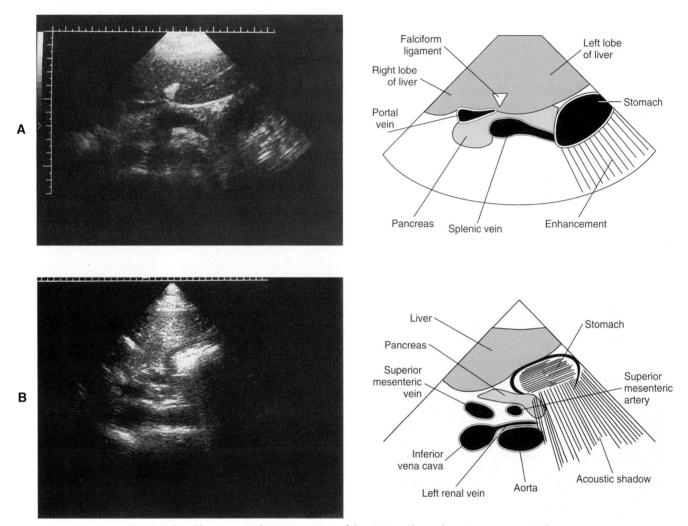

Figure 4-24 The sonographic appearance of the GI tract depends on its contents. **A,** The stomach is fluid filled and appears anechoic. Note the posterior acoustic enhancement. **B,** The stomach lumen appears highly echogenic from either gas or air (its size is too large to be collapsed). Note the hypoechoic appearance and size of the stomach wall. Also note the shadow cast posteriorly.

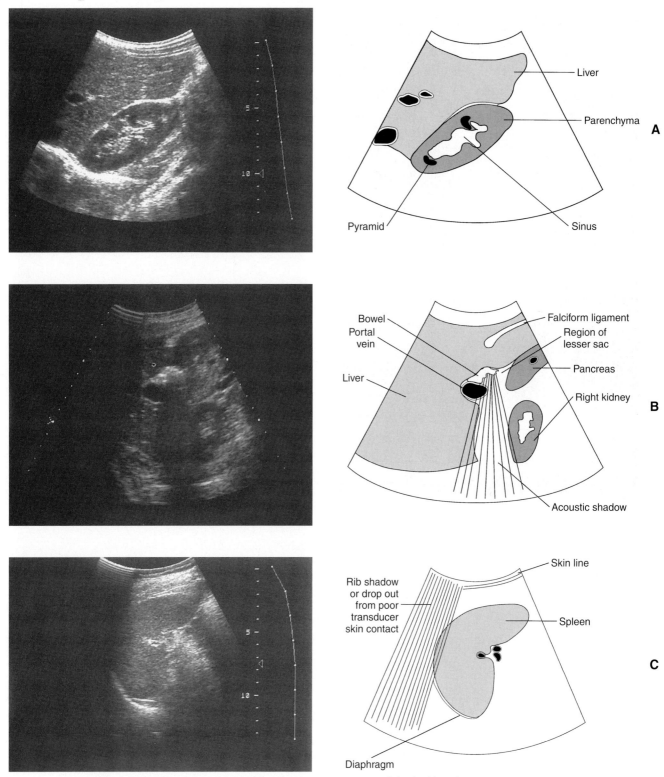

Figure 4-25 Fat, ligaments, and the diaphragm are some of the highly echogenic structures in the body. Note how hyperechoic they are to adjacent structures. **A,** The renal sinus is composed primarily of fat, which causes this highly echogenic appearance. Note how hyperechoic the sinus is to the adjacent renal cortex. **B,** Ligaments are composed of either folds of peritoneum or fibrous cording, which cause this highly echogenic appearance. Note the hyperechoic appearance of the falciform ligament compared with the surrounding liver. **C,** The diaphragm is a very thick, highly echogenic section of muscle. Note its hyperechoic appearance compared with the adjacent spleen.

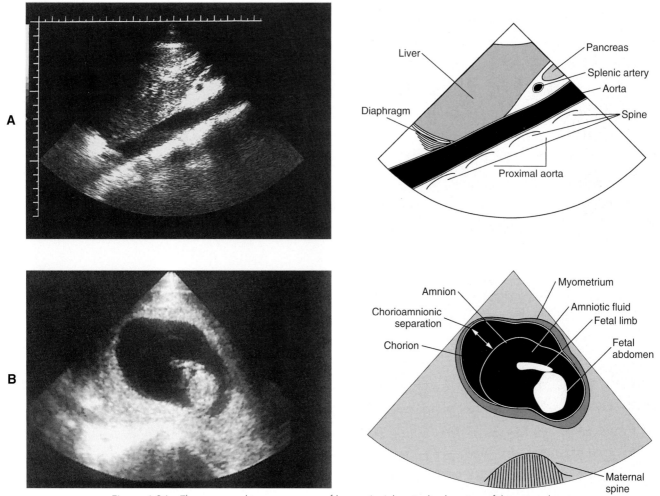

Figure 4-26 The sonographic appearance of bone. **A,** A longitudinal section of the spine showing its highly reflective surface. **B,** A transverse section of the maternal spine demonstrating its reflective surface and the shadow it casts.

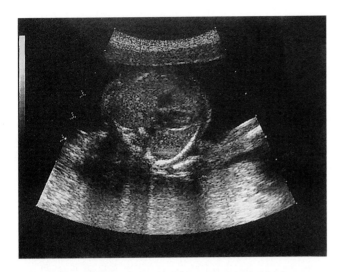

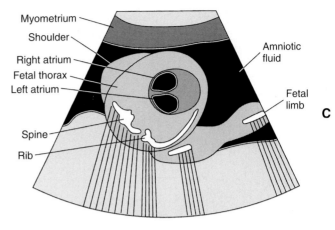

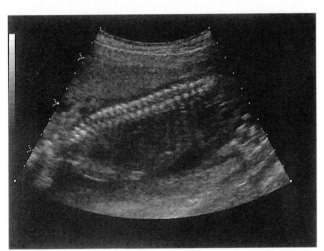

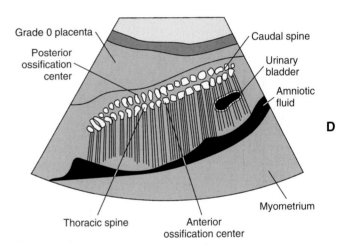

Figure 4-26, cont'd C, In the fetus, the bones are easily recognized because of their highly echogenic appearance and characteristic shadowing. D, The echogenic fetal spine and the shadow it casts.

BIBLIOGRAPHY

April EW: *Anatomy,* Media, PA, 1984, Harwal.

Dorland's pocket medical dictionary, ed 24, Philadelphia, 1982, WB Saunders.

Grant JCB: *An atlas of anatomy,* ed 9, Baltimore, 1991, Williams & Wilkins.

Gray H: *Anatomy: descriptive and surgical,* ed 15, New York, 1977, Crown.

Hagen-Ansert SL: *Textbook of diagnostic ultrasonography,* ed 5, St Louis, 2001, Mosby.

Heap SW: Cross sectional anatomy of the vessels and ducts of the upper abdomen, *Austral Radiol* 24:32, 1980.

Jones B, Braver JM: *Essentials of gastrointestinal radiology,* Philadelphia, 1982, WB Saunders.

Kawamura DM: *Diagnostic medical sonography,* vol 3, Philadelphia, 1992, JB Lippincott.

Lane A, Sharfaei H: *Modern sectional anatomy,* Philadelphia, 1992, WB Saunders.

Lane A: Sectional anatomy: standardized methodology, *J Int Soc Plastination* 4:16, 1990.

Lane A: Using plastinated specimens to teach the body layering concept correlated with ultrasound scans, *J Int Soc Plastination* 19:2, 1994.

Lane A: Sectional anatomy: strategy for mastery. Banvard RA et al, editors: The second Visible Human Project Conference Proceedings, 1998, National Library of Medicine. Available from http://www.nlm.nih.gov/research/visible/vhpconf98/AUTHORS/LANE/LANE. HTM

Lane A: Prescribed sequence labeling method: a strategy for mastery of sectional anatomy using plastinated specimens (abstract) *J Int Soc Plastination* 16, 2001.

Mittelstaedt CA: *Abdominal ultrasound,* New York, 1987, Churchill Livingstone.

Williams P: *Anatomy of the human body,* ed 38, Oxford, 1995, Churchill Livingstone.

SECTION III

Abdominal Sonography

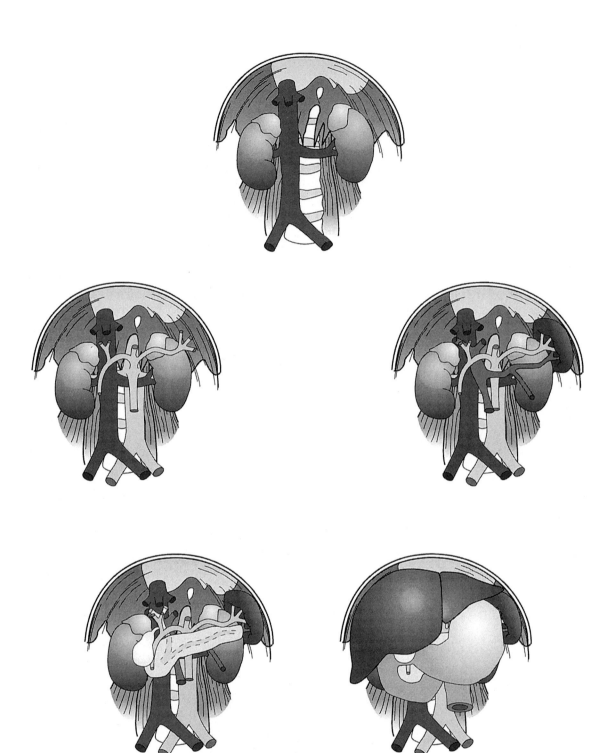

The abdominal aorta and surrounding anatomic layers. See Figure 4-3, **C, D, E, G,** and **I** for more details.

CHAPTER 5

The Abdominal Aorta

VIVIE MILLER AND CANDYCE JAMES

OBJECTIVES

Discuss the embryologic development of the aorta and its major branches.
Describe the normal location, course, and size of the aorta.
Describe the layers (gross anatomy) of an artery.
Describe the location of the aortic branches and the organs supplied by those branches.
Discuss the function of the aorta.
Describe the sonographic appearance of the aorta and its branches.
Describe the associated laboratory values and diagnostic tests.
Define the key words.

KEY WORDS

Aorta	Left gastric artery
Celiac artery	Proper hepatic artery
Common hepatic artery	Renal artery
Common iliac arteries	Splenic artery
Gastroduodenal artery	Superior mesenteric artery
Gonadal arteries	Suprarenal artery
Inferior mesenteric artery	Tunica media

Although all body vessels are important, the aorta is especially vital because the blood flowing to the abdominal organs and lower extremities must pass through at least some part of this vessel to reach its destination. Thus, because of the large volume of blood that it transports, the aorta is considered one of the two great vessels of the abdomen.

PRENATAL DEVELOPMENT

The cardiovascular system is the first system to begin to function in the embryo. This is necessary to provide an adequate supply of nutrients and oxygen to the other body systems as they develop. The vascular portion of the cardiovascular system develops from mesodermal cells, the angioblasts, during the third week. At this time, all vessels are composed of endothelium; thus the location of vessels in relation to the heart determines which vessels are arteries and which vessels are veins. During the third week, there are two dorsal aortas, which are extensions of the two endocardial heart tubes (Figure 5-1). The aortas quickly fuse into a single vessel after this period.

The single aorta has several branches. Numerous intersegmental arteries branch posteriorly and feed the embryo. Eventually many of these arteries become the lumbar arteries (see Figure 5-1). In addition, the common iliac arteries and the median sacral artery develop from intersegmental arteries. The vitelline artery complex branches anteriorly from the aorta and extends into the yolk sac. The celiac artery (CA), superior mesenteric artery (SMA), and inferior mesenteric artery (IMA) develop from this complex. The umbilical arteries branch off the inferior aspect of the anterior aorta and return the deoxygenated blood to the placenta. The umbilical arteries eventually give rise to the internal iliac arteries and superior vesical artery. The majority of the remaining vessels develop from the primitive vascular network by forming channels connecting the organ systems to existing capillaries and vessels.

LOCATION

The aorta is a retroperitoneal structure coursing in a superior-to-inferior direction along the left side of the spine. This tubular structure originates from the heart at the left ventricular outflow tract and follows a candy cane–shaped loop down into the thoracic cavity. This portion, considered the thoracic aorta, is not visualized when an abdominal sonogram is performed. After the aorta passes posteriorly to the diaphragm at the aortic hiatus on the posterior superior portion of the diaphragm, it is

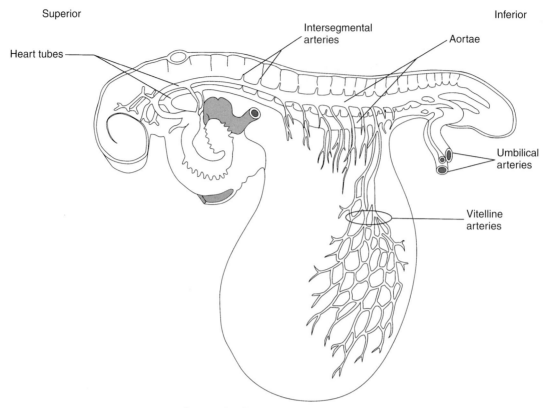

Figure 5-1 Representation of aortic development at approximately the third embryologic week.

termed the abdominal aorta (AO). It continues to course inferiorly, giving off several branches, many of which can be visualized by sonography. The AO bifurcates into the **common iliac arteries** slightly to the left of the umbilicus (Figure 5-2). The aorta is lateral and to the left of the spinal column. It is posterior to the left lobe of the liver, body of the pancreas, pylorus of the stomach, splenic artery, splenic vein, and left renal vein. It is anterior to the musculature of the back.

The AO has many branches (Figures 5-3 and 5-4). There is considerable variation in the origin and course of these vessels; therefore only the most common configurations will be discussed.

Directly after the aorta passes posteriorly to the diaphragm, the inferior phrenic arteries branch off the anterior-lateral aspect of the aorta and course superiorly to supply the underside of the diaphragm. At approximately the same level, the celiac trunk (also known as the **celiac artery** or **celiac axis**) branches anteriorly from the aorta. The CA, often measuring less than 1 cm, further branches into the left gastric (LGA), splenic (SPA), and common hepatic arteries (CHA). The **left gastric artery** courses superiorly and to the left. It doubles back to supply the left side of the lesser curvature of the stomach and eventually anastomoses with the right gastric artery. The **splenic artery** supplies the spleen, pan-

creas, and left side of the greater curvature of the stomach as it courses horizontally to the left with a slight inferior-to-superior angulation. The pancreas is supplied primarily via the main, dorsal, caudal, and great pancreatic arteries, which branch from the SPA. The left side of the greater curvature of the stomach is supplied by the left gastroepiploic artery, which branches from the distal end of the SPA. The **common hepatic artery** pursues a horizontal course to the right and branches into the gastroduodenal (GDA) and proper hepatic artery (PHA). The **gastroduodenal artery** courses inferiorly, supplying the right side of the greater curvature of the stomach via the right gastroepiploic artery and the pancreatic duodenal area via the superior-anterior and superior-posterior pancreatic duodenal arteries. The **proper hepatic artery** courses superiorly, supplying the liver via the right, middle, and left hepatic arteries. The cystic artery feeds the gallbladder after it branches from the right hepatic artery. The right gastric artery, which supplies the right side of the lesser curvature of the stomach, commonly originates from the GDA, CHA, or PHA. The CA and its branches are of extreme importance in supplying the majority of the abdominal organs, the stomach, and the duodeum.

The origin of the next most inferiorly located branch of the aorta varies. The suprarenal arteries commonly

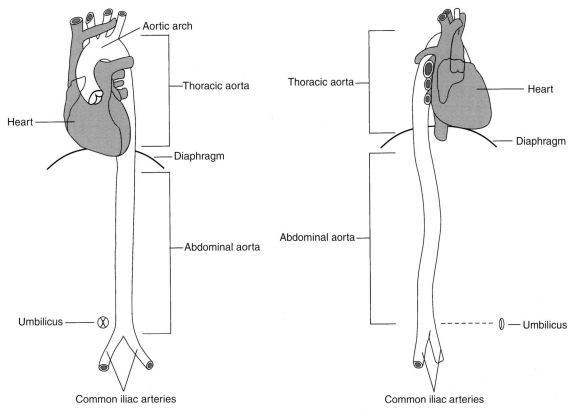

Figure 5-2 Anterior and lateral views of the aorta.

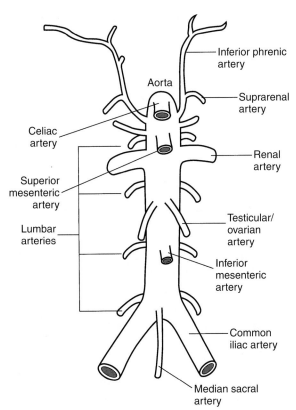

Figure 5-3 Initial branches of the abdominal aorta.

originate from the level of the CA to the level of the SMA, which is located a few centimeters inferior to the CA. The **suprarenal arteries,** also termed the adrenal arteries, originate bilaterally from the lateral aspect of the aorta and course horizontally to the adrenal glands.

Moving inferiorly, the **superior mesenteric artery** branches from the anterior aspect of the aorta within centimeters of the CA. The SMA continues an anterior-inferior course and divides into several arteries that supply the largest portion of the small intestine and the ascending colon and part of the transverse colon. In addition, the inferior-anterior pancreatic duodenal artery and the inferior-posterior pancreatic duodenal artery originate from the SMA and feed the pancreatic head and duodenal area. Within a few centimeters of the origin of the SMA, the right and left **renal arteries** branch from the lateral aspect of the aorta. Both arteries course horizontally and supply the kidneys; however, the right renal artery (RRA) has a longer course than the left renal artery (LRA) because the aorta sits on the left side, which forces the RRA to travel a greater distance. In addition, it should be noted that the RRA normally courses posteriorly to the inferior vena cava (IVC) to reach the right kidney.

Inferior to the superior mesenteric artery and renal arteries, the **gonadal arteries** originate from the ante-

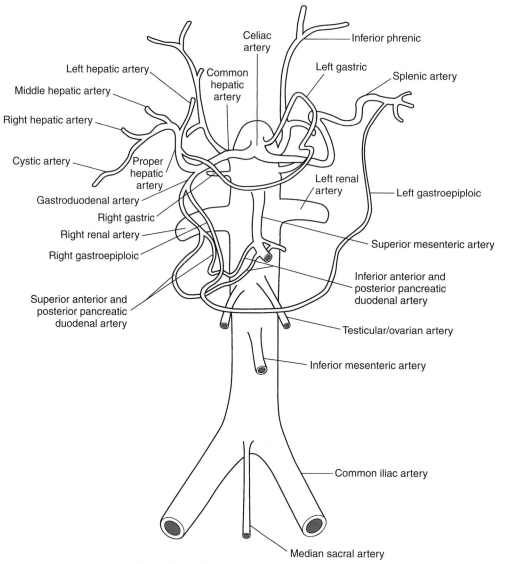

Figure 5-4 Branches of the abdominal aorta.

rior aspect of the aorta and course inferiorly to their respective organs. The left artery often originates slightly superiorly to the right artery. The male gonadal arteries are termed the testicular arteries, and the female gonadal arteries are termed the ovarian arteries.

The **inferior mesenteric artery** is the next major artery that branches from the aorta. It originates from the anterior aspect of the aorta and pursues the anterior-inferior course dividing into several other smaller arteries supplying the transverse colon, descending colon, and rectum.

The median sacral artery supplies the sacrum and is the most inferior branch of the aorta; however, the aorta bifurcates at this point into the common iliac arteries, which, along with their branches, supply the pelvis and lower extremities. One should also note that lumbar ar-

teries originate bilaterally from the lateral aspect of the aorta throughout the entire length of the aorta.

SIZE

Although the size of the vessel varies depending on body habitus, it is accepted that the average anterior-posterior diameter of the normal aorta is 2 cm at the most superior portion of the abdomen. Coursing inferiorly, it decreases in size with an average measurement of 1.5 cm at its bifurcation into the iliac arteries. This vessel should not exceed 3 cm at any level. It has been suggested that the best method to decrease observer variation when measuring the aorta is to take the anterior-posterior measurement in the longitudinal plane. One should always be consistent in the technique used to measure this vessel to ensure consistent results.

GROSS ANATOMY

The aorta, like other vessels, has three layers: tunica intima, tunica media, and tunica adventitia (Figure 5-5). Their thickness varies. Arteries often have a thicker **tunica media** to allow for greater elasticity.

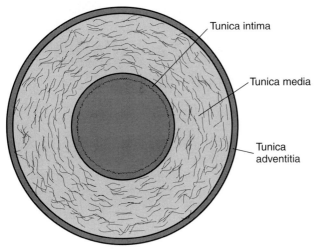

Figure 5-5 Cross-section of an arterial wall.

PHYSIOLOGY

The primary function of the aorta and its branches is to channel blood to organs and tissues to ensure oxygenation and metabolism. The arterial system also serves other functions.

Although the arteriole-capillary system is primarily responsible for other functions such as blood pressure maintenance and assisting in the control of bleeding, the aorta does participate in these functions. The venous system is capable of maintaining blood pressure through its valves; however, valves are not present in the arterial system. Thus the aorta and large arteries use a different mechanism to maintain blood flow during diastole. As the ventricles contract during systole, blood is quickly sent into the aorta, forcing the expansion of the vessel wall. As a result, potential energy is stored in the vessel wall. When the aortic valve in the heart closes and diastole ensues, the arterial wall recoils to release the stored potential energy. The wall recoil forces blood to continue its forward movement; thus the blood pressure is maintained. In addition, multiple nerve and chemical receptors are present throughout the arterial system that respond to various stimuli. The many local and systemic chemical and neurologic events can cause vasoconstriction or vasodilatation. For instance, renin is released from the kidney in the event of bleeding. Renin acts on angiotensin II, which initiates vasoconstriction; thus blood pressure is maintained through vasoconstriction. In addition, chemical-humoral reactions allow for vasoconstriction of certain arterial segments, which can result in increased organ perfusion or heat dissipation. As is evident, the aorta and its branches play a critical role in homeostasis.

SONOGRAPHIC APPEARANCE

Arterial vasculature should normally display an anechoic center with echogenic walls that clearly delineate it from adjacent structures. Larger vessels will often display significant pulsatility, which will assist in proper identification. In the longitudinal plane, the aorta is a tubular, highly pulsatile structure slightly anterior and to the left of the spine. The proximal portion of the aorta is often seen as a curvilinear structure as it courses from posterior to anterior after piercing the diaphragm. The aorta continues to course anteriorly until it bifurcates; however, this slight degree of posterior-to-anterior angulation results in the mid and distal aorta displaying more of a linear configuration than the proximal portion (Figure 5-6). Note that the aorta is often tortuous; thus identification of a significant portion in the longitudinal plane can be difficult. Although it is not always possible, one should attempt to identify the layers of the vessel to assist in excluding pathology. The tunica intima often appears as a bright echogenic line on the innermost portion of the vessel wall. The tunica media is believed to be represented by the echo-free area between the echogenic tunica intima and tunica adventitia. The tunica adventitia is the fibrous outermost section of the vessel that appears as a moderately echogenic line separating the vessel from other structures.

Although the aorta has many branches, the branches that are demonstrated with reasonable consistency are the CA, SMA, renal arteries, and common iliac arteries. The CA is most easily seen in the transverse plane slightly superior to the pancreas. The vessel is recognizable as it branches anteriorly from the aorta by displaying the characteristic shape of a seagull (Figure 5-7). The SPA and the CHA represent the wings of the bird. The CA will appear as a short tubular structure branching anteriorly from the aorta (Figure 5-8).

The SMA can also be identified in the longitudinal plane as a linear structure branching anteriorly from the aorta slightly inferior to the CA (see Figure 5-8). The SMA courses posteriorly to the pancreas and can usually be identified more easily in the transverse plane as a circular, anechoic structure surrounded by echogenic parapancreatic fat directly posterior to the splenic vein (Figure 5-9).

The renal arteries are usually most easily seen in the transverse plane as small-diameter curvilinear structures branching laterally from the aorta (Figure 5-10). Although the LRA is difficult to identify in the longitudinal plane, the RRA can usually be identified in the longitudinal plane directly posterior to the IVC (Figure 11-11). The IMA is the next most inferiorly located vessel; however, it is not consistently demonstrated.

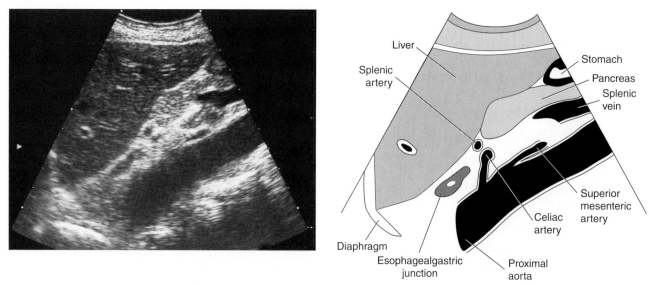

Figure 5-6 Longitudinal section of the proximal aorta.

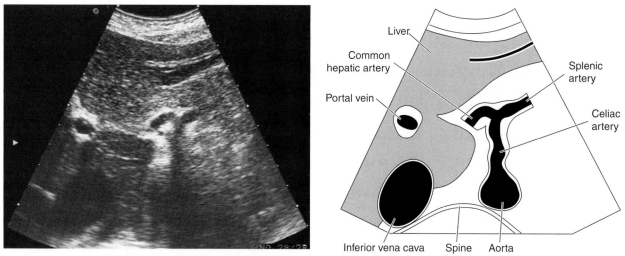

Figure 5-7 Transverse section of the aorta, celiac artery, common hepatic artery, and splenic artery.

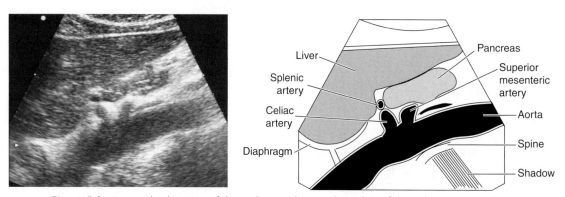

Figure 5-8 Longitudinal section of the mid aorta showing branches of the celiac artery and superior mesenteric artery.

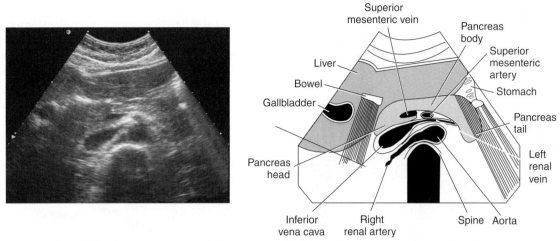

Figure 5-9   Transverse section of the mid aorta displaying the superior mesenteric artery branch.

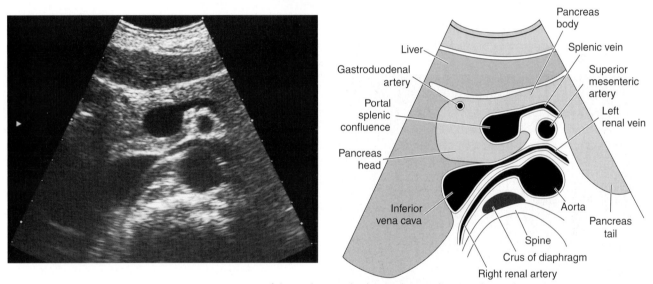

Figure 5-10   Transverse section of the mid aorta displaying the curvilinear right renal artery.

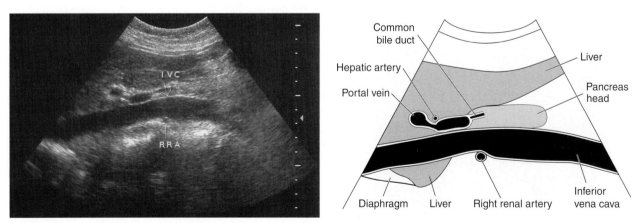

Figure 5-11   Longitudinal section of the inferior vena cava delineating the right renal artery.

As was discussed, the aorta bifurcates into the common iliac arteries at the level of the umbilicus. This bifurcation is most easily demonstrated in the transverse plane. One will see the single aorta divided into two separate vessels as the transducer is angled or moved inferiorly (Figures 5-12 to 5-14).

SONOGRAPHIC APPLICATIONS

The aorta and its branches are primarily evaluated to detect aneurysms and stenosis. Fusiform, saccular, and dissecting aneurysms can be readily identified. Stenosis of the CA, SMA, renal artery , and iliac artery can also be identified with the aid of Doppler sonography. Stenosis

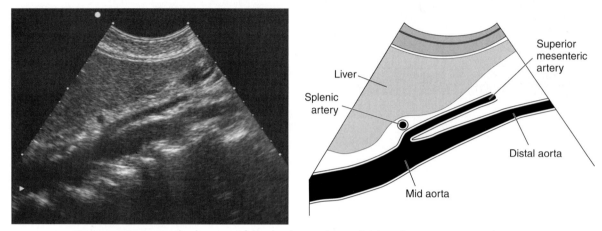

Figure 5-12 Longitudinal section of the distal aorta *(arrows)*. Note decrease in aortic diameter.

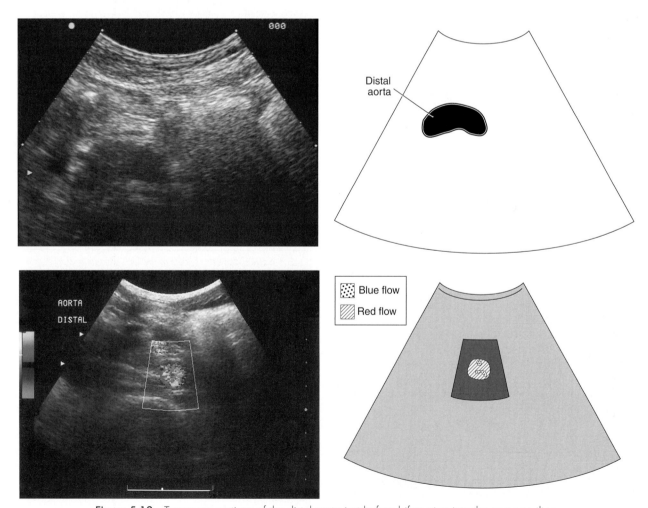

Figure 5-13 Transverse sections of the distal aorta just before bifurcation into the common iliac arteries. (See Color Plate 3.)

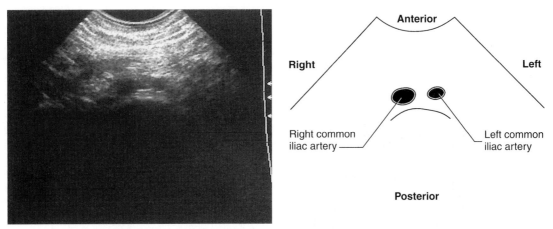

Figure 5-14 Transverse image of the common iliac arteries distal to the bifurcation.

is often the causative factor in other disease states such as bowel ischemia resulting from SMA stenosis or renovascular hypertension caused by renal artery stenosis. In addition, grafts can be evaluated for patency and complications using Doppler sonography.

NORMAL VARIANTS

Nonapplicable.

REFERENCE CHARTS

■ ■ ■ ASSOCIATED PHYSICIANS

Many physicians may be involved in care of the patient with a disorder of the aorta or its branches, depending on the organ affected. The vascular surgeon, who specializes in the surgical treatment of the vasculature, is the primary physician who treats the arterial system.

■ ■ ■ COMMON DIAGNOSTIC TESTS

Diagnostic tests to evaluate the arterial system include duplex Doppler sonography, color-flow Doppler, plethysmography, segmental blood pressures, arteriography, computed tomography, and magnetic resonance imaging.

Duplex Doppler Sonography: Duplex Doppler sonography can indicate flow patterns within the vasculature, and these abnormalities indicate certain disease states such as stenosis and aneurysms. (This chapter includes only a limited discussion of Doppler sonography as an aid in evaluating the aorta and its branches.) The normal Doppler waveform may be a low-resistance waveform, a high-resistance waveform, or a combination waveform. A low-resistance waveform occurs when there is no reverse flow and significant diastolic flow is present throughout the cardiac cycle. This is generally seen when the diastolic flow is approximately one third of the normal peak systolic flow. A low-resistance waveform should be present in arteries that feed low-resistance beds such as the brain, kid-

neys, and abdominal organs (Figure 5-15). A normally high-resistance waveform will exhibit a sharp systolic upstroke along with reduced diastolic flow, and it may display reverse flow. High-resistance waveforms will be seen in the external carotid artery, extremities, and the preprandial SMA (Figure 5-16). A combination waveform will show attributes of both low- and high-resistance waveforms. This type of waveform is seen in the common carotid artery and abdominal aorta (Figures 5-17 and 5-18). In addition, most waveforms should not exhibit spectral broadening. Spectral broadening can be detected as excessive echoes within the window of the waveform. Various abnormalities within these waveforms such as increased peak systolic velocities, increased diastolic velocities, significant spectral broadening, flow reversal, and other findings assist one in ascertaining the presence of pathology in the vessel or the organ supplied by the vessel. (It should be noted that this discussion does not explain Doppler sonography sufficiently to allow one to interpret Doppler waveforms.) A sonographer or vascular technologist performs this examination and often presents a preliminary impression. A physician, usually a radiologist or vascular surgeon, interprets the sonogram.

Color Flow Doppler: Color flow Doppler or color imaging often gives similar results to duplex sonography; however, its main use is to facilitate in locating vessels for duplex sonography or to ascertain the presence and location of flow in a structure (Figures 5-19 and 5-20). Recent improvements in equipment may shortly allow for color imaging to be used much like duplex sonography. Personnel responsible for performing and interpreting duplex sonography have similar functions in this examination.

Plethysmography and Segmental Blood Pressure: Although plethysmography and segmental blood pressures are primarily used to evaluate vascular disease of the extremities, they can assist in determining the presence and extent of occlusive aortic disease. There are several types of plethysmographs; the function of each is to measure volume changes within an area. Thus one can ascertain the volume of blood and extent of arterial disease within that particular area. In addition, segmental blood pressures

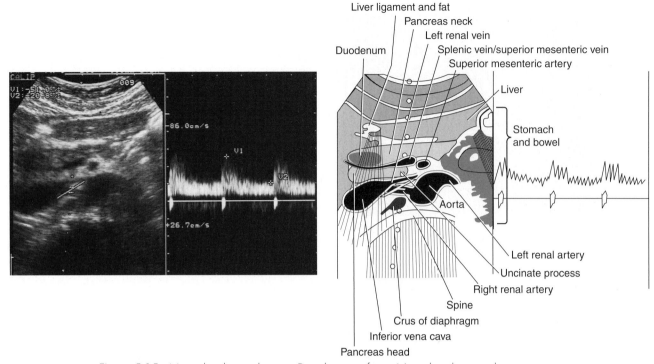

Figure 5-15 Normal right renal artery Doppler waveform. Note that this is a low-resistance waveform (the diastolic flow is approximately one third of the peak systolic flow, indicating a low resistance vascular bed).

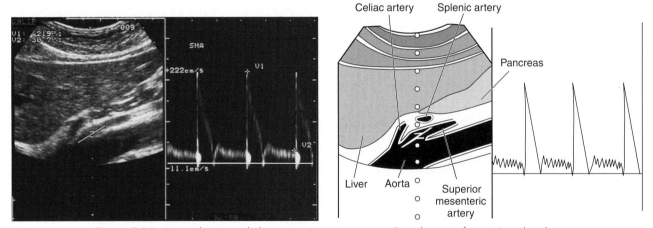

Figure 5-16 Normal preprandial superior mesenteric artery Doppler waveform. Note that the diastolic flow, as compared with the low-resistance renal artery waveform, is much less in relation to the peak systolic flow. The preprandial superior mesenteric artery waveform is considered a high-resistance waveform.

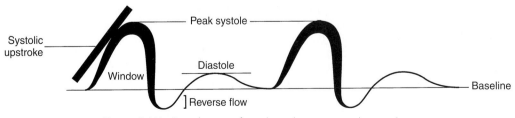

Figure 5-17 Doppler waveform throughout two cardiac cycles.

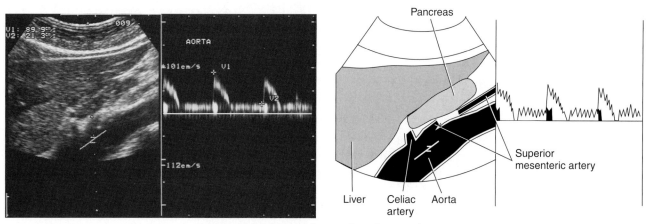

Figure 5-18   Normal aortic Doppler waveform.

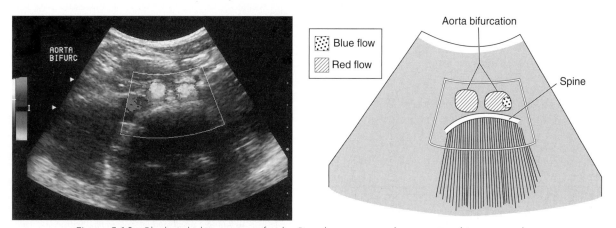

Blue flow
Red flow

Figure 5-19   Black-and-white version of color Doppler sonogram demonstrating the common iliac arteries. (See Color Plate 4.)

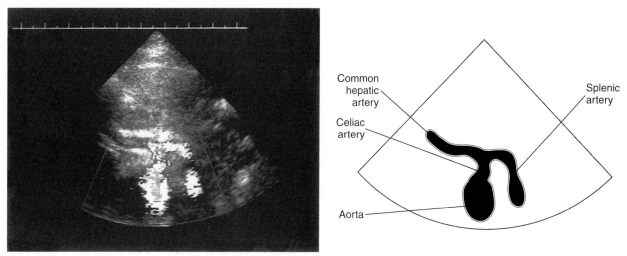

Figure 5-20   Black-and-white version of color Doppler sonogram demonstrating flow within the aorta, celiac artery, splenic artery, and common hepatic artery. (See Color Plate 5.)

can be used in conjunction with plethysmography or separately to ascertain blood flow to an area. When compared with normal values, the pressure information can also indicate the presence or severity of disease. A sonographer or vascular technologist performs this examination and often provides a preliminary impression. A vascular surgeon usually interprets the examination.

Arteriography: Arteriography is most often considered the gold standard when evaluating the aorta and its branches. In the arteriogram, dye is injected into the vessel supplying the target area and several radiographs are then taken. A radiologist assisted by a radiologic technologist performs this examination. The radiologist interprets this examination.

Computed Axial Tomography (CT scan): CT is often utilized to evaluate the aorta. This examination consists of a series of sequential radiographs taken over the target area. The images are computer reconstructed in two or three dimensions, enabling excellent identification and differentiation of structures. Structures can be evaluated with or without the aid of contrast material. A radiologic technologist performs this examination and a radiologist interprets it.

Magnetic Resonance Imaging (MRI): MRI is rapidly increasing in applications, which now include the vascular area. The images are similar in format to those of CT. The resolution is often superior, however, the image being created by magnetic field, not by radiation. A magnetic resonance imaging technologist or radiologic technologist performs this procedure, and a radiologist interprets the examination.

■ ■ ■ LABORATORY VALUES

Many laboratory values are based on the arterial system, most of which indicate the functioning of other organs. Hematocrit (the percentage of red blood cells to whole blood) is used to measure possible bleeding from the arterial system; measurement of red blood cells aids in this determination. An abnormal decrease in red blood cells may also point to bleeding. Levels of cholesterol and lipids may indicate the potential for pathology or suggest the current arterial disease state; however, they cannot directly measure either. The arterial vascular system is complex. One should be well acquainted with its anatomy, physiology, sonographic appearance, and associated tests to ensure that the patient receives the highest quality of care.

■ ■ ■ NORMAL MEASUREMENTS

The diameter of the normal aorta measures 2 cm at its most superior aspect in the abdomen, diminishing to approximately 1.5 cm as it courses inferiorly. The normal aorta should not exceed 3 cm at any point.

■ ■ ■ VASCULATURE

Aorta → inferior phrenic
Aorta → celiac axis—left gastric
                —splenic—left gastroepiploic
                —common hepatic—proper hepatic
                                —left hepatic
                                —right hepatic
    —gastroduodenal—left gastroepiploic
    (branch of   —superior, anterior and posterior
    right hepatic) pancreatic duodenal artery
                —inferior anterior and posterior
                 pancreatic duodenal artery
Aorta → superior mesenteric
Aorta → gonadals
Aorta → inferior mesenteric
Aorta → common iliacs

■ ■ ■ AFFECTING CHEMICALS

Nonapplicable

BIBLIOGRAPHY

Anderhub B: *Manual of abdominal sonography,* Baltimore, 1983, University Park Press.

Ganong WF: *Review of medical physiology,* ed 12, Los Altos, 1985, Lange Medical Publications.

Gay W-R, Rothenburger A: *Color atlas of physiology,* ed 4 (Trans Joy Wieser). New York, 1991, Thieme.

Mittelstaedt CM: *Abdominal ultrasound,* New York, 1987, Churchill Livingstone.

Moore KL: *The developing human: clinically oriented embryology,* ed 6, Philadelphia, 1998, WB Saunders.

Netter FH: *The CIBA collection of medical illustrations,* vol 5, Heart, Summit, NJ, 1978, CIBA Division of CIBA-Geigy.

Yucel EK, Fillmore DJ, Knox TA, et al: Sonographic measurement of abdominal aortic diameter: intraobserver variability, *J Ultrasound Med* 10:681-683, 1991.

Zweibel WJ, editor: *Introduction to vascular ultrasonography,* ed 4, Philadelphia, 2000, WB Saunders.

CHAPTER 6

The Inferior Vena Cava

VIVIE MILLER AND CANDYCE JAMES

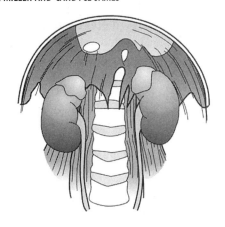
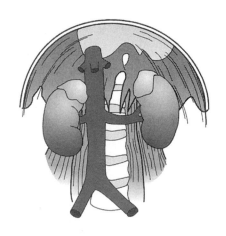
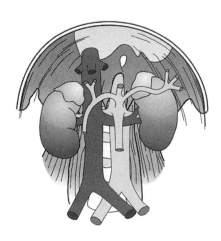
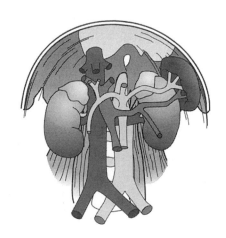
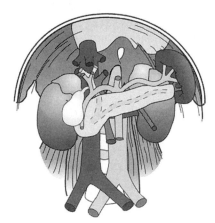
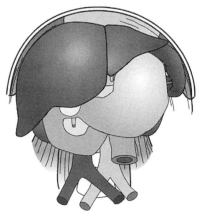

The inferior vena cava and surrounding anatomic layers. See Figure 4-3, B, C, D, E, G, and I for more details.

The **inferior vena cava** (IVC) is one of the two great abdominal vessels. Like all other veins, the IVC transports blood toward the heart. Thus the sonographer must have a full understanding of this vasculature to adequately evaluate the abdomen during a sonographic examination.

PRENATAL DEVELOPMENT

The development of the IVC is complex, which predisposes it to multiple anatomic variations. The IVC and its tributaries are formed from a portion of the **vitelline vein** and portions of the **cardinal venous system** within the embryo (Figures 6-1 and 6-2). The posterior cardinal veins (PCVs), subcardinal veins, and supracardinal veins are formed during the sixth, seventh, and eighth weeks of embryonic development, respectively. The PCVs regress during this period and do not evolve into a portion of the IVC; however, they do serve as a base for the development of the subcardinal and supracardinal

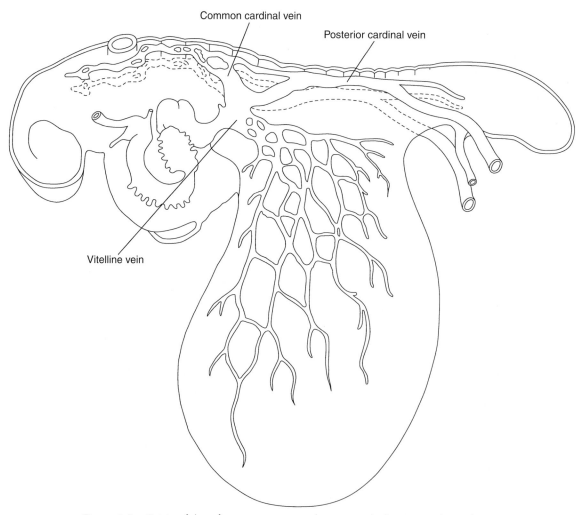

Figure 6-1 Origin of the inferior vena cava and associated tributaries in the embryo.

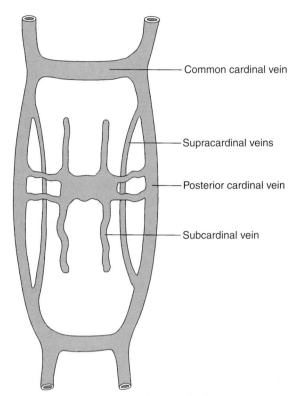

Figure 6-2   Anterior view of the cardinal venous system.

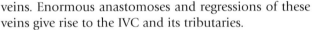

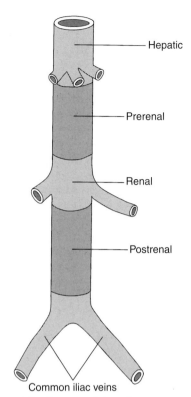

Figure 6-3   Sections of the inferior vena cava.

veins. Enormous anastomoses and regressions of these veins give rise to the IVC and its tributaries.

The IVC is considered to have four sections (Figure 6-3). Beginning superiorly, the first area encountered is the hepatic section, located directly posterior to the liver where the **hepatic veins** empty into the IVC. The hepatic section of the IVC and hepatic veins develop from the proximal vitelline vein. The next section is termed the prerenal section. It extends from just inferior to the hepatic veins to slightly superior to the **renal veins** and is derived from a subcardinal vein. The renal section is the next most inferiorly located area of the IVC. The renal veins and multiple tributaries are located within this section, which terminates almost immediately after the branching of the renal veins. The subcardinal and supracardinal veins undergo multiple anastomoses to form this level. The final section is the postrenal section, which is formed from a supracardinal vein. The postrenal section of the IVC extends from just inferior to the renal veins until the **common iliac veins** converge into the IVC.

LOCATION

The IVC is formed by the convergence of the common iliac veins, which empty the lower extremities and pelvis. The IVC continues to course superiorly through the retroperitoneum along the anterior lateral aspect of the spine and to the right of the aorta. One should be

cognizant that the IVC can have many possible congenital variations, including double IVC, IVC located on the left, absence of certain portions of the IVC, or a combination of these. This is because of its complex development, as previously discussed. Many tributaries, including the **lumbar veins,** right gonadal vein, renal veins, and hepatic veins, will empty into the IVC as it continues its superior course and pierces the diaphragm at the caval hiatus to enter the right atrium of the heart. The IVC is located posterior to the intestines and the body of the liver. It is medial to the right kidney. The IVC is located more posteriorly as it courses superiorly.

The IVC has many tributaries; however, several contain multiple configurations or are not suitable for sonographic evaluation. Thus only major tributaries will be discussed (Figure 6-4). As previously mentioned, the IVC is formed from the convergence of the common iliac veins, which empty the lower extremities and pelvis at approximately the level of the umbilicus. The lumbar veins, which empty into the lateral aspect of the IVC, are the next most superior branch. These horizontally coursing veins empty the posterior abdominal wall and are located bilaterally. In addition, there is usually more than one pair that continues emptying into the IVC to the level of the renal veins.

Moving superiorly, the right gonadal vein, which courses parallel to the IVC, empties into the anterior lateral aspect of the IVC. Within a few centimeters

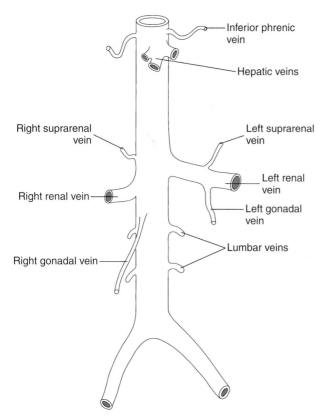

Figure 6-4 The inferior vena cava and its major tributaries.

superiorly, the renal veins empty into the IVC. Although the right renal vein generally empties only the right kidney or sometimes the right adrenal gland via the right suprarenal vein, the left renal vein has additional tributaries that it assists in draining. The left gonadal vein courses parallel and lateral to the IVC and empties into the left renal vein. In addition, the left suprarenal vein follows a course similar to that of the left renal vein, into which it eventually empties. Many smaller tributaries may also drain into the left renal vein. Note that the normal right renal vein is much shorter than the left renal vein. The left renal vein passes anteriorly to the aorta and posteriorly to the superior mesenteric artery as it courses from the left kidney. The right suprarenal vein often empties into the IVC slightly superior to the right renal vein. The next major tributaries are the hepatic veins. There are most commonly three hepatic veins, which course from the inferior aspect, deep within the liver, to the superior aspect of the liver where they empty into the IVC. Generally, the right hepatic vein empties the right lobe of the liver, the middle hepatic vein empties the caudate lobe, and the left hepatic vein empties the left lobe of the liver. The most superior branches of the IVC are the inferior phrenic veins, which course in a superior-to-inferior direction, draining the diaphragm and emptying into the lateral aspect of the IVC. One should note that several vein locations parallel the locations of their sister arteries.

SIZE

The diameter of the IVC will increase during a Valsalva maneuver or inspiration and commonly decrease during expiration. Asking the patient to "sniff" will cause the IVC to momentarily collapse. Although it varies, the diameter of the IVC is approximately 2.5 cm.

GROSS ANATOMY

In general, venous walls are thinner because their tunica media is thin compared with that of the arterial system. This is because a highly tensile vessel is not needed because the venous network is a low-pressure system.

PHYSIOLOGY

The IVC and its associated tributaries have the primary function of returning deoxygenated blood to the heart. Because the pressure on the venous side of the circulatory system is low compared with the arterial side, the venous circulation contains valves, which prevent backflow of blood during diastole.

The momentum of the blood during systole forces the valves open. Once the momentum decreases and the blood is not pushed forward, the valve closes and prevents retrograde flow. In various diseases, the valves may not function, and this will cause retrograde blood flow. Blood is also moved forward by a decrease in thoracic pressure, which pulls the blood into the right atrium. In this case, the IVC simply acts as a transportation vehicle.

SONOGRAPHIC APPEARANCE

Venous vasculature should normally display an anechoic center with thin, hyperechoic walls. During real-time examination, one will note that the IVC displays significant variation in diameter compared with the arterial vasculature. In addition, small moving echoes are often noticed within the lumen of the IVC. The reason for these echoes is debated; however, it is agreed that they are related to the flow of blood within the vessel.

As the transducer is longitudinally placed in the epigastric area, the hepatic section of the IVC can be seen as a tubular, elastic structure located directly posterior to the liver (Figure 6-5). In some instances, the IVC may appear to be coursing through the liver parenchyma, especially in the most superior section of the liver. The hepatic veins can often be seen at this level as linear structures originating in the liver and emptying into the IVC (Figure 6-6). It is evident that the hepatic veins increase in diameter as they approach the IVC. In the transverse plane, the hepatic veins can once again be seen as anechoic linear struc-

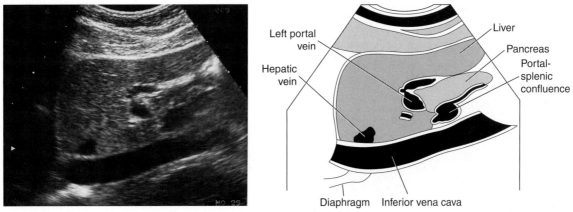

Figure 6-5 Longitudinal image of the inferior vena cava.

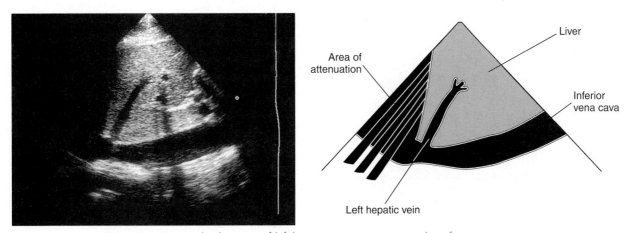

Figure 6-6 Longitudinal section of left hepatic vein emptying into the inferior vena cava.

tures, whose walls are not obvious, emptying into the IVC (Figure 6-7, *A*). One often notices a characteristic "bunny ear" pattern with this image. Figure 6-7, *C* shows a color image of the hepatic veins emptying into the IVC. The renal veins are the next most inferiorly located venous structures that are consistently recognized. The left renal vein is seen as a curvilinear structure emptying into the lateral aspect of the IVC as it courses anterior to the aorta and posterior to the superior mesenteric artery from its origin in the left kidney (Figure 6-8). The right renal vein is also seen as a curvilinear structure emptying into the lateral aspect of the IVC at this level. The gonadal vein and lumbar veins are not consistently imaged. However, the common iliac veins are most easily visualized in the transverse plane at approximately the umbilicus immediately before they converge to form the IVC.

SONOGRAPHIC APPLICATIONS

The IVC and its visible branches are primarily evaluated to detect intraluminal thrombosis and tumor invasion. The thrombosis may be the result of numerous causes. Tumor invasion most commonly occurs in the renal veins and often extends into the IVC. The venous system can be evaluated by many diagnostic modalities. However, sonography is continually increasing in diagnostic accuracy and acceptance by medical professionals. Thus sonographers must have a complete understanding of this system to ensure that each patient receives the best care possible.

NORMAL VARIANTS

Variations of the IVC can occur because of its complex formation. There may be a double IVC or a left-positioned IVC, or a portion of the vessel may be absent. However, these are not common.

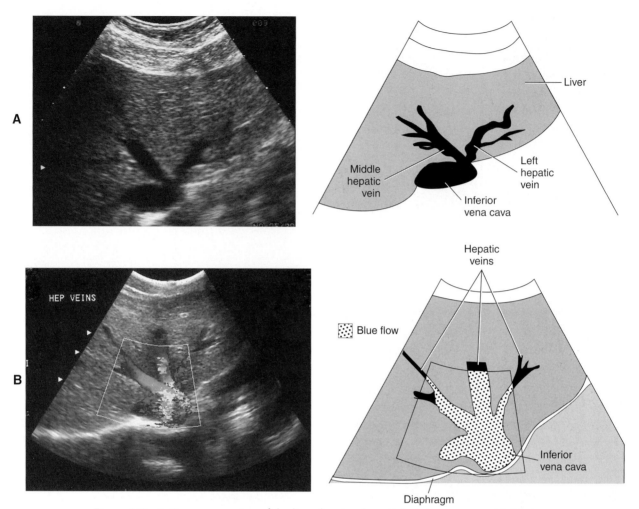

Figure 6-7 **A,** Transverse section of the liver showing the middle hepatic vein and left hepatic vein emptying into the inferior vena cava. **B,** Black-and-white version of color image showing hepatic veins emptying into the inferior vena cava. (See Color Plate 6.)

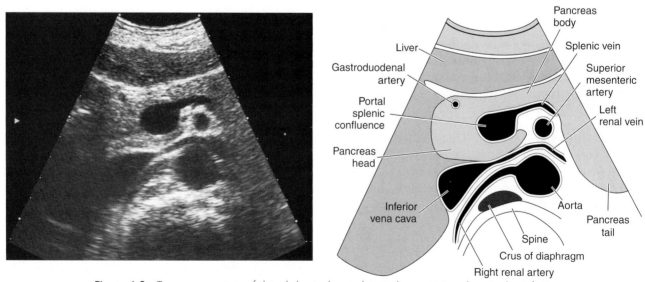

Figure 6-8 Transverse section of the abdominal vasculature demonstrating the circular inferior vena cava, aorta, and superior mesenteric artery along with the curvilinear left renal vein coursing posterior to the superior mesenteric artery and anterior to the aorta. Note the right renal artery.

REFERENCE CHARTS

■ ■ ■ ASSOCIATED PHYSICIANS

Generally, vascular surgeons treat the patient whose disorder involves the venous system. However, other physicians are often involved depending on the other organs or organ systems involved. In addition, internists—internal medicine practitioners—often render care to patients who do not require surgery.

■ ■ ■ COMMON DIAGNOSTIC TESTS

The following diagnostic tests are commonly used to evaluate the venous system: duplex Doppler sonography, color Doppler, continuous wave Doppler sonography, impedance flow plethysmography, venography, computed tomography, and magnetic resonance imaging.

Duplex Doppler Sonography: Although veins of the extremities can be evaluated with B-mode imaging and compression, one also needs to assess the flow dynamics of the area. Thus duplex Doppler is necessary to ensure an adequate examination. A normal venous flow pattern should be spontaneous and phasic (change with respiration). Proximal compression and distal augmentation are also used to assess venous flow. Abnormalities often suggest disease. The abdominal venous system displays characteristic Doppler waveforms (Figure 6-9). A sonographer, vascular technologist, or nurse performs this examination and often provides a preliminary impression. A physician, usually a radiologist or a vascular surgeon, interprets the findings.

Color Flow Doppler: Color Doppler can often assist in determining flow characteristics in the abdomen and extremities by quickly identifying flow and turbulence. Continuous wave Doppler is also helpful in determining the status of extremity veins. The Doppler signal is amplified by a loudspeaker, which allows the examiner to hear an audible

signal. Abnormalities in this signal indicate disease. The same personnel who perform and interpret duplex sonography also perform and interpret this examination.

Impedance Flow Plethysmography: Impedance flow plethysmography is the technique of measuring the blood volume change of an area. Strain gauge plethysmography is generally used when evaluating veins. Bilateral inflatable cuffs are placed on the proximal portion of the extremities along with gauges that measure change in extremity size. As the cuffs are inflated, the flow of blood toward the heart is stopped and blood accumulates distal to the cuff, causing the extremity to increase in size. Next, the cuffs are deflated, allowing the blood to rush from the extremity back toward the heart. The strain gauge presents a readout of this rate of volume change. The results between extremities are compared as well as to established normals. If the flow of blood toward the heart is abnormally slow, some type of blockage should be considered; this test should be done in conjunction with B-mode imaging, continuous wave sonography, and/or duplex sonography to ensure accuracy. The same personnel who perform and interpret duplex and color sonography also perform and interpret this examination.

Venography: Venography is considered by many the gold standard when detecting venous disease. Dye (contrast material) is injected into the target vein and serial radiographs are taken. Defects in filling indicate the presence of disease. This is a highly invasive test, and reactions to the injected dye are of great concern. This procedure is performed by a radiologist assisted by a radiologic technologist. The radiologist interprets this examination.

Computed Axial Tomography (CT Scan): CT is sometimes done to evaluate the abdominal venous system; however, it is rarely used to determine the disease state of extremities. This examination consists of a series of sequential radiographs, which are computer reconstructed to identify various structures. A radiologic technologist performs this examination and a radiologist interprets the findings.

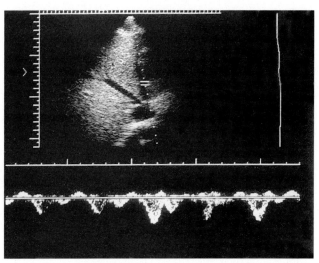
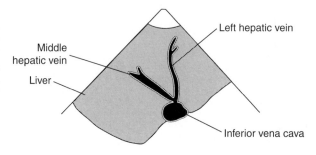

Figure 6-9 Transverse section of the liver demonstrating a normal spontaneous and phasic Doppler pattern from the left hepatic vein.

Magnetic Resonance Imaging (MRI): MRI is infrequently called on to evaluate the venous system. Furthermore, it is not utilized to assess the extremity veins. The images are similar in format to those of CT; however, the images are generated using a strong magnetic field instead of radiation as in CT. A magnetic resonance imaging technologist or radiologic technologist performs this examination and a radiologist interprets the examination.

■ ■ ■ LABORATORY VALUES

Almost all blood laboratory values are taken from the venous system; however, the majority of examinations indicate the status of other organs or body systems. As with the arterial system, the percentage of red blood cells to whole blood (hematocrit) indicates possible bleeding from the venous system.

■ ■ ■ NORMAL MEASUREMENTS

The IVC will vary with respiration; however, it should not exceed 3.7 cm.

■ ■ ■ VASCULATURE

IVC → inferior phrenic veins
IVC → hepatic veins
IVC → renal veins
IVC → gonadal veins
IVC → lumbar veins
IVC → iliac veins

■ ■ ■ AFFECTING CHEMICALS

Nonapplicable.

BIBLIOGRAPHY

Mittelstaedt CM: *Abdominal ultrasound,* New York, 1987, Churchill Livingstone,.

Moore KL: *The developing human: clinically oriented embryology,* ed 6, Philadelphia, 1998, WB Saunders.

Netter FH: *The CIBA collection of medical illustrations,* vol 5, Heart, Summit, NJ, 1978, CIBA Division of CIBA-Geigy.

Zwiebel WJ, editor: *Introduction to vascular ultrasonography,* ed 4, Philadelphia, 2000, WB Saunders.

CHAPTER 7

The Portal Venous System

VIVIE MILLER AND CANDYCE JAMES

OBJECTIVES ■■■

Discuss the embryologic development of the portal vein.
Discuss the normal location, course, and size of the portal vein.
Discuss the normal location of the portal vein tributaries.
Describe the function of the portal venous system.
Describe the sonographic appearance of the portal vein and its tributaries.
Discuss associated diagnostic tests.
Define the key words.

KEY WORDS ■■■

Inferior mesenteric vein	Right portal vein
Left portal vein	Splenic vein
Main portal vein	Superior mesenteric vein
Portal triad	

The portal venous system is unique because it is the system that supplies blood to the liver for metabolic processes. This blood originates from organs within the gastrointestinal tract, including the stomach, small intestine, large intestine, and spleen. Disruption to the flow can cause multiple adverse effects. Therefore it is imperative that the sonographer understand the many factors associated with the portal system.

PRENATAL DEVELOPMENT

The portal vein develops during approximately the eighth embryologic week. The vitelline veins undergo several anastomoses, forming a vascular network that gives rise to the main portal vein (Figure 7-1). The venous tributaries are also formed from the primitive vascular network, and they join the main portal vein at its inferior aspect.

LOCATION

The portal vein is an intraabdominal structure normally measuring less than 13 mm. It is formed by the confluence of the splenic vein and the superior mesenteric vein directly posterior to the head of the pancreas (Figure 7-2). The **splenic vein** drains the spleen and courses from lateral to medial directly posterior to the pancreas. The **superior mesenteric vein** courses from inferior to superior and drains the small intestine and portions of the large intestine via several smaller branches. The **inferior mesenteric vein** also courses from inferior to superior as it drains the large intestine via several smaller branches. This vessel most often empties blood into the splenic vein; however, there is considerable variance regarding where the inferior mesenteric vein joins the portal system. Several other tributaries empty into the portal vein, including the left and right gastric veins, pancreaticoduodenal veins, and gastroepiploic veins. There is significant variability regarding where these vessels enter the system.

After the main portal vein forms, it continues to course superiorly approximately 5 to 6 cm. At this point it divides into right and left branches. The left branch continues to course horizontally and branches into medial and lateral subdivisions. The left lateral subdivision feeds the left lobe of the liver. The right branch of the portal vein continues to course to the right and branches into anterior and posterior subdivisions. Both right and left portal veins give off multiple subdivisions, and variations in location are commonplace.

SIZE

The portal vein is an abdominal structure normally measuring up to 13 mm.

GROSS ANATOMY

Refer to location.

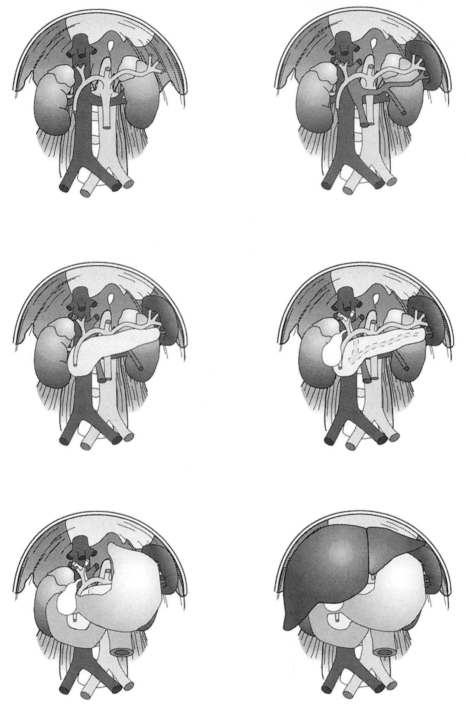

The portal venous system and surrounding anatomic layers. See Figure 4-3, **D, E, F, G, H,** and **I** for more details.

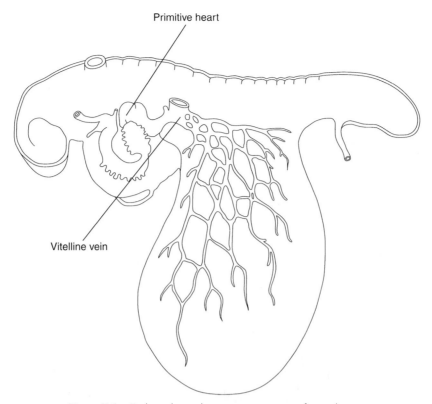

Figure 7-1 Early embryo demonstrating origin of portal vein.

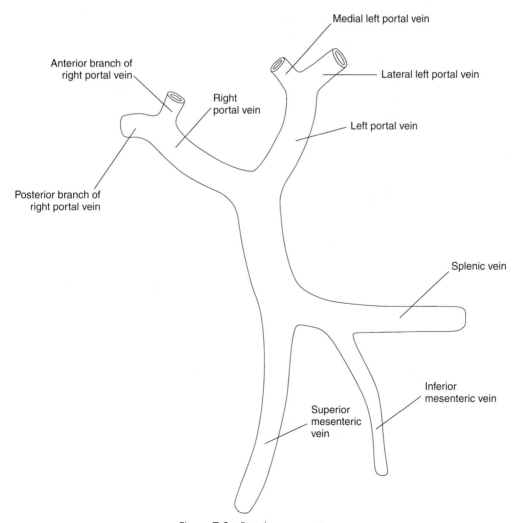

Figure 7-2 Portal venous system.

PHYSIOLOGY

The function of the portal vein and its tributaries is to deliver blood from the spleen and gastrointestinal tract (esophagus, stomach, and small and large intestines) to the liver for metabolism and detoxification. This system is much different from the arterial supply to the liver or the systemic venous supply, which empties the liver after the arterial and portal venous blood has been delivered to the organ. As noted, this is a vital and unique function.

SONOGRAPHIC APPEARANCE

The portal veins are one portion of the **portal triad** (made up of the hepatic arteries, bile ducts, and portal veins) located throughout the liver. However, the portal veins can generally be distinguished from other structures, especially hepatic veins, by their highly echogenic walls. This echogenicity is a result of the high collagen content in the walls of the portal veins (Figure 7-3).

In transverse section, one visualizes the beginning of the **main portal vein** as an oval, anechoic structure, where the splenic vein and superior mesenteric vein join directly posterior to the neck of the pancreas (Figure 7-4). Superiorly to this location, the main portal vein can be seen as it branches into right and left portal veins (Figure 7-5). The **left portal vein** can often be followed further to the left and be seen branching into its medial and lateral subdivisions (Figure 7-6). The left lateral branch is more commonly visualized than the medial branch, and the lateral branch feeds the traditional left lobe of the liver. The **right portal vein** can be seen in the transverse plane as a linear horizontal structure coursing to the right. It shortly bifurcates into its anterior and posterior branches (Figure 7-7).

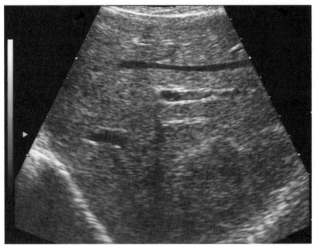 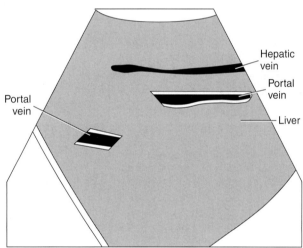

Figure 7-3 Longitudinal section, right lobe of the liver, showing a hepatic vein without echogenic walls and a portal vein with echogenic walls.

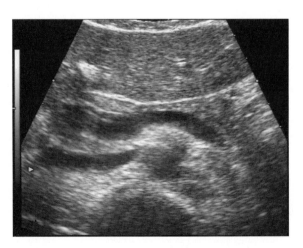 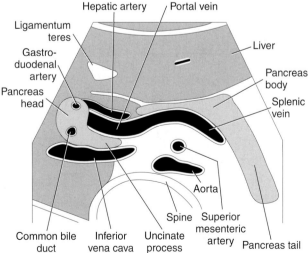

Figure 7-4 Transverse section of the epigastric area demonstrating the linear anechoic splenic vein joining the portal vein.

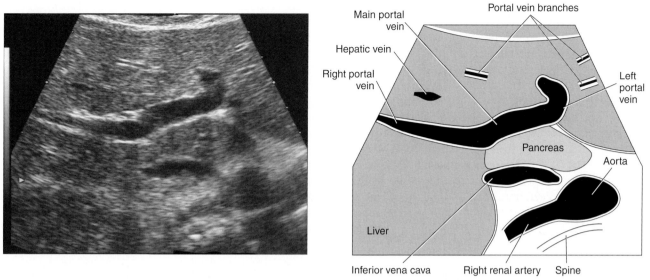

Figure 7-5 Transverse section showing the division of the main portal vein into the right portal vein and left portal vein.

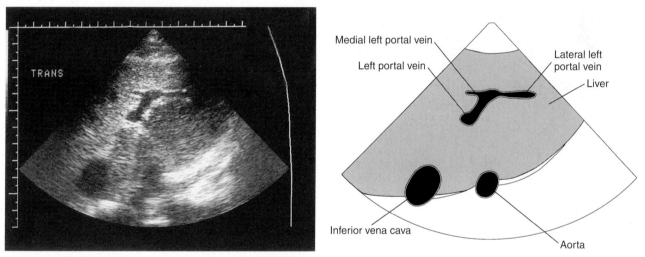

Figure 7-6 Transverse section of the left lobe of the liver demonstrating the left portal vein dividing into its medial and lateral subdivisions.

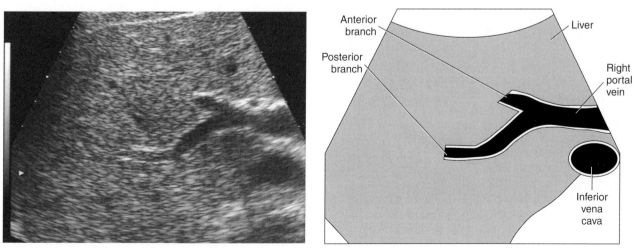

Figure 7-7 Transverse section of the right lobe of the liver demonstrating the division of the right portal vein into its anterior and posterior divisions.

In a longitudinal plane, the main portal vein can be seen as a linear anechoic structure directly posterior to the pancreatic neck as it joins the superior mesenteric vein (Figure 7-8). Moving laterally, the right portal vein can be imaged. The bile ducts are generally imaged as linear anechoic structures located anterior to the circular right portal vein (Figure 7-9). One can often see smaller echogenic portal vein tributaries throughout the liver parenchyma that are routinely imaged in this section. In the left lobe of the liver, it is often more difficult to image the normal portal vein. However, it appears as small anechoic circular structures with echogenic walls when imaged (Figure 7-10).

SONOGRAPHIC APPLICATIONS

Because the portal vein can be consistently imaged with sonography, it is often evaluated to detect tumor invasion and thrombosis. In addition, the most common reason for examination of the portal vein is to uncover portal vein hypertension. However, this pathology involves more structures than the portal vein, including the abdominal cavity, spleen, and liver. These organs are often more indicative of portal vein hypertension. Furthermore, evaluating the portal vein with color Doppler and duplex Doppler is far superior as a diagnostic tool than evaluating the structure with only B-mode imaging. Figure 7-11 shows a normal pulsed wave Doppler of the portal vein. Figure 7-12 (Color Plate 7) shows color

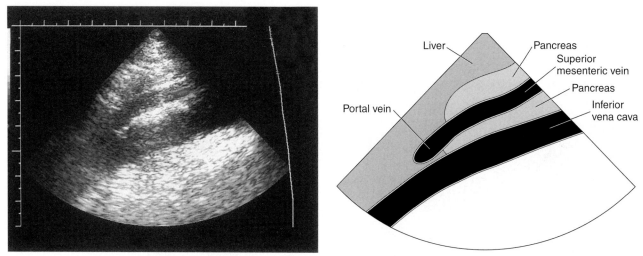

Figure 7-8 Longitudinal oblique section of the epigastric area demonstrating the joining of the superior mesenteric vein to the main portal vein. Note the pancreatic tissue visible anterior and posterior to the portal vein, superior mesenteric vein, and inferior vena cava.

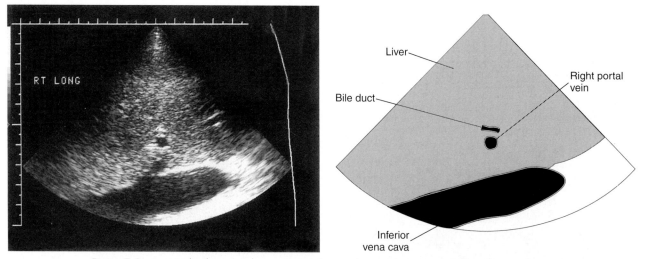

Figure 7-9 Longitudinal section demonstrating the circular anechoic section of a right portal vein with echogenic walls. A linear anechoic duct with hyperechoic walls is located directly anterior to the right portal vein.

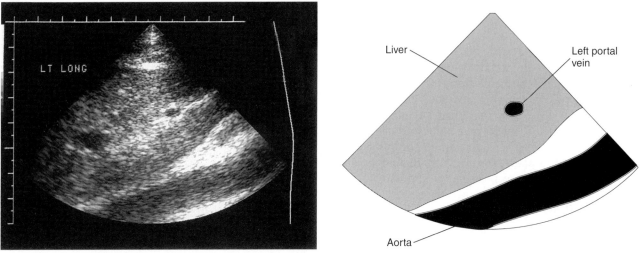

Figure 7-10 Longitudinal section of the left lobe of the liver demonstrating a left portal vein branch, which appears as a circular anechoic structure with echogenic walls.

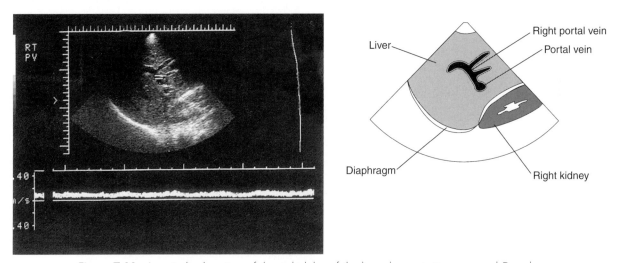

Figure 7-11 Longitudinal section of the right lobe of the liver demonstrating a normal Doppler waveform of the right portal vein. Note the phasic flow (variation) of the Doppler signal in response to respiration. In addition, note that the flow is above baseline. In this case, blood is flowing into the liver, which is normal.

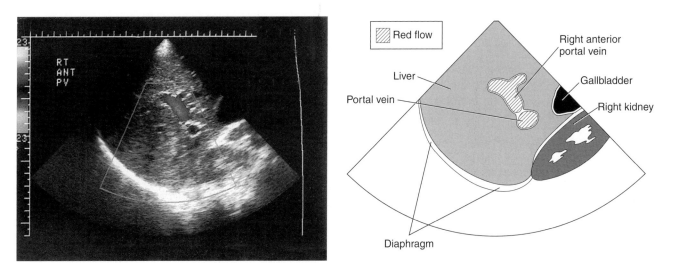

Figure 7-12 Longitudinal section of the right lobe of the liver demonstrating the black-and-white version of the normal color flow Doppler. Note that flow toward the transducer is indicated in red. Thus the flow is toward the transducer (into the liver) in this case. (See Color Plate 7.)

flow into the liver toward the transducer and therefore is red in color.

As stated earlier, the portal system is unique because it carries blood and nutrients from the bowel and abdominal organs to the liver for metabolism and detoxification. Thus pathologies that affect other organs are often the reason for portal vein pathology. Therefore one needs to have a good understanding of this system to ensure that the patient receives the highest quality sonographic examination possible.

NORMAL VARIANTS
Nonapplicable.

REFERENCE CHARTS

■ ■ ■ ASSOCIATED PHYSICIANS

Various physicians may be involved in caring for the patient who has a disorder of the portal vein, depending on the problem. A physician who specializes in internal medicine may treat the patient whose portal vein hypertension is due to cirrhosis of the liver or one who is not a surgical candidate or does not require surgery. Various surgical specialists may treat the patient who requires surgery.

■ ■ ■ COMMON DIAGNOSTIC TESTS

Diagnostic tests may include duplex Doppler sonography, color sonography, venography, computed tomography, and magnetic resonance imaging.

Duplex Sonography: Duplex sonography can detect the direction and magnitude of flow within a portal vein. Flow should be toward the liver from the portal vein, and the portal venous system should display phasic flow in response to respiration (Figure 13-11). This examination and the color flow examination provide extremely valuable information in a short time period and without the use of ionizing radiation. Thus duplex sonography and color flow sonography are often utilized. A sonographer or vascular technologist usually performs this examination and often provides a preliminary impression. A radiologist interprets the findings.

Color Flow Sonography: Color flow sonography reveals information similar to that derived from duplex sonography. However, color flow imaging can often yield this information much faster (Figure 13-12). The same personnel who perform and interpret duplex sonography also perform and interpret color flow sonography.

Direct Portal Venography: Although not usually done given today's technological environment, direct portal venography can be carried out by injecting contrast material (dye) into the splenic or portal vein and taking radiographs of the area as the contrast agent is transported throughout the system. This examination provides information related to portal vein anatomy and intraluminal contents. A radiologist assisted by a radiologic technologist performs this examination. The radiologist interprets it.

Computed Axial Tomography (CT Scan) and Magnetic Resonance Imaging (MRI): CT and MRI can also be done to evaluate the portal vein. In CT, a series of sequential radiographs are taken over the area of interest. The information is stored in a computer, which converts the data into a two- or three-dimensional image. CT is not the best method, since it may be difficult to ascertain intraluminal contents. MRI, although not widely utilized, can often distinguish subtle differences in tissues within the portal system. In MRI, a magnetic field generates data, and a computer converts the information into a diagnostic image. Although MRI is nonionizing, it has several limitations because of the magnetic field. A radiologic technologist performs the CT and MRI examinations. A radiologist interprets the findings.

Benefits of Sonography: Clinical data often suggest portal vein pathology. Sonography can easily verify the intraluminal contents and the direction of flow, in addition to indicating other pathological findings of the abdomen. Thus sonography is often used as a diagnostic tool in evaluating the system.

■ ■ ■ LABORATORY VALUES

Generally, laboratory values do not directly indicate portal vein pathology. However, a tumor, or cirrhosis of the liver, for example, will produce various laboratory and clinical data that could point to portal vein involvement in the disorder.

■ ■ ■ NORMAL MEASUREMENTS

The main portal vein should measure les than 13 mm.

■ ■ ■ VASCULATURE

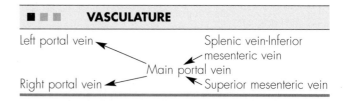

Left portal vein Splenic vein-Inferior
mesenteric vein
Main portal vein
Right portal vein Superior mesenteric vein

■ ■ ■ AFFECTING CHEMICALS

Nonapplicable.

BIBLIOGRAPHY

Mittelstaedt CM: *Abdominal ultrasound,* New York, 1987, Churchill Livingstone.

Moore KL: *The developing human; clinically oriented embryology,* ed 6, Philadelphia, 1998, WB Saunders.

Netter FH: *The CIBA collection of medical illustrations,* vol 3, digestive system, part iii: liver, biliary tract and pancreas,. Summit, NJ, 1978, CIBA Division of CIBA-Geigy.

Weinreb I, et al: Portal vein measurements by real-time sonography, *Am J Radiol* 139:497, 1982.

CHAPTER 8

Abdominal Vasculature

MARSHA M. NEUMYER

OBJECTIVES

Describe the anatomy of the vasculature of the liver, spleen, mesenteric, and renal systems.

Describe the function of the hepatoportal, mesenteric, and renal arterial systems.

Define the role of duplex scanning and color flow imaging for evaluation of abdominal vascular disease.

Describe the sonographic appearance of the hepatoportal, mesenteric, and renal vascular systems.

Define the hemodynamic patterns and spectral waveforms found in the normal abdominal vasculature.

Define key words.

KEY WORDS

Biphasic
Doppler spectral waveform
Duplex ultrasonography
Hepatofugal
Hepatopetal
High-resistance vascular bed
Low-resistance vascular bed
Spectral bandwidth
Spectral broadening
Systolic window
Triphasic

The past two decades have yielded technical advances in ultrasound imaging. The introduction of low-frequency, broad bandwidth pulsed Doppler transducers and color, power, and compound imaging has allowed pursuit of hemodynamic information from the abdominal vasculature. Encouraged by the facility and accuracy of duplex ultrasound interrogation of the cerebrovascular and peripheral arterial and venous systems, investigators have validated Doppler velocity criteria for the hepatoportal, mesenteric, and renal vascular systems.

PRENATAL DEVELOPMENT

This section was discussed in Chapters 5, 6, and 7.

THE ABDOMINAL ARTERIAL SYSTEM
Location

The abdominal arterial system consists of the segment of the abdominal aorta from the level of the diaphragm to the aortic bifurcation; the celiac axis; the common hepatic, splenic, superior mesenteric, inferior mesenteric, and renal arteries; and the vessels of the renal parenchyma (Figure 8-1).

The celiac, superior, and inferior mesenteric arteries originate from the anterior wall of the aorta (Figure 8-2). The celiac axis is located 1 to 3 cm below the diaphragm. This vessel divides into three major branches, the common hepatic, splenic, and left gastric arteries, approximately 1 to 2 cm from its origin. The celiac artery and its branches supply blood to the stomach, liver, spleen, and small intestine.

The superior mesenteric artery (SMA) originates from the aorta 1 to 2 cm distal to the origin of the celiac axis. This artery anastomoses to the celiac artery by way of the superior and inferior pancreaticoduodenal arteries, which serve as major collateral pathways in the presence of occlusive disease of the SMA or celiac artery. The SMA supplies blood to the small intestine, cecum, and ascending and transverse colon.

The inferior mesenteric artery originates from the anterolateral aortic wall approximately 4 cm proximal to the aortic bifurcation. This vessel lies in close proximity to the aorta along the first several centimeters of its course and may be difficult to interrogate with Doppler ultrasound. The artery supplies blood to the descending and sigmoid flexures of the colon and the greater part of the rectum.

The renal arteries originate from the lateral wall of the aorta below the SMA just posterior to the left renal

121

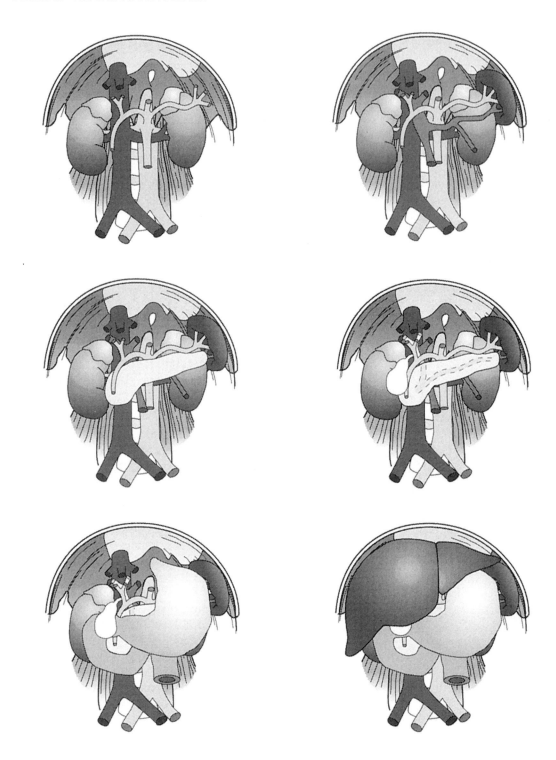

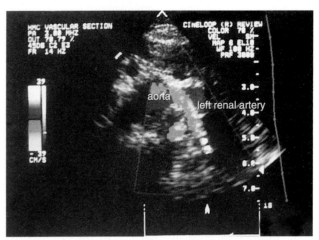

Figure 8-3 Transverse color flow image of the abdominal aorta showing the origin of the left renal artery. (See Color Plate 9.)

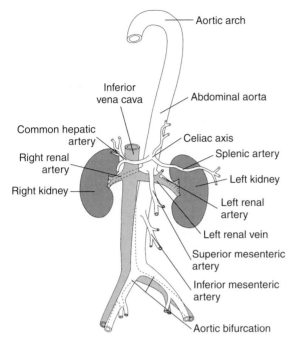

Figure 8-1 Diagram of the visceral arterial system.

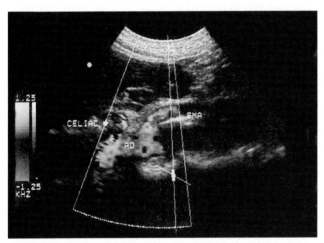

Figure 8-2 Longitudinal Doppler color flow image of the abdominal aorta and the origins of the celiac and superior mesenteric arteries from the anterior wall of the aorta. (See Color Plate 8.)

vein. The right renal artery is longer than the left because it must pass behind the inferior vena cava (IVC) to enter the hilum of the right kidney. The left renal artery originates from the aortic wall somewhat higher than the right (Figure 8-3).

Before entering the hilum of the kidney, each renal artery divides into four or five branches, the greater number of which most often lie between the renal vein and the ureter. The vessels further branch to form the interlobar and arcuate arteries, which pass between the medullary pyramids of the renal parenchyma (see Chapter 12).

Occasionally accessory renal arteries are noted originating from the aortic wall. These may enter the upper or lower poles of the kidney rather than enter the organ at the hilum.

Size of the Visceral Arteries

The average diameter of each of the visceral arteries is:

Aorta	2.0 to 2.5 cm
Celiac	0.70 cm
SMA	0.60 cm
Inferior mesenteric artery	0.30 cm
Renal arteries	0.40 to 0.50 cm

Sonographic Appearance

The abdominal aorta commences at the aortic opening of the diaphragm, lying slightly to the left of the vertebral column. It terminates on the body of the fourth lumbar vertebra, at which point it bifurcates into the common iliac arteries. The vessel diameter tapers slightly from its proximal to distal segments.

The abdominal aorta is bordered anteriorly by the stomach, pancreas, celiac axis, splenic vein, and superior mesenteric artery and vein, and on its right by the IVC. It lies anterior to the vertebral column.

The celiac artery lies anterior to the abdominal aorta. It is bordered on its left side by the cardiac end of the stomach and rests on the upper border of the pancreas.

The SMA lies anterior to the aorta, being covered at its origin by the splenic vein and pancreas. In its proximal segment, it lies between the pancreas and the transverse portion of the duodenum.

The inferior mesenteric artery lies anterolateral to the distal abdominal aorta at its origin. It then descends to the left iliac fossa, anterior to the left common iliac artery, to enter the pelvis as the superior hemorrhoidal artery.

The renal arteries originate from the lateral wall of the aorta immediately below the SMA. In their proximal segment, the renal arteries follow the crus of the diaphragm.

On the right, the renal artery is posterior to the right renal vein and IVC in its mid to distal segments. On the left, the renal artery lies posterior to the left renal vein.

Hemodynamic Patterns

The suprarenal abdominal aorta supplies the largest portion of its blood flow to branch vessels that feed **low-resistance vascular beds.** The liver, spleen, and kidneys all have high metabolic rates and demand constant forward blood flow. In contrast, the stomach and small intestine offer a **high-resistance vascular bed** to the SMA. Blood flow through the suprarenal aorta therefore meets little resistance to runoff, and forward flow is noted throughout the cardiac cycle (Figure 8-4, *A*). The peak aortic systolic velocity decreases with age, perhaps as a result of vessel wall compliance. The infrarenal aortic blood supply is principally to the high-resistance peripheral arterial system of the lower extremities and lumbar arteries. The pressure wave noted in this segment of the aorta therefore resembles the velocity waveforms recorded from peripheral arteries (Figure 8-4, *B*).

The celiac axis supplies low-resistance end organs—the liver and spleen—through its branch vessels—the hepatic, left gastric, and splenic arteries. Like the flow patterns seen in the suprarenal aorta, constant forward flow is documented throughout the vascular tree supplied by the celiac artery (Figure 8-5).

The SMA supplies the tissues of the stomach, small intestine, and colon. Flow in the SMA varies, depending on the activity of these organs and their metabolic status. In the fasting state, there is relatively high resistance to arterial flow to the tissues of the gut (Figure 8-6, *A*). After ingestion of a meal, remarkable changes occur in the flow patterns in the SMA, reflecting the metabolic demands imposed by the digestive process. There is an increase in the diameter of the SMA, peak systolic and end-diastolic velocities, and volume flow to the small bowel. Constant forward flow should be observed throughout the cardiac cycle, reflecting the flow demands of the postprandial vascular bed (Figure 8-6, *B*).

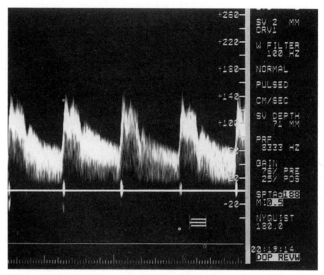

Figure 8-5 Doppler velocity waveform from the celiac axis. Note constant forward diastolic flow.

The kidneys, like the brain, eyes, liver, and spleen, are low-resistance organs that demand constant blood flow to moderate their metabolic activity. Hemodynamic flow patterns in normal renal arteries supplying nondiseased kidneys demonstrate high diastolic flow (Figure 8-7). In patients with chronic renal disease, the vascular resistance of the kidney increases. This increase in renovascular resistance of the end organ may be expressed in the flow patterns from the renal artery as a decrease in the diastolic flow component.

Doppler Velocity Spectral Analysis

The Doppler velocity waveform from the suprarenal abdominal aorta demonstrates an absence of reversed diastolic flow, reflecting the low vascular resistance of its end organs (see Figure 8-4, *A*). In contrast, the signals from the infrarenal aorta are **triphasic,** consistent with a vessel feeding a high-resistance peripheral arterial tree (see Figure 8-4, *B*). Occasionally a **biphasic** flow pattern is present. The absence of a forward diastolic flow cycle

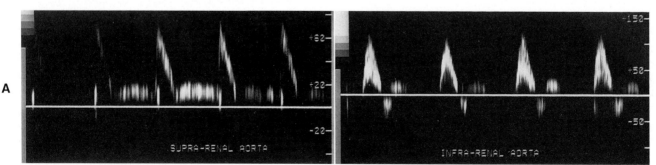

Figure 8-4 **A,** Doppler time-velocity waveform from the suprarenal abdominal aorta. Note forward diastolic flow. **B,** Doppler spectral waveform from the infrarenal aorta demonstrating the triphasic velocity waveform consistent with a vessel feeding a high-resistance vascular bed.

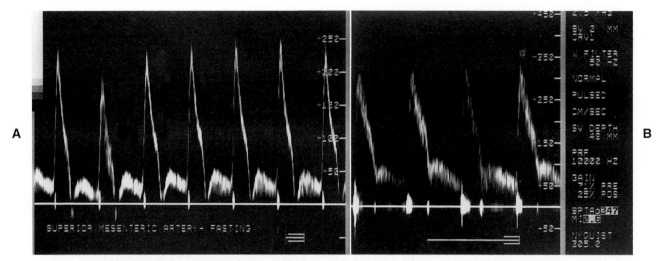

Figure 8-6 **A,** Velocity spectral waveform recorded from the fasting superior mesenteric artery. **B,** Postprandially, the superior mesenteric artery diastolic flow component increases twofold to threefold in response to the metabolic demands imposed by digestion.

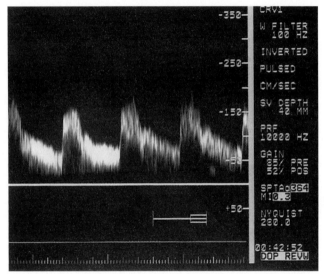

Figure 8-7 Doppler time-velocity waveform from the normal renal artery. The high diastolic flow component is consistent with a vessel feeding a low-resistance end organ.

reflects the relative decrease in arterial wall compliance or elasticity. This flow pattern may be seen in the elderly population and in patients with diabetic medial calcification of the arterial wall.

The **Doppler spectral waveforms** from the celiac, hepatic, and splenic arteries demonstrate forward diastolic flow compatible with high flow demands of the liver and spleen (see Figure 8-5). Peak systolic velocity in the celiac artery normally is less than 200 cm/sec. The splenic artery is frequently tortuous, and **spectral broadening** may be noted in the quasi-steady waveform recorded from this vessel.

In the fasting state, the Doppler spectral waveform from the SMA demonstrates low or reversed flow during the diastolic portion of the cardiac cycle (see Figure 8-6, A). Peak systolic velocity normally is less than 275 cm/sec in the fasting state. Postprandially, the peak systolic velocity increases in the normal artery, and a twofold to threefold increase in end-diastolic flow may be documented (see Figure 8-6, B). Because of the collateral potential expressed in the mesenteric arterial system, disease in one of the three major mesenteric arteries can result in increased flow and velocity in the others.

The inferior mesenteric artery may be difficult to accurately identify by duplex or color flow imaging. In the fasting state, its Doppler spectral waveform mimics that of the fasting SMA exhibiting low diastolic flow. Age-matched peak systolic velocities have not been well validated for the inferior mesenteric artery. Postprandially, there is little immediate change in the diastolic flow value.

The signature Doppler velocity waveform from the renal arteries resembles that from other vessels that feed organs with high flow demand (see Figure 8-7). The normal waveform from the proximal renal artery usually demonstrates a clear **systolic window,** with broadening of the spectrum of velocities evident in the mid to distal segments of the vessel. This increase in **spectral bandwidth** occurs because the sample volume size used to monitor the flow is normally large in relation to the lumen of the vessel, or it increased in size during the study to encompass the entire lumen of a poorly visualized artery. Normally, the renal artery peak systolic velocity is less than 120 cm/sec.

Because the normal kidney has high metabolic demands and low vascular resistance, the Doppler spectral waveform from the interlobar and arcuate arteries of the renal medulla and cortex should demonstrate significant diastolic flow (Figure 8-8, A). With increased renovascular resistance caused by intrinsic renal pathology,

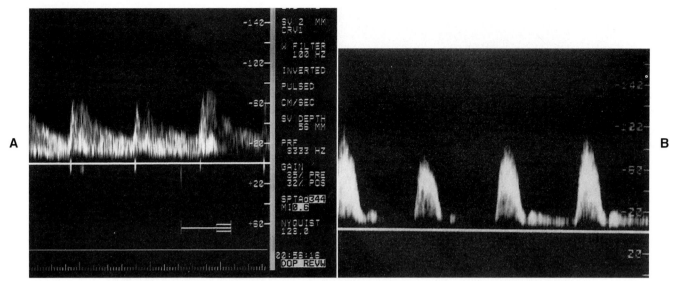

Figure 8-8 A, Doppler velocity waveform recorded from the normal renal parenchyma. **B,** Diastolic flow component of the renal parenchymal Doppler velocity signal decreases as renovascular resistance increases because of intrinsic renal pathology.

the end-diastolic flow component decreases throughout the vascular tree of the kidney, and the velocity waveform becomes markedly pulsatile (Figure 8-8, *B*).

THE ABDOMINAL VENOUS SYSTEM
Location

The abdominal venous system consists of the IVC from the level of its bifurcation into the common iliac veins to the diaphragm and the inferior and superior mesenteric, splenic, portal, hepatic, and renal veins (Figure 8-9). Because the hepatic artery shares a partnership with the ve-

nous circulatory supply of the liver, it will be considered in the discussion of the abdominal venous system.

The IVC is formed by the confluence of the common iliac veins, which drain the lower extremities and pelvis. The IVC normally courses through the retroperitoneum, lying to the right of the abdominal aorta and anterolateral to the vertebral processes. The vessel courses posteriorly in the abdomen as it advances superiorly. It lies medial to the right kidney and posterior to the liver before coursing through the diaphragm to enter the right atrium of the heart.

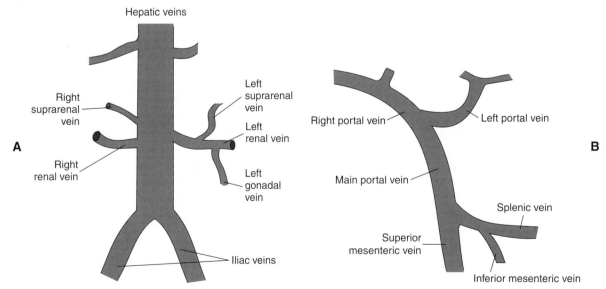

Figure 8-9 A, Diagram of abdominal venous system showing major branches. **B,** Diagram of portal venous system.

A number of anatomic anomalies have been recognized. The most common of these include duplication of the entire length or short segments of the IVC, segmental absence of portions of the vessel, and anatomic relocation of the suprarenal segment, infrarenal segment, or entire length of the IVC to the left of the aorta.

Although the IVC gives rise to multiple tributaries, only those accessible to sonographic evaluation and included as part of the vascular ultrasound examination of the hepatoportal and renal systems will be discussed.

The renal veins return blood from the kidneys to the systemic circulation, emptying into the IVC immediately superior to the level of the renal arteries. The left renal vein is longer than the right renal vein, coursing anterior to the aorta to lie between the aortic wall and the SMA (Figure 8-10). The left renal vein receives the left gonadal and suprarenal veins (see Figure 8-9, *A*). These smaller veins are not included in the routine evaluation of the renal venous system. The right renal vein is shorter than the left renal vein and may receive the right suprarenal vein.

The hepatic veins empty into the IVC superior to the location of the renal veins. Normally there are three major hepatic veins—the right, middle, and left—that give rise to multiple branches within the parenchyma of the liver. The right and left hepatic veins empty the right and left lobes of the liver, respectively, and the middle hepatic vein drains the caudate lobe.

The portal vein and its branches are intraabdominal vessels. The portal vein is formed by the confluence of the superior mesenteric and splenic veins (see Figure 8-9, *B*). It is located posterior to the head of the pancreas where the splenic vein can be found in a posterolateral or posteromedial position. The splenic vein may receive the inferior mesenteric vein before emptying into the portal vein. The superior mesenteric vein returns blood from the small intestine and segments of

the large intestine, where it courses superiorly with the inferior mesenteric vein. The main portal vein courses superiorly and laterally for several centimeters before entering the liver through the porta hepatis. It divides into the left and right portal veins (Figure 8-11). The left portal vein courses horizontally to supply the left lobe of the liver, giving rise to several primary medial and lateral branches. The right portal vein courses to the right lobe of the liver and gives rise to anterior and posterior branches.

The hepatic artery is one of the three primary branches of the celiac trunk. From its origin, it courses superiorly and laterally to enter the porta hepatis (Figure 8-12, *A*) with the portal vein and common bile duct (Figure 8-12, *B*). It branches into the right and left trunks, which have multiple subdivisions that carry arterial blood flow to the right and left lobes of the liver.

Size of the Abdominal Veins

The size of the abdominal veins varies with respiration. The diameters indicated below are associated with expiration:

IVC	35 mm
Renal veins	4.0 to 6.0 mm
Hepatic veins	4.0 to 7.0 mm
Superior mesenteric vein	6.0 to 7.0 mm
Splenic vein	4.0 to 6.0 mm
Portal vein	13 mm

Sonographic Appearance

The sonographic appearance of the abdominal veins is covered in Chapters 6 and 7.

Hemodynamic Patterns and Doppler Spectral Display

The IVC and its tributaries drain the lower extremities, large and small intestines, kidneys, and liver. In contrast

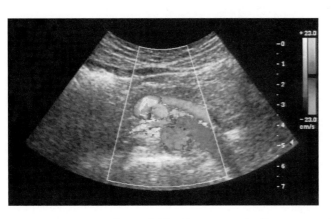
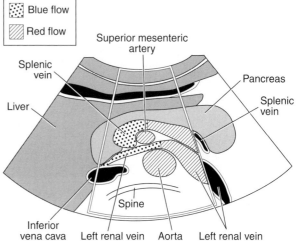

Figure 8-10 Transverse color flow image of abdominal aorta. (See Color Plate 10.)

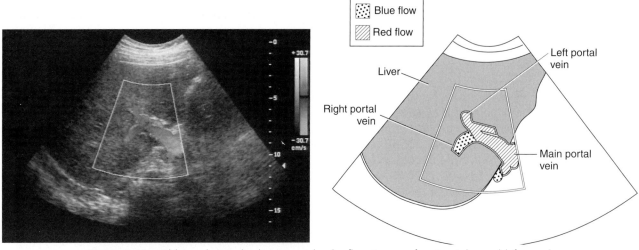

Figure 8-11 Oblique, longitudinal, intercostal color flow image of main, right, and left portal veins. (See Color Plate 11.)

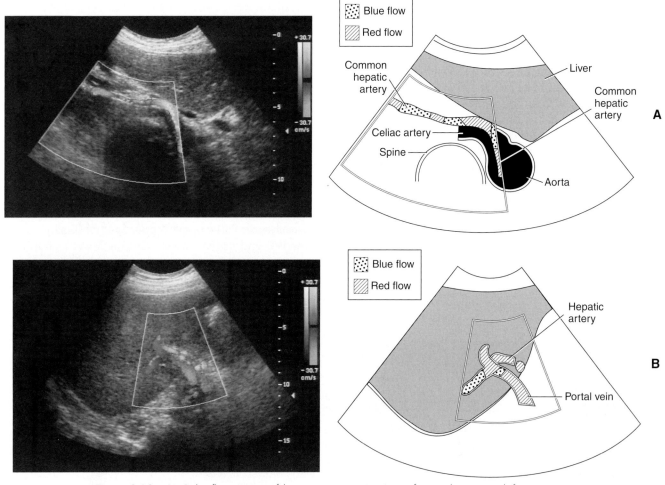

Figure 8-12 A, Color flow image of hepatic artery at its origin from celiac artery bifurcation. B, Color flow image of hepatic artery as it courses with portal vein in the porta hepatis. (See Color Plates 12 and 13.)

to other systemic veins, the portal venous system supplies, rather than empties, a major organ system.

The IVC demonstrates complex flow patterns in its proximal segment as a result of variations in intraabdominal pressure associated with respiration and regurgitation of blood from the right atrium during atrial systole (Figure 8-13, *A*). Distally, the IVC flow pattern reflects the phasic flow patterns seen in the peripheral veins (Figure 8-13, *B*).

The renal veins carry blood from tributaries within the renal medulla and cortex and empty into the IVC. Their flow patterns are influenced by the systemic circulation. For this reason, they do not exhibit pulsatility associated with atrial or ventricular contraction (Figure 8-14).

In contrast, the hepatic veins exhibit pulsatility, a reflection of cardiac and respiratory activity (Figure 8-15). Characteristically, the normal hepatic venous flow pattern is similar to that seen in the proximal IVC. The right, middle, and left hepatic veins should demonstrate three phases of flow. The first two are toward the heart and represent reflections of right atrial and ventricular

diastole. The third phase is represented by systolic flow reversal and is caused by contraction of the right atrium. Flow direction is **hepatofugal,** or away from the liver. Flow should be found throughout all segments of the right, middle, and left hepatic veins without significant disturbance at the hepatocaval confluence.

Intraabdominal pressure effects associated with respiration are transmitted through the liver to the portal and splanchnic veins, causing an undulating flow pattern in the portal venous system (Figure 8-16). The portal vein and its tributaries are responsible for approximately 70% of the oxygenated blood supply of the liver. Normally the high-volume portal venous flow pattern is characterized by continuous, slightly disordered flow with low peak and mean velocities. Flow direction should be **hepatopetal,** or toward the liver. Portal venous flow normally accelerates during expiration and decelerates during inspiration. Portal venous flow is affected by posture, exercise, and dietary state. Exercise and postural changes usually cause a decrease in portal venous flow, whereas eating will increase flow as a result

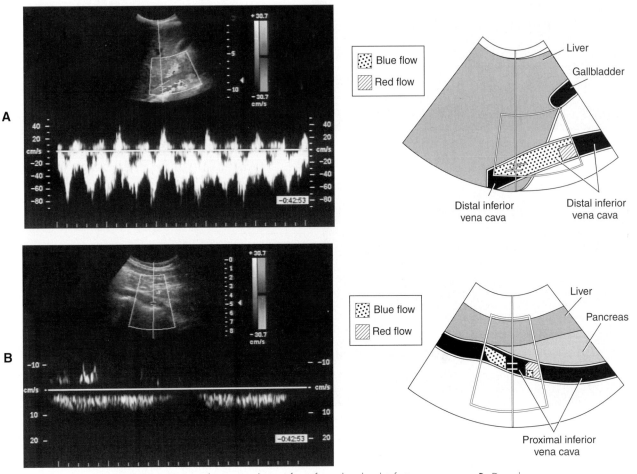

Figure 8-13 **A,** Doppler spectral waveform from the distal inferior vena cava. **B,** Doppler spectral waveform from the proximal inferior vena cava. (See Color Plates 14 and 15.)

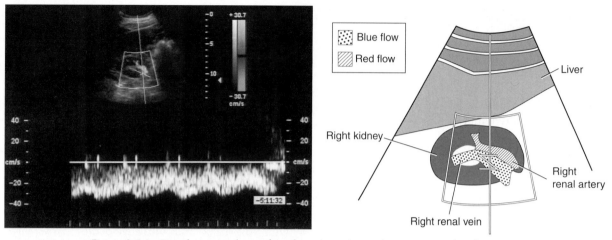

Figure 8-14 Doppler spectral waveform from the right renal vein. (See Color Plate 16.)

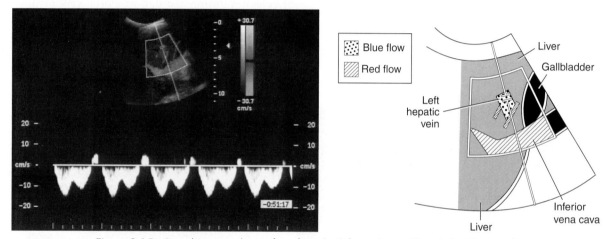

Figure 8-15 Doppler spectral waveform from the left renal vein. (See Color Plate 17.)

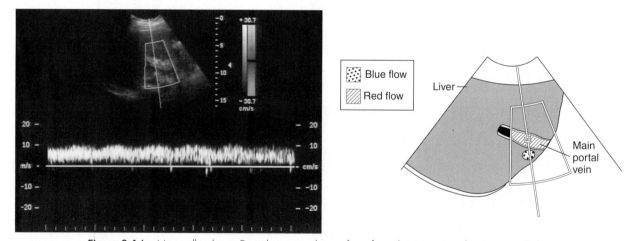

Figure 8-16 Minimally phasic Doppler spectral waveform from the main portal vein. (See Color Plate 18.)

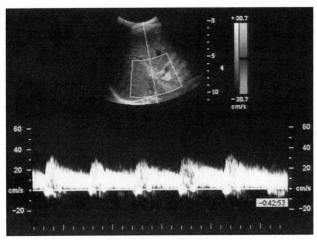
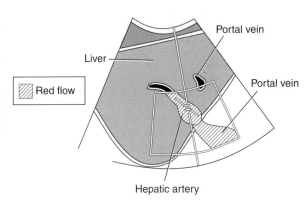

Figure 8-17 Low-resistance Doppler spectral waveform pattern from hepatic artery. (See Color Plate 19.)

of splanchnic vasodilation and hyperemia. To control variations in flow, patients should be examined in the supine or left lateral decubitus position after an 8-hour fast.

The hepatic artery is normally responsible for approximately 30% of the oxygenated blood supply to the liver. Because the liver is a low-resistance end organ, the Doppler spectral waveform pattern from the hepatic artery is characterized by constant forward flow throughout the cardiac cycle (Figure 8-17). Peak systolic velocity is normally less than 100 cm/sec. When portal venous flow is compromised, velocity will most often increase in the hepatic artery as a result of collateral compensatory mechanisms.

REFERENCE CHARTS

■ ■ ■ **ASSOCIATED PHYSICIANS**

Vascular Surgeon: Specializes in the surgical treatment of abdominal vascular disorders.
Gastroenterologist: Specializes in the treatment of disorders involving the gastrointestinal system.
Nephrologist: Specializes in treatment of disorders involving the kidneys.

■ ■ ■ **COMMON DIAGNOSTIC TESTS**

Vascular Angiography: A contrast medium is injected into an artery or vein, and radiographic films are taken at specific intervals to observe blood flow patterns in vessels and organ vasculature. Performed by angiographers (radiologists) and radiologic technologists and interpreted by radiologists and vascular surgeons.

■ ■ ■ **LABORATORY VALUES**

Nonapplicable.

■ ■ ■ **NORMAL MEASUREMENTS**

Average Diameter of Visceral Arteries
Aorta 2.0-2.5 cm	IMA 0.30 cm
Celiac 0.70 cm	Renal arteries 0.40-0.50 cm
SMA 0.60 cm	

Average Diameter of Visceral Veins
IVC 35 mm	Superior mesenteric vein
Renal veins 4.0-6.0 mm	6.0-7.0 mm
Hepatic veins 4.0-7.0 mm	Splenic vein 4.0-6.0 mm
	Portal vein 13 mm

■ ■ ■ **VASCULATURE**

See Chapters 5, 6, and 7 for a discussion of the AO, IVC, PV, and related structures.

■ ■ ■ **AFFECTING CHEMICALS**

Nonapplicable.

BIBLIOGRAPHY

Bernstein EF, editor: *Vascular diagnosis*, ed 4, St Louis, 1993, Mosby.
Gill KA, editor: *Abdominal ultrasound: a practitioner's guide*, Philadelphia, 2001, WB Saunders.
Kremkau FW: *Doppler ultrasound principles and instrumentation*, Philadelphia, 2000, WB Saunders.
Mittelstaedt CM: *General ultrasound*, New York, 1992, Churchill Livingstone.

Netter FH: *Atlas of human anatomy,* ed 3, Teterboro, NJ, 2003, ICON Learning Systems.

Neumyer MM, Wengrovitz M, Ward T, et al: The differentiation of renal artery stenosis from renal parenchymal disease by duplex ultrasonography, *JVT* 13:205-216, 1989.

Pick TP, Howden R, editors: *Gray's anatomy,* New York, 1977, Bounty Books.

Scoutt LM, Zawin ML, Taylor KJW: Doppler US: clinical applications. *Radiology* 174:309-319, 1990.

Strandness DE Jr: *Duplex scanning in vascular disorders,* New York, 1990, Raven Press.

Taylor KJW, Burns PN, Woodcock JP, et al: Blood flow in deep abdominal and pelvic vessels: ultrasonic pulsed-Doppler analysis, *Radiology* 154:487-493, 1985.

Zweibel WJ, editor: *Introduction to vascular ultrasonography,* ed 4, Philadelphia, 2000, WB Saunders.

CHAPTER 9

The Liver

MARILYN DICKERSON

OBJECTIVES

Identify the principal functions of the liver.

Describe the location of the liver.

Describe the size of the liver.

Describe and identify the vasculature of the liver.

Identify the ligaments, segments, and fissures of the liver.

Describe the sonographic appearance of the liver.

Differentiate between carbohydrate, protein, and fat metabolism in the liver.

Describe the associated physicians, diagnostic tests, and laboratory values related to the liver.

Define the key words.

KEY WORDS

Albumin	Ligamentum venosum
Bare area	Main lobar fissure
Caudate lobe	Main portal vein
Cholesterol	Middle hepatic vein
Coronary ligament	Papillary process
Couinaud's liver segmentation	Porta hepatis
	Portal confluence
Diverticulum	Portal triad
Ductus venosus	Prothrombin
Falciform ligament	Quadrate lobe
Fibrinogen	Reidel's lobe
Gastrohepatic ligament	Right hepatic vein
Glisson's capsule	Right lobe
Hemopoiesis	Right triangular ligament
Hepatic segments	Round ligament (ligamentum teres)
Hepatocytes	
Hepatoduodenal ligament	Septum transversum
Hilus	Subhepatic space
Kupffer cells	Subphrenic (subdiaphragmatic)
Left hepatic vein	
Left intersegmental fissure	TIPS
Left lobe	Transverse fissure
Left triangular ligament	Umbilical veins
Lesser omentum	Vitelline veins

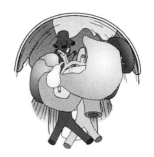

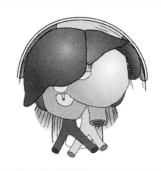

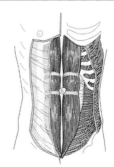

The liver and surrounding anatomic layers. See Figure 4-3, **H**, **I**, and **J** for more details.

The liver is a powerhouse among abdominal organs, the largest parenchymal organ in the body. Its bulky mass displaces gas-filled components of the digestive system and provides an acoustic window for visualization of upper abdominal and upper retroperitoneal structures. Liver structures include the portal veins; the hepatic veins, arteries, and ducts; and the hepatic ligaments and fissures. On ultrasound images, many of these structures help divide the liver into easily identifiable segments.

PRENATAL DEVELOPMENT

The primitive gut is formed during the fourth week of embryonic life and is composed of three parts: a foregut, a midgut, and a hindgut. The liver develops from the foregut (Figure 9-1).

The distal or caudal foregut outpouches between the layers of the ventral mesentery. The head of the outpouch demonstrates a superior **diverticulum** (a circumscribed sac), also known as the extrahepatic biliary ducts. The diverticulum tissue moves into the septum transversum and divides to form the right and left hepatic lobes.

The endodermal cells of the diverticulum give rise to the liver parenchymal cells, the **hepatocytes.** These cells become arranged in a series of branching and anastomosing plates. Hepatic cells are corded within and join the blood sinuses of the umbilical and vitelline veins to complete the formation of hepatic parenchyma.

The **umbilical veins** bring oxygenated blood from the embryonic portion of the placenta to the embryonic tubular heart, whereas the **vitelline veins** return blood from the yolk sac to the heart. The liver tissue sequentially moves into the vitelline veins and then the umbilical veins. As the liver tissue moves into the vitelline veins their midsection becomes capillarized, whereas their caudal ends become the primitive portal veins and their cranial ends become the early hepatic veins.

The right umbilical vein and part of the left umbilical vein degenerate. The remaining left umbilical vein portion carries all the blood from the placenta to the fetus. The **ductus venosus** concurrently develops as a large shunt within the liver to connect the umbilical vein to the inferior vena cava (IVC), thus allowing some blood to bypass the liver and flow directly from the placenta to the heart. Postnatally the umbilical vein becomes the ligamentum teres, and the ductus venosus becomes the **ligamentum venosum.**

The hepatic parenchyma is composed of hepatocytes interspersed with **Kupffer cells** and organized into lobules approximately 1×2 mm in size. Typically approximately 1 million lobules are found in the liver. Peripherally around each lobule are several **portal triads,** each containing portal venules, bile ductules, and hepatic arterioles.

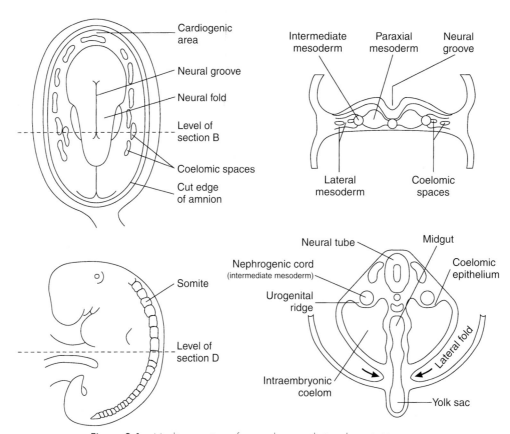

Figure 9-1 Median section of an embryo outlining the primitive gut.

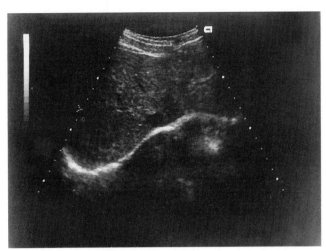

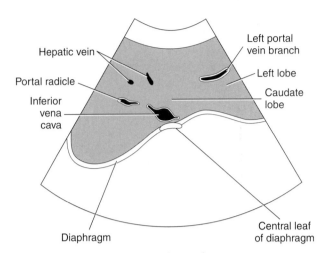

Figure 9-2 Transverse view of the diaphragmatic undersurface and the posterosuperior liver surface.

The **septum transversum** is a mesodermal structure that becomes the connective tissue of the liver. The Kupffer cells and the fibrous and hematopoietic tissue are derived from the splanchnic mesenchyme of the septum transversum.

The liver grows rapidly and bulges into the midportion of the abdominal cavity. **Hemopoiesis**—the formation and development of blood cells—begins during the sixth week of embryonic life and is primarily responsible for the liver's large size.

The inferior portion of the hepatic diverticulum enlarges to form the gallbladder. The common bile duct is derived from the stalk, which connects the hepatic and cystic ducts to the duodenum.

Anomalies of the liver include the left-sided liver (situs inversus), congenital cysts, congenital hemangioma, and intrahepatic biliary duct atresia or stenosis.

LOCATION

The liver occupies a major portion of the right hypochondrium. Normally it extends inferiorly into the epigastrium and laterally into the left hypochondrium. Superiorly it reaches the dome of the diaphragm, and posteriorly it borders the bony lumbar region of the muscular posterior abdominal wall. The bulk of the liver lies beneath the right costal margin (Figure 9-2).

The superior surface, anterior surface, and a portion of the posterior surface of the liver are in contact with the diaphragm. The inferior or visceral surface of the liver rests on the upper abdominal organs (Figure 9-3).

The right lobe of the liver lies close to the anterolateral abdominal wall. Its square, convex right lateral surface is the base of its pyramid (Figure 9-4). The right lobe is related to the right lateral undersurface of the diaphragm along the right midaxillary line from the seventh to the eleventh ribs. On the lateral right side, the liver is related to the diaphragmatic recess and the descending fibers of the diaphragm.

The left lobe of the liver is closely related to the undersurface of the diaphragm. The smallest lobe, the caudate, is related to the lumbar region of the posterior abdominal wall and to the lower posterior thoracic wall. The anterior boundary of the caudate lobe is marked by the posterior surface of the left portal vein, and the posterior boundary is the IVC. The lateral margin projects into the superior recess of the lesser sac, and the caudal border forms the cephalad margin of the epiploic foramen of Winslow.

The IVC courses through the **bare area** of the liver, which lies between the leaflets of the anterior inferior and posterior superior **coronary ligaments.** The right kidney and right adrenal gland lie near the bare area laterally and inferiorly. The boundaries of the bare area include the falciform ligament, right anterior inferior and right posterior superior coronary ligaments, **right triangular ligament, gastrohepatic ligament,** left anterior and left posterior coronary ligaments, and the **left triangular ligament** (Figure 9-5).

The major relations of the right posterosuperior surface are the right posterior fibers of the diaphragm, the upper posterior abdominal wall, the right kidney, and

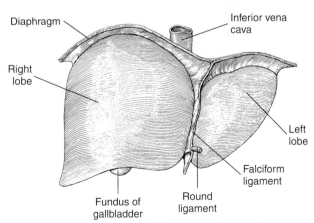

Figure 9-3 Depiction of the anterior liver surface.

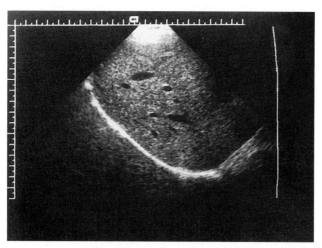

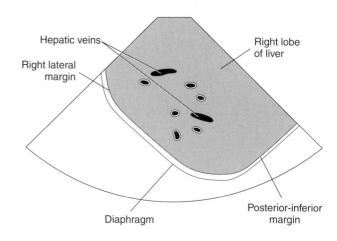

Figure 9-4 Longitudinal scan of the right lateral margin of the liver illustrating the base of the liver pyramid.

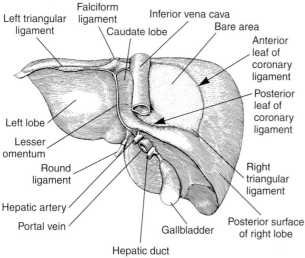

Figure 9-5 Depiction of the posterior surface outlining boundaries of the bare area of the liver.

the right adrenal gland. The inferior segment of this surface below the inferior leaf of the coronary ligament communicates with the upper end of the right lumbar paracolic gutter and the visceral surface of the liver.

The bony and muscular posterior abdominal wall protects the posterior surface of the liver. The border between the anterior aspect of the liver and the visceral surface is the inferior margin.

The inferior surface of the liver is marked by indentations from organs in contact with its surface. Right-sided inferior indentations occur at the right hepatic flexure of the colon, the right kidney and adrenal gland, the first part of the duodenum, and the gallbladder. The left side of the inferior surface contains a gastric indentation, and the posterior surface is marked by the groove that surrounds the IVC (Figure 9-6).

The inferior (visceral) surface is related to the gallbladder, pylorus, duodenum, right colon, right hepatic

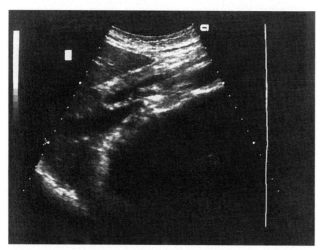

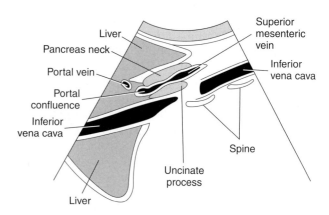

Figure 9-6 Longitudinal image of the left inferior margin of the left hepatic lobe. Note the superior mesenteric vein merging into the portal confluence and the emerging main portal vein anterior to the inferior vena cava.

flexure of the colon, right third of the transverse colon, right adrenal gland, and right kidney. The anterior midportion of the inferior surface is the medial portion of the left lobe of the liver. This portion is also referred to as the **quadrate lobe** of the liver. The left lateral boundary of this portion is the falciform ligament, noted just to the right of the midline (Figure 9-7).

The posterior midportion of the inferior surface, below the **porta hepatis,** marks the location of the **caudate lobe.** The posterior portions of the left and caudate lobes form a portion of the anterior boundary of the lesser sac. The lesser sac lies anterior to the pancreas and posterior to the stomach.

The left hepatic lobe varies in size and shape and may extend deeply into the left upper quadrant. The free inferior margin of the left lobe is closely related to the gastric body and antrum of the stomach. It frequently lies anterior to the body of the pancreas, the splenic vein, and the splenic artery.

SIZE

In men, the liver weighs between 1400 and 1800 g, and in women, it weighs between 1200 and 1400 g. The length of the right lobe and the size of the lateral segment of the left lobe determine the contours of the liver.

The **right lobe** is larger than the left, containing approximately two thirds of the parenchymal tissue. Along the midclavicular line, the normal longitudinal measurement of the right lobe is 13 cm or less. This measurement has also been stated to be 15 to 17 cm.

The **left lobe** is more varied in size. It may be atrophic if interference with the left portal venous supply occurs as the ductus venosus closes at birth. A larger left lobe helps in visualization of the pancreas and left upper quadrant.

GROSS ANATOMY

The liver is divided into three lobes: a right lobe, a left lobe, and a caudate lobe. The right and left lobes are subdivided into four segments: anterior and posterior segments on the right, and lateral and medial segments on the left. The caudate lobe is a midline structure on the posterior aspect of the liver that separates a portion of the right and left hepatic lobes. The caudate lobe is separated from the left hepatic lobe by the proximal portion of the left hepatic vein and the fissure for the ligamentum venosum. This fissure contains the ligamentum venosum and a portion of the lesser omentum (Figure 9-8).

The anterior midportion of the inferior surface of the liver is sometimes called the quadrate lobe. It is not an anatomically distinct lobe but is more correctly identified as the medial segment of the left lobe. The **left intersegmental fissure** divides the medial and lateral segments of the left hepatic lobe. The falciform ligament and the ligamentum teres (round ligament) are located within this fissure. The inferior surface of the liver presents a characteristic H pattern of anatomic lobar segmentation (Figure 9-9). The anterior portion of the H depicts the gallbladder on the right, dividing the anterior right lobe from the medial left lobe. On the left anteriorly, the **ligamentum teres** divides the medial from the lateral left lobe. Posteriorly on the right, the IVC separates the right lobe and the caudate lobe, whereas on the left, the ligamentum venosum divides the caudate from the lateral left lobe. The crossbar of the H depicts the porta hepatis.

The hepatic veins drain blood from the segments and lobes of the liver. They are interlobar and intersegmental. The **right hepatic vein** separates and drains the anterior and posterior segments of the right lobe. The **left hepatic vein** separates and drains the medial and lateral

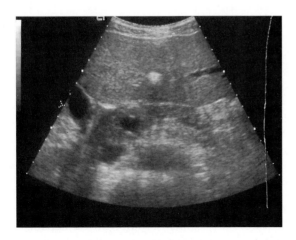

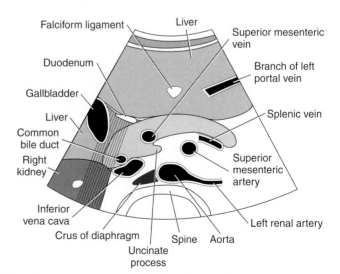

Figure 9-7 Transverse scan of liver. The falciform ligament appears as a bright echogenic focus demarcating the lateral border of the quadrate lobe. The gallbladder fossa is located at the right border of the main lobar fissure and indents the medial left and anterior right hepatic lobes.

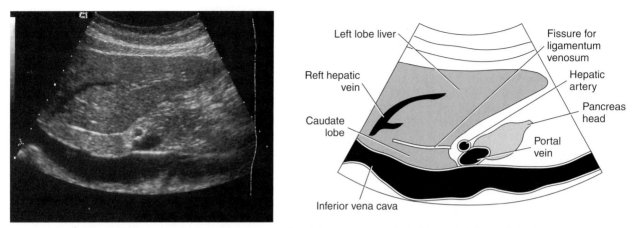

Figure 9-8 Longitudinal image of the caudate lobe posterior to the left hepatic lobe and the ligamentum venosum. The left hepatic vein courses anterosuperiorly toward the inferior vena cava.

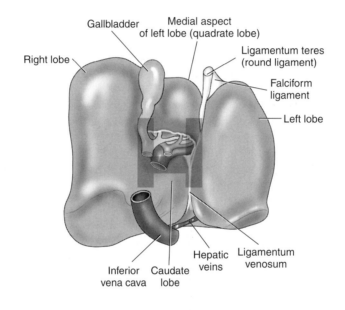

Figure 9-9 The inferior surface of the liver depicting the **H** pattern of lobar segmentation.

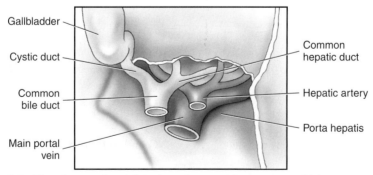

segments of the left lobe of the liver. The **middle hepatic vein** separates and drains the right and the medial left liver lobes (Figures 9-10 and 9-11). The hepatic veins subdivide into superior and inferior groups. The smaller inferior veins drain the caudate lobe and the posteromedial portion of the right lobe.

The portal veins course within and supply the hepatic lobes and segments. Although the hepatic veins usually divide the liver segments, the left portal vein serves as an intersegmental boundary between the medial and lateral segments of the left lobe on caudal transverse scans of the left hepatic lobe.

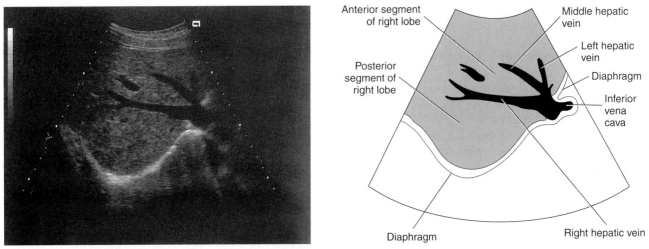

Figure 9-10 Transverse scan of the hepatic veins draining into the inferior vena cava. Anterior and posterior segments of the right hepatic lobe are prominently displayed. Recall that the right hepatic vein separates the anterior liver segments 5 and 8 from the posterior segments 6 and 7.

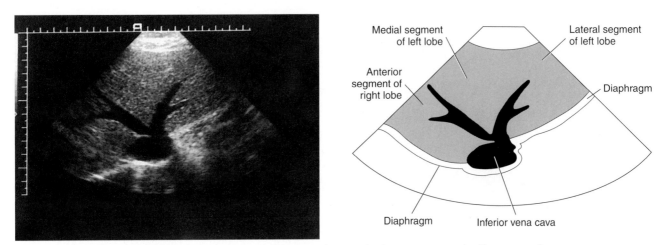

Figure 9-11 Transverse scan of the liver showing the hepatic veins in the "bunny sign."

The branching patterns of the portal vein, the hepatic artery, and the bile ducts and their divisions are central to the functional segmentation of the hepatic lobes, originally described by Couinaud. This pattern of anatomic segmentation provides the basis for surgical resections of the liver. **Couinaud's liver segmentation** is based on venous anatomy, with either hepatic or portal veins dividing the liver. When using the portal vein as the dividing basis, there is always a central portal vein within the segment, whereas a hepatic vein will course at its periphery in the plane between adjacent portal divisions. Segments are thus defined by the portal venous branches that lead into them and by the hepatic veins that separate them.

The liver is divided into a right and left hemiliver via a plane known as the Rex-Cantlie line, which runs from the gallbladder fossa toward the IVC and passes through a portion of the caudate lobe. This is the plane we refer to as the **main lobar fissure.** Each hemiliver is further subdivided into an anterior and posterior segment. On the right, the anterior and posterior segments are each subdivided into inferior and superior segments, whereas on the left, only the left anterior segment is divided into superior and inferior segments.

The caudate lobe represents segment 1 (see Figure 9-15). The caudate lobe is bordered posteriorly by the IVC and anteriorly by the left portal vein. Moving in a counterclockwise direction, segment 1 is separated from segment 2 by the ligamentum venosum. The left hemiliver contains segments 2 through 4. Segments 2 and 3 are found to the left of the ligamentum venosum and the **falciform ligament.**

The falciform ligament separates segment 3 from segment 4. Segment 4 is separated from segment 1 by the left portal vein, and the middle hepatic vein and the main lobar fissure separate segments 5 and 8. The right hepatic vein separates the anterior segments 5 and 8 from the posterior segments 6 and 7 (see Figure 9-10). Segments 5 through 8 are part of the right hemiliver. Each of these eight segments of the liver is distinct in having a central portal triad independent of the other segments, thus providing an important factor in segmental hepatic surgical resections.

The portal system supplies 75% of total blood flow to the liver and has three main tributaries to its confluence: the splenic vein, the superior mesenteric vein, and the inferior mesenteric vein, which may join the splenic vein on its course to the portal confluence.

The **main portal vein** enters the porta hepatis and divides into left and right branches. These veins then branch into medial and lateral divisions on the left and anterior and posterior divisions on the right, and become intrasegmental. The main and right portal veins traverse and supply the bulk of the liver centrally. The left portal vein ascends anteriorly, proximal to the falci-

form ligament. In patients with severe portal hypertension, the left portal vein enters the falciform ligament and communicates with the recanalized ligamentum teres, which had been the postnatally obliterated umbilical vein. The caudate lobe is supplied with blood from the right and left portal veins (Figures 9-12 to 9-15).

The anterosuperior surface of the liver fits snugly into the dome of the diaphragm, separated from the overlying pleural cavities and pericardium. On the right, it rises to the level of the fourth rib interspace on full expiration. The thin edge of the superior surface of the left lobe reaches the level of the fifth rib on full expiration. The anterosuperior surface runs superiorly, then posteriorly, to the anterior leaf of the coronary ligaments on the right. On the left, it runs posteriorly to the left triangular ligament. The right anterosuperior surface of the liver is closest to the anterolateral abdominal wall and is palpable most often when the organ is enlarged.

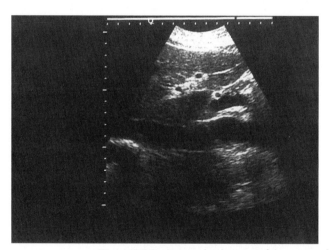
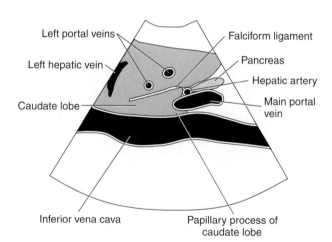

Figure 9-12 Longitudinal image of the origin of the main portal vein. Note the papillary process of the caudate lobe.

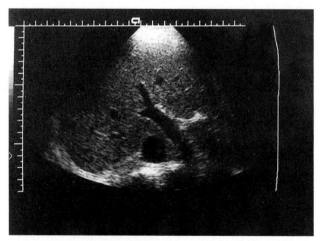
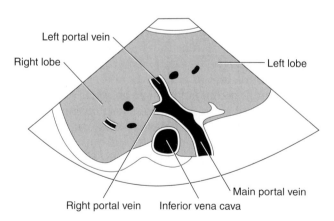

Figure 9-13 Main portal vein entering the porta hepatis just anterior to the inferior vena cava and dividing into right and left branches.

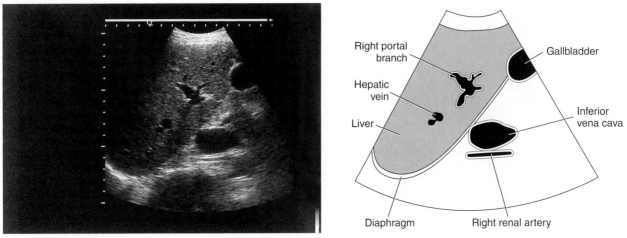

Figure 9-14 Transverse scan of the right portal vein. Note the right renal artery coursing linearly posterior to the short axis inferior vena cava.

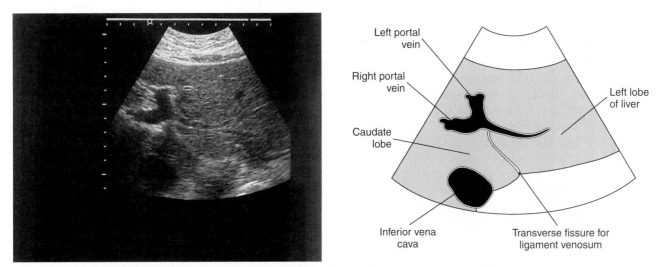

Figure 9-15 Transverse scan of the left portal vein demonstrating Couinaud's liver segments 1 through 4. The umbilical portion of the left portal vein branches to liver segments 2, 3, and 4. Note the caudate lobe (segment 1) anterior to the inferior vena cava and posterior to the left portal vein at this level.

The liver is enclosed by a tight, fibrous capsule known as **Glisson's capsule** and is largely covered by the peritoneum of the greater sac. The caudate lobe is covered by the peritoneum of the lesser sac. To the left of the midline, the posterosuperior surface of the liver is covered by the peritoneum of the greater sac. A portion of the posterior surface of the liver is without a peritoneal covering and is called the bare area. This is in direct contact with the diaphragm.

Peritoneal ligaments connect the liver to upper abdominal structures. The coronary ligament connects the posterosuperior surface of the liver to the diaphragm at the margins of the bare area. The bare area separates and lies between the right posterior subphrenic space above the posterior **subhepatic space** (Morison's pouch) below (Figure 9-16). The upper layer of the coronary ligament extends from the superior liver surface to the inferior surface of the diaphragm. The lower layer extends from the posterior surface of the right lobe of the liver to the right kidney, the right adrenal gland, and the IVC.

The right triangular ligament is formed by an extension of the coronary ligament inferiorly to the right. It begins at the right margin of the bare area and connects the posterior surface of the right lobe to the right undersurface of the diaphragm. The posterior subphrenic and posterior subhepatic spaces, separated by the bare area medially, become continuous, lateral to the right triangular ligament.

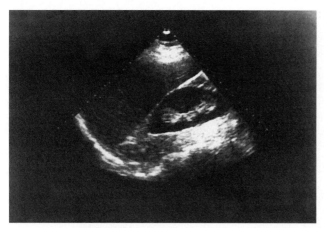
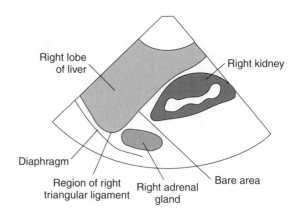

Figure 9-16 Longitudinal scan of the right kidney and the right adrenal gland in contact with the bare area of the liver.

The left triangular ligament is an extension of the falciform ligament to the left. As the falciform ligament passes over the liver dome, it divides into two leaflets. The left leaflet forms a portion of the left triangular ligament. The right leaflet merges with the coronary ligament. It connects the posterior surface of the left lobe to the left aspect of the diaphragm. The triangular and coronary ligaments are not normally visualized on ultrasound examinations.

The falciform ligament connects the liver to the anterior abdominal wall and to the diaphragm. The attachment extends from the superior surface of the liver at the umbilical notch to the inferior surface at the porta hepatis (Figure 9-17). The right, anterior, and superior surfaces unite to form the convex upper surface of the liver. The posterior surface is a continuation of that surface.

The **lesser omentum** is a mesentery or double layer of peritoneum that joins the lesser curvature of the stomach and the proximal duodenum to the liver. The lesser omentum contains the gastrohepatic and hepatoduodenal ligaments.

The gastrohepatic ligament is the portion of the lesser omentum that extends across the **transverse fissure** (fissure for the ligamentum venosum) of the liver at the porta hepatis to the lesser curvature of the stomach. The lesser omentum separates the lesser sac from the gastrohepatic recess.

The ligamentum venosum marks the left anterolateral border of the caudate lobe. The lateral segment of the left lobe is separated from the caudate lobe by the fissure for the ligamentum venosum. The ligamentum venosum is a remnant of the fetal ductus venosus, which shunted oxygenated blood from the umbilical vein to the IVC (Figure 9-18). The fissure for the ligamentum venosum contains the gastrohepatic ligament.

The **hepatoduodenal ligament** is the portion of the lesser omentum that extends as the right free border of

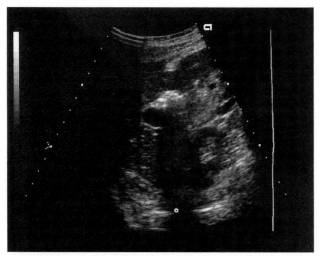
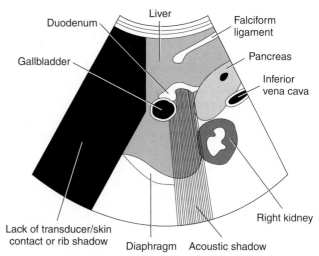

Figure 9-17 Longitudinal scan of the falciform ligament coursing toward the umbilicus and the anterior abdominal wall. Note the characteristic sickle shape.

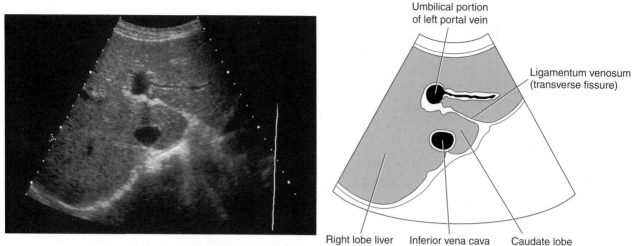

Figure 9-18 *Transverse scan of the caudate lobe. The transverse fissure (ligamentum venosum) courses toward the left portal vein, marking the anterior border of the caudate.*

the gastrohepatic ligament to the proximal duodenum and the right hepatic flexure of the colon. The hepatoduodenal ligament marks the right ventral border of the lesser omentum. Portions of the common bile duct and the hepatic artery are often visualized on transverse scans at the level of the hepatoduodenal ligament, just cephalad to the head of the pancreas and adjacent to the porta hepatis. The porta hepatis is the opening of the liver through which the portal veins and hepatic arteries enter and the hepatic ducts exit. The common bile duct and hepatic artery course anterior to the portal vein in the portal triad at this level. The common bile duct is the anterolateral vessel. It then passes posterior to the duodenum and enters the pancreas (Figure 9-19).

PHYSIOLOGY

The liver is a primary center of metabolism, supporting multiple body systems and activities. In support of the digestive and excretory systems, the liver metabolizes fats, carbohydrates, and proteins and forms bile and urea.

Principal functions of the liver may be categorized as metabolic, protective, secretory, formative, and miscellaneous.

Metabolic functions of the liver involve uptake of body nutrients, such as carbohydrates, amino acids or proteins, fats, and vitamins. The liver serves as a storage site for these substances, performs metabolic conversions of these substances into nutrients, and subsequently releases them into the blood and bile vessels.

The liver absorbs intestinal splanchnic and venous blood received from the portal veins, which drain the digestive tract, the pancreas, and the spleen, and receives a second supply of arterial blood from the hepatic artery, a branch of the superior mesenteric artery.

The venous blood contains products of digestion, such as amino acids and glucose. The liver uses glucose

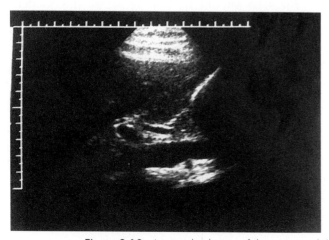

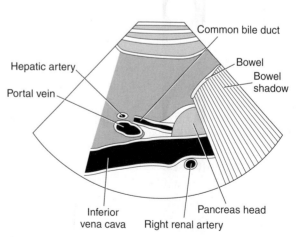

Figure 9-19 *Longitudinal scan of the common bile duct coursing into the head of the pancreas at the level of the hepatoduodenal ligament.*

to metabolize carbohydrates. For carbohydrate metabolism, the liver breaks down, stores, and manufactures simple sugars, which the body uses as a primary source of energy.

Carbohydrate metabolism in the liver involves the processes of glycogenesis, the formation and storage of glycogen, a polysaccharide; glycogenolysis, the conversion of glycogen into its essential nutrient, glucose; and the release of glucose into the bloodstream. Diabetes mellitus is a commonly identified disease characterized by high levels of glucose measured in the blood.

Protein metabolism results in the synthesis of amino acids into proteins. Proteins serve a variety of functions in the structure and metabolism of the body. Structural proteins are found in hair, muscle, and connective tissue. Enzymes such as those that act as biological catalysts in metabolic reactions are proteins, as are molecules such as hemoglobin that transport vital nutrients.

Fat metabolism in the liver is a process involving the synthesis of fatty acids from carbohydrates. Fat is absorbed from fatty acids and desaturated in the liver. Ketones are intermediary products formed during this process. Fat metabolism results in the formation of cholesterol and phospholipids. Phospholipids are structural components of cell membranes that protect the cell's contents from its environment.

Cholesterol is a major component of the bile that is secreted by the liver and serves to emulsify fats. Cholesterol is a steroid present in many food products, such as eggs, dairy products, oils, fats, and meats, and is present in all tissues, most abundantly in nervous and glandular tissue and the brain.

The presence of cholesterol in the bile is a result of its solubility in the presence of bile salts and the phospholipid lecithin. These substances, along with the bile pigments bilirubin (reddish) and biliverdin (greenish), are the primary components of bile. If either the bile salts or lecithin is deficient, cholesterol may precipitate, or separate, out of solution and form gallstones, which may accumulate in the gallbladder or obstruct the common bile duct. In patients with bile duct obstruction, excessive bile pigments may appear in the blood and result in jaundice, a yellow discoloration of the skin, sclerae of the eyes, and mucous membranes. Approximately 1 pint of bile is secreted each day.

The secretion of bile comprises a major secretory function of the liver. Bile is secreted continuously by the liver and passes from the liver through the hepatic ducts into the common bile duct and empties into the duodenum as food is digested. When the duodenum is empty, bile backs up into the gallbladder, where the organic substances are concentrated and stored.

Additional metabolic functions of the liver include the storage of minerals and vitamins, formation of vitamin A, metabolism of steroid hormones, and degradation and detoxification of drugs such as alcohol and barbiturates.

Detoxification of poisonous and harmful substances absorbed by the intestine is also a protective function of the liver. Other protective functions include the conversion of harmful substances, such as ammonia, a waste product of protein metabolism, into useful or excretable substances, such as the amino acid arginine and urea. Arginine is a useful amino acid, and urea is a waste product that is excreted. The Kupffer cells of the liver are protective specialized cells of the liver that play a major phagocytic role in the body's defense against invading organisms, such as bacteria, viruses, and parasites.

The liver synthesizes the blood proteins **albumin, fibrinogen, prothrombin,** and globulins. The synthesis of blood plasma proteins, which include albumin and various globulins, is a formative function of the liver. Prothrombin and fibrinogen are blood-clotting factors. The synthesis of heparin, an anticoagulant, also takes place in the liver.

The liver is a contributor to the lymphatic system by the formation of lymph fluid. Lymph fluid from the liver is rich in proteins formulated from hepatocytes. The liver supplies the major portion of lymph entering the lymphatic system via its principal lymph duct, the thoracic duct.

The liver also stores vitamins and other metabolic substances, detoxifies harmful chemicals, regulates blood volume, and is a major source of body heat.

Miscellaneous functions of the liver include its usefulness as a reservoir for blood that is released as the liver regulates blood volume and blood flow through the body. An important function the liver provides is a major source of body heat that results from the many hepatocellular chemical reactions taking place within it.

SONOGRAPHIC APPEARANCE

The liver should be homogeneous and moderately echogenic throughout. A boundary between the left and right hepatic lobes can be imagined along a line coursing posteriorly from the gallbladder fossa to the groove for the IVC. This line is the main lobar fissure. This fissure is identified on most sonograms along the right oblique plane and extends a varying and short distance between the long axis neck of the gallbladder and a cross-section of the portal vein. The fissure does not extend cephalad to the plane of the right portal vein. The reflection is hyperechoic and appears as a thin line connecting the gallbladder neck to the portal vein (Figure 9-20).

Many landmark structures are visible on a longitudinal scan through the long axis of the IVC. Cephalad (superiorly) to caudad (inferiorly), one should see, anterior

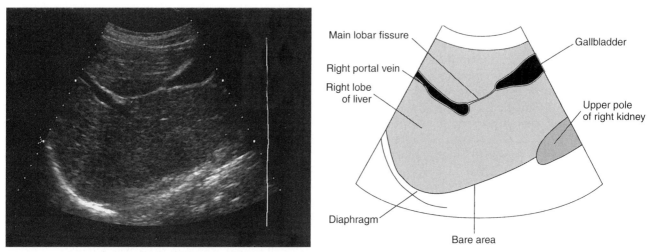

Figure 9-20 Longitudinal scan of the main lobar fissure seen as an echogenic line connecting the neck of the gallbladder to the right portal vein.

to the IVC, the following structures: the right atrium, the central leaf of the diaphragm superior to the left hepatic lobe, the middle hepatic vein as it enters the vena cava, the caudate lobe of the liver separated from the lateral left lobe by the ligamentum venosum, the extrahepatic main portal vein in cross-section, and the head of the pancreas. The superior mesenteric vein may be seen coursing toward its junction with the splenic vein at the **portal confluence.** The left portal vein may be visualized on its C-shaped superior course, proximal to the falciform ligament.

Ligaments and fissures are demonstrated as highly echogenic because of the presence of collagen and fat within and around these structures. The attachment of the falciform ligament from the upper surfaces of the liver to the diaphragm and the upper abdominal wall

appears to divide the right and left lobes. It represents the lower margin of peritoneum surrounding the ligamentum teres, or round ligament, of the liver. The falciform ligament is highly echogenic on longitudinal and transverse scans, appearing sickle shaped on longitudinal scans and pyramidal on transverse scans (Figure 9-21).

The **round ligament** (ligamentum teres) is the obliterated umbilical vein, a fibrous cord that extends upward from the diaphragm to the anterior abdominal wall. On transverse scans, it most often is identifiable coursing within the lower margin of the falciform ligament. These structures lie close to the anterior midline surface of the body and within the near field of the transducer. They are displayed on the upper midportion of the screen.

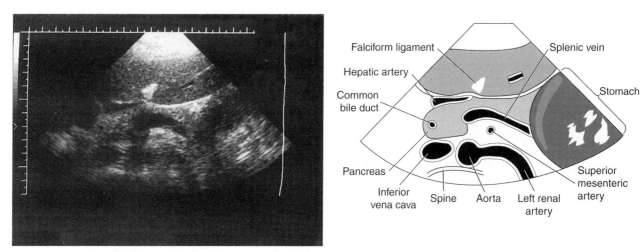

Figure 9-21 Transverse scan of the falciform ligament. Note its characteristic pyramidal shape. The echogenic focus is also referred to as the round ligament or ligamentum teres at this level.

The echogenic falciform ligament courses anteriorly and inferiorly from the left portal vein toward the umbilicus. Transverse scans through the liver frequently demonstrate an echogenic focus in the area of the falciform ligament. This structure correlates the sonographic appearance of the falciform ligament with its appearance on computed tomography (CT) scans, although it may be prominent enough to raise the suspicion of a solid mass. The presence of a recanalized umbilical vein within the falciform ligament should be looked for in patients with portal hypertension.

The main portal vein is visualized at its origin, posteroinferior to the neck of the pancreas. Identification of the porta hepatis is possible with visualization of the main portal vein lying anterior to the IVC. This point of contact is also an indicator for the **hilus** of the liver. Once the main portal vein enters the porta hepatis, it divides into a smaller, more anterior and more superior left portal vein and a larger, more posterior and more inferior right portal vein. Portal veins decrease in size as they approach the diaphragm.

The junction of the right and left portal veins is noted on a superiorly angled transverse scan just inferior to the plane that demonstrates the convergence of the three hepatic veins on the IVC. This level identifies the location of the union of the left and right hepatic ducts to form the common hepatic duct. The right portal vein is followed medially to detect the common hepatic duct crossing linearly anterior to it. The common hepatic duct should be measured at this location anterior to the right portal vein. Any measurement greater than 5 mm raises the possibility of biliary obstruction.

The hepatic veins increase in size as they drain toward the diaphragm and IVC. Any large vein in the liver near the diaphragm may be considered a hepatic vein. There are several features that distinguish hepatic veins from portal veins. Hepatic veins course between lobes and segments, whereas portal veins course within segments. Hepatic veins drain toward the right atrium and usually have anechoic borders, except near the IVC, where the venous walls are more reflective. The positions of the hepatic veins can therefore be used to identify the segments of the liver and provide precise descriptions of focal lesions.

Identification of **hepatic segments** is important in localizing potentially resectable lesions of the liver. Lesions of this type include primary hepatic neoplasms, single metastatic lesions, and some nonmalignant hepatic abnormalities (Figure 9-22).

Posterior to the IVC on parasagittal scans, the anechoic right renal artery is seen in short axis, anterior to the right linear crus of the diaphragm noted with midlevel echoes.

Any other solid-appearing mass posterior to the IVC and inferior to the liver suggests the presence of enlarged lymph nodes or adrenal lesions.

SONOGRAPHIC APPLICATIONS

Ultrasound examinations of the liver are indicated for suspected liver enlargement, hepatic or perihepatic masses, abscesses, and obstructive or metastatic lesions. Cystic, solid, and complex masses are readily identifiable because they distort the smooth contour of the liver. Abnormal lesions usually are increased or decreased in echogenicity when compared with the moderate echo strength of the liver parenchymal reflectors. The liver parenchyma is normally homogeneous and should be carefully examined to exclude small focal lesions. Pleural effusions may be visualized in the **subdiaphragmatic (subphrenic)** region superior to the liver capsule. Ascites

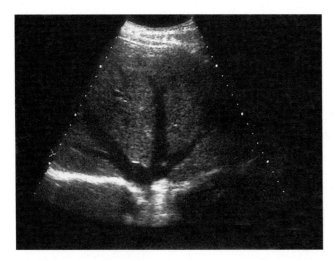
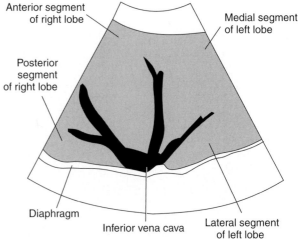

Figure 9-22 Transverse scan of hepatic veins draining into the inferior vena cava, providing for sonographic segmentation of hepatic lobes.

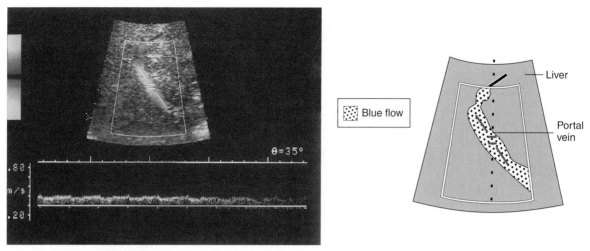

Figure 9-23 Color flow Doppler image showing the characteristic waveform of a normal portal vein. Note that the blood flow is in the direction of the liver toward the transducer. (See Color Plate 20.)

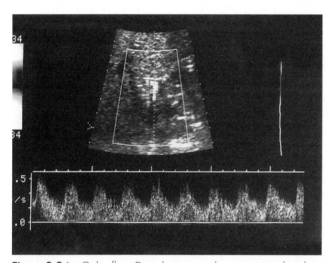

Figure 9-24 Color flow Doppler image demonstrating the characteristic arterial waveform of the normal hepatic artery. (See Color Plate 21.)

is identifiable when fluid collects in the subcapsular or intraperitoneal spaces surrounding the liver.

Vascular structures of the liver and porta hepatis are evaluated using duplex abdominal and color flow Doppler techniques (Figures 9-23 and 9-24). The presence, direction, and blood flow velocity in a sample volume are assessed with these examinations.

The portal vein, the hepatic arteries and veins, and the splenic artery and vein are the upper abdominal vessels normally evaluated.

The usual indications for color Doppler liver sonography include suspected portal hypertension, portal or hepatic vein thrombosis, and preoperative and postoperative hepatic surgery.

For example, in some patients with esophageal varices, interventional radiologists surgically place a permanent shunt between the hepatic vein and intrahepatic portal vein. This placement is designed to divert blood around the liver, thereby relieving portal hypertension by reducing portal vein pressure. The procedure is known as placement of a **TIPS** (transjugular intrahepatic portosystemic) shunt. Color Doppler ultrasound evaluation of the direction and flow of the portal vein in a patient with a TIPS shunt is commonly performed before and after the procedure (Figures 9-25 to 9-27).

NORMAL VARIANTS

Reidel's lobe is a tonguelike inferior extension of the right lobe, as far caudally as the iliac crest (Figure 9-28). It has the same sonographic appearance as normal liver parenchyma. On ultrasound this variant can be identified when liver tissue extends well below the inferior pole of the right kidney during normal respiration.

The caudate lobe may have a distal **papillary process** that may be confused with an enlarged lymph node or another extrahepatic lesion. This process appears as a rounded prominence on the anteroinferior aspect of the caudate lobe. The papillary process may appear as a separate structure on longitudinal and transverse sections. It has the same sonographic appearance as normal liver parenchyma.

Another variation is an elongated left lobe with a tip that may extend laterally to the spleen. Sonographic appearance is the same as the normal liver.

NORMAL MEASUREMENTS

Nonapplicable.

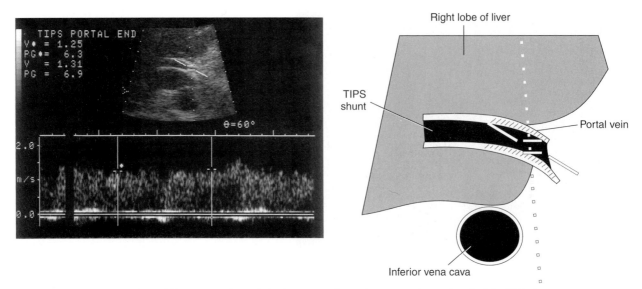

Figure 9-25 Oblique scan through the liver to evaluate the proximal portal end of the TIPS shunt after placement.

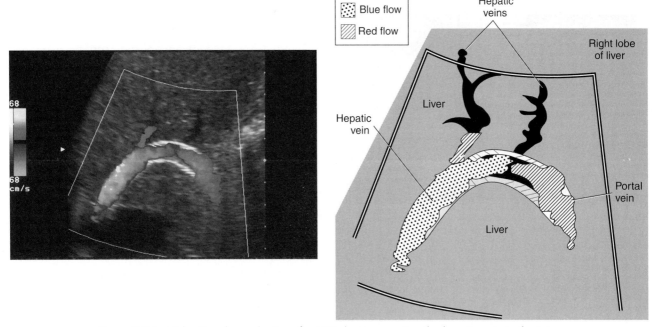

Figure 9-26 Color Doppler evaluation of a TIPS shunt connecting the hepatic vein to the intrahepatic portal vein. Note that the color blue represents flow away from the transducer (hepatic vein) and the color red represents flow moving toward the transducer (portal vein). (See Color Plate 22.)

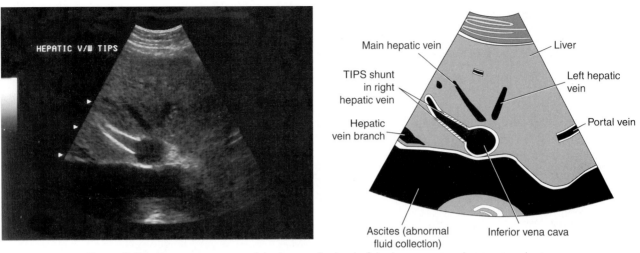

Main hepatic vein

Liver

TIPS shunt
in right
hepatic vein

Left hepatic
vein

Hepatic
vein branch

Portal vein

Ascites (abnormal
fluid collection)

Inferior vena cava

Figure 9-27 Transverse section of the liver at the level of the hepatic veins draining into the inferior vena cava. Note the highly reflective terminal end of the TIPS shunt within the right hepatic vein.

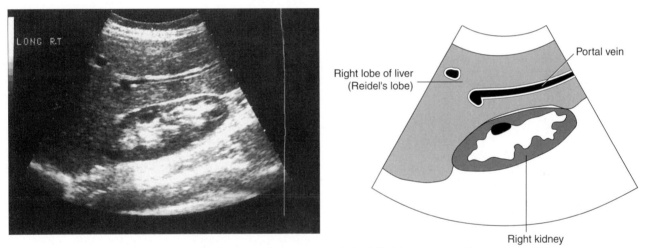

Portal vein

Right lobe of liver
(Reidel's lobe)

Right kidney

Figure 9-28 Longitudinal image of a woman with Reidel's lobe, a tonguelike extension. This lobe extends inferiorly to the iliac crest.

REFERENCE CHARTS

■ ■ ■ ASSOCIATED PHYSICIANS

Gastroenterologist: Specializes in treating diseases of the gastrointestinal tract, including the stomach, small and large bowel, gallbladder, and bile ducts.

Internist: Specializes in studying the physiology and pathology of internal organs and diagnosing and treating disorders of those organs.

Oncologist: Specializes in the study and treatment of tumors and malignancies.

Radiologist: Specializes in the diagnostic interpretation of imaging modalities that assess the liver.

Vascular specialist: Studies and treats disorders of blood vessels.

Surgeon: Utilizes operative procedures to treat diseases, trauma, and organ deformity.

■ ■ ■ COMMON DIAGNOSTIC TESTS

Examination	Use
COMPUTED TOMOGRAPHY (CT)	Focal lesions Tumor masses Bone displacement Fluid accumulation Biopsy

This x-ray examination utilizes a narrow collimated beam of x-rays that rotate around the patient in a continuous 360-degree arc in order to image the body in cross-sectional slices. The image is created by a digital computer that calculates attenuation or tissue absorption of the x-ray beams. Very small differences in density of body structures may be demonstrated and are displayed on x-ray film. The examination is performed by radiologic technologists who specialize in computed tomography and is interpreted by radiologists.

Examination	Use
ANGIOGRAPHY	Focal lesions Myocardial infarction Vascular occlusion Portal hypertension Renal tumors Pulmonary emboli Mass characterization Vascular anatomy Therapy

This examination utilizes x-rays to visualize the internal structure of the heart and blood vessels after the injection of a contrast medium into an artery or vein. A catheter is used to insert the contrast material into a peripheral artery, and threaded through the vessel to a visceral site. Angiograms are performed by radiologists and assisted by radiologic technologists. The examination is interpreted by the radiologist.

Examination	Use
MAGNETIC RESONANCE IMAGING (MR, MRI)	Focal lesions Tumors Brain functions Body chemistry Heart disease 3-D imaging

The MR scanner surrounds the patient with powerful electromagnets that create a magnetic field. Hydrogen atoms in the patient's body are disturbed by this field. The atoms' protons become aligned in the direction of the magnetic field's poles. The computers process and measure the speed and volume with which the protons return to their normal state, and display a diagnostic image of striking clarity on a monitor. Intravenous contrast materials may be given to enhance image definition. MR produces cross-sectional and sagittal soft tissue images. The examinations are performed by registered radiologic technologists and interpreted by radiologists. Physicists assist radiologists in the MR laboratory because of the complexity of the MR equipment.

Examination	Use
RADIONUCLIDE SCINTIGRAPHY	Focal lesions Tumors Cysts Abscesses Vascular anatomy

Scintigraphy utilizes a gamma camera to detect radioactive substances given intravenously or by mouth. Scintigraphy commences when the radioisotope reaches optimum activity in the part being examined. For liver studies this begins immediately after injection. A technetium sulfur colloid is the radionuclide used in liver studies. Recording devices convert voltage impulses received from the scanner into a paper or x-ray film record of a series of dots that reflect the radiation intensities received. Abnormalities are indicated by an absence of activity. The examinations are performed by certified nuclear medicine technologists. They are interpreted by radiologists or nuclear physicians.

Examination	Use
LIVER BIOPSY	Hepatitis Liver cell carcinoma

A needle is inserted into the RUQ to remove a sample of liver tissue for microscopic evaluation. Used to assess severity of liver cell damage. The examination is performed by a radiologist.

■ ■ ■ LABORATORY VALUES

LIVER FUNCTION TESTS

Test	Normal	Increase	Decrease
Albumin	3.3-4.5 g/dl	Liver damage, hemolytic anemia	
Bilirubin	Adult indirect ≤1.1 mg/dl	Jaundice, liver damage, obstruction	
	Adult direct <0.5 mg/dl		
Alkaline phosphatase (ALP)	1.5-4.5 BU/dl	Metastases	
	0.8-2.9 BLB	Obstruction	
	Unit	Lesions	
		Jaundice	
AST (SGOT)	5-30 U/L	Hepatitis	
		Liver injury	
		Jaundice	
		Cholestasis	
		Myocardial infarction	
		Muscle disease	
		Cirrhosis	
		Metastases	
		Fatty liver	
		Lymphoma	
ALT (SGPT)	6-37 U/L	Jaundice	
		Hepatitis	
Beta globulin	0.7-1.2 g/dl	Fatty liver	Liver disease
Cholesterol	140-200 mg/dl		Cancer
Gamma globulin	0.5-1.6 g/dl		
Lactic dehydrogenase (LDH)	100-225 U/L	Liver disease	
	180-280 U/L	Cancer	
Protein	6.6-7.8 g/dl	Chronic liver disease	
Prothrombin			
Time (PTT)	11-15 seconds	Liver disease	
1—Forward			
2—Reverse			

■ ■ ■ NORMAL MEASUREMENTS

Nonapplicable.

■ ■ ■ VASCULATURE

ARTERIAL SYSTEM

Vessel	Branch of	Supplies
Common hepatic artery	Celiac artery	Liver
Proper hepatic artery	Common hepatic	Liver
Right hepatic artery	Proper hepatic	Right lobe, Right caudate
Left hepatic artery	Proper hepatic (may arise from left gastric artery)	Left lobe, Quadrate lobe, Left caudate

VENOUS SYSTEM

Vessel	Tributary to	Drains
Central veins	Hepatic veins	Sinusoids
Right hepatic vein	Inferior vena cava	Right lobe
Middle hepatic vein	Inferior vena cava	Right lobe, Caudate lobe
Left hepatic vein	Inferior vena cava	Left lobe, Quadrate lobe

PORTAL SYSTEM

Vessel	Tributary to	Drains
Main portal vein		Gastrointestinal tract
Superior mesenteric vein	Portal vein	Gastrointestinal tract
Inferior mesenteric vein	Splenic vein	Gastrointestinal tract
Splenic vein	Portal vein	Spleen
	Pancreas	

■ ■ ■ **AFFECTING CHEMICALS**

Nonapplicable.

BIBLIOGRAPHY

Anderhub B: *Manual of abdominal sonography*, Baltimore, 1983, University Park Press.

Applegate EJ: *The sectional anatomy learning system: concepts*, ed 2, Philadelphia, 2002, WB Saunders.

April EW: *Anatomy*, Media, PA, 1984, Harwal.

Bartrum RJ, Crow HC: *Real-time ultrasound: a manual for physicians and technical personnel*, Philadelphia, 1983, WB Saunders.

Basmajian JV, Slonecker CE: *Grant's method of anatomy*, ed 11, Baltimore, 1989, Williams & Wilkins.

Becker CD, Cooperberg PL: Sonography of the hepatic vascular system, *Am J Radiol* 150:999-1005, 1988.

Bernardino ME: The liver: anatomy and examination techniques. In Tavares JM, Ferruchi IT, editors: *Radiology: diagnosis-imaging-intervention*, vol 4, Philadelphia, 1988, JB Lippincott, pp 1-8.

Bisset RA, Khan AN: *Differential diagnosis in abdominal ultrasound*, London, 1990, Bailliere Tindall.

Bockus HL: *Gastroenterology*, ed 2, vol 3, Philadelphia, 1965, WB Saunders.

Carlsen EN, Filly RA: Newer ultrasonographic anatomy in the upper abdomen. I. The portal and hepatic venous anatomy, *J Clin Ultrasound* 4:85-90, 1976.

Cooperberg PL, Rowley VA: Abdominal sonographic examination technique. In Tavares JM, Ferruchi JT, editors: *Radiology: diagnosis-imaging-intervention*, vol 4, Philadelphia, 1988, JB Lippincott, pp 1-11.

Cosgrove DO, Arger PH, Coleman BG: Ultrasonic anatomy of hepatic veins, *J Clin Ultrasound* 15:231-235, 1987.

Dodds WJ, Erickson SJ, Taylor AJ, et al: Caudate lobe of the liver: anatomy, embryology, and pathology, *AJR Am J Roentgenol* 154:87-93, 1990.

Donoso L, Martinez-Noguera A, Zidan A, et al: Papillary process of the caudate lobe of the liver: sonographic appearance, *Radiology* 173:631-633, 1989.

Haskal, ZJ, Rees CR, Ring EJ, et al: (1997) Reporting Standards for Transjugular Intrahepatic Portosystemic Shunts, Society of Cardiovascular & Interventional Radiology, Technology Assessment Committee. Retrieved October 11, 2001 from the Society of Cardiovascular & Interventional Radiology Web site: HYPERLINK http://www.scvir.org/clinical/T64.htm

Hillman BJ, D'Orsi CJ, Smith EH, et al: Ultrasonic appearance of the falciform ligament, *Am J Radiol* 132:205-206, 1979.

Holt DR, Thiel DV, Edelstein S, et al: Hepatic resections, *Arch Surg* 135(11):1353-1358, 2000.

Kane RA, Lavery M: Techniques of liver examination, *Semin Ultrasound* 2:198-201, 1981.

Kane RA: Sonographic anatomy of the liver, *Semin Ultrasound* 2:190-196, 1981.

Lafortune M, Madore F, Patriquin H, et al: Segmental anatomy of the liver: a sonographic approach to the Couinaud nomenclature, *Radiology* 181:443-448, 1991.

LeMay HE, Beall H, Robblee KM, et al: Chemistry: connections to our changing world, Upper Saddle River, NJ, 1996, Prentice-Hall.

Linder HH: *Clinical anatomy*, Norwalk, CT, 1989, Appleton & Lange.

Marks WM, Filly RA, Callen PW: Ultrasonic anatomy of the liver: a review with new applications, J Clin Ultrasound 7:137-146, 1979.

Mittelstaedt CA: *Abdominal ultrasound*, New York, 1987, Churchill Livingstone.

Miyal K: Structure-function relationship of the liver in health and disease. In Gitnick GL, editor: *Principles and practice of gastroenterology and hepatology*, ed 2, East Norwalk, 1994, Appleton & Lange, pp 679-696.

Moore KL: *The developing human: clinically oriented embryology*, ed 4, Philadelphia, 1988, WB Saunders.

Moore KL, Persaud TVN: *The developing human: clinically oriented embryology*, ed 6, Philadelphia, 1998, WB Saunders.

Netter FH: *The CIBA collection of medical illustrations*, vol 3, The Digestive System. Summit, NJ, 1977, CIBA Pharmaceutical, CIBA-Geigy.

Pagani JJ: Intrahepatic vascular territories shown by computed tomography (CT), *Radiology* 147:173-178, 1983.

Parulekar SG: Ligaments and fissures of the liver: sonographic anatomy, *Radiology* 130:409-411, 1979.

Rubenstein WA, Auh YH, Whalen JP, et al: The perihepatic spaces: computed tomographic and ultrasound imaging, *Radiology* 149:231-239, 1983.

Sarti DA: *Diagnostic ultrasound: text and cases*, ed 2, Chicago, 1987, Year Book.

Sexton CC, Zeman RK: Correlation of computed tomography, sonography, and gross anatomy of the liver, *Am J Radiol* 141:711-718, 1983.

Steen EB, Montagu A: *Anatomy and physiology*, vol 1, ed 2, New York, 1984, Harper & Row.

Strasberg S: Terminology of liver anatomy and liver resections: coming to grips with hepatic babel, *J Am Coll Surg* 184:413-434, 1997.

CHAPTER 10

The Biliary System

VIVIE MILLER AND CANDYCE JAMES

OBJECTIVES ■

Describe the gross anatomy of the biliary system.
Describe the basic function of the biliary system.
Describe the ultrasound appearance of the biliary system.
Describe other imaging modalities that may be used to examine the biliary system.
Define the key words.

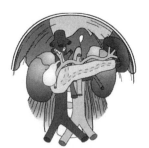

KEY WORDS ■

Ampulla of Vater	Hartmann's pouch
Bilirubin	Hepatic ducts
Cholecystectomy	Hilum/hilus
Cholecystitis	Infundibulum
Cholecystokinin	Intrahepatic
Cholelithiasis	Pancreatic duct
Common bile duct	Polyps
Common hepatic duct	Porta hepatis
Cystic duct	Proper hepatic artery
Extrahepatic	Sludge
Fossa	Sphincter of Oddi
Fundus	Spiral valve of Heister
Gallbladder	

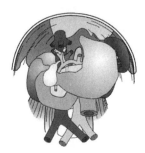

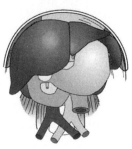

The biliary system is intimately associated with the liver and pancreas. It consists of the **gallbladder,** acting as a reservoir for bile, and the ducts that drain the liver of bile. For our purpose, we will not include the pancreatic ducts as part of the biliary system, although in many people, the two do join to form the ampulla of Vater before opening into the duodenum. The pancreas and associated ducts will be the focus of Chapter 11.

The basic function of the biliary system is to drain the liver of bile and to store the bile until it is needed to aid in the digestive process. As mentioned, the gallblad-

The biliary system and surrounding anatomic layers. See Figure 4-3, **F, G, H,** and **I** for more details.

der acts as the storage receptacle for bile, and the various ducts provide a place to which the bile flows. The gallbladder concentrates the bile by secreting mucus and absorbing water. For a review of bile production, see Chapter 9.

PRENATAL DEVELOPMENT

The liver, gallbladder, bile ducts, and part of the pancreas are formed by a ventral diverticulum, or sac, which turns into the septum transversum. This process begins at approximately 4 weeks or when the embryo is approximately 2.5 mm in length. The gallbladder is present in the fetus and is often noted on sonography. It is nonfunctional until birth.

LOCATION

Gallbladder

A **fossa** (or indentation) is located on the posterior and inferior portion of the right lobe of the liver where the gallbladder is situated. This fossa or bed is closely related to the main lobar fissure of the liver (Figure 10-1). Even though the gallbladder is typically not totally surrounded by hepatic tissue, it is possible for this to occur. An **intrahepatic** gallbladder will be totally (or almost totally) enclosed in liver tissue.

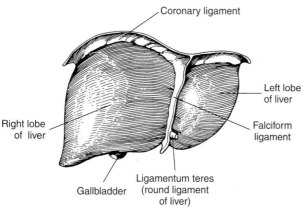

Figure 10-1 Location of gallbladder in relation to anterior view of the liver.

Following the main portal vein as it courses toward the right side of the body will usually reveal the gallbladder to be just inferior to the level of the right portal vein in longitudinal slices. In a transverse cut of the abdomen, finding the portal vein (or portal-splenic confluence) and following it to the right will reveal (in typical order of appearance) the portal vein, head of the pancreas, duodenum, liver, gallbladder, and, again, liver (Figure 10-2). The right kidney may also be typically noted on transverse and longitudinal imaging with the gallbladder immediately anterior.

The gallbladder will change location as the patient changes position. A gallbladder found to be just at the inferior border of the right lobe of the liver with the patient supine may then be found to have shifted closer to the midline when the patient is placed on the left side with the right side raised.

Some imagers believe that by simply bending the right arm 90 degrees at the elbow and then placing that hand over the midline the location of the gallbladder may be estimated. The gallbladder will probably be near the area of the wrist. This method is not particularly accurate, but it does give a rough idea of the location of the gallbladder.

Hepatic Ducts

Bile from the liver reaches the gallbladder through the hepatic and cystic ducts. The left and right **hepatic ducts** join at approximately the level of the liver **hilum** (also called the **porta hepatis** or doorway) to form the **common hepatic duct** (CHD). The CHD will eventually become the **common bile duct** (CBD), entering the duodenum near the head of the pancreas (Figure 10-3).

The right and left hepatic ducts are considered intrahepatic because they are completely enclosed by liver

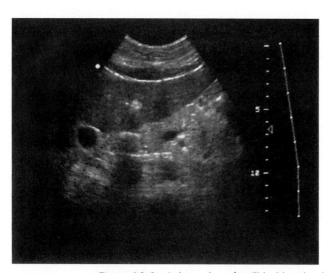

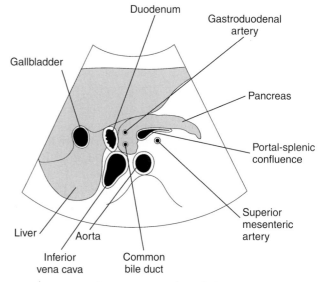

Figure 10-2 Relationship of gallbladder, duodenum, and pancreas. A transverse cut through the abdomen may reveal the above relationship. Note that the gallbladder is just lateral to the duodenum, which is just lateral to the head of the pancreas.

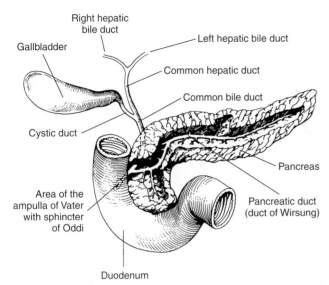

Figure 10-3 The biliary system, including the pancreas and pancreatic duct.

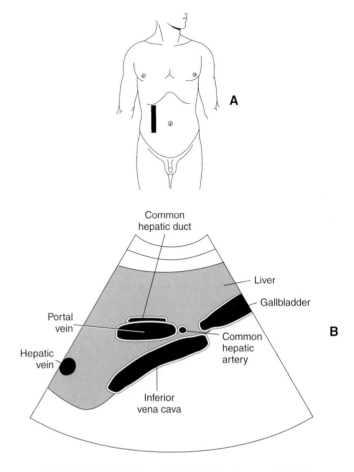

tissue. On longitudinal cuts of the cadaver abdomen, the CHD will most likely be located just anterior to the right portal vein (Figure 10-4). It is often mistaken for the CBD, which is generally more closely associated with the main portal vein than the right branch. However, there are always variations, so it is possible to see the CBD and the right portal vein at the same time. To make matters more interesting, the cystic artery is also located near the portal veins and may appear as a bile duct. Careful examination should reveal that the bile duct is usually more lateral to the portal vein, whereas the cystic artery is usually more medial.

Cystic Duct

The **cystic duct** connects the gallbladder to the CHD. Bile flowing from the liver via the hepatic ducts must pass through the cystic duct to finally reach the gallbladder. It is sometimes difficult to distinguish a short cystic duct from the neck of the gallbladder. Once the cystic duct joins the CHD at approximately the level of the gallbladder, the CHD is then called the CBD.

Common Bile Duct

The common bile duct extends from the point where the cystic duct joins the CHD all the way to the duodenum. It has a close association with the main portal vein and is usually located slightly lateral and anterior to the main portal vein. The hepatic artery is usually found medial and also slightly anterior to the main portal vein. The portal vein, CBD, and hepatic artery form the portal triad, which has become known as Mickey's sign when viewed in a transverse section. The portal vein is the "face" of the famous mouse, whereas the hepatic artery forms the left "ear" and the CBD forms the right "ear" (Figure 10-5).

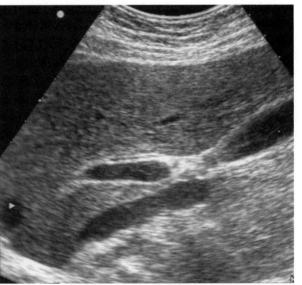

Figure 10-4 Common hepatic duct and portal vein relationship. Longitudinal diagram demonstrates the relationship between the right portal vein, common hepatic duct, and the gallbladder. The common hepatic duct is often mislabeled as the common bile duct, which is located more inferiorly and is more closely associated with the main portal vein. **A,** Position of transducer on patient. **B,** Diagram of relationship. **C,** Sonogram of common hepatic duct (cursor "+").

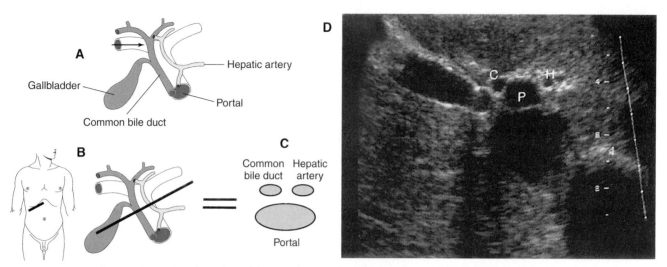

Figure 10-5 A, Relationship of the portal vein to the hepatic artery and common bile duct. Note that the common hepatic duct is just anterior to the right portal vein *(arrow)*. **B,** Taking an image at approximately the angle of the solid line (approximately the same as the right costal margin angle) may produce the relationship demonstrated in **C.** The common bile duct and the hepatic artery have approximately equal diameter. **D,** Sonogram of Mickey's sign. *P,* Portal vein; *H,* hepatic artery; *C,* common bile duct.

When referring specifically to the CBD, anatomists use terms that relate its position to the duodenum. The part of the CBD superior to the duodenum is the supraduodenal section. As the names imply, the portion posterior to the duodenum is the retroduodenal section; the infraduodenal portion is inferior to the duodenum; and the part of the CBD within the duodenum is the intraduodenal portion (Figure 10-6). The infraduodenal portion of the CBD may lie within a groove on the head of the pancreas or may travel through an opening in the head. It continues on to enter the duodenum at the **ampulla of Vater,** sometimes called the hepatopancreatic ampulla. A muscle sheath, known as the **sphincter of Oddi** or Oddi's muscle, surrounds the CBD (joined at times by the **pancreatic duct**) at the ampulla of Vater. The sphincter of Oddi aids in regulating bile flow into the duodenum.

SIZE
Gallbladder
The overall length of the normal gallbladder is highly variable, depending on the amount of bile within and the normal variants. There are times when the gallbladder is simply difficult to see, not because of some structural variation, but because of physiology. As an example, a patient who has fasted since midnight before an ultrasound examination may present with a full, easily visualized gallbladder. A patient who has eaten, smoked, chewed gum, or had coffee with cream and sugar (to name just a few examples) may present with a small gallbladder or may even appear, at first, to completely lack a gallbladder. However, when the gallbladder is visualized, it is found to have a length of approximately 8 to 9 cm in many patients, as measured from the neck to the fundus. It is approximately 3 cm in diameter and holds up to approximately 40 ml of fluid. To put this amount in perspective, a teaspoon typically holds approximately 5 ml of fluid; therefore the gallbladder holds approximately 8 teaspoons of fluid. Recall that 2.5 cm equals 1 inch; this provides a better picture of the sizes involved when visualizing the biliary system. With experience, the sonographer discovers that the gallbladder has a wide variety of shapes, sizes, and locations.

Common Hepatic Duct
The length and inside diameter of the CHD are variable. Schwartz reports a CHD length of 3 to 4 cm. A fairly widely accepted upper limit for the inner diameter of the CHD is 4 mm. Cosgrove has reported the diameter to range from approximately 1 to 7 mm in the normal patient, depending on age, previous surgery, and gallbladder function or disease. It is typical for an individual sonographic practice to set an acceptable upper limit on duct size based on criteria used by referring physicians, especially surgeons.

Cystic Duct
The diameter of the cystic duct is approximately 3 mm. The length is highly variable, ranging from 1.0 to 3.5 cm. An average length of 4 cm has been reported at surgery. The apparent large difference in these figures is common and holds little significance on sonography.

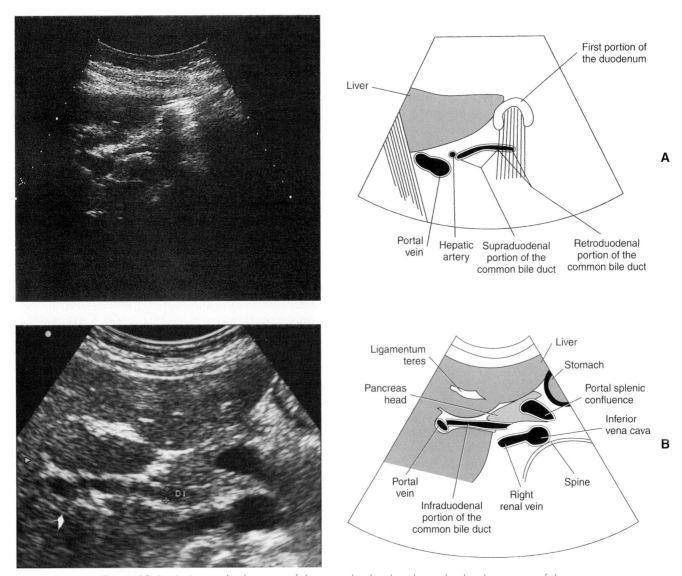

Figure 10-6 **A,** Longitudinal section of the supraduodenal and retroduodenal segments of the common bile duct. **B,** Longitudinal section of the infraduodenal segment of the common bile duct.

Common Bile Duct

The length of the CBD is also highly variable, determined by the junction of the cystic duct and the CHD. A range in length of 8 to 11.5 cm has been suggested. The diameter has been reported to be 1 to 7 mm in the normal patient and up to 10 mm in a patient after **cholecystectomy** (surgical removal of the gallbladder). As before, individual practices will set an upper limit that is appropriate to their particular patient population.

GROSS ANATOMY
Gallbladder

The gallbladder is perfused by the hepatic artery, which is a branch of the celiac trunk, off of the abdominal aorta. The hepatic artery, or common hepatic artery as it

is called, divides into the proper hepatic and gastroduodenal arteries. The **proper hepatic artery** supplies the gallbladder and the liver. The cystic artery usually originates from the right branch of the proper hepatic artery. It passes posterior to the CHD and anterior to the cystic duct, to the superior portion of the neck of the gallbladder. Here it travels inferiorly and divides into superficial and deep branches. The cystic artery may sometimes originate directly from the common hepatic artery and rarely from the gastroduodenal artery.

Venous drainage of the gallbladder is by way of the hepatic portal system. This system includes all the veins draining the gastrointestinal tract, including the spleen, pancreas, and gallbladder. Blood is conveyed from these organs via the portal vein to the liver. The portal vein subdivides until the blood reaches the hepatic sinusoids. Blood therefore passes through two sets of "exchange" vessels: the capillaries within the organs of the gastrointestinal tract, the spleen, pancreas, and gallbladder, and the hepatic sinusoids. From the sinusoids, blood converges into hepatic veins and finally the inferior vena cava (IVC) before returning to the heart. The gallbladder is drained by tributaries of the hepatic portal venous system, which carry blood to the IVC. Portal circulatory route is the term used to describe venous blood that passes through two capillary exchange systems before reaching the heart. Portal comes from the Latin word *porta* and means gateway. The portal vein is the gateway for blood returning from the gastrointestinal tract and accessory organs to pass before the blood returns to the heart.

The normal gallbladder appears a bit like a partially filled water balloon because it is slightly more oval than round. A gallbladder that appears round (spherical) may indicate the presence of disease, especially those conditions that cause obstruction of the lower portion of the biliary system. The shape of the gallbladder has also been likened to that of a pear, which has a narrow "neck" and a round "bottom." The walls are generally only a few millimeters thick, up to approximately 3 mm. This wall thickness is important to note. Certain conditions, such as **cholecystitis** (inflammation of the gallbladder), may cause the walls to appear edematous and perhaps even greatly thickened. Localized thickening of the gallbladder wall may indicate the presence of a mass or other condition that would call for further investigation. As would be expected, the wall thickness is slightly less when the gallbladder is full (the walls are stretched) as compared with an empty gallbladder, when the walls are slightly thicker.

There are three distinct layers to the gallbladder wall. The inner layer is the mucosa; the middle is the fibro-muscular layer; and the outer is the serous layer. Inside the gallbladder are many minute inward folds or rugae. These folds aid in concentrating the bile through absorption of water and secretion of mucus.

The gallbladder may be divided into three major sections: fundus, body, and neck. The **fundus** is the "bottom" of the pouch (Figure 10-7). It is important to notice the location of the fundus in relation to gravity. Gallstones and **sludge** (thick bile) may find their way to the fundus, but only if the fundus is the portion of the gallbladder closest to gravity. The exception, of course, is "floating" stones. The part of the gallbladder that is closest to gravity is called the dependent portion. The dependent portion will change with a change in the position of the patient.

The middle and main portion of the gallbladder is called the body, whereas the more narrow area leading into the cystic duct is called the neck (Figure 10-8). A small sacculation (outpouching) may be seen in some patients in the area of the gallbladder neck. This has been called **Hartmann's pouch** after Henri Hartmann, a French surgeon who lived from 1860 to 1952. The term **infundibulum** is also applied to this dilatation of the gallbladder neck area. Some consider this sacculation an abnormality, whereas others consider it an oddity. It must be carefully screened to detect coexisting abnormalities, such as **cholelithiasis** (gallstones) (Figure 10-9).

Hepatic Ducts

The intrahepatic bile ducts run alongside portal veins and hepatic arteries in portal triads, surrounded by connective tissue and radiating through the lobes and segments of the liver. The intrahepatic ducts join to form the right and left main hepatic ducts, and, as previously mentioned, the right and left main hepatic ducts join at approximately the level of the porta hepatis to form the CHD.

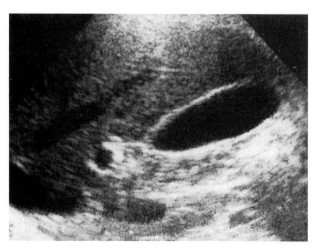

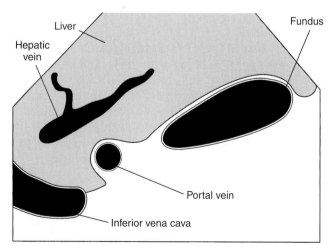

Figure 10-7   Longitudinal section of the gallbladder fundus.

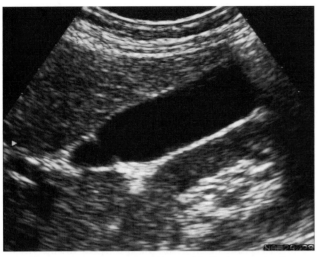

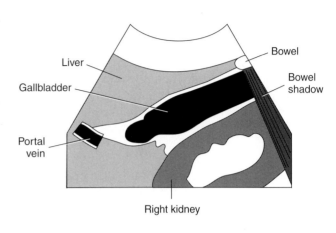

Figure 10-8 Longitudinal section of the gallbladder neck and body.

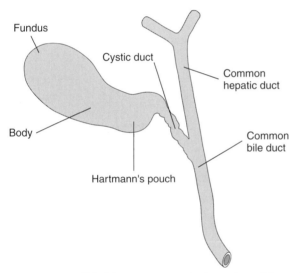

Figure 10-9 Gallbladder anatomy and relationship of the gall-bladder to the ductal system. Also note Hartmann's pouch, a di-latation located in the neck of the gallbladder. This slight saccu-lation is also known as the infundibulum and is considered by some as merely an oddity, although others believe it is a possi-ble abnormality. In either case, it should be examined carefully for related disease, such as gallstones.

Cystic Duct

The cystic duct connects the gallbladder to the CHD; where the cystic duct and CHD join, they form the CBD. The lumen of the cystic duct contains a series of mu-cosal folds, the spiral valves of Heister. Even though it is common to call this area of folds a valve, it is mis-named. There does not seem to be any valve or flow control action; bile flows freely in both directions through the cystic duct. Pressure differences in the bil-iary system along with the stimulated contraction of the gallbladder seem to govern the flow of bile, and the **spi-**

ral valves of Heister prevent the cystic duct from overdistending or collapsing.

Common Bile Duct

Formed by the junction of the cystic duct and CHD, the CBD courses inferiorly along the right border of the lesser omentum, then along the hepatoduodenal liga-ment and posterior to the first part of the duodenum, passing on or through the head of the pancreas just an-terior to the IVC. The duct terminates at the posterome-dial aspect of the descending portion of the duodenum. The CBD, the cystic duct, and part of the CHD are **ex-trahepatic** (not enclosed by liver tissue) ducts. They are lined with subepithelial connective tissue and some smooth muscle fibers.

PHYSIOLOGY

Bile is produced by the liver and carried to the gastroin-testinal system by the biliary ducts. The sphincter of Oddi, located in the duodenum, regulates the passage of bile into the duodenum and at the same time prevents re-flux of gastrointestinal fluids into the biliary system. When closed, the sphincter of Oddi forces the gallblad-der to fill with bile. When fats and amino acids are in-gested, the duodenal mucosa releases **cholecystokinin** (CCK), a peptide hormone. CCK stimulates the gallblad-der to contract and the sphincter of Oddi to relax, and in-creases hepatic production of bile. An injectable form of CCK has been used to stimulate the gallbladder during sonographic examination for a type of function test.

The gallbladder is actually more than just a storage area for bile. Related blood vessels and lymphatics con-centrate the stored bile through absorption of water and inorganic salts. Bile in the gallbladder is much more concentrated than hepatic bile. Bile is composed mostly of water (82%) and bile acids (12%). The remaining constituents include cholesterol, **bilirubin** (bile pigment), proteins, electrolytes, and mucus.

SONOGRAPHIC APPEARANCE

Much of the biliary system is readily appreciated on sonography. It is especially common for the gallbladder, CHD, and CBD to be imaged. In the absence of disease, the other portions of the biliary system may prove difficult to appreciate because they are small.

Gallbladder

The sonographic appearance of the gallbladder is that of an anechoic or nearly anechoic pear-shaped structure in the right upper quadrant of the abdomen (Figure 10-10). As mentioned, there is wide variation in shape and size of the gallbladder. The walls tend to be well defined, regular, and echodense, especially when the gallbladder is distended. In the "empty" gallbladder, the walls are thicker and may appear more irregu-lar, with the central portion containing a few random echoes (Figure 10-11). The wall thickness is usually 3 mm or less and may be difficult to measure when the gallbladder is in its partially distended, normal state. Inadequate examination may lead to a false diagnosis of thickened walls or cholelithiasis. The nature of ultrasound tends to obscure one or both of the leading edges of the anterior (or proximal) wall of the gallbladder, making it difficult to determine where to place the measurement cursors.

The fundus may be difficult to visualize because of the close relationship of the gallbladder to the bowel. The bowel often creates a shadow that partially obscures the fundus. Changing patient position or angling the transducer may be necessary to examine the entire gallbladder. Floating stones, **polyps** (protruding masses from the inner wall of the gallbladder), and other masses may be present in the fundus of the gallbladder and easily missed on casual examination.

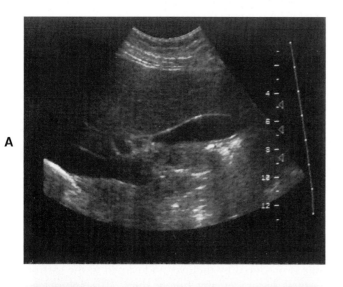

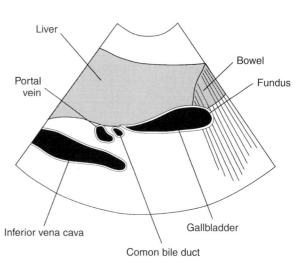

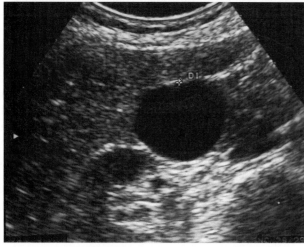

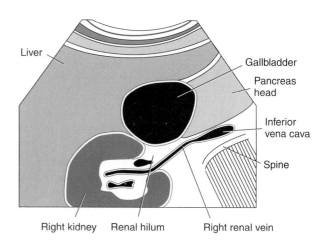

Figure 10-10 **A,** Longitudinal section of the gallbladder. Note that the fundus is partially obscured by bowel. **B,** Transverse section of the gallbladder. Note the posterior right kidney.

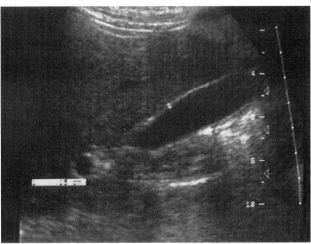

Figure 10-11 *Gallbladder wall thickness. The thickness of the gallbladder wall is usually less than 3 mm and should be noted on each study. Cholecystitis and carcinoma are just two examples of pathologic states that may alter the thickness and appearance of the gallbladder wall. Care must be taken not to falsely thicken the walls through too high gain or power settings.*

Three landmarks may be helpful in locating the gallbladder on longitudinal imaging: the portal vein, the main lobar fissure, and the right kidney. The main lobar fissure may also be demonstrated just at the level of the gallbladder because it helps to form the "bed" in which the gallbladder lies. The main lobar fissure is considerably more difficult to consistently appreciate than the portal vein, but it is of value. Moreover, the portal vein must be located in a longitudinal sonogram to measure the CHD (Figure 10-12). Some sonographers locate the right kidney as an aid in locating the gallbladder. In most patients, the gallbladder fundus is anterior to the superior pole of the right kidney.

An additional landmark for the gallbladder is the duodenum. In a transverse image taken at the level of the head of the pancreas, on a single plane drawn from midline to the right, the portal-splenic confluence, the head of the pancreas, the duodenum, probably a portion of the liver, and then the gallbladder are seen (see Figure 10-2). This common relationship is important because each anechoic structure can be eliminated as a possible gallbladder while scanning. The IVC is just posterior to the head of the pancreas and may be mistaken for an extremely posteriorly lying gallbladder. Additionally, the appearance of the duodenum changes depending on when and how much fluid the patient has ingested. Reference to all the landmarks will make locating the gallbladder easier.

At times, regardless of technique, the gallbladder simply will not be visualized. Nonvisualization may occur for a number of reasons. If the gallbladder fails to develop (agenesis), there will be nothing to image. This

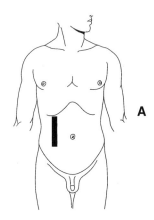
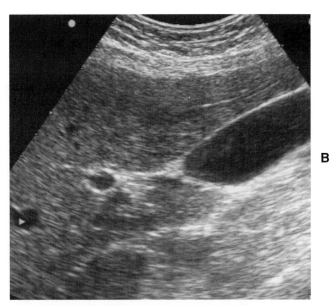
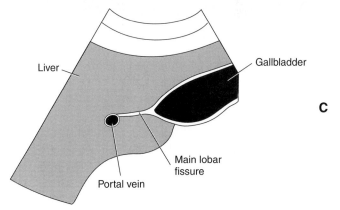

Figure 10-12 *Relationship of the gallbladder to the main lobar fissure of the liver.* **A,** *Transducer position on patient.* **B,** *Longitudinal sonogram of main lobar fissure and gallbladder.* **C,** *Diagram of main lobar fissure and gallbladder.*

cause of nonvisualization is rare, however. A small tube-like (vermiform or wormlike) gallbladder may appear as a bile duct and be missed on sonography. As has been noted, an empty gallbladder may be small and can be overlooked.

Shadows and other minor distortions related to the edge of the gallbladder walls and distal to the spiral valves of Heister are common. High-frequency sound produces a particularly striking shadow from these areas because it is more easily reflected than the lower frequencies (Figure 10-13). Each shadow must be explored to determine whether it is natural or associated with disease. An acoustic shadow should be followed to its origin to learn whether it begins slightly more anteriorly and interrupts the representation of the wall. If it interrupts the wall, the shadow may indicate abnormal anatomy and deserves further study.

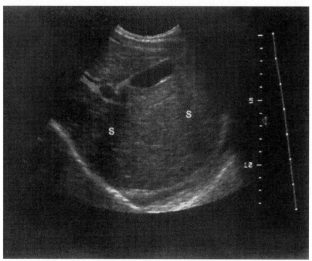

Figure 10-13 Normal wall shadowing from the gallbladder. With higher frequency transducers it is common to find some shadowing ("S") from the walls of the gallbladder and the area of the spiral valve of Heister.

Ductal System

In the normal patient, bile ducts other than the common ducts are small and usually not appreciated. The CHD and CBDs are larger in diameter and can be seen associated with the portal venous system. The CHD is usually located anterior to the right portal vein, and on a longitudinal sonogram it may be noted as two echogenic short parallel lines separated by just 1 mm or so of anechoic space (see Figure 10-4). The gallbladder is usually nearby, as is the main lobar fissure.

As noted, the CBD may be observed as part of Mickey's sign when traversed. On scans taken at a transverse oblique angle, it appears as a small round anechoic structure just anterior and slightly lateral on the right of the main portal vein. A perfectly round, ane-

choic duct structure will not be visualized consistently. Cutting the duct at an angle other than perfectly transverse may produce an oval structure (see Figure 10-5).

SONOGRAPHIC APPLICATIONS

For most patients sonography is the method of choice for examining the biliary system. Some specific applications of sonographic examination of the biliary system include:

Measuring the CHD
Measuring the CBD
Measuring the general volume of the gallbladder
Assessing the gallbladder and adjacent liver masses
Assessing possible obstruction of the biliary ductal system
Presence of stones in the gallbladder (cholelithiasis)
Presence of stones in the ductal system (choledocholithiasis)
Ruling out masses, including cysts, associated with the biliary system
Postsurgical follow-up evaluation (i.e., cholecystectomy)

NORMAL VARIANTS

The biliary system may not develop normally, and deviation can occur. Deviations are of special interest to the sonographer because they may challenge adequate examination. For example, what appears to be a septated gallbladder (a gallbladder with divisions or septations) may simply be one folded onto itself. If the patient's position is changed, the gallbladder may unfold to reveal no septation (Figure 10-14). Other variations may be considered pathologic or may contribute to the development of disease. For instance, a gallbladder attached to the liver by a particularly long mesentery can mimic a "floating" gallbladder that is prone to torsion (twisting) as opposed to a gallbladder that is partially embedded in liver tissue.

Gallbladder

Congenital abnormalities of the gallbladder are relatively common. In addition to the floating gallbladder, there may be hypoplasia (underdevelopment) or agenesis (complete failure of the gallbladder to develop). Both of these conditions are relatively rare but must be ruled out as possible reasons for nonvisualization on sonography and other imaging modalities. At the opposite end of the scale is duplication of the gallbladder, with or without duplication of the cystic duct.

More common are variations in gallbladder shape. It may be bilobed (hourglass), septated, or folded into any of several shapes. Septations tend to be associated with gallstone formation resulting from the stasis of gallbladder contents. Septations may make it difficult to identify cholelithiasis. The most common variation in gallbladder shape is that of a Phrygian cap. In this case,

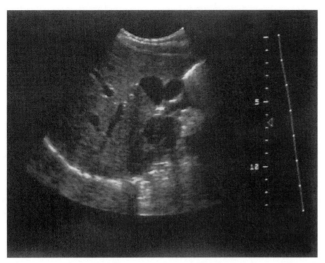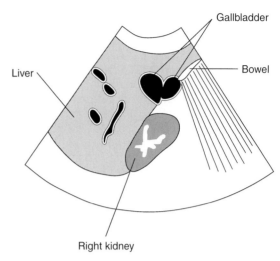

Figure 10-14 False appearance of a gallbladder variation. In this longitudinal section, it appears that a septation is present in the gallbladder. However, when the patient's position was changed, the gallbladder was observed folded onto itself. It is imperative that the patient be placed in at least two different positions during sonographic examination.

the gallbladder is partially folded onto itself, so that it appears similar to the Phrygian cap worn by the early Roman freed slaves and later by French revolutionaries as a symbol of liberty (Figure 10-15).

Biliary Ducts

Variations in the extrahepatic biliary ducts are common and may appear in almost any combination. As an example, the cystic duct may join the CHD at almost any point from the porta hepatis to the duodenum. With a low juncture, the cystic duct may run parallel to the CHD for some distance. Accessory hepatic ducts are also fairly common and on sonographic examination may present as an "extra" tubular structure. Such variations should not be an obstacle, although they may make it more difficult to identify every structure on the imaging screen.

A more easily recognized variation is the choledochal (or choledochus) cyst. Of the three types—congenital

cystic dilation, intraduodenal (choledochocele), and congenital diverticulum—the first is the most common. A choledochal cyst is a localized dilatation of the CBD. When caused by a congenital diverticulum, it may appear as a separate or loosely connected structure to the CBD. The choledochocele (or intraduodenal) is formed by a section of the CBD that has entered the duodenum and enlarged. This is similar to the process involved in the formation of a ureterocele.

Biliary atresia (congenital closure) may be diffuse or focal in the extrahepatic ducts, or intrahepatic. Diffuse extrahepatic biliary atresia is the most common.

REFERENCE CHARTS

■ ■ ■ ASSOCIATED PHYSICIANS

Surgeon: Involved in the diagnosis of biliary disease as well as surgical intervention.
Internist: Involved in the diagnosis and medical treatment of biliary disease.
Radiologist: Performs and interprets the various imaging tests used to diagnose biliary disease.

■ ■ ■ COMMON DIAGNOSTIC TESTS

Oral Cholecystogram (OCG): A contrast material (dye) is ingested by the patient the night before the test. Information on structure and function of the gallbladder is obtained. This test is performed by a radiologist assisted by a radiologic technologist, and is interpreted by the radiologist.
Nuclear Medicine (HIDA Scan): A minute amount of a radiopharmaceutical is injected. It passes through the bloodstream to the liver, then to the biliary system and eventually

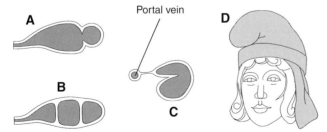

Figure 10-15 Typical gallbladder variations. Some possible shapes of the gallbladder: **A,** Bilobed gallbladder. **B,** True septated gallbladder. **C,** Gallbladder folded onto itself in what has been called the Phrygian gallbladder. **D,** One possible shape of an early Phrygian cap. This cap was worn by the early Roman freed slaves and later by French revolutionaries as a symbol of liberty.

into the duodenum. Functional information is the primary focus of this test, and some structural information is also obtained. This test is performed by a nuclear medicine technologist and interpreted by the radiologist.

Computed Axial Tomography (CT Scan): A radiologic examination in which cross-sectional x-ray images of the biliary system and other abdominal structures are obtained. A contrast medium may be administered to differentiate between disease and normal anatomy. Structural information is the primary focus of this test, but some functional information may be obtained. It is performed by a radiologic technologist and is interpreted by the radiologist.

Cholangiography: A contrast material is injected into the biliary system either by catheter (i.e., T-tube cholangiogram) or by needle (transhepatic cholangiogram) under radiographic guidance. This yields structural information about the entire biliary system, especially about obstruction. It may be performed before, during, or after surgery. Surgeons, surgical assistants, radiologists, and radiologic technologists are involved in the procedure, and it is interpreted by the radiologist.

Endoscopic Retrograde Cholangiopancreatography (ERCP): In this endoscopic, radiographically guided examination, the ampulla of Vater is cannulized through a tube inserted into the patient's upper gastrointestinal tract. Contrast material is then injected to fill and delineate the pancreatic and bile ducts. Information on obstructive processes is the objective. This type of endoscopy is usually performed by the gastroenterologist assisted by the radiologist. The gastroenterologist interprets the endoscopic results and the radiologist interprets the radiologic findings.

■ ■ ■ LABORATORY VALUES

Serum Bilirubin: Adult: direct (conjugated): <0.5 mg/dl
indirect (unconjugated): ≤1.1 mg/dl
urine: negative
Infant: total: 1 to 12 mg/dl
Urobilinogen: Fecal: 50 to 300 mg/24 hours
Urine: Men: 0.3 to 2.1 Ehrlich units/2 hours
Women: 0.1 to 1.1 Ehrlich units/2 hours[19]

■ ■ ■ NORMAL MEASUREMENTS

Gallbladder (note that the shape of the gallbladder may be more important):
Length: 8 to 9 cm as measured from the neck to the fundus of a completely bile-filled gallbladder.
Diameter: about 3 cm
Common hepatic duct:
Length: highly variable
Diameter: 1 to 4 mm, in some normal persons up to 7 mm
Cystic duct:
Length: 1 to 3.5 cm
Diameter: up to 3 mm
Common bile duct:
Length: variable
Diameter: 1 to 7 mm, up to 10 mm postcholecystectomy

■ ■ ■ VASCULATURE

Common hepatic artery
—Proper hepatic artery
—Cystic artery
—Gallbladder
Gallbladder
—Cystic veins
—Hepatic veins
—IVC

■ ■ ■ AFFECTING CHEMICALS

Nonapplicable.

BIBLIOGRAPHY

Bisset RAL, Khan AN: *Differential diagnosis in abdominal ultrasound,* London, 1990, Bailliere Tindall, pp 58, 63, 65-66.

Cohen L, Atwood R, Newelt M: Ultrasound of the normal fetal chest, abdomen, and pelvis, *Obstet Gynecol* 1(1):240, 1991.

Cosgrove DO, McCready VR: *Ultrasound imaging: liver-spleen-pancreas,* New York, 1982, Wiley, pp 226-227.

Dorland WA: *Dorland's illustrated medical dictionary,* ed 29, Philadelphia, 2000, WB Saunders, p 787.

Ford RD, editor: *Diagnostic tests handbook,* Springhouse, PA, 1987, Springhouse, pp 61, 217-219, 673.

Gray H: *Anatomy, descriptive and surgical,* 1901 ed, Philadelphia, 1974, Running Press, p 942.

Hagen-Ansert S: *Textbook of diagnostic ultrasonography,* ed 5, St Louis, 2001, Mosby.

Harrison M: *The history of the hat,* London, 1960, William Oowes, p 22.

Kawamura DM: *Diagnostic medical sonography,* vol III, Philadelphia, 1992, JB Lippincott.

McPhee MS, Greenberger NJ: Diseases of the gallbladder and bile ducts. In Harrison TR, editor: *Principles of internal medicine,* New York, 1987, McGraw-Hill, pp 1358-1359.

Mittelstaedt C: *Abdominal ultrasound,* New York, 1989, Churchill Livingstone, pp 86-87.

Netter F: *Digestive system. The CIBA collection of medical illustrations,* Summit, NJ, 1975, CIBA Pharmaceutical, CIBA-Geigy, pp 3(111):22-23, 123.

Picken M: *The fashion dictionary,* New York, 1957, Funk and Wagnalls, pp 49-50.

Price S, Wilson LM: *Pathophysiology,* ed 3, New York, 1986, McGraw-Hill, p 299.

Romanes GJ: *Cunningham's textbook of anatomy,* ed 11, London, 1972, Oxford University Press, pp 61, 459-460.

Schoenfield U: Gallstones and other biliary diseases, *Clinical Symposia* CI8A, (34,4):32, 1982.

Schwartz SI: Gallbladder and extrahepatic biliary system. In *Principles of surgery,* ed 5, New York, 1989, McGraw-Hill, pp 1381-1382.

Thibodeau GA, Patton KT: *Anatomy and physiology,* ed 4, St Louis, 1999, Mosby, p 576.

Wilcox RT: *The mode in hats and headdress,* New York, 1945, Scribner's, pp 6-15.

Williams PL: *Gray's anatomy,* ed 38, New York, 1995, Churchill Livingstone.

Wilson SA, Gosnick BB, vanSonnenberg E: Unchanged size of dilated common bile duct after a fatty meal: results and significance, *Radiology* 160:29-31, 1986.

CHAPTER 11

The Pancreas

REVA ARNEZ CURRY, BETTY BATES TEMPKIN, VIVIE MILLER, AND CANDYCE JAMES

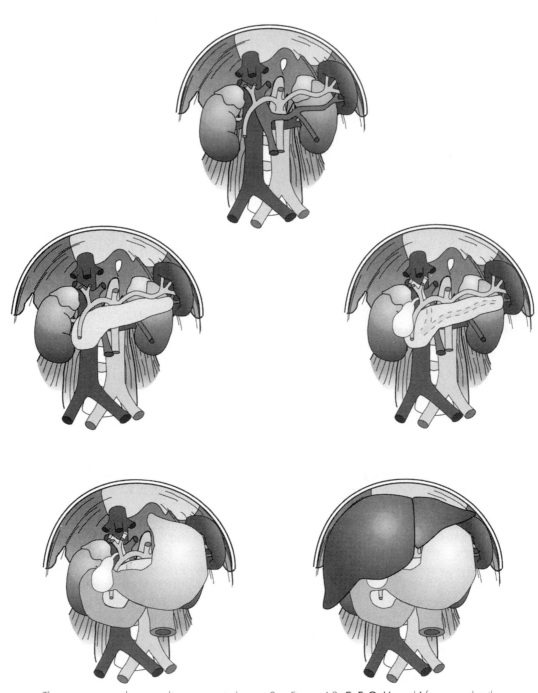

The pancreas and surrounding anatomic layers. See Figure 4-3, **E, F, G, H,** and **I** for more details.

The pancreas has been and continues to be a most interesting challenge to image using sonography. Its close relationship to the stomach, duodenum and proximal jejunum of the small intestine, transverse colon of the large intestine, and their contents may affect sound beam transmission and obscure pancreatic structures. This is especially true for patients who have been poorly prepped. Despite these obstacles, sonography has become useful for the evaluation and early detection of diseases of the pancreas.

PRENATAL DEVELOPMENT

The pancreas gland is formed from ventral and dorsal diverticula of the primitive foregut. The diverticula rotate and fuse, with the ventral portion forming most of the head of the pancreas and the dorsal portion forming the entire body and tail. The ductal system drains into the dorsal duct, the duct of Wirsung, which empties into the duodenum or common bile duct. The ventral duct, the duct of Santorini, is an accessory duct, which is small and sometimes absent. It enters the duodenum separately from Wirsung's duct.

LOCATION

When describing the location of the pancreas, we move from the head on the right, through the neck and body, to the tail on the left. The pancreas is situated in the epigastrium and left hypochondrium. Position of the gland is variable, but usually it lies at the level of the first or second lumbar vertebra, extending from the C-loop of the duodenum to the splenic hilum. It lies horizontally across the aorta and is shaped like an upside down U—the ends of the U appear to have been pulled outward. The shape of the pancreas has also been described as dumbbell, tadpole, sausage, and comma-shaped with the head being the larger portion. Most of the pancreas is retroperitoneal; however, a small portion of the head is surrounded by peritoneum. Behind the pancreas are connective prevertebral tissue, the inferior vena cava, aorta, and diaphragm. Anterior to the pancreas are the stomach and transverse colon. The pancreas is closely related to the biliary tree and the portal venous system. The main pancreatic duct usually joins the common bile duct before both vessels enter the duodenum (Figure 11-1). (For a description of the biliary tree, see Chapter 10.) The **portal splenic confluence** is the area where the splenic vein meets the superior mesenteric vein (Figure 11-2). Together, posterior to the neck of the pancreas, these veins form the portal vein. The inferior mesenteric vein also drains into the splenic vein before the latter receives the superior mesenteric vein. Understanding surrounding vessel anatomy is essential to locating the pancreas.

SIZE

The length of the pancreas ranges between 12 and 18 cm. It is approximately 2.5 cm thick, 3 to 5 cm wide, and weighs between 60 and 80 g. It is important to note the overall contour of the gland along with its size. Is the contour smooth, well defined, and without localized enlargement that appears to be out of place compared with the rest of the gland? This is important because a portion of the gland may be enlarged yet fall within normal limits. Therefore an assessment of glandular contour is essential when evaluating size.

Anterior posterior measurements of the head, neck, body, and tail vary widely. The head ranges between 2 and 3 cm, although some as long as 4 cm have been noted. Some question whether the uncinate process (a medial extension of the head) may contribute to these wide ranges. The size of the neck is between 1.5 and 2.5 cm; the body is between 2 and 3 cm; and the tail is between 1 and 2 cm. According to one reference, the "top

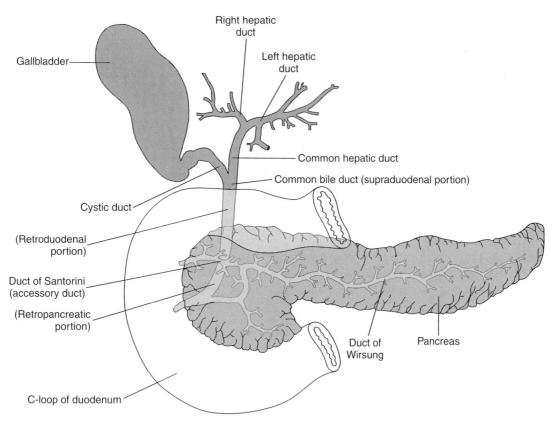

Figure 11-1 Relationship of the pancreas, duodenum, and biliary system. Note that the head of the pancreas is partially surrounded by the C-loop of the duodenum. The union of the main pancreatic duct and distal common bile duct is shown.

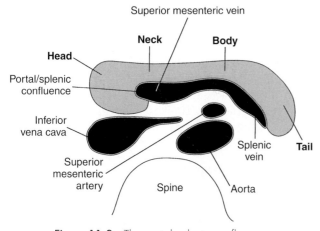

Figure 11-2 The portal splenic confluence.

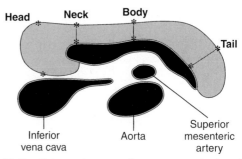

Figure 11-3 Caliper placement for measuring the head, neck, body, and tail of the pancreas.

GROSS ANATOMY

As previously mentioned, the pancreas is 12 to 18 cm long, and although it is not actually segmented, it is described in segments: the head, neck, body, and tail.

Head

The **head** of the pancreas lies to the right of the superior mesenteric vein, cradled in the C-loop of the duodenum, anterior to the inferior vena cava. Two vessels may be identified in the head of the pancreas: the **common bile duct** in the posterolateral portion, and the more

normal" measurements for the adult pancreas were 3 cm for the head, 1 cm for the neck, 2.2 cm for the body, and 2.8 cm for the tail. Figure 11-3 shows caliper placement to measure the segments of the pancreas. Note the use of the epigastric vessels as landmarks. The splenic vein should be seen in its entirety to accurately measure the tail. As with many abdominal organs, the size of the pancreas gland normally decreases with age.

anterolateral **gastroduodenal artery.** The common bile duct courses inferomedially, running behind the first part of the duodenum on its way to the head of the pancreas. It either passes through the pancreatic head or runs along a groove on its posterior surface to meet with the main pancreatic duct. Joined together or separately, the ducts enter the duodenum at the ampulla of Vater (see Figure 11-1). The gastroduodenal artery is the first branch of the common hepatic artery, which originates from the celiac axis. It courses along the anterior aspect of the head just to the right of the neck, where it divides into the anterior and posterior superior pancreatico-duodenal branches. It supplies blood to the head of the pancreas and the duodenum (Figure 11-4). The **uncinate process** is a posteromedial projection of the head that lies directly posterior to the superior mesenteric vein. One way to visualize this area is to draw an imaginary line from the middle of the portal splenic confluence to the middle of the inferior vena cava on a transverse scan (longitudinal view) of the pancreas. The tissue located to the right of the imaginary line is most likely the uncinate process (Figure 11-5). Variable in size, it can extend as far left as the aorta and superior mesenteric artery.

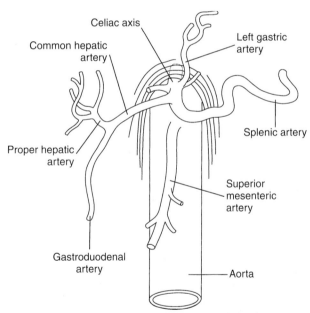

Figure 11-4 Celiac axis and branches. Note the gastroduodenal artery, the first branch of the proper hepatic artery.

Neck

The **neck** of the pancreas is found immediately anterior to the superior mesenteric vein. Slightly superior to that level, the neck lies anterior to the portal splenic confluence. One part of the confluence, the **splenic vein,** carries blood from the splenic hilum along the posterior aspect of the pancreas, whereas the second part of the confluence, the **superior mesenteric vein,** drains the small bowel and proximal colon as it runs posterior to

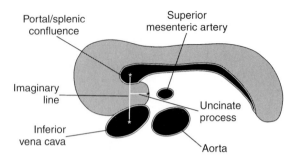

Figure 11-5 Transverse section showing a line drawn from the middle of the portal splenic confluence to the middle of the inferior vena cava to locate the uncinate process.

the lower pancreas neck and anterior to the uncinate. Both veins meet at the confluence to form the **portal vein.** Structurally, the neck is located between the pancreatic head and body. Some sonographers do not consider the neck to be an individual structure but rather include it as part of either the head or the body.

Body

The **body** of the pancreas lies anterior to the aorta, superior mesenteric artery, and splenic vein. The splenic vein runs along the posterior superior surface of the body and tail, closely following the shape of the gland (see Figure 11-2). The pancreas body is bordered on the right by the neck, on the left by the tail (but exactly where is not definite), and anteriorly by the posterior wall of the stomach. Although its anteroposterior dimension is small, the body is considered the largest portion of the pancreas.

Tail

The pancreas **tail** generally begins just to the left of the spine and extends to the hilum of the spleen. It lies between the stomach anteriorly and left kidney posteriorly. The splenic vein courses along its posterior superior surface. Usually, the tail lies even with the body, but in some patients, it may be at a higher or lower level.

VASCULAR ANATOMY

The arterial supply of the pancreas includes blood from **pancreaticoduodenal arteries** and branches of the splenic artery. The anterior and inferior pancreaticoduodenal arteries supply the head and part of the duodenum. These arteries comprise part of the **pancreatic arcades**—the vascular connections between the hepatic, splenic, and superior mesenteric arteries that supply the head of the pancreas.

The **splenic artery** supplies the body and tail of the pancreas and consists of four sections: **suprapancreatic** (the first 3 cm of the artery as it originates from the celiac axis), **pancreatic, prepancreatic** (before it leaves the pancreas), and **prehilar** (before it enters the spleen). The **dorsal pancreatic artery** originates from the suprapancreatic section; the **pancreatica magna,** or great, **artery** originates from the pancreatic section; and the **caudal pancreatic artery** originates from the prepancreatic or prehilar sections (Figure 11-6). As the splenic artery originates from the celiac axis it courses along the superior edge of the pancreas body and tail parallel to the splenic vein. If the artery is tortuous, it may run anterior to the lateral portion of the tail.

The venous drainage of the pancreas is through tributaries of the splenic vein and superior mesenteric vein.

PHYSIOLOGY

The pancreas is a digestive **(exocrine)** and hormonal **(endocrine)** gland. The gland is mostly exocrine: only 2% of the gland's weight is endocrine tissue. The exocrine function is carried out by the **acini cells** of the pancreas, which can produce up to 2 L of pancreatic juice per day. Acini cells resemble grape clusters with small areas of endocrine tissue interspersed between.

Pancreatic juice is composed of enzymes that help digest fats, proteins, carbohydrates, and nucleic acids. Pancreatic enzymes that aid in digestion include amylase, which digests carbohydrates; lipase, which digests fat; trypsin, chymotrypsin, and carboxypepidase, which digest proteins; and nucleases, which digest nucleic acids. The largest component of pancreatic juice is sodium bicarbonate, a substance needed to neutralize hydrochloric acid produced in the stomach. Cells lining the pancreatic duct produce bicarbonate (Table 11-1).

Chyme (partially digested food) in the duodenum stimulates the release of hormones, which act on pan-

creatic juice formation. These hormones are cholecystokinin, gastrin, acetylcholine, and secretin. The first three stimulate acini cells to produce digestive enzymes; the last-named hormone, secretin, stimulates production of sodium bicarbonate.

Pancreatic juice moves into the duodenum through the main pancreatic duct, the **duct of Wirsung,** a vessel approximately 2 mm in diameter. In approximately 77% of cadavers, the duct of Wirsung meets the common bile duct before both enter the duodenum through the **ampulla of Vater.** An accessory duct, the **duct of Santorini,** is a normal variant that enters the duodenum approximately 2 cm superior to the main duct (see Figure 11-1). The sphincter of Oddi, a muscle surrounding the ampulla, relaxes to allow pancreatic juice (and, if the gallbladder has been stimulated, bile) to flow into the duodenum.

The endocrine portion of the pancreas is located in the alpha, beta, and delta cells in the **isles of Langerhans.** **Beta cells** comprise 60% to 70% of the endocrine cells and produce **insulin,** a hormone that causes glycogen

■ ■ ■ **Table 11-1** Components of Pancreatic Juice

Enzyme	Acts on
Amylase	Carbohydrates
Lipase	Fats
Trypsin, chymotrypsin, carboxypeptidase	Proteins
Nucleases	Nucleic acids
Sodium bicarbonate	Hydrochloric acid

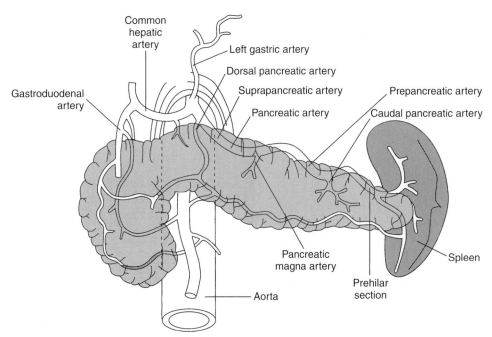

Figure 11-6 The suprapancreatic, pancreatic, prepancreatic, and prehilar sections of the splenic artery are shown. Note the origin of the dorsal pancreatic, pancreatic magna, and caudal pancreatic arteries from the splenic artery.

formation from glucose in the liver. It also enables cells with insulin receptors to take up glucose. Hence blood sugar decreases. **Alpha cells** comprise 15% to 20% of endocrine tissue and produce **glucagon,** a hormone that causes the opposite effect—cells release glucose to meet the immediate energy needs of the body. Glucagon also stimulates the liver to convert glycogen to glucose, thus increasing blood sugar levels. **Delta cells** comprise an even smaller percentage of endocrine tissue and produce a substance called **somatostatin.** This hormone inhibits the production of insulin and glucagon. The pancreatic hormones are released in minute quantities directly into the bloodstream (Table 11-2).

■ ■ ■ **Table 11-2** Pancreatic Hormones

Hormone	Type of Cell	Action
Insulin	Beta	Glucose → Glycogen
Glucagon	Alpha	Glycogen → Glucose
Somatostatin	Delta	Alpha/beta inhibitor

SONOGRAPHIC APPEARANCE

When evaluating the pancreas, the parenchymal texture, contour, shape, and echopattern and the size of the various portions of the gland and the pancreatic duct must be examined. Echogenicity of the pancreas varies, depending on the amount of interlobular fat. Generally the pancreas is expected to have a slightly more echodense (hyperechoic) appearance than the typical liver, although the texture is not as homogeneous. The borders of the pancreas are usually well defined with a smooth, curvilinear contour. The main pancreatic duct, or duct of Wirsung, can be seen as two short, highly reflective lines, about 2 mm apart, within the body of the pancreas. These reflective lines may also be observed in the head, neck, and tail of the pancreas. When identifying the pancreatic duct, care should be taken not to mistake the splenic vein, splenic

artery, or posterior wall of the stomach for the duct. The splenic vein can be followed to its portal vein junction if there is a question. The splenic artery can be followed back to its origin in the celiac axis, and by having the patient drink fluid, the stomach can easily be identified.

On transverse views, the long axis and other longitudinal sections of the pancreas are seen surrounded by epigastric vessels. The head contains two small, circular, anechoic structures: the posterolateral common bile duct and the anterolateral gastroduodenal artery (Figures 11-7 and 11-8). Anterior to the portal splenic confluence is the pancreatic neck. The gland is thinner at this point and merges into the body, located anterior to the superior mesenteric artery and aorta. These vessels appear anechoic with reflective borders (Figures 11-9 and 11-10). Note the relationships of the different vessels in this area as they relate to the pancreas (Figures 11-11 to 11-13). The splenic vein marks the tail and body of the pancreas and can be seen coursing from the hilum of the spleen to the confluence at the neck. It is anechoic, curvilinear, and follows closely along the posterior border of the pancreas (Figures 11-14 and 11-15). The splenic vein enlarges at the confluence, marking the entrance of the superior mesenteric vein.

Sagittal views of the pancreas show the gland in transverse sections. The head can be seen posteroinferior to the homogeneous liver and anterior to the elongated, anechoic inferior vena cava (Figure 11-16). Just medial to this, another transverse section shows the head and uncinate process separated by the elongated, anechoic superior mesenteric vein (Figure 11-17). A more medial section shows a transverse view of the neck. A smaller amount of tissue may be noted in this view (Figure 11-18). The transverse section of the body of the pancreas is seen anterior to the anechoic splenic vein, superior mesenteric artery, and aorta (Figures 11-19 to 11-21). The traversed, circular, anechoic splenic vein demarcates the posterior portion of the tail of the pancreas. In some

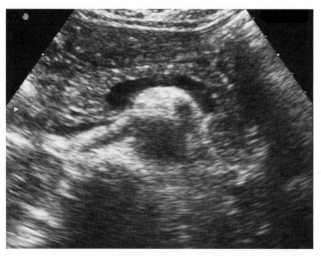
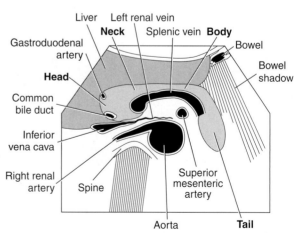

Figure 11-7 A transverse image showing the common bile duct and gastroduodenal artery in the head of the pancreas.

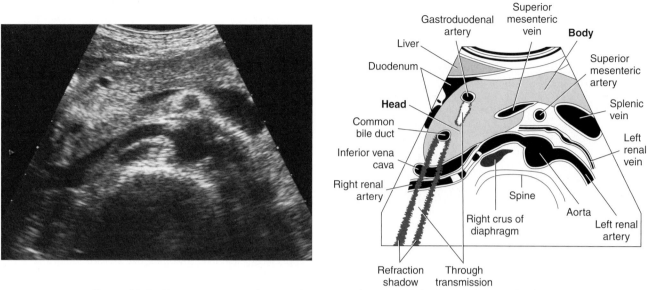

Figure 11-8 Transverse image showing the traversed common bile duct and gastroduodenal artery in the head of the pancreas (note that transverse images show longitudinal sections of the pancreas).

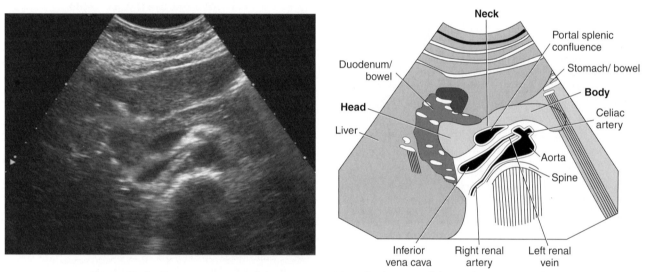

Figure 11-9 Transverse image of the pancreas. Note the location of the neck, anterior to the portal splenic confluence, and the body, anterior to the aorta.

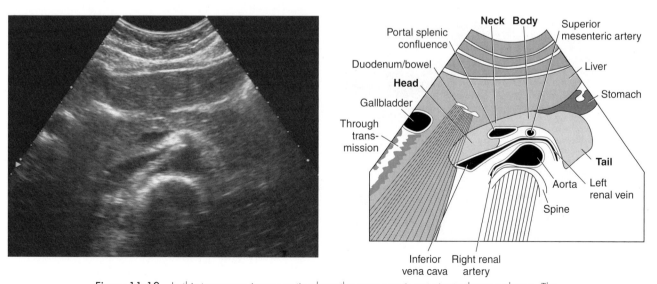

Figure 11-10 In this transverse image notice how the pancreas is anterior to the vasculature. The head and uncinate lie in front of the inferior vena cava. The neck is anterior to the confluence, and the body lies in front of the superior mesenteric artery and aorta.

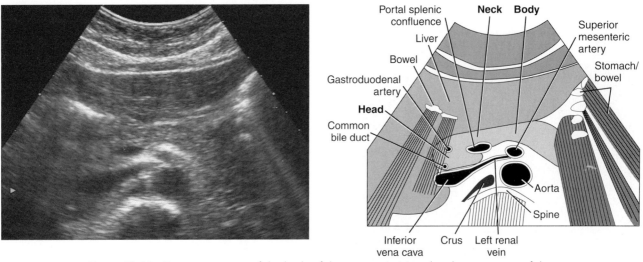

Figure 11-11 Transverse image of the body of the pancreas. Note the close proximity of the pancreas to the vasculature.

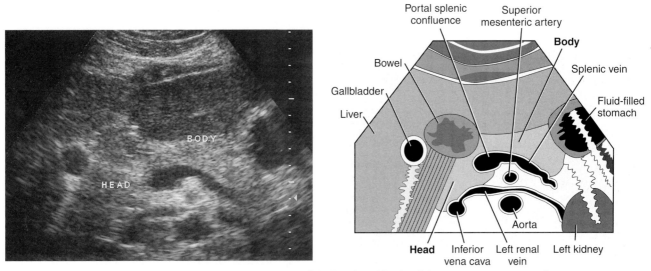

Figure 11-12 Enlarged, transverse image of the head and body of the pancreas. Respectively, the left renal vein, superior mesenteric artery, splenic vein, pancreas body, and liver lie in front of or anterior to the aorta. Right lateral to the confluence, the pancreas head lies anterior to the inferior vena cava.

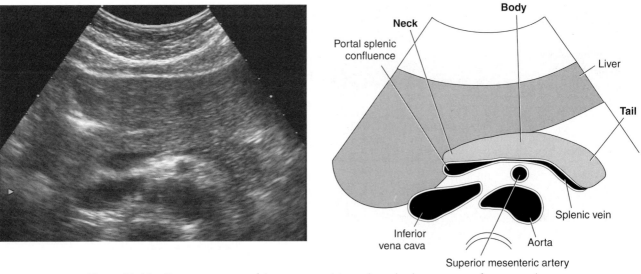

Figure 11-13 Transverse image of the pancreas. Notice how this long section of pancreas lies in front of the splenic vein and confluence. Directly behind the confluence is the inferior vena cava. Posterior and medial to the splenic vein lie the superior mesenteric artery and aorta.

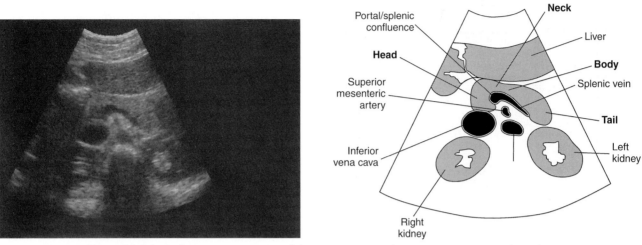

Figure 11-14 In this transverse image of the pancreas note the posterior position and curvilinear shape of the splenic vein. (Image courtesy Jeanes Hospital, Philadelphia, PA.)

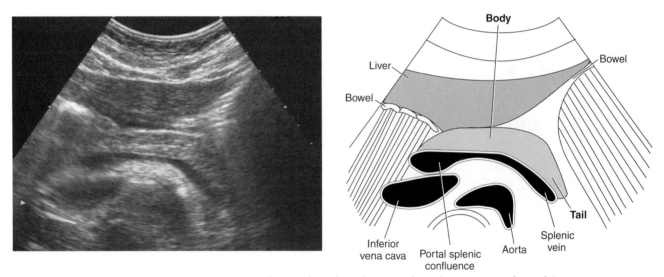

Figure 11-15 Transverse image showing how the splenic vein hugs the posterior surface of the tail and body along its course to the confluence.

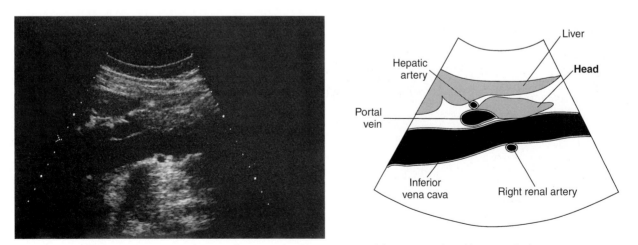

Figure 11-16 Sagittal image showing a transverse section of the pancreas head between the liver anteriorly and inferior vena cava posteriorly. (Image courtesy Jeanes Hospital, Philadelphia, PA.)

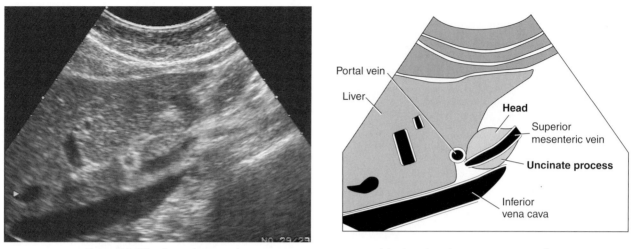

Figure 11-17 Sagittal image showing a transverse section of the head and uncinate process of the pancreas.

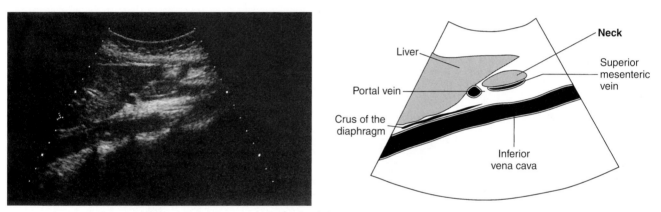

Figure 11-18 Sagittal image of the neck of the pancreas. (Image courtesy Jeanes Hospital, Philadelphia, PA.)

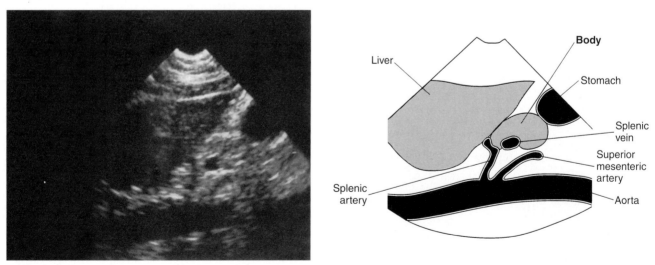

Figure 11-19 Sagittal image showing the transverse section of the body of the pancreas between the celiac axis and superior mesenteric artery. Note the circular section of splenic vein immediately posterior to the body.

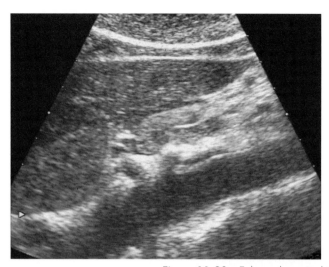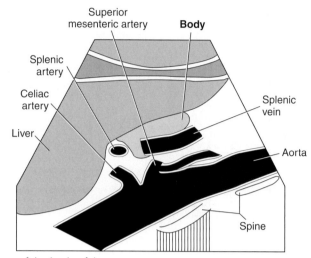

Figure 11-20   Enlarged, sagittal image of the body of the pancreas.

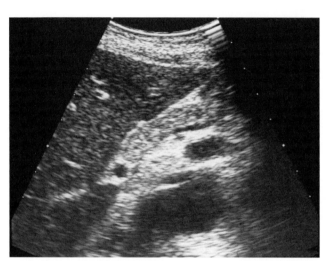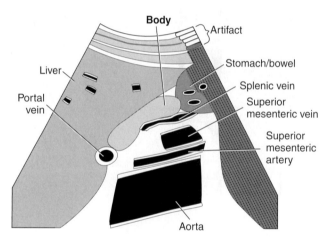

Figure 11-21   Enlarged, sagittal image of the body of the pancreas. Note the splenic artery superior to the body.

transverse sections, the left kidney is noted posterior to the tail and splenic vein. See Figures 11-22 and 11-23 for an enlarged view of the tail.

SONOGRAPHIC APPLICATIONS
Some uses of pancreatic sonography include:
Structural measurements
Distal biliary tree measurements
Identification of pancreatic masses
Identification of epigastric masses
Main pancreatic duct measurements
Adjacent associated biliary masses
Biliary obstruction
Diagnosis and follow-up evaluation of acute and chronic pancreatitis
Diagnosis and follow-up evaluation of pancreatic pseudocysts

NORMAL VARIANTS
Annular pancreas is a condition in which a ring of pancreatic tissue surrounds the second portion (C-loop) of the duodenum.

Ectopic (heterotopic, aberrant) pancreas is tissue that has no vascular or structural connection to the body of the pancreas. Because ectopic tissues may be as small as 1 cm in size, the condition is extremely difficult to detect using sonography.

Partial duplication of the tail of the pancreas is rare. On transverse images, the tail may appear to be grossly enlarged (Figure 11-24).

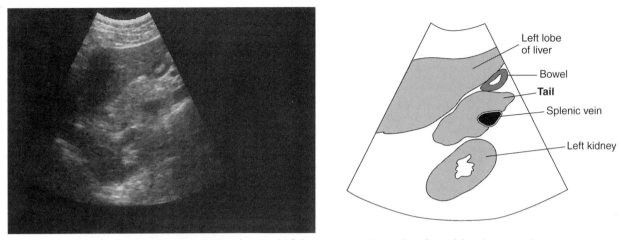

Figure 11-22 Sagittal image of the tail of the pancreas. Note that the tail lies between the bowel and the left kidney. (Image courtesy Jeanes Hospital, Philadelphia, PA.)

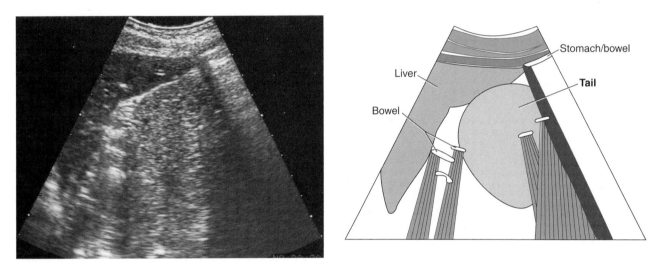

Figure 11-23 Enlarged sagittal image of the tail of the pancreas.

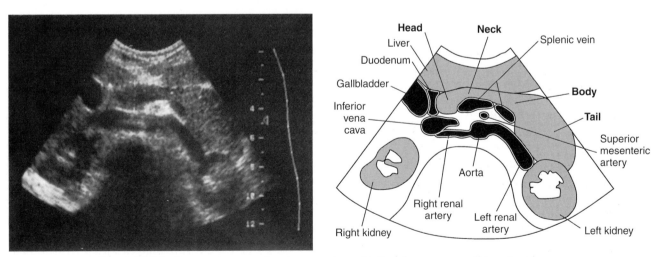

Figure 11-24 Transverse image showing an enlarged tail of the pancreas. This patient has a congenital malformation in which the tail is partially duplicated.

REFERENCE CHARTS

■ ■ ■   ASSOCIATED PHYSICIANS

Surgeon: Involved in surgery of the pancreas.

Internal Medicine: Involved in diagnosing and treating pancreatic disease.

Radiologist: Performs and interprets most of the tests used to diagnose pancreatic and related diseases.

■ ■ ■   COMMON DIAGNOSTIC TESTS

General Radiography: Except for the appearance of calcifications, plain radiography is not very revealing for pancreatic disease. An upper gastrointestinal (UGI) series, a study in which the patient swallows barium to outline the stomach and duodenum, detects pancreatic masses or enlargement through displacement of the C-loop of the duodenum by the mass. The UGI series is performed by a radiologist assisted by a radiologic technologist. The radiologist interprets the examination.

Endoscopic Retrograde Cholangiopancreaticoduodenography (ERCP): A tube is placed into the duodenum via the esophagus and stomach. Within the tube are fiberoptics to allow visualization of the anatomy and a means for inserting a catheter. The catheter tip is placed in the end of the common bile duct (or the pancreatic duct, depending on the anatomic configuration). A contrast medium is injected into the biliary system, which visualizes structures retrogradely (in the reverse direction). This examination is usually performed and interpreted by a gastroenterologist and a radiologist. Radiologic technologists may assist physicians in performing this procedure.

Computed Axial Tomography (CT Scan): A contrast material may or may not be administered. An x-ray beam passes through the patient to be detected by a series of devices that provide an electrical signal to a computer. The computer then arranges the data into a sectional image of the body. Structural and some functional information may be obtained. This examination is performed by a radiologic technologist and is interpreted by a radiologist.

Magnetic Resonance Imaging (MRI): Images are similar in format to those of a CT scan; however, the images are generated using a strong magnetic field instead of radiation as in CT. A magnetic resonance imaging technologist or a radiologic technologist performs the examination and a radiologist interprets the study.

Angiography: A contrast material is injected into an epigastric vessel to visualize the vascularity of the pancreas of a suspected lesion. This examination is performed by a radiologist assisted by a radiologic technologist. The radiologist interprets the study.

■ ■ ■   LABORATORY VALUES

Serum Tests:
Amylase: 60-80 units
Lipase: <1.5 U/ml
Glucose (fasting): 65-110 mg/dl
        (all sugars): 80-120 mg/dl
Urine Tests:
Amylase (2 hr): 35-260 units/hr
Alkaline phosphatase: <3.5 U/8 hr

Byrne CJ, Saxton DF, Pelikan PK, Nugent PM: *Laboratory tests: implications for nursing care.* Reading, 1986, Addison-Wesley, Appendix C.

■ ■ ■   NORMAL MEASUREMENTS

Total length: 12.5-15 cm
Approximate anterior posterior measurements:

Head: 2.00-3 cm	**Body:** 1.20-2.8 cm
Neck: 1.00-2 cm	**Tail:** 2.00-2.8 cm

■ ■ ■   VASCULATURE

Arterial Supply to the Head and Neck of the Pancreas:
Gastroduodenal artery—Pancreaticoduodenal arteries—
    Pancreatic arcades
Arterial Supply to the Body and Tail of the Pancreas:
Splenic artery—Suprapancreatic artery—Pancreatic artery—
    Prepancreatic artery—Prehilar artery

■ ■ ■   AFFECTING CHEMICALS

Prolonged alcohol ingestion over a period of years (alcoholism) is toxic to the pancreas.

BIBLIOGRAPHY

Balthazar EJ: CT diagnosis and staging of acute pancreatitis, *Radiol Clin North Am* 27(1):19-24, 1989.

Byrne CJ, Saxton DF, Pelikan PK, et al: *Laboratory tests: implications for nursing care*, Reading, 1986, Addison-Wesley, Appendix C.

Craig M: *Pocket guide to ultrasound measurements*, Philadelphia, 1988, JB Lippincott, p 30.

Federle MP, Burke VD: Pancreatitis and its complications: computed tomography and sonography, *Semin Ultrasound CT MR* 5:414-418, 1984.

Frick H, Leonhardt H, Starck D: *Human anatomy 2: special anatomy: viscera and nervous system, classification of muscles and vessels, organization of lymphatics and nerves*, New York, 1991, Thieme Medical, pp 139-141.

Friedman AC, Birns MT: Embryology, anatomy, histology, and physiology. In Friedman AC, editor: *Radiology of the liver, biliary tract, pancreas and spleen*, Baltimore, 1987, Williams & Wilkins, pp 619-641.

Guyton AC: *Textbook of medical physiology*, ed 10, Philadelphia, 2000, WB Saunders.

Hole JW: *Essentials of human anatomy and physiology*, ed 3, Dubuque, 1989, Wm C Brown.

Mittelstaedt CA: *Abdominal ultrasound*, New York, 1987, Churchill Livingstone.

O'Rahilly R: *Anatomy: a regional study of human structure*, ed 5, Philadelphia, 1986, WB Saunders.

Rubin E, Farber JL: *Pathology*, Philadelphia, 1988, JB Lippincott.

Schmidt RF, Thews G, editors: *Human physiology*, New York, 1989, Springer-Verlag.

Thibodeau GA, Patton KT: *Anatomy and physiology*, ed 4, St Louis, 1999, Mosby.

van DeGraaff KM: *Concepts of human anatomy and physiology*, ed 2, Dubuque, 1989, Wm C Brown, pp 882-884.

CHAPTER 12

The Urinary System

REVA ARNEZ CURRY, BETTY BATES TEMPKIN, VIVIE MILLER, AND CANDYCE JAMES

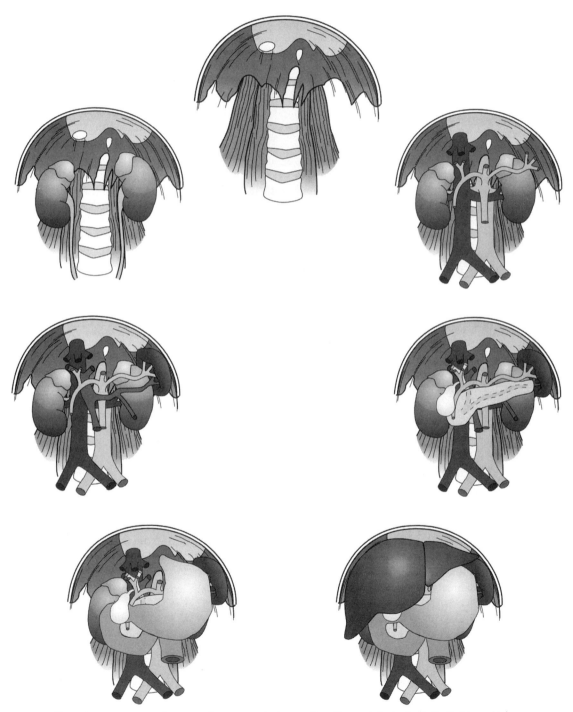

The urinary system and surrounding anatomic layers. See Figure 4-3, A, B, D, E, G, H, and I for more details.

179

Describe the function of the urinary system.

Describe the location of the kidneys, ureters, urinary bladder, and urethra.

Describe the size of the kidneys, ureters, urinary bladder, and urethra.

Describe the sonographic appearance of the urinary system.

Compare the appearance and size of the adult kidney with the kidney in the fetus, neonate, and child.

Describe associated physicians, diagnostic tests, and laboratory values.

Define the key words.

Afferent arteriole	Minor calyces
Aldosterone	Morison's pouch
Antidiuretic hormone	Nephron
Arcuate arteries	Renal capsule
Bowman's capsule	Renal corpuscle
Blood urea nitrogen (BUN)	Renal cortex
Columns of Bertin	Renal hilum
Creatinine (Cr)	Renal medulla
Efferent arteriole	Renal pelvis
Erythropoietin	Renal sinus
Gerota's fascia	Renal tubule
Glomerulus	Renin
Homeostasis	Specific gravity
Infundibulum	Ureters
Loop of Henle	Urethra
Major calyces	Urinary bladder

The urinary system includes two kidneys, a ureter for each kidney, a urinary bladder, and a urethra. The kidneys are excretory organs that maintain the body's chemical equilibrium through the excretion of urine, a waste product. Each kidney has a ureter that carries the urine to the urinary bladder for temporary storage. Urine is excreted from the bladder to outside of the body through the urethra, a membranous canal. Detoxification, blood pressure regulation, and the maintenance of the correct balance of pH, minerals, iron, and salt levels in the blood are functions of the urinary system.

PRENATAL DEVELOPMENT

The kidneys pass embryonically through three developmental stages. The pronephros and mesonephros appear in the fourth to fifth week of gestation and are precursors to the metanephros. The embryonic kidneys are drained by the mesonephric (wolffian) ducts. The paramesonephric ducts are located alongside the mesonephric ducts

(para = next to). It is from this site that the reproductive organs will develop. The permanent kidney—the metanephros—appears toward the end of the fifth week of gestation. It is derived from the mesodermal tissue of the embryo and is not functional until the end of the eighth week. The kidneys initially lie in the pelvic cavity. As the embryo grows, the kidneys move up into the abdomen.

Congenital defects in renal development include ectopic kidney (located away from the normal position), renal agenesis (unilateral or bilateral absence of the kidney[s]), and horseshoe kidney (both kidneys joined together at their superior or inferior poles). Variants in the renal vasculature and ureters may also occur. For example, multiple renal arteries occur in 25% of the U.S. population. Variations of the ureter occur much less frequently, in 2% of that population. Seventy-five percent of these variations consist of partial bifurcation of the ureter, with the remaining 25%, total duplication of the ureter along its entire length.

LOCATION

The kidneys are bean-shaped, retroperitoneal organs that lie one on each side of the spine between the peritoneum and the back muscles. The kidney has a lateral convex and a medial concave border. The liver displaces the right kidney inferiorly; hence it is located lower than the left kidney and has a slightly shorter ureter. The kidneys and ureters comprise the upper urinary tract, and the urinary bladder and urethra form the lower urinary tract. The kidneys lie in the lower thoracic and lumbar area, between the twelfth thoracic and fourth lumbar vertebrae. Deep inspiration causes the kidneys to descend (Figure 12-1).

Anterior to the right kidney are the right adrenal gland, right lobe of the liver, second part of the duodenum, hepatic flexure of the colon, and jejunum or ileum of the small bowel (Figure 12-2). Table 12-1 describes portions of the right kidney covered by these structures.

Anterior to the left kidney are the tail of the pancreas, the left adrenal gland, the spleen, the jejunum, the stomach, and the splenic flexure of the colon (see Figure 12-2). Table 12-2 describes portions of the left kidney covered by these structures.

Posterior to both kidneys are the diaphragm, the psoas muscle, the transversus muscle, and the quadratus lumborum muscle (Figure 12-3). Table 12-3 lists structures posterior to the kidneys.

The **ureters** are tubular, retroperitoneal structures that begin as an expanded area, the **renal pelvis,** in the hilum of each kidney. The ureters extend inferiorly along the psoas muscle. They travel from the renal hilum into the abdominopelvic cavity, and finally enter the urinary bladder posteriorly (see Figure 12-1, C).

The right ureter is posterior to the duodenum, termi-

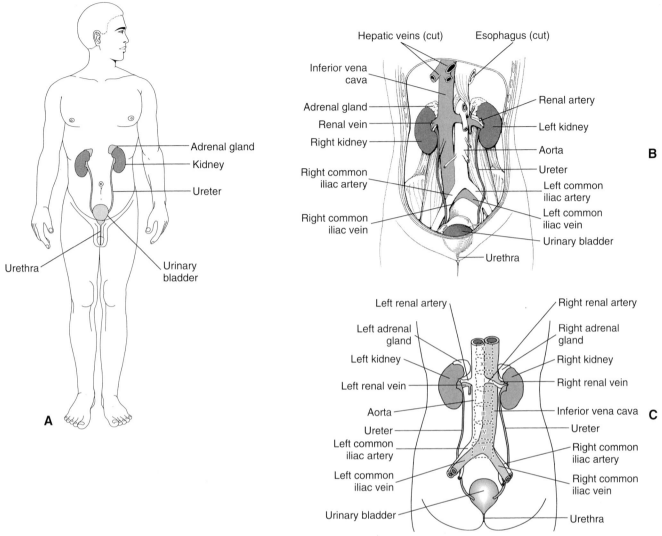

Figure 12-1   The urinary tract. **A,** Adrenal glands, kidneys, ureters, urinary bladder, and urethra. **B,** Frontal view of the urinary system shows how the ureters cross the iliac vessels anteriorly. **C,** Posterior view shows the urinary tract from behind. Note frontal placement of the ureters.

■ ■ ■ **Table 12-1**   Anterior Structures That Cover the Right Kidney

Structure	Portion of Kidney Covered
Right adrenal	Superior-medial
Right lobe of liver	Lateral
Second part of duodenum	Medial
Hepatic flexure of colon and jejunum or ileum of small bowel	Inferior

nal ileum, and right colic, ileocolic, and gonadal vessels. The left ureter is posterior to the colon and the left colic and left gonadal (testicular or ovarian) vessels.

The abdominal portion of both ureters passes anteriorly to the psoas muscle and the bifurcation of the com-mon iliac arteries. The pelvic portions of the ureters pass posteriorly to the ductus deferens in the male and uter-ine artery in the female.

Both ureters empty posteriorly into the **urinary blad-der,** a hollow, muscular, retroperitoneal organ that is posterior to the symphysis pubis. The male urinary bladder is anterior to the seminal vesicles and the rec-tum, and superior to the prostate gland. The ductus def-erens, on its superior, slightly lateral course from the scrotum, crosses the ureter anteriorly, before descending into the prostate gland (Figure 12-4). The female uri-nary bladder is anterior to the vagina, posterior cul-de-sac, and rectum (Figure 12-5).

The **urethra** is a membranous canal that conveys urine out of the urinary bladder. It exits inferiorly via the neck of the urinary bladder. The male urethra is

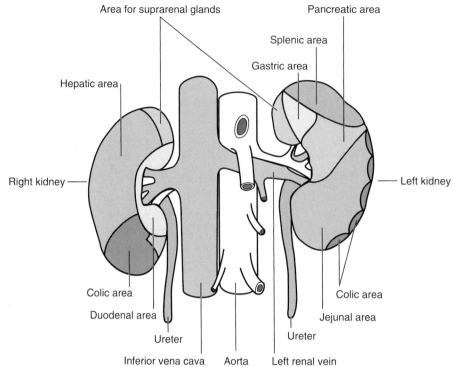

Figure 12-2 Frontal view of the kidneys delineating the portions of the kidneys covered by the overlying adrenal glands, liver, duodenum, hepatic flexure, jejunum, stomach, splenic flexure, spleen, and pancreatic tail (see Tables 12-1 and 12-2).

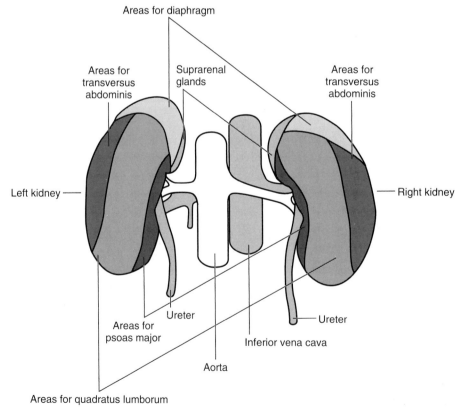

Figure 12-3 Posterior view of the kidneys delineating the portions of the kidneys covered by the overlying diaphragm, quadratus lumborum, psoas, and transversus muscles (see Table 12-3).

■ ▨ ▨ **Table 12-2** Anterior Structures That Cover
the Left Kidney

Structure	Portion of Kidney Covered
Tail of pancreas	Medial
Left adrenal gland	Superior-medial
Spleen	Superior-lateral
Jejunum	Inferior
Stomach	Superior
Splenic flexure of colon	Lateral

■ ▨ ▨ **Table 12-3** Structures Posterior to Kidneys

Structure	Portion of Kidney Covered
Diaphragm	Superior
Psoas muscle	Medial
Transversus muscle	Lateral
Quadratus lumborum muscle	Between lateral and medial portions

much longer than the female urethra, and also functions as a pathway for seminal fluid.

SIZE

The normal adult kidney is approximately 9 to 12 cm in length, 2.5 to 4 cm in depth, and 4 to 6 cm in diameter. The kidney may shrink due to atrophic changes associated with age, circulatory insufficiency, or renal disease. If only one kidney is present (i.e., congenital absence of a kidney), it may be larger than normal, due to hypertrophy necessary to accommodate the increased workload.

The neonatal kidney measures 3.3 to 5.0 cm in length, 1.5 to 2.5 cm in depth, and 2 to 3 cm in diameter. The pediatric kidney is proportionately larger than the adult kidney and may extend inferiorly to the iliac crest.

The ureters are hollow, narrow tubes ranging from 25 to 30 cm in length. The diameter ranges between 4 and 7 mm. In a cadaver, the diameter is a uniform 5 mm

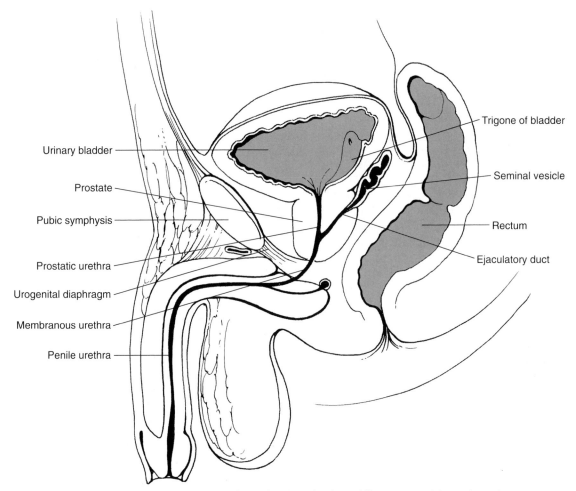

Figure 12-4 Lower urinary tract in the male. Note the three different parts of the male urethra.

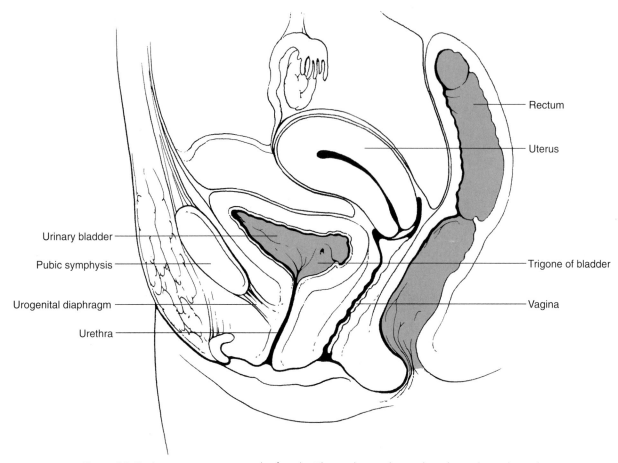

Figure 12-5 Lower urinary tract in the female. The urethra is shorter than the male urethra, although it also pierces the urogenital diaphragm.

throughout the length. The ureters transport urine to the bladder through peristaltic action. The urinary bladder is a symmetric hollow organ, whose size depends on the quantity of contained urine. The wall of a distended bladder will normally measure 3 to 6 mm, depending on the degree of bladder distension. The male urethra is 20 cm in length; the female is considerably shorter, approximately 3.5 cm in length.

GROSS ANATOMY

Upper Urinary Tract

The kidney consists of an upper, a middle, and a lower pole. It has several protective coverings, which cushion and protect the entire organ (Figure 12-6). First, it is covered with a tough, fibrous capsule that is closely applied but not adherent to the parenchyma. Second, a layer of perirenal fat surrounds the encapsulated kidney and is continuous with the fat in the renal sinus. The third layer, the renal fascia or **Gerota's fascia,** surrounds the kidney and perirenal fat. Gerota's fascia is surrounded by yet another layer of fat, called pararenal fat. This layer is especially thick posterior to Gerota's fascia. The renal fascia anchors the kidneys and limits

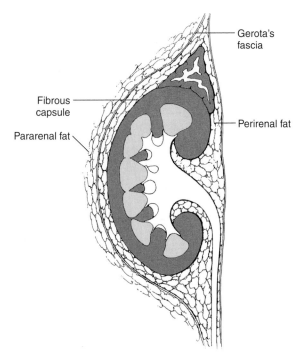

Figure 12-6 Four layers surrounding the kidney: fibrous capsule, perirenal fat, Gerota's fascia, and pararenal fat.

■ ■ ■ **Table 12-4** Common Names for Tissues
Covering Kidneys

Perinephric fat = adipose capsule = packing fat of
Zuckerkandl
Perirenal fascia = perinephric fascia = fascia of Gerota
Pararenal fat = pararenal body
Renal capsule = true capsule = fibrous capsule

any infection arising from them. The double layer of renal fat (perirenal and pararenal) accommodates kidney movement during respiration. Table 12-4 lists some common alternative terms given to the tissues that cover the kidneys.

The kidney is composed of two distinct areas, the renal parenchyma and the renal sinus. A dissected view of the kidney is shown in Figure 12-7.

The renal parenchyma consists of two areas. The outer portion of the parenchyma is the **cortex** (see Figure 12-7). It contains the renal corpuscle and the proximal and distal convoluted tubules of the nephron. The inner portion of the parenchyma is called the **medulla;** it contains the **loop of Henle** (also called renal loops). Thus filtration takes place in the renal cortex, and reabsorption occurs in the medulla. The medulla consists of eight to eighteen medullary pyramids, which contain the loops of Henle (see Figure 12-13).

The medullary pyramids are triangular structures with a narrow tip, called the apex, and a broad base. The apex of a pyramid sits within a minor calyx located in the renal sinus. From the apex, the pyramid expands and extends laterally to its base, which abuts the renal cortex. Pyramids are separated from each other by bands of cortical tissue called **columns of Bertin.** Therefore the base and sides of each pyramid are surrounded by the cortex (see Figure 12-7). Pyramids are also one of the components that comprise a renal lobe. Renal lobes are referred to as those portions of the kidney that consist of a single pyramid, bordered on both sides by interlobar arteries and veins, with cortical tissue at its base (Figure 12-8).

The function of the pyramids is to convey urine to the minor calyces. Thus the number of renal pyramids will equal the number of **minor calyces,** which form the border of the renal sinus (see Figure 12-7).

The **renal sinus** is the central portion of the kidney. It contains the collecting system, composed of the **infundibulum** (minor and major calyces) and renal pelvis. The sinus also houses the renal artery and vein, fatty fibrous tissue, nerves, and lymphatics. There are usually two to three **major calyces** that receive urine from the minor calyces. The major calyces convey urine to the upper, expanded end of the ureter, the renal pelvis. The **hilum** is the portion of renal sinus where the renal artery enters the kidney and the renal vein and ureter exit (see Figure 12-7).

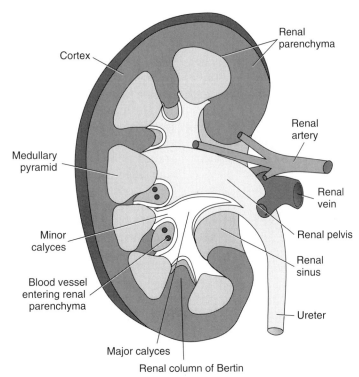

Figure 12-7 Section of internal kidney anatomy. Notice how the number of medullary pyramids equals the number of minor calyces, and also how the minor calyces form the border of the renal sinus. Observe how the ureter begins in the kidney as the renal pelvis.

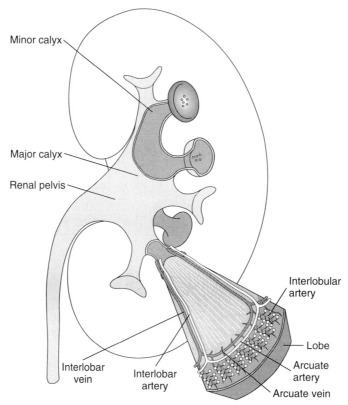

Figure 12-8 Renal lobe. Note that the lobe is triangular and bordered by the interlobar vasculature. The arcuate and interlobular vessels and the surrounding cortical tissue form the base of the lobe.

The ureters begin in the kidney as the renal pelvis. They are composed of three layers of tissue: an inner mucosal layer, a medial layer of longitudinal and circular smooth muscle, and an outer fibrous layer. Ureteral peristalsis transports urine to the urinary bladder. The ureters enter the bladder posteriorly at the trigone area. Urine is carried into the urinary bladder between intervals of several seconds and several minutes, depending on the state of hydration. Blood is supplied to the ureters by branches from the renal, internal spermatic, hypogastric, and inferior vesical arteries.

Lower Urinary Tract

The urinary bladder consists of four layers of tissues: an inner mucosa, a submucosa, the muscularis, and the outer serosa. The mucosa folds when the bladder is empty, and distends and becomes smooth when the bladder is full. The muscularis layer is comprised of three layers of smooth muscle called the detrusor muscle. The outermost layer of the bladder, the serosa, is located at the superior portion of the bladder. It is an extension of pelvic peritoneum (Figure 12-9).

The inferior portion of the urinary bladder is comprised of a posterior base (the trigone area) and the neck, which communicates with the urethra. The inferolateral surfaces of the bladder meet anteriorly, and are in contact with the pelvic floor muscles (see Figure 12-9).

The anterior portion of the urinary bladder lies behind the pubic bone and the symphysis pubis. Only the superior portion of the urinary bladder is covered by an extension of peritoneum. The location of the superior portion is variable, depending on the amount of urine in the bladder (Figure 12-10).

The urinary bladder is anchored to the pelvis by ligaments. Ligaments extending anteriorly from the bladder neck attach to the pubic bones. These ligaments are called pubovesical in the female, and puboprostatic in the male. Laterally, ligaments extend to fuse with the tendinous arch of the obturator internus muscles. These attachments are called lateral ligaments. Blood is supplied to the urinary bladder by the superior, middle, and inferior vesicles derived from the anterior trunk of the hypogastric artery. The obturator and inferior gluteal arteries also supply small visceral branches to the bladder, and additional branches in the female are derived from the uterine and vaginal arteries.

The urethra consists of a membranous, hollow canal that conveys urine from the bladder to the outside. The male urethra is approximately 20 cm in length, compared with the female urethra, which is approximately 3.5 cm in length. The male urethra is composed of three parts. The first portion, the prostatic urethra, receives secretions from the prostate gland. The second part is the short membranous urethra, which pierces the urogenital diaphragm.

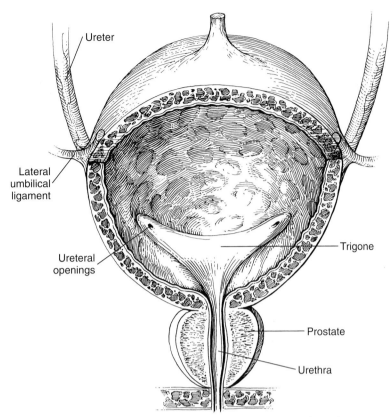

Figure 12-9 Urinary bladder. Note the triangular area, the trigone, where the ureters enter. Also shown is the lateral umbilical ligament.

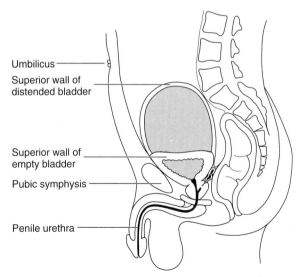

Figure 12-10 Difference between the appearance of an empty and distended urinary bladder. Note how the superior portion of the distended bladder moves toward the umbilicus.

The third, and longest, portion is the penile urethra, which extends the entire length of the penis. The female urethra is composed of the membranous urethra, which also pierces the urogenital diaphragm. Male and female urethras are shown in Figures 12-4 and 12-5.

PHYSIOLOGY

As the primary excretory organs (see Chapter 3), the kidneys have as their principal functions urine production and **homeostasis** (maintenance of normal body physiology). The kidneys excrete metabolic waste products and maintain blood volume, and function independently. A unilateral condition (complete obstruction, congenital absence of a kidney, trauma, or removal of a kidney) will not affect the remaining kidney's function; the healthy kidney will accommodate the increased workload. Failure of both kidneys, however, will lead to uremia, a toxic and fatal condition if untreated.

The kidneys filter approximately 1200 ml of blood per minute and produce on average 1500 ml of urine daily. The excreted urine is 95% water and 5% nitrogenous waste and inorganic salts. Nitrogenous waste consists of the byproducts of metabolism. The amount of nitrogenous waste is measured by **blood urea nitrogen (BUN)** and **creatinine (Cr)** laboratory tests, which measure the kidneys' ability to get rid of waste. Normal ranges for BUN and Cr are 26 mg/dl and 1.1 mg/dl, respectively. Another laboratory test that can assess the kidneys' ability to concentrate urine is specific gravity. **Specific gravity** is a measure of how much dissolved material is present in the urine. The higher the quantity of dissolved solutes, the higher the specific gravity. For example, specific gravity is higher when the kidneys must preserve water (e.g., during exercise) to compensate for water lost in sweat. The volume of urine therefore is decreased. The normal range of specific gravity is 1.101 to 1.025. (The specific gravity of distilled water, which has no solutes, is 1.000.)

The functional unit of the kidney is the **nephron.** There are over a million microscopic nephrons in each kidney. The nephron functions by moving metabolic products from areas of high concentration to areas of low concentration. This is accomplished through osmosis, the passive transport of cellular material. Another method is active transport, which uses cellular energy to move material from one area to another.

There are two types of nephrons, named for their location in the kidney and the length of their loops. (The loop of Henle is discussed later in this chapter.) Juxtamedullary nephrons originate in the inner third of the

renal cortex and have longer loops of Henle than cortical nephrons located in the outer two thirds of the renal cortex (Figure 12-11).

The nephron consists of a **renal corpuscle,** which includes **Bowman's capsule** and the glomerulus, and a **renal tubule,** which includes the proximal convoluted tubule, loop of Henle (with descending and ascending branches), distal convoluted tubule, and a collecting duct (Figure 12-12). The medulla contains the loop of Henle and collecting duct. The renal cortex contains the renal corpuscle and the proximal and distal convoluted tubules.

Blood reaches the nephron in the following manner. Blood enters the kidney through the renal artery, a branch of the aorta. The renal artery forms interlobar arteries, which travel between the renal pyramids. The interlobar arteries branch into **arcuate arteries,** located at the base of the renal pyramids. From the arcuate arteries, the interlobular arteries travel into the renal cortex. The

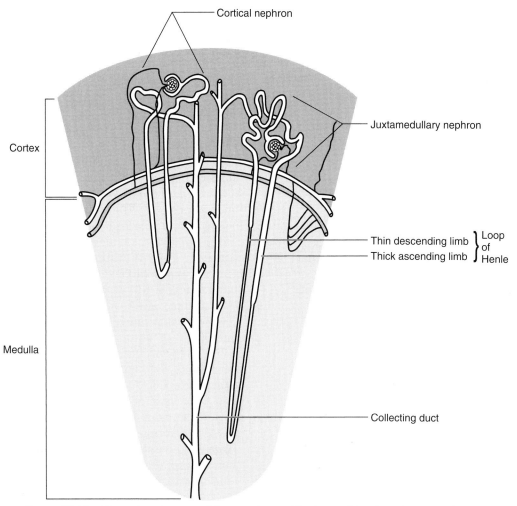

Figure 12-11   Cortical and juxtamedullary nephrons. The loop of Henle is longer in the juxtamedullary nephron.

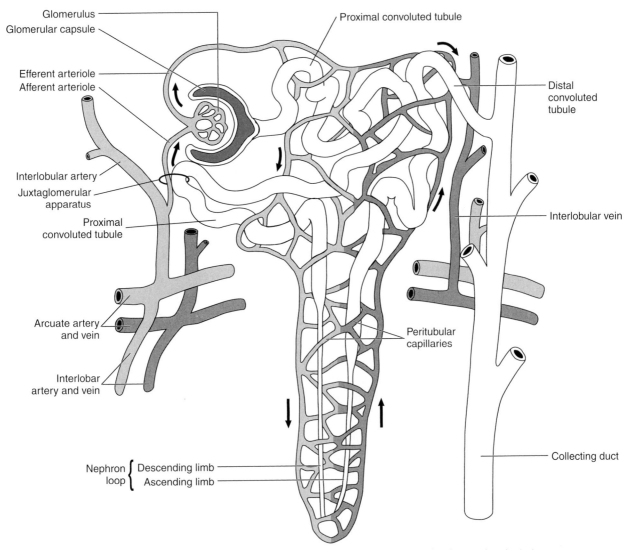

Figure 12-12 *Enlarged view of nephron. Glomerulus, proximal and distal convoluted tubules, loop of Henle, and collecting duct are shown. Note juxtaglomerular apparatus.*

interlobular arteries branch into **afferent arterioles,** which carry blood into the glomerulus of the nephron.

How the Nephron Works

The filtration, which takes place in the **glomerulus,** is the first step in urine formation. As blood enters the glomerulus, afferent arterioles carrying the blood branch into capillaries. As the vessels narrow, the blood pressure in the vessels increases. Most capillaries have a blood pressure of approximately 25 mm Hg (mercury). However, in the glomerulus, the pressure is 60 to 90 mm Hg. This higher blood pressure forces a plasmalike fluid from the blood to filter into Bowman's capsule. This "nephric filtrate" contains water, salts, glucose, urea, and amino acids. Proteins and cells, which are too large to pass through the semipermeable walls of the glomerular capillaries, remain in the blood.

Osmotic pressure forces water to return to the blood. This pressure is created by the difference in protein content of the fluid in the proximal convoluted tubule and the plasma in the glomerular capsule. The protein concentration in the proximal convoluted tubule is 2 to 5 mg/100 ml compared with the capsule concentration of 6 to 8 mg/100 ml. This concentration gradient creates osmotic pressure, which returns water from the proximal convoluted tubule back to the plasma in the glomerular capsule, where it is returned into the blood.

The fluid that enters the glomerulus is called ultrafiltrate. The volume of filtrate produced per minute is 115 ml for women and 125 for males. This means that the body's entire blood volume is filtered approximately every 40 minutes. Ninety-nine percent of the blood volume is returned, and 1% is excreted.

Tubular reabsorption is the process by which substances in the plasma solute that are useful to the body are reabsorbed into the bloodstream. These substances include water, glucose, vitamins, amino acids, bicarbonate ions, and chloride salts of magnesium, sodium, calcium, and potassium. Reabsorption takes place in the proximal convoluted tubule and the descending and ascending loop of Henle. Sixty-five percent of the salt and water in the ultrafiltrate is reabsorbed from the proximal convoluted tubule, and 20% is reabsorbed from the loop of Henle. The amount of reabsorption of the remaining ultrafiltrate depends on hormonal influence and takes place in the distal convoluted tubule. Tubular resorption takes place through active transport and expends a large amount of energy. It has been estimated that 6% of total calories consumed by the body at rest (no physical activity) may be required for tubular resorption.

Blood from the **efferent arteriole** supplies the peritubular capillaries, which in turn supply the proximal and distal convoluted tubules, and the vasa recta (see Figure 12-12). The vasa recta are a series of intertwining capillary loops that surround the juxtamedullary nephron (see Figure 12-11). Through osmotic pressure, the vasa recta trap salt and urea in the medulla and move water back into the blood. This mechanism is called the countercurrent multiplier system and helps the kidneys maintain homeostasis.

Blood from the peritubular capillaries drains into the interlobular veins, which, in turn, drain into arcuate veins. The arcuate veins drain into the interlobar veins, which convey blood back to the renal veins. The renal veins carry blood to the inferior vena cava.

Tubular secretion is the process whereby waste substances, including ammonia, drugs, hydrogen, and potassium, are secreted into the distal convoluted tubule. The secretion process is controlled through active transport. Urine exits the distal convoluted tubule into the collecting tubule or duct. The collecting ducts convey urine to the renal pyramids. The apex of the pyramid lies within the minor calyx, which is part of the collecting system for urine. Several minor calyces empty urine into each major calyx; several major calyces empty urine into the renal pelvis (Figure 12-13). The urine is emptied from the renal pelvis into the ureter, and by peristalsis is carried to the urinary bladder.

Protective Mechanisms That Preserve Nephron Function

The kidneys are sensitive to changes in blood volume and have the capacity to alter blood volume to maintain homeostasis. This is necessary because the kidneys need a large volume of blood for urine production and to nourish the cells lining the nephron. The latter are especially sensitive to anoxia (lack of O₂), and prolonged decrease in blood oxygen may result in irreversible cel-

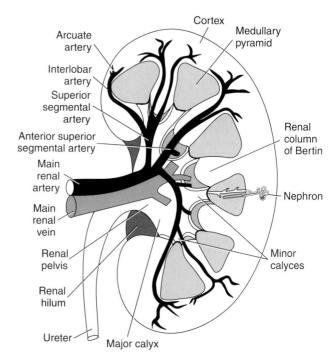

Figure 12-13 Dissected view of the kidney. Observe how the apex of the medullary pyramid lies within the minor calyx and how several minor calyces empty urine into a single major calyx. Also, notice how the urine would empty from all of the major calyces into the renal pelvis and down the ureter on its way to the urinary bladder.

lular death. Thus there are several protective mechanisms that enable the kidneys to regulate blood volume and guard against anoxia.

A decrease in blood volume stimulates receptors in the left atrium of the heart and the lungs. This activates the release of **antidiuretic hormone (ADH)** from the posterior pituitary gland. ADH increases the quantity of water returned from the distal collecting tubule to the bloodstream. As a result, urine volume decreases and blood volume increases. Another hormone that affects blood volume is **aldosterone,** which is produced by the adrenal cortex and acts on the distal convoluted tubule. A decrease in blood volume stimulates the release of aldosterone. Aldosterone causes salt and water to be reabsorbed from the nephron into the bloodstream, which increases blood volume.

A third mechanism affecting blood volume is the juxtaglomerular apparatus. This system is located at the point where the afferent and efferent arterioles and distal convoluted tubule come into contact (Figure 12-14). Granular cells in the afferent arteriole detect a decrease in blood volume. The granular cells release **renin,** which acts on angiotensinogen in the blood to increase systemic pressure. Cells in the distal convoluted tubule in contact with the afferent and efferent arterioles are

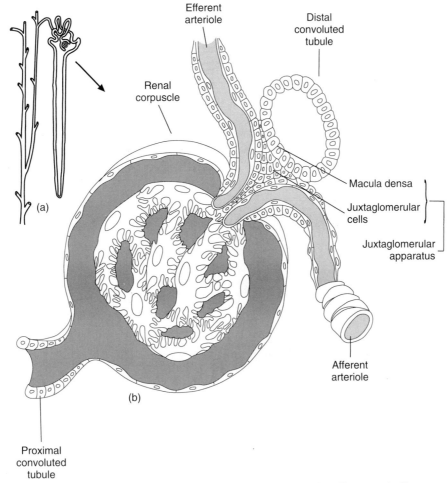

Figure 12-14 Juxtaglomerular apparatus. Note granular cells in the afferent and efferent arterioles. The macula densa are located in the distal convoluted tubule.

called macula densa (see Figure 12-14). It is believed that the macula densa can inhibit renin secretion when the blood volume returns to normal.

The kidneys produce another hormone that affects blood volume. **Erythropoietin** is released in response to a decrease in oxygen (e.g., due to hemorrhage). Erythropoietin acts on bone marrow, causing red blood cells to be produced. It also causes mature red blood cells stored in the bone marrow to be released into the bloodstream. This mechanism increases the number of

red cells in the blood, thus enhancing the ability of the blood to carry oxygen.

Another protective mechanism takes place during prolonged anoxia. Blood is shunted from the outer cortex to the inner cortex to maintain renal function. The kidneys are also able to decrease resistance in the renal capillary bed (increasing the blood supply to the kidneys), when systemic pressure drops.

See Table 12-5 for a summary of the kidneys' protective mechanisms.

■ ▨ ▨ **Table 12-5** Protective Mechanisms

Source	Functions	Effect
Kidney	1. Decreases renal capillary bed resistance	Increases blood supply to kidneys
	2. Moves blood from outer cortex to inner cortex	Preserves renal function in severe blood loss
	3. Makes erythropoietin	Increases amount of red blood cells to carry oxygen
Juxtaglomerular apparatus of kidney	Makes renin	Increases systemic pressure
Adrenal cortex	Secretes aldosterone	Increases blood volume
Posterior pituitary gland	Secretes antidiuretic hormone	Increases blood volume

SONOGRAPHIC APPEARANCE
Kidneys

In a longitudinal section the normal adult kidney appears as a heterogeneous, smooth contoured, elliptical structure (Figure 12-15). In a transverse section the kidney also appears heterogeneous with a smooth contour, but is rounded and broken medially by the renal hilum. The renal vein and artery can be visualized in this hilar region (Figure 12-16).

A detailed description of the sonographic pattern of normal renal anatomy follows (see Figures 12-15 and

12-16). The descriptions begin with the outer edge, the renal capsule, and end at the center of the kidney, the renal sinus.

Renal Capsule. This fibrous **capsule** appears as a thin, continuous, highly reflective line visualized along the periphery of the kidney; it is hyperechoic to the adjacent renal cortex.

Renal Cortex. The **renal cortex** presents as mid-gray or medium- to low-level, homogeneous echoes that are less than or equal to the density of the liver or spleen. Extensions of the cortex seen between the medullary

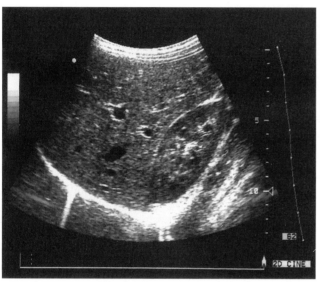
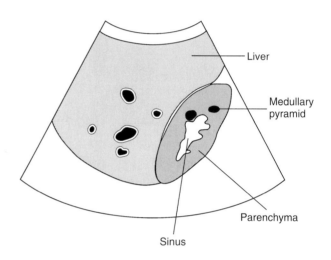

Figure 12-15 Sagittal scan and longitudinal view of the right kidney. The liver is superoanterior to the kidney. The curvilinear, highly echogenic line between the liver and right kidney is **Morison's pouch,** a peritoneal space. Note the anechoic areas within the renal parenchyma representing the renal pyramids. The hyperechoic area in the center of the kidney represents the renal sinus.

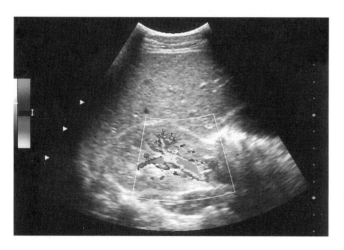
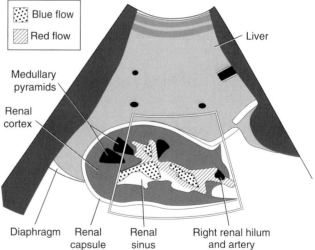

Figure 12-16 Color Doppler image of the right renal hilum. Transverse section of the right kidney shows the rounded pole. The liver is anterior. Note the hilar area, where the renal artery and vein are located. (See Color Plate 23.)

pyramids are referred to as the columns of Bertin. The discrete, hyperechoic dots that may be seen at the corticomedullary junction are the arcuate vessels; they serve as a marker for evaluation of cortical thickness.

Renal Medulla. The **renal medullae** of the parenchyma, or medullary pyramids, appear as triangular, round, or blunted hypoechoic areas compared with the more urine-filled anechoic areas. They are 1.2 to 1.5 cm thick. Anechoic pyramids have a distinctive and readily identifiable appearance; their echo-free presentation is in sharp contrast to the highly echogenic sinus and medium gray cortex.

Renal Sinus. The **renal sinus** presents as the echodense, ovoid center of the kidney with irregular borders. The sinus is markedly echogenic due to the fat and fibrous tissue it contains. It also houses the collecting system, lymphatics, and renal vessels. The renal pelvis and infundibulum of the collecting system are not seen if collapsed; otherwise they appear anechoic from being filled with urine. In most cases, normal lymphatics are not visualized.

Figures 12-17 through 12-20 show longitudinal views of the right and left kidneys. Transverse views of both kidneys are shown in Figures 12-21 through 12-24.

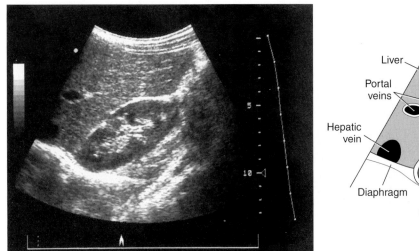
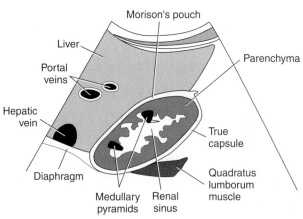

Figure 12-17 Sagittal scan and longitudinal view of the right kidney. Note the highly reflective, hyperechoic sinus. The renal parenchyma can be described as heterogeneous because the otherwise homogeneous cortex is interrupted by anechoic medullary pyramids. Also, notice that the renal cortex is hypoechoic to the liver parenchyma and that they are separated from each other by the hyperechoic Morison's pouch.

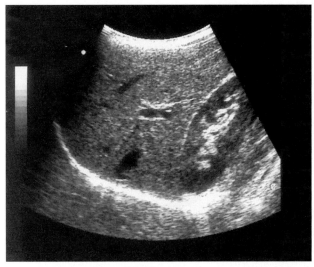
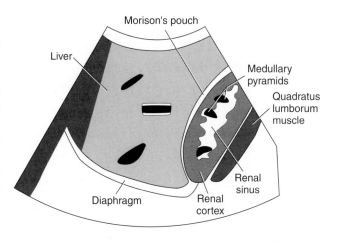

Figure 12-18 Sagittal scan and longitudinal view of the right kidney. Again, notice the hyperechoic renal sinus and Morison's pouch. Observe how the liver is slightly hyperechoic compared with the renal cortex.

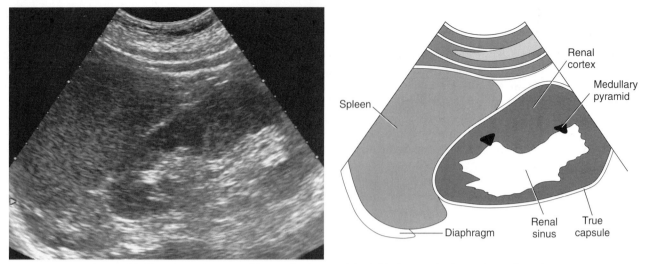

Figure 12-19 Coronal scan and longitudinal view of the left kidney and spleen. Notice how the renal cortex is hypoechoic compared with the spleen. Also note the anechoic pyramids adjacent to the hyperechoic sinus.

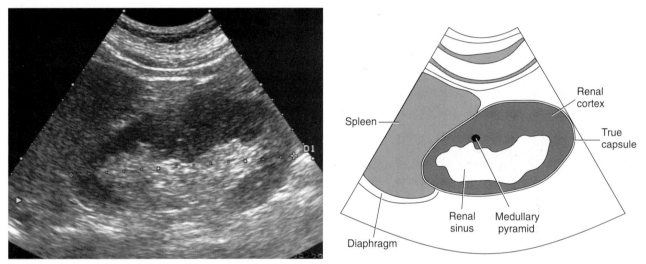

Figure 12-20 Coronal scan and longitudinal view of the left kidney. The long axis (longest length) of the left kidney is visualized. Note the well-defined, hyperechoic renal sinus.

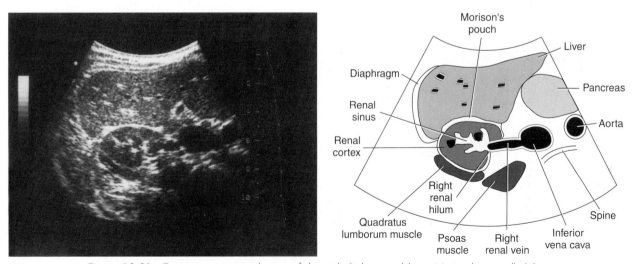

Figure 12-21 Transverse scan and view of the right kidney and liver. Notice how well delineated Morison's pouch is on this view. Observe how the anechoic right renal vein exits the renal hilum and enters the anechoic inferior vena cava. The anechoic aorta can be identified immediately left lateral to the inferior vena cava. Also, note how the psoas and quadratus lumborum muscles are hypoechoic compared with the renal cortex and sinus.

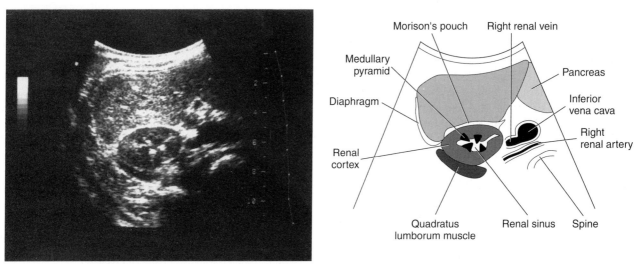

Figure 12-22 Transverse scan and view of the right kidney. Notice the distinctive shape of this short axis of the kidney. The kidney is seen between the anterior liver and posterior quadratus lumborum muscle. Observe how the homogenous columns of Bertin extend between the anechoic pyramids to meet the hyperechoic renal sinus. Note the portion of anechoic right renal vein and inferior vena cava just medial to the kidney.

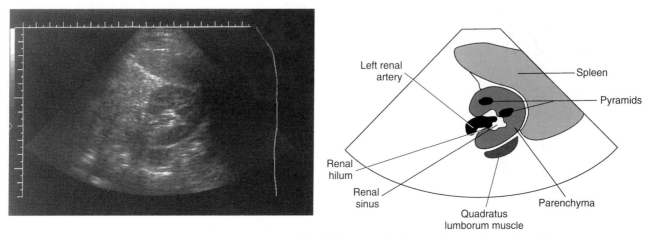

Figure 12-23 Transverse scan and view of the left kidney and spleen. Observe the anechoic left renal artery entering the renal hilum. Note the anechoic pyramids lateral to the highly reflective sinus.

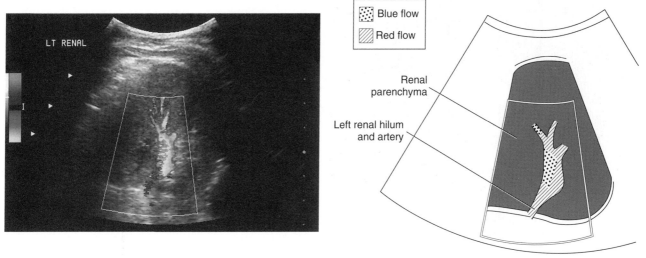

Figure 12-24 Transverse scan with color Doppler of the renal hilum of the left kidney. (See Color Plate 24.)

Renal vasculature is identified as anechoic lumens surrounded by hyperechoic walls, which can be followed to their origin (Figure 12-25).

Caliper placement for renal measurements is shown in Figure 12-26. Compare the size of the adult kidney shown in Figure 12-26 with the kidney size in the fetus, neonate, and child shown in Figure 12-27. Normal renal length in children can range from approximately 4.48 cm in the neonate to the normal adult size of 9 to 12 cm by the time the child reaches adolescence.

Next, compare the ultrasound appearance of the adult kidney shown in Figure 12-26 with the kidneys shown in Figure 12-27. Note that the renal cortex in the normal pediatric kidney is hyperechoic to the cortex in the adult kidney. Also, the renal pyramids in the pediatric kidney are more visible than the pyramids in the adult kidney. The pediatric renal pyramids are so readily distinguishable that a novice sonographer may mistake them for cystic masses within the kidney.

Ureters

The ureters are not normally visible. However, the effect of the ureters ejecting urine into the bladder, called ureteral jets, can be observed on real-time examination (Figure 12-28).

Urinary Bladder

In a transverse section the bladder appears somewhat squared by the laterally lying psoas muscles. The anechoic urine in the urinary bladder provides an excellent medium to visualize urinary bladder filling. The trigone, the area where the ureters enter the urinary bladder, is located along the posterior border of the bladder. Squirts of urine can be seen entering the urinary bladder in this area. This action, called ureteral jets, can be seen in as little as 20 minutes after ingestion of large amounts of water in a well-hydrated patient (see Figure 12-28).

In a longitudinal section the posterior surface of the bladder may be somewhat indented by an anteverted uterus or an enlarged prostate (Figure 12-29). Ureteral jets can also be seen in this image. The size and shape of the bladder vary due to the quantity of urine stored. Nevertheless, the distended bladder should appear symmetric.

The bladder lumen is not visible if it is collapsed; otherwise it appears anechoic. The distended bladder wall appears as a smooth, hyperechoic line compared with the urine-filled anechoic lumen.

Urethra

The urethra, when visualized, appears hyperechoic to surrounding structures.

Renal Doppler may be used to assess arterial and venous blood flow in kidneys. It is also used in assessing blood flow in renal transplant patients. However, research has shown that renal Doppler alone cannot effectively evaluate transplant patients for signs of acute rejection. Renal Doppler has also been used to detect vascularity in renal tumors and atriovenous malformations.

The Adrenal Glands

The adrenal glands are only briefly discussed in this section, because in the adult they are difficult to visualize sonographically. The glands are much more readily detected in fetuses and young children. This has been attributed to adrenal size. The infant adrenal is proportionately larger than the adult adrenal. At birth, the adrenal is one third the size of the kidney, whereas in the adult, it is one thirteenth the size of the kidney. Normally, the adult adrenal glands appear as distinct hypoechoic structures. In some cases, only the highly reflective fat that surrounds them is seen. In the neonate, the adrenals are characterized by a thin hyperechoic core surrounded by a thick anechoic zone.

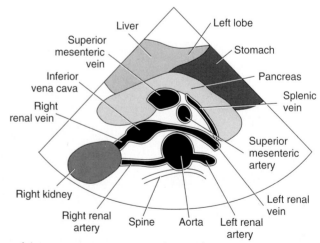

Figure 12-25 Renal vasculature. Transverse scan of the epigastric region. Note the renal veins anterior to the renal arteries.

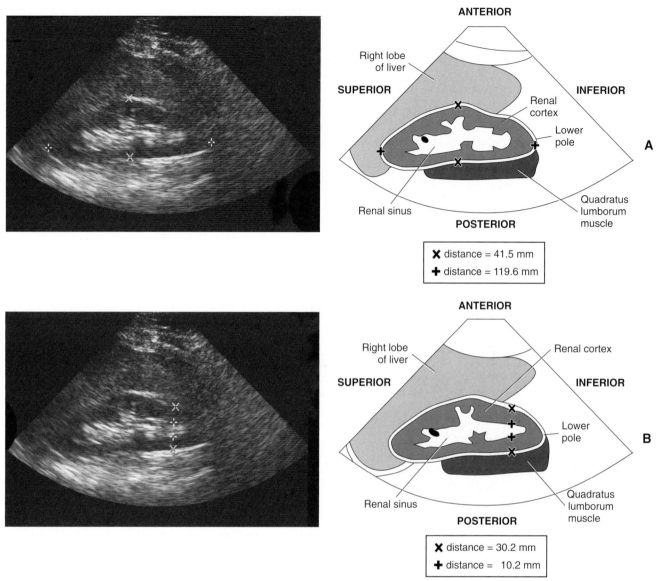

Figure 12-26 **A,** Long axis measurement of the right kidney. The length (superior to inferior) and anteroposterior dimensions are measured and are within normal limits. **B,** Longitudinal view of the right kidney demonstrating the renal sinus measurement compared with the anteroposterior measurement. The anteroposterior renal sinus measurement is approximately ⅓ that of the anteroposterior measurement. Note that a cortical thickness measurement can be obtained by subtracting the anteroposterior renal sinus measurement from the anteroposterior kidney measurement.

This section will take a brief look at the anatomy and physiology of the adrenal gland.

The adrenals are paired endocrine organs located at the superior and medial border of the kidneys. They are approximately 2 inches in length, 1.1 inch in diameter, and 0.4 inch in depth. The glands are enclosed with the kidneys in Gerota's fascia and are surrounded by fat. Each gland consists of an outer cortex and an inner medulla (Figure 12-30). The cortex and medulla function independently; thus the adrenal is actually two hormonal glands in one.

The cortex contains three areas called zones. Each zone produces steroid hormones, commonly called corticoids. The zone at the outermost portion of the cortex is called the zona glomerulosa. It produces mineralocorticoids, of which the most important is aldosterone; aldosterone regulates sodium and potassium levels. The next zone is called the zona fasciculata. It produces glucocorticoids. Cortisol is its primary substance; it regulates glucose metabolism. The innermost zone is called the zona reticularis. It supplements the sex hormones produced by the reproductive organs, the ovaries and testes.

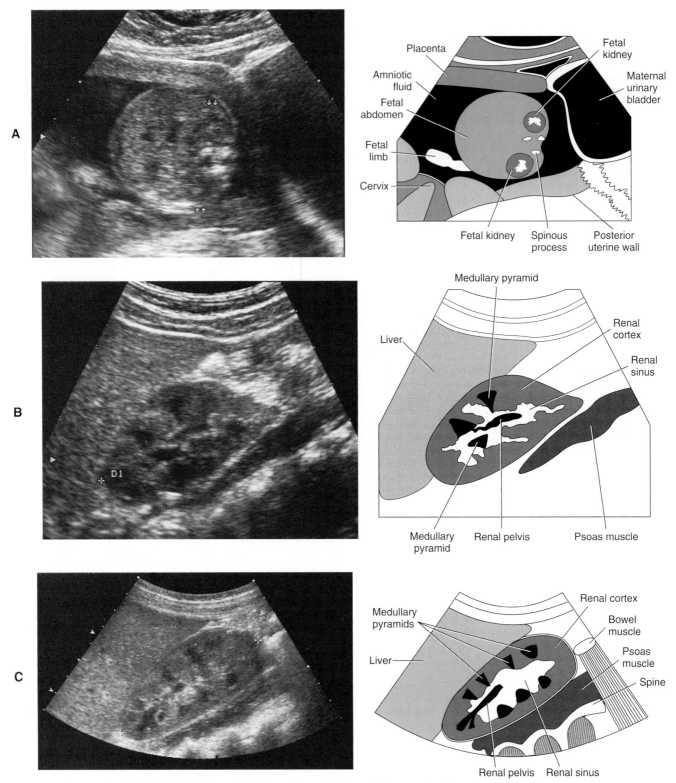

Figure 12-27 Pediatric kidneys in chronologic order by age in different patients. **A,** Fetal kidneys. **B,** A 3-week-old neonate. **C,** A 7-year-old child.

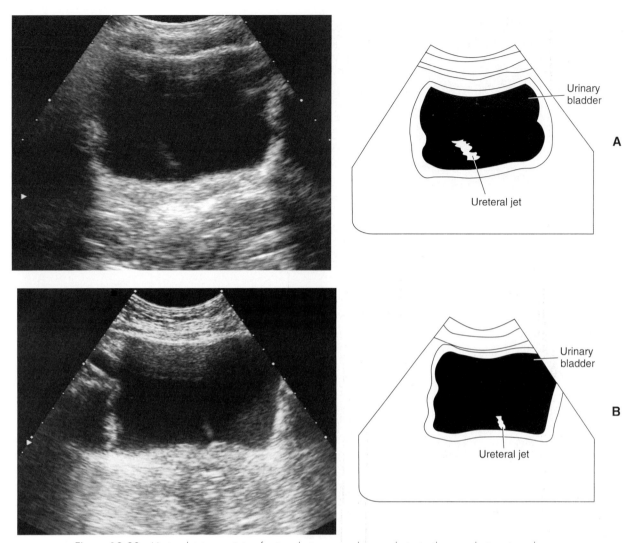

Figure 12-28 Ureteral jets are jets of urine that appear hyperechoic to the anechoic urine already within the bladder because the ureteral jets are visualized in motion as the urine squirts into the bladder from the ureter(s). **A**, Ureteral jet from the left ureter entering the distended bladder. **B**, Hyperechoic ureteral jet seen squirting into the anechoic urine-filled bladder.

The adrenal medulla is composed of chromaffin cells. They secrete epinephrine and norepinephrine. The adrenals produce four times as much epinephrine as norepinephrine. These hormones are responsible for the "flight or fight" response. Their effects include an increase in heart and respiratory rates and dilatation of the coronary blood vessels.

The adrenals are supplied with blood from the suprarenal arteries (Figure 12-31). The right suprarenal artery originates slightly inferior to the superior mesenteric artery and slightly superior to the right renal artery. The left suprarenal artery is a branch of the inferior phrenic artery, which arises directly from the aorta. The origin of the inferior phrenic artery is more superior than the origin of the right suprarenal artery. The left phrenic artery originates slightly inferior to the celiac axis and slightly superior to the origin of the superior mesenteric artery.

The adrenals are drained by the suprarenal veins (see Figure 12-31). The left suprarenal vein drains into the left renal vein, which then drains into the inferior vena cava, while the right suprarenal vein drains directly into the inferior vena cava.

SONOGRAPHIC APPLICATIONS

Sonography is used to evaluate several aspects of the urinary system. Common considerations include:
Renal size
Detection and composition of renal masses and
    cysts
Urinary system obstruction
Renal abscess

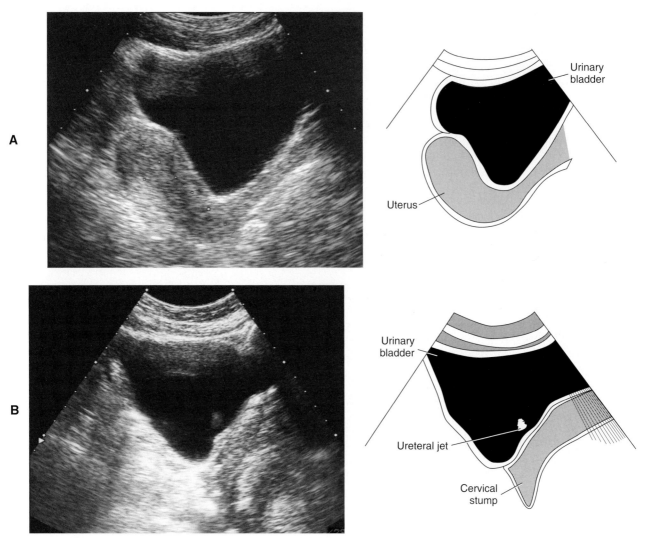

Figure 12-29 Urinary bladder. Note the highly reflective, hyperechoic walls compared with the anechoic, urine-filled lumen. **A,** Distended urinary bladder. Note the uterus posterior to the bladder. **B,** Sagittal scan and longitudinal view showing a right ureteral jet.

Renal hematoma
Enlarged ureters
Urinary bladder masses
Renal transplantation
Doppler evaluation of renal blood flow abnormalities
Ultrasound-guided biopsies of renal parenchyma or
    masses
Ultrasound-guided fluid aspirations

NORMAL VARIANTS

The following normal variants can be observed on ultrasound (Figure 12-32).

Dromedary Hump

A dromedary hump is a localized bulge(s) on the lateral border of the kidney. It has the same sonographic appearance as a normal renal cortex (see Figure 12-32, *A*).

Hypertrophied Column of Bertin

A hypertrophied column of Bertin occurs in varying degrees of size and may indent the renal sinus of the kidney. It has the same sonographic appearance as normal renal cortex (see Figure 12-32, *B*).

Double Collecting System

A double collecting system occurs when the renal sinus is divided (see Figure 12-32, *C*). Each sinus has a renal pelvis. A bifid (double) ureter may also be present.

Horseshoe Kidneys

A horseshoe kidney occurs when the kidneys are connected, usually at the lower poles (see Figure 12-32, *D*). It has the same sonographic appearance as normal renal tissue. However, the junction between the two kidneys can be visualized on sonography.

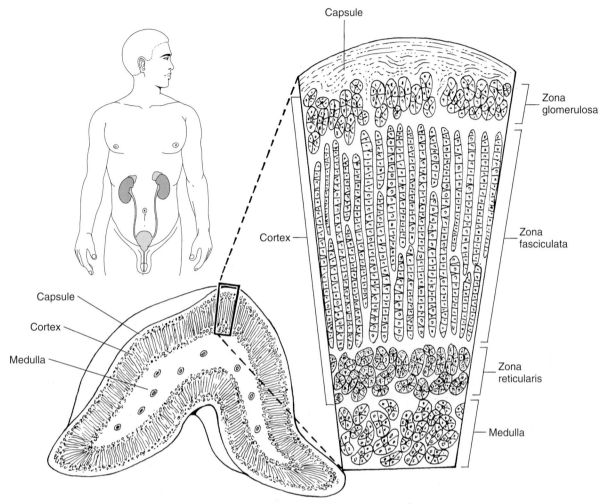

Figure 12-30 Zones of the adrenal cortex, zona glomerulosa, zona fasciculata, and zona reticularis. Also depicted is the adrenal medulla.

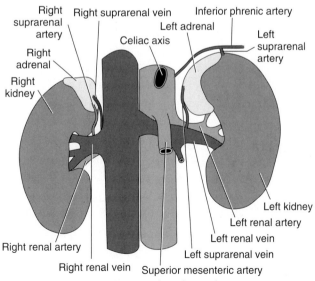

Figure 12-31 Adrenal vasculature.

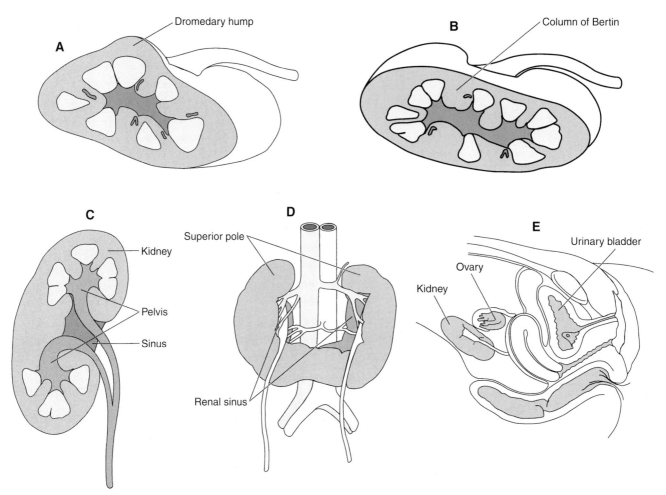

Figure 12-32 Renal variants. **A,** Dromedary hump. **B,** Column of Bertin. **C,** Double collecting system with double renal pelvis and partially bifid ureter. **D,** Horseshoe kidney connected at the lower poles. **E,** Sagittal adnexal section of the pelvis demonstrating an ovary and pelvic kidney.

Renal Ectopia

Renal ectopia occurs when one or both kidneys occur outside the normal renal fossa. Locations include the lower abdominal and pelvic region (see Figure 12-32, *E*). Other ectopic locations (e.g., intrathoracic) are rare.

REFERENCE CHARTS

■ ■ ■ ASSOCIATED PHYSICIANS

Urologist: Specializes in surgical diseases of the urinary system in the female and genitourinary tract in the male.
Nephrologist: Specializes in diseases of the kidney.
Radiologist: Specializes in the diagnostic interpretation of imaging modalities that assess renal disease.

■ ■ ■ COMMON DIAGNOSTIC TESTS

Intravenous Pyelogram (IVP): A radiologic examination in which a contrast medium ("dye") is injected into a vein

and x-ray films are taken at specific intervals to observe kidney function and urinary system anatomy. This test is performed by a radiologic technologist and radiologist. The examination is interpreted by the radiologist.
Computed Axial Tomography (CT scan): A radiologic examination in which cross-sectional x-ray images are obtained of the kidneys and other urinary system structures to assess anatomy. A contrast medium may be administered to differentiate between pathology and normal anatomy. This test is performed by a radiologic technologist and radiologist. The examination is interpreted by the radiologist.

■ ■ ■ LABORATORY VALUES

Blood Urea Nitrogen (BUN): Used to asses renal function. Normal BUN is 26 mg per dl. Elevation of this value may indicate renal disease.
Creatinine (Cr): Used to assess renal function. Normal Cr is 1.1 mg per dl. Elevation of this value may indicate renal disease.

■ ■ ■ NORMAL MEASUREMENTS

Adult Kidney: 9 to 12 cm in length; 4 to 6 cm in diameter; 2.5 to 4 cm in depth.
Neonatal Kidney: 3.5 to 5.0 cm in length; 2 to 3 cm in diameter; 1.5 to 2.5 cm in depth.
Ureters: 28 to 34 cm in length; 6 mm in diameter.
Distended Urinary Bladder Wall: 3 to 6 mm in depth.
Female Urethra: 4 cm in length.
Male Urethra: 20 cm in length.

■ ■ ■ VASCULATURE

Aorta→Renal artery—Interlobar artery—Arcuate artery—Interlobular artery—Afferent arterioles—Glomerulus—Efferent arteriole—Peritubular capillaries—Interlobular vein—Arcuate vein—Interlobar vein—Renal vein—Inferior vena cava.

■ ■ ■ AFFECTING CHEMICALS

Aldosterone: A hormone that increases salt and water reabsorption by the kidneys.
Renin: A hormone that helps the kidneys maintain blood pressure.
Antidiuretic Hormone (ADH): A hormone that increases water reabsorption.

BIBLIOGRAPHY

Abu-Yousef MM, Narayana AS, Brown RC, et al: Urinary bladder tumors studied by cystosonography, part II: staging, *Radiology* 153:227-231, 1984.

Alcamo IE: *Anatomy coloring workbook,* State University of New York, New York, 1997, Random House.

Anthony CP, Thibodeau G: *Textbook of anatomy and physiology,* ed 14, St Louis, 1983, Mosby.

Bo WJ, Wolfman NT, Krueger WA, et al: *Basic atlas of sectional anatomy with correlated imaging,* ed 3, Philadelphia, 1998, WB Saunders.

Clements CD: *Anatomy: a regional atlas of the human body,* ed 2, Baltimore, 1981, Urban & Schwarzenberg.

Coleman B: *Genitourinary ultrasound,* New York, 1988, Igaku-Shoin.

Craig TS, Madsen KM: Anatomy of the kidney. In Brenner BM, Rector FC, editors: *The kidney,* ed 3, Philadelphia, 1986, Ardmore.

Drake DG, et al: Doppler evaluation of renal transplants in children: a prospective analysis with histopathologic correlation, *Am J Radiol* 154:785-787, 1990.

Fong E, et al: *Body structures and functions,* ed 6, New York, 1984, Delmar.

Frick H, Leonhardt H, Starck D: *Human anatomy two,* New York, 1991, Thieme.

Friedland GW, Cunningham J: The elusive ectopic ureterocele, *Am J Radiol* 116:792-811, 1972.

Gosling A, Dixon S, Humpherson JR: *Functional anatomy of the urinary tract,* Baltimore, 1982, University Park.

Gray H, Goss M: *Anatomy of the human body,* ed 27, Philadelphia, 1965, Lea & Febiger, pp 1337-1345.

Guyton, AC: *Textbook of medical physiology,* ed 10, Philadelphia, 2000, WB Saunders.

Jacob W, Francone CA: *Elements of anatomy and physiology,* ed 2, Philadelphia, 1989, WB Saunders.

Kier R, et al: Renal masses: characterization with Doppler ultrasound, *Radiology* 176:703-707, 1990.

Langebartel DA: *The anatomical primer: an embryological explanation of human gross morphology,* Baltimore, 1977, University Park Press.

Marsh DJ: *Renal physiology,* New York, 1981, Raven Press.

Martini F: *Fundamentals of anatomy and physiology,* ed 2, Englewood Cliffs, 1992, Prentice Hall.

McInnis AN, Felman AH, Laude JV, et al: Renal ultrasound in the neonatal period, *Pediatr Radiol* 12:15, 1982.

Mittelstaedt C: *Abdominal ultrasound,* New York, 1987, Churchill Livingstone.

Moore K: *Before we are born: essentials of embryology and birth defects,* ed 5, Philadelphia, 1998, WB Saunders.

Perrella RR, et al: Evaluation of renal transplant dysfunction by duplex Doppler sonography: a prospective study and review of the literature, *Am Kidney Dis* 20(6):544-550, 1990.

Rogers AW: *Textbook of anatomy,* New York, 1992, Churchill Livingstone.

Rosenbaum DM, Korngold E, Teele RL: Sonographic assessment of renal length in normal children, *Am J Radiol* 142:467-469, 1984.

Scanlon V, Sanders T: *Essentials of anatomy and physiology,* Philadelphia, 1991, FA Davis.

Scott JES, et al: Ultrasound measurement of renal size in newborn infants, *Arch Dis Child* 65:361-364, 1990.

Snell RS: *Clinical anatomy for medical students,* ed 2, Boston, 1981, Little, Brown.

Spitz L, Wurnig P, Angerpointer TA: Surgery in solitary kidney and corrections of urinary transport disturbances, *Prog Pediatr Surg* vol 23, 1989.

Takebayashi S, Aida N, Matsul K: Arteriovenous malformations of the kidneys: diagnosis and follow-up with color Doppler sonography in six patients, *Am J Radiol* 157:991-995, 1991.

VanDeGraaff KM, Fox SI: *Concepts of human anatomy and physiology,* ed 3, Dubuque, 1992, Wm C Brown.

Vander AJ: *Renal physiology,* ed 2, New York, 1980, McGraw-Hill.

Walsh C, Gittes RF, Perlmutter AD, Stamey A: *Campbell's urology,* ed 7, Philadelphia, 1998, WB Saunders.

Weill FS, Rohmer P, Zeltner F: *Renal sonography,* ed 2, New York, 1987, Springer-Verlag.

Wolfman NT, Bechtold RE, Watson NE: Chap 4. In Resnick L, Rifkin M, editors: *Ultrasonography of the urinary tract,* Baltimore, 1991, Williams and Wilkins.

■ **CHAPTER 13**

The Spleen

VIVIE MILLER AND CANDYCE JAMES

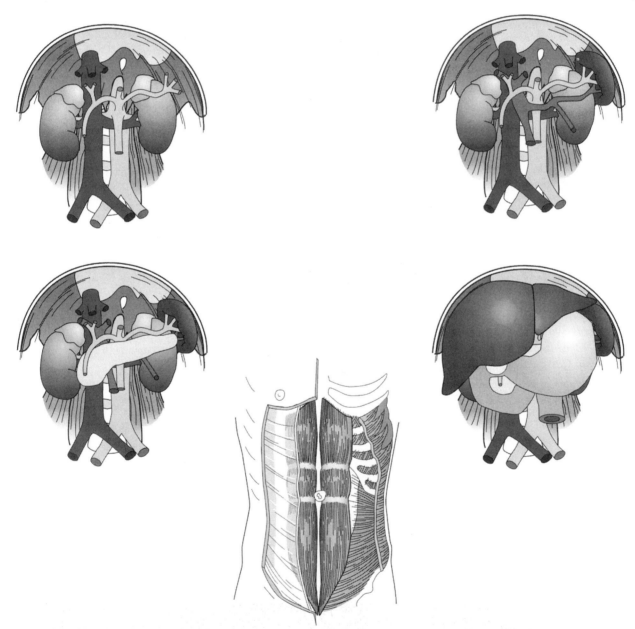

The spleen and surrounding anatomic layers. See Figure 4-3, **D, E, F, I,** and **J** for more details.

OBJECTIVES

Describe the function of the spleen.
Describe the location of the spleen.
Define size relationships of the normal spleen.
Describe the sonographic appearance of the normal spleen.
Describe the associated physicians, diagnostic tests, and laboratory values relevant to the normal spleen.
Define the key words.

KEY WORDS

Culling	Red pulp
Erythrocyte	Reticuloendothelial
Hematopoietic	Splenic artery
Hemoglobin	Splenic hilum
Hemosiderin	Splenic vein
Phagocytosis	White pulp
Pitting	

The spleen is an intraperitoneal organ that lies in the left upper quadrant of the abdominal cavity. It is part of the **reticuloendothelial** system. This system has the responsibility of **phagocytosis** (engulfing and destroying) of damaged or old cells and their debris, foreign materials, and pathogens, taking them out of the circulating blood. The spleen is composed primarily of lymph tissue. Although the spleen is a component of the body's defense system, it is not essential to life and can be removed without adverse effects (Figure 13-1).

PRENATAL DEVELOPMENT

Development of the spleen begins at about the fifth week of gestation, and arises from mesodermal cells. It begins as a thickening in the mesenchyme on the left side of the mesogastrium, or the omentum bursa. These mesenchymal cells differentiate into two types of cells—reticular cells, and primitive free cells that resemble adult lymphocytes. The spleen is separated from the stomach by the gastrolienal ligament and from the left kidney by the lienorenal ligament. The fetal spleen is normally quite lobulated (Figure 13-2).

During embryonic life, the spleen is important in producing red and white blood cells. It begins to perform this **hematopoietic,** or blood cell–producing, function by approximately the eleventh week of gestation. This activity is a result of tissue-myeloid functions. These functions generally end shortly after birth, but may reactivate in certain pathologic conditions. In adult life the spleen will continue to produce lymphocytes and monocytes.

By the fifth or sixth month of gestation, the spleen begins to assume its smooth ovoid adult shape and its adult functions. Its **white pulp,** which contains malpighian corpuscles, performs the lymphocytic functions. This distinct portion of the spleen begins to form late in fetal development.

The **red pulp** carries out various functions. The splenic cords house reticular cells, which are responsible for the reticuloendothelial functions of the spleen. This portion does not develop until after birth, when primary fetal blood cell formation ceases. The purpose of the red pulp is to destroy the degenerating red blood cells. This process is called phagocytosis.

LOCATION

The spleen lies in the left hypochondrium, with its longest axis along the tenth rib. It lies posterolateral to the body and fundus of the stomach, posterolateral to the tail of the pancreas, and posterior to the left colic flexure. The left kidney is located posteroinferior to the medial portion of the spleen. Posterior to the spleen are the diaphragm; the lung; and the ninth, tenth, and eleventh ribs. The spleen is covered by peritoneum, with the exception of the hilum. This portion of the spleen, located medially, is where the vasculature enters and exits (Figure 13-3).

SIZE

The size of the spleen varies in different individuals, and at different times it can vary in the same individual. Its longest dimension superior to inferior should be no greater than 12 or 13 cm. The largest transverse dimension (anterior to posterior) should be no larger than 7 or 8 cm.

The spleen is generally smooth in contour, with a convex superior surface and a concave inferior surface.

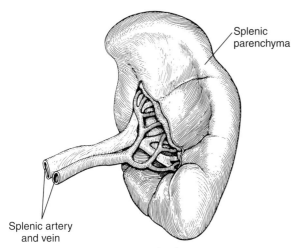

Splenic parenchyma

Splenic artery and vein

Figure 13-1 Normal splenic anatomy.

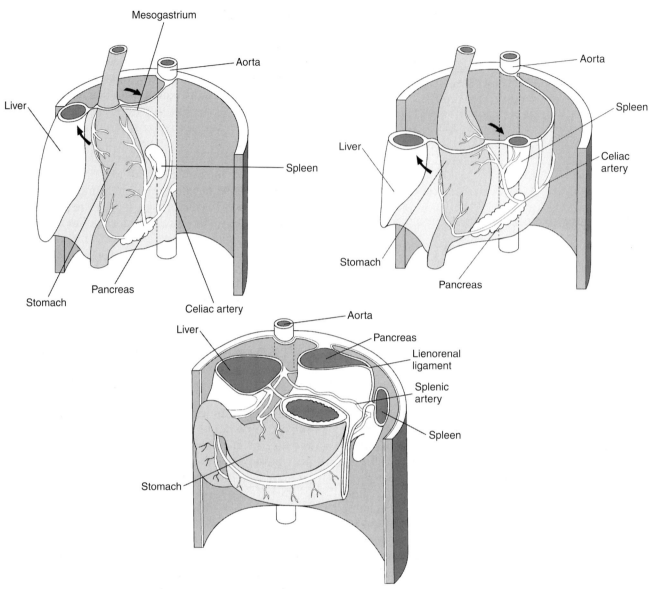

Figure 13-2 Early prenatal development of the spleen.

GROSS ANATOMY

The spleen is a highly vascular mass of lymphoid tissues located in the left upper quadrant of the abdomen. It is ovoid and has a convex superior surface and a concave inferior surface. The spleen is entirely covered by the peritoneum except at the hilum, where all vessels enter and leave. The **splenic vein** exits the hilum and courses along the gastrolienal ligament to its confluence with the superior mesenteric vein to form the portal vein. The **splenic artery,** which originates at the celiac trunk of the aorta, often branches into two or more smaller arteries before entering the hilum (see Figure 13-6).

The spleen's posterior location gives it the protection of the ribs. Consequently, the spleen is usually not palpable unless it is pathologically enlarged.

As described earlier, the spleen is composed of red pulp and white pulp. The white pulp consists of lymphatic tissue that surrounds and follows the smaller splenic arteries. The primary components of this portion of the spleen are the malpighian corpuscles. The red pulp, which is looser and more vascular, consists of the splenic sinuses and splenic cords. The sinuses are long, slender channels lined with epithelial cells. It occupies all of the space not filled by white pulp or splenic cords (see Figure 13-3, *C*).

PHYSIOLOGY

Four major functions of the spleen include defense, hematopoiesis, red blood cell and platelet destruction, and service as a blood reservoir. Functioning as a defense

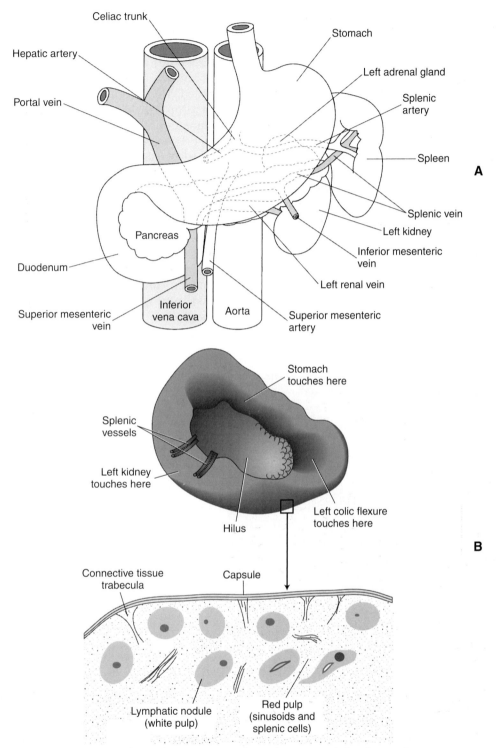

Figure 13-3 **A,** Surrounding splenic anatomic relationships. **B,** Medial surface and microscopic organization of the spleen.

mechanism, the spleen aids in the destruction and removal of microorganisms by phagocytosis. In the white pulp, lymphocytes and monocytes are continually produced and are active in ingesting and digesting harmful pathogens that enter the bloodstream. These cells are able to recognize foreign harmful substances and turn themselves into antibody-producing plasma cells and memory cells. The plasma cells destroy the invading microorganism by creating antibodies to that particular pathogen. The memory cells "remember" that particular pathogen and should it attack the body again, the antibodies to destroy it are quickly activated. This is called the "immune response."

The spleen in its hematopoiesis function produces red blood cells (and white blood cells) in the growing fetus. In the adult, however, red blood cell production is performed only in cases of severe hemolytic anemia.

Worn out and abnormal red blood cells and platelets are taken out of the bloodstream by the spleen. Blood passes through the red pulp and into the splenic sinuses. This portion of the spleen is a filter that aids in phagocytosis of degenerating red blood cells. The **hemoglobin** (iron-containing pigment) in these cells is broken down. The iron is either used immediately to produce new red blood cells or is transported via the portal vein to the liver and bone marrow for storage. The globin is used to break down other proteins for use in the body. The most abundant pigment released is **hemosiderin.** Iron can be stored in hemosiderin until it is needed to make more hemoglobin. Heme, also a pigment, is not needed and is turned into bilirubin and excreted by the liver in bile.

The ability of the spleen to store red blood cells (blood reservoir) is due to its high smooth-muscle content. The red pulp of the spleen with its venous sinuses holds a considerable volume of blood that can be quickly released into the circulatory system if needed. The spleen's average volume of about 350 ml can drop quickly and dramatically after sympathic stimulation that causes the smooth muscle to constrict. However, if the number of cells stored becomes excessive, splenomegaly will develop.

In summary, splenic functions can be divided into those related to the reticuloendothelial system and its functions as an organ. The reticuloendothelial system produces lymphocytes and plasma cells, as well as antibodies, and stores iron and metabolites.

As an organ, the spleen has the following functions: **erythrocyte,** or red blood cell surface, maturation; a reservoir; **culling** (removing the nuclei from red blood cells); **pitting** (removing senescent or abnormal red blood cells); and regulation of platelet and leukocyte life span.

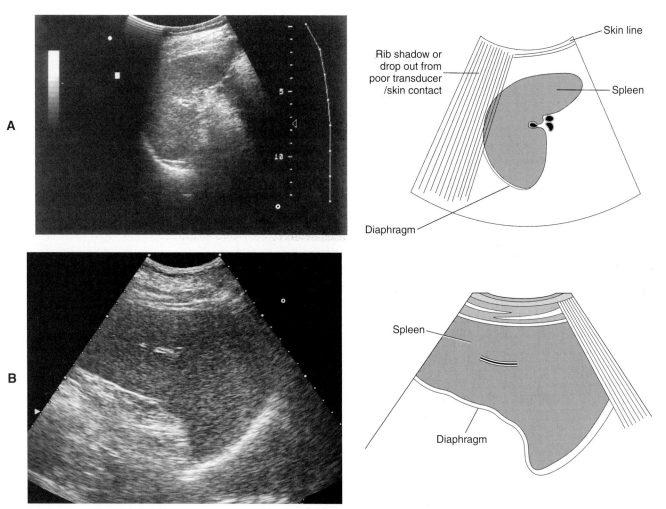

Figure 13-4 **A,** Normal spleen, coronal longitudinal approach. **B,** Normal spleen, a transverse left approach.

SONOGRAPHIC APPEARANCE

The spleen appears to be homogeneous in texture. It is very smooth and medium gray in color. It should be the same or less echogenic than the liver. Echogenic reflections may be seen that represent calcifications of small arterial walls or calcified granulomatous inclusions. The significance of the latter varies according to patient history. The organ may be difficult to visualize due to gas in the adjacent bowel and to the overlying ribs. It is often easiest to scan the spleen intercostally from a coronal approach. It is more readily visualized ultrasonically when pathologically enlarged (Figure 13-4).

SONOGRAPHIC APPLICATIONS

The most common use of sonography in imaging the spleen is to detect its enlargement.

Previously, when articulated arm B scanning was in wide use, the rule of thumb was that if the spleen was visualized anterior to the aorta, it was pathologically enlarged. Today, with real time scanning, the determination of splenomegaly has become basically a subjective judgment. The more experience the sonographer and interpreting physician have, the more accurate their judgment will be.

Ultrasound can help assess splenic masses. Primary splenic masses are quite rare. Ultrasound is also useful in assessing splenic damage from blunt trauma, such as rupture or hemorrhage.

NORMAL VARIANTS

Accessory Spleen

Accessory spleen is found in up to 10% of the general population. These islands of tissue are usually less than 1 cm in diameter. More than one accessory spleen may be present, most often near the splenic hilum or attached to the tail of the pancreas (Figure 13-5).

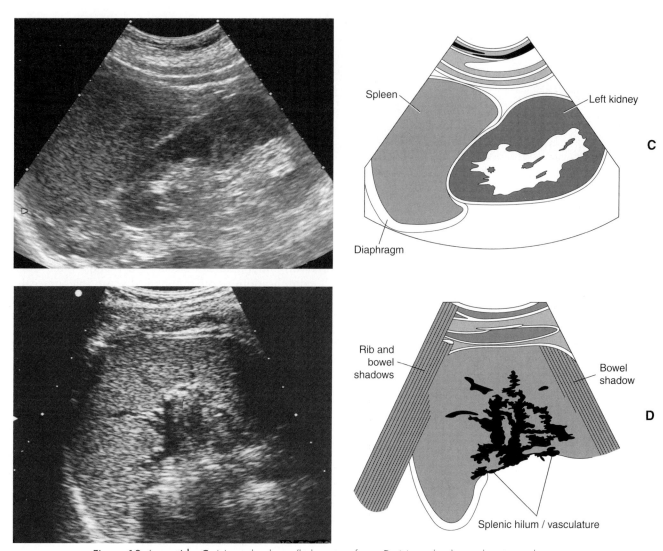

Figure 13-4, cont'd   C, Normal splenic/kidney interface. D, Normal spleen, showing splenic hilum.

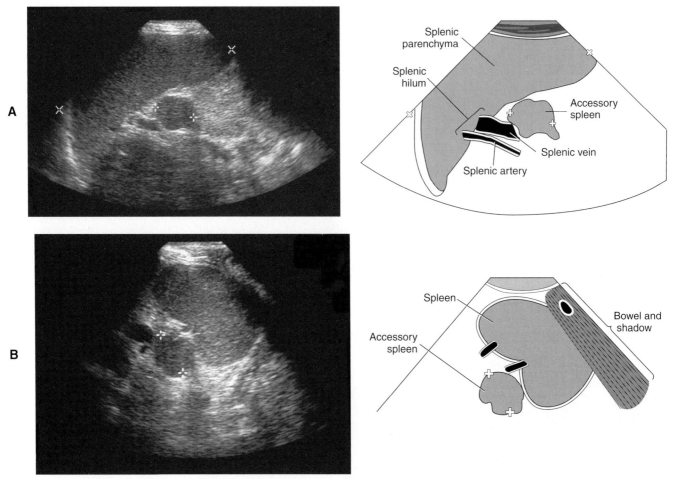

Figure 13-5 **A,** Longitudinal view of splenomegaly with an accessory spleen. **B,** Transverse left approach of same patient showing splenomegaly with an accessory spleen.

Asplenia

This rare congenital abnormality may be associated with a congenital heart defect. If solitary, there are no complications. The liver may be visualized more distinctly to the left of the midline than usual.

Splenomegaly

This pathologic finding is included because it is the most common splenic abnormality. It is most often due to complications of other organic disease. Splenomegaly is noted as a mass in the left upper quadrant. It may be due to recent trauma, portal venous congestion, systemic infection, or a blood disorder such as anemia.

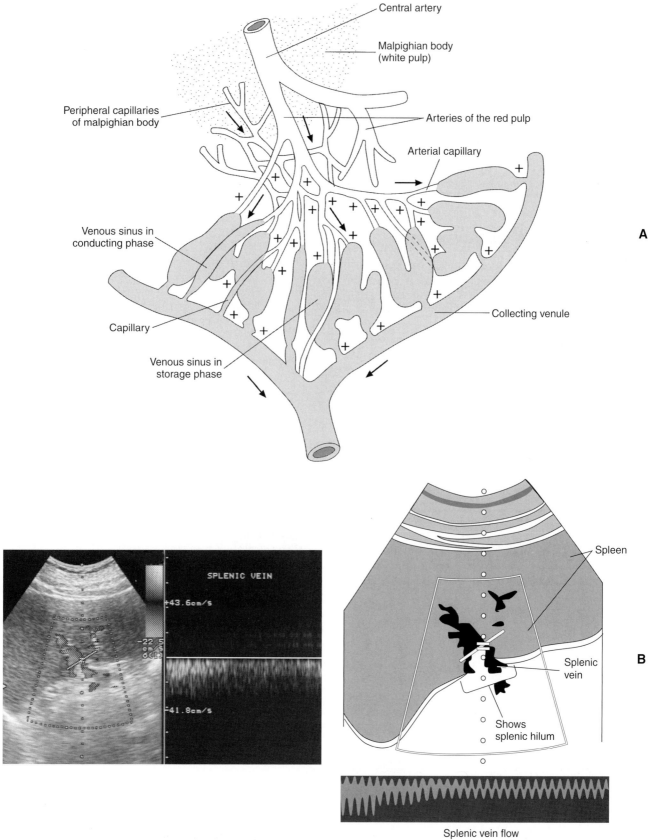

Figure 13-6 **A,** Vascular anatomy of the spleen. **B,** Normal splenic hilum showing splenic vein and Doppler tracing.

REFERENCE CHARTS

■ ■ ■ ASSOCIATED PHYSICIANS

Family Physician: Often serves as referring physician, coordinating patient care. In this capacity, the physician recommends referral to specialists when necessary.

Internist: Specializes in the diagnosis and treatment of internal disorders.

Surgeon: Specializes in performing surgical procedures.

Radiologist: Specializes in interpreting diagnostic imaging procedures.

Hematologist: Specializes in treating diseases of blood.

■ ■ ■ COMMON DIAGNOSTIC TESTS

X-Ray: In this test, ionized electromagnetic waves create photographic images, which are then "read" and interpreted. It is performed by a radiologic technologist and interpreted by a radiologist.

Ultrasound: Nonionized sound waves generate diagnostic images in this test. The sound waves do not penetrate bone or air. The test is performed by a sonographer and interpreted by a radiologist.

Nuclear Medicine: This test involves intravenous injection of radionuclides to create diagnostic images. The radionuclides "tag" specific cells, so that the resulting image is specific to the area of interest. This test is performed by a nuclear medicine technologist and interpreted by a radiologist.

Computed Axial Tomography (CT Scan): The ionized waves create a cross-sectional x-ray image of the body. This test is performed by a radiologic technologist who is certified for "CT" or "CAT scan," and is interpreted by a radiologist.

■ ■ ■ LABORATORY VALUES

Hematocrit: The hematocrit reading indicates the percentage of red blood cells per volume of blood. Normal values for men are 40% to 54%, for women, 37% to 47%. An abnormally low hematocrit points to internal bleeding.

Bacteremia: The presence of bacteria within the blood system, also known as sepsis. Symptoms include chills, fever, and possibly the presence of abscesses.

Leukocytosis: An increase in the number of circulating leukocytes (above 10,000 per cu mm). This finding is indicative of an infection of the blood. It may occur in hemorrhage, following surgery, in malignancies, during pregnancy, and in toxemia, and may be due to leukemia.

Leukopenia: An abnormally low number of leukocytes in the blood (below 5000 per cu mm). This may develop due to certain drugs, or to a bone marrow disorder.

Thrombocytopenia: An abnormal decrease in the number of circulating platelets. The normal range is 150,000 to 350,000 per cu mm. The decrease may be due to internal hemorrhage.

■ ■ ■ NORMAL MEASUREMENTS

The adult spleen is normally 12 or 13 cm in the superior to inferior axis; 6 or 7 cm in the medial to lateral axis; and 5 or 6 cm in the anterior to posterior plane.
Average volume is approximately 350 ml.

■ ■ ■ VASCULATURE

The splenic venous sinuses unite to form venules, which in turn merge to become the large splenic vein. The vein exits the hilum medially, coursing along the posterior border of the body and tail of the pancreas.

The spleen receives most of its blood supply through the splenic artery. This artery originates at the celiac axis from the aorta and courses laterally, serving as the superior border of the tail and body of the pancreas. The artery enters the splenic hilum medially, then branches into smaller arteries.

The smaller splenic arteries terminate in tiny capillaries that anastomose with the venous sinuses. The capillaries are permeable, which means that red blood cells can pass through them. This provides for the filtering functions of the spleen (Figure 13-6).

■ ■ ■ AFFECTING CHEMICALS

Anticoagulants: Thin the blood in patients whose blood tends to clot abnormally, or patients who are at high risk for developing thromboemboli. Patients receiving such treatment are more likely to experience internal hemorrhage or bleeding from small cuts that does not clot in a normal manner. The patient's hematocrit should be monitored.

BIBLIOGRAPHY

Moore KL, Persaud TVN: *The developing human: clinically oriented embryology,* ed 6, Philadelphia, 1998, WB Saunders.

Rumack CM, Charboneau W, Wilson SR: *Diagnostic ultrasound,* ed 2, St Louis, 1998, Mosby.

CHAPTER 14

The Gastrointestinal System

MARILYN DICKERSON

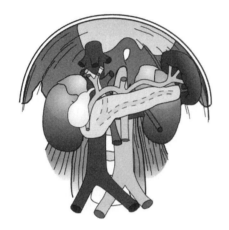

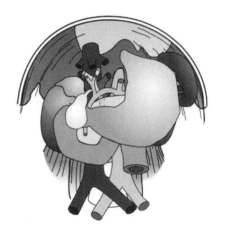

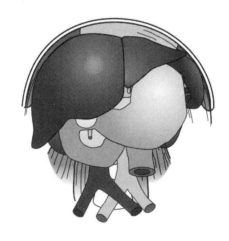

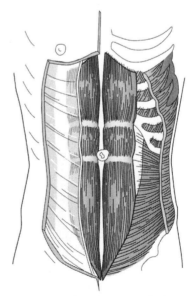

The gastrointestinal (GI) tract and surrounding anatomic layers. (See Figure 4-3, **G, H, I,** and **J** for more details.)

The gastrointestinal (GI) tract includes the mouth, pharynx, esophagus, stomach, and small and large intestines. It is also known as the **alimentary canal** (Figure 14-1).

The GI tract comprises a major portion of the digestive system. Food is ingested through the mouth and chewed. The salivary glands in the mouth release enzymes that initiate the breakdown of the food particles into small digestible molecules. The particles are then conveyed through the pharynx and esophagus to the stomach. In the stomach, food is mixed and the principal chemical changes occur; here food is reduced and converted to solution, stored, and then propelled into the small bowel.

Most of the digestive processes take place in the small bowel. Carbohydrates, proteins, fats, vitamins, and some fluids including water and electrolytes are digested and absorbed in the small bowel. The large bowel absorbs much of the remaining fluid and finally eliminates the undigested products.

PRENATAL DEVELOPMENT

The primitive gut develops from the posterior portion of the yolk sac during the fourth week of embryonic development. It is divided into four parts: the foregut, the midgut, the hindgut, and the tailgut.

A portion of the mouth, all of the pharynx, esophagus, stomach, and proximal duodenum originate from the **foregut** and are supplied with blood from the celiac axis artery. The remainder of the duodenum, the small bowel, and the colon as far as the middle and left thirds of the transverse colon originate from the **midgut.** Blood supply to the midgut is from the superior mesenteric artery. The **hindgut** gives rise to the remainder of the colon, supplied with blood from the inferior mesenteric artery. In the adult, these regions retain the same blood supply. The tailgut is resorbed.

The mouth and pharynx develop from the cranial part of the foregut. The tracheoesophageal septum divides the cranial portion of the foregut into the laryngotracheal tube and the esophagus.

The stomach originates as a fusiform dilatation of the caudal portion of the foregut. It is suspended from the dorsal wall of the abdominal cavity by the dorsal mesentery and attaches, along with the duodenum, to the developing liver and the ventral abdominal wall by the ventral mesentery. The liver, growing into the ventral mesentery, divides the mesentery into the falciform ligament and the lesser (gastrohepatic) omentum. The dorsal mesentary bulges ventrally as the greater omentum; the spleen appears in its craniolateral portion.

The final position of the stomach is the result of two rotations. The first rotation is 90 degrees around a vertical axis, moving the dorsal mesogastrium to the left and creating the **omental bursa** (lesser peritoneal cavity). The second rotation is around an anteroposterior axis, moving the pylorus to the right and superiorly and the proximal portion of the stomach to the left, resulting in the gastric cavity running from superior left to inferior right.

During embryogenesis, the midgut herniates out of and then back into the abdominal cavity (Figure 14-2). While outside, the midgut rotates 270 degrees counterclockwise and then returns to the abdomen. Thus the root of the mesentery becomes fixed, with one end at the ligament of Treitz and the other in the right iliac fossa. The colon returns next; distal bowel first and cecum, last. The colon wraps around the central small bowel and becomes fixed around the edge of the abdomen. This creates a "picture frame" for the small bowel.

The duodenum develops from both the caudal portion of the foregut and the cranial portion of the midgut, forming a C-shaped loop that projects ventrally. The lumen of the duodenum becomes reduced and may

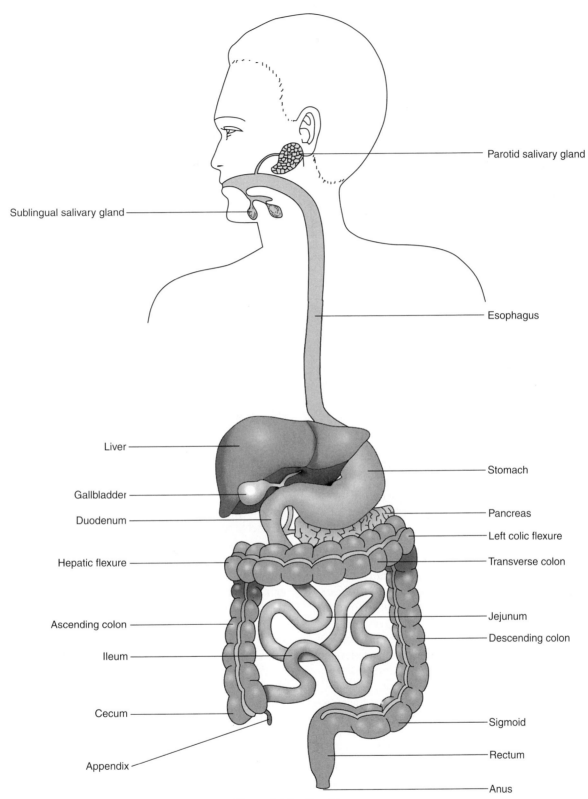

Parotid salivary gland

Sublingual salivary gland

Esophagus

Liver

Stomach

Gallbladder

Pancreas

Duodenum

Left colic flexure

Hepatic flexure

Transverse colon

Ascending colon

Jejunum

Descending colon

Ileum

Cecum

Sigmoid

Rectum

Appendix

Anus

Figure 14-1 The GI tract.

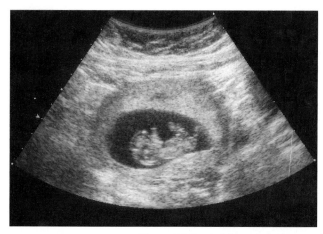
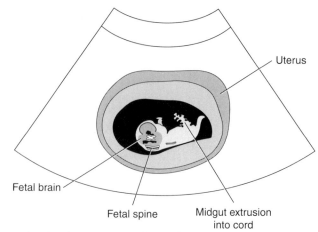

Uterus

Fetal brain

Fetal spine

Midgut extrusion
into cord

Figure 14-2 A 10-week-old fetus with normal midgut herniation into the cord.

be obliterated by epithelial cells. Normally the duodenum recanalizes and the lumen is restored.

The embryonic duodenum is the site of origin of the liver and pancreas; thus the excretory ducts of these two organs discharge into the developed structure.

The intestines project into the umbilical cord during the fifth week of embryonic development and return to the abdomen, coiling, during the tenth week, when the abdominal cavity has enlarged. Peristalsis occurs by the eleventh week and swallowing begins at week 12, and the intestines begin to fill with meconium. By the twentieth week the GI tract has reached its normal configuration and relative size.

The anal canal opens during week 7, when a membrane that separates the rectum from the exterior ruptures.

LOCATION

The mouth is placed at the origin of the alimentary canal, bound ventrally by the lips, laterally by the cheeks, anteriorly by the hard and soft palate, and posteriorly by the tongue. It communicates posteroinferiorly with the pharynx.

The pharynx is placed behind the nose, mouth, and larynx. It extends from the undersurface of the skull to the level of the cricoid cartilage in front and to the intervertebral disk between C5 and C6 behind.

Superiorly, the pharynx contacts the body of the sphenoid and basilar process of the occipital bone; inferiorly, it is continuous with the esophagus. Posteriorly, the pharynx is connected with the cervical portion of the vertebral column and the longus colli muscles. Anteriorly, it forms attachments to the lower jaw, the tongue, the hyoid bone, and the thyroid and cricoid cartilages. Laterally, the pharynx is in contact with the common and internal carotid arteries and the internal jugular veins.

The esophagus begins at the level of the cricoid cartilage of the neck, which is the level of the sixth cervical vertebra. The esophagus is a continuation of the pharynx and ends at the stomach, after passing through the left

dome of the diaphragm at the T10 level. It courses posterior to the trachea from the C7-T4 vertebral bodies.

As the esophagus continues through the thorax, it courses through the posterior portion of the middle **mediastinum** and is in contact with the aorta and its branches, the tracheobronchial tree, the heart, the lungs, and the interbronchial lymph nodes. Descending below the bifurcation of the trachea, it is in contact with the left atrium (base) of the heart.

The esophagus lies anterior to vertebral bodies C7 through T8. It courses inferiorly to the right of and slightly anterior to the descending aorta to enter the left diaphragmatic dome at T10.

The terminal part of the esophagus lies in a groove on the posterior aspect of the left lobe of the liver. It connects with the cardiac region of the stomach. The entrance of the esophagus into the stomach occurs at the **cardiac (esophageal) orifice.** This orifice marks the juncture of the greater and lesser curvatures of the stomach. The orifice is anterior to and slightly to the left of the abdominal aorta (Figure 14-3).

Above and to the left of the esophageal (cardiac) orifice, the fundus of the stomach curves superiorly to the left undersurface of the diaphragm.

The stomach lies in the left upper quadrant, within the left hypochondrium and epigastric regions. Its lower aspect lies on the transpyloric plane as it crosses the midline to reach its terminal point at the duodenum of the small intestine.

The left hemidiaphragm separates the stomach from the pleura of the left lung and the apex of the heart.

The anterior surface of the stomach is in contact with the diaphragm; the thoracic wall formed on the left by the seventh, eighth, and ninth ribs; the left lobe of the liver; and the anterior abdominal wall.

The stomach is suspended within the peritoneal cavity. The posterior surface of the stomach is related to the diaphragm, the gastric surface of the spleen, the left adrenal gland, the superior portion of the left kidney, the

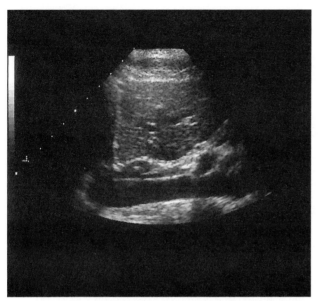
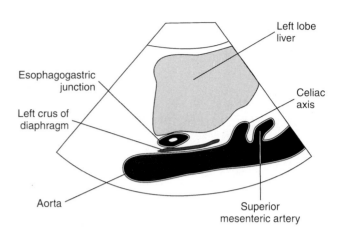

Figure 14-3 Longitudinal section just to the left of the midline, demonstrating the esophagogastric junction posterior to the left lobe of the liver.

anterior surface of the pancreas, the splenic flexure of the colon, and the ascending layer of the transverse mesocolon. These structures form a shallow bed on which the stomach rests. A small portion of the stomach, proximal to the cardiac orifice and in contact with the diaphragm and left adrenal gland, is not covered by peritoneum.

Posteroinferior to the stomach are the lesser sac, the pancreas, the left adrenal gland, the transverse colon, and the spleen.

The lesser curvature of the stomach marks the right border of the organ, extending between the esophageal (cardiac) and pyloric orifices.

The greater curvature marks the left border, descending in front of the left crus of the diaphragm along the left side of the eleventh and twelfth thoracic vertebrae.

This curvature crosses the first lumbar vertebra as it courses to the right and ascends to the pylorus.

The body of the stomach is in contact on the left with the left costal margin and the anterior abdominal wall. Inferiorly, it descends to the midlumbar vertebral level.

The antrum of the pylorus is near the midline and begins as a slight dilatation at the angular incisure in the lesser curvature. The antrum ascends, blending into the pyloric canal, which lies on the transpyloric plane between L1 and L2 vertebral bodies.

The pyloric orifice communicates with the duodenum. With the stomach empty, the pylorus is just to the right of the midline at the L1 vertebral level (Figure 14-4). A fully distended stomach may cause the pylorus to become situated 5 to 8 cm to the right of midline (Figure 14-5).

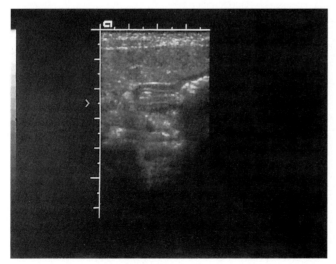
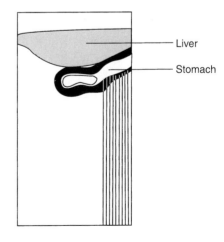

Figure 14-4 Transverse section demonstrating the long axis of the pylorus.

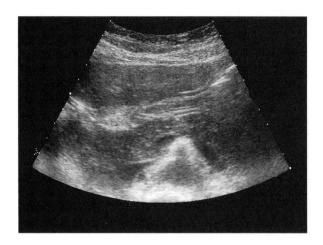

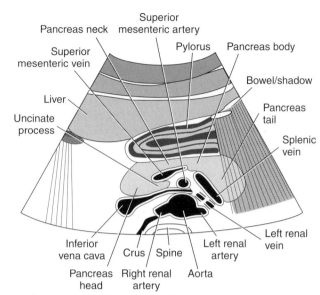

Figure 14-5 Transverse epigastric section showing the stomach wall anterior to the pancreas.

The small bowel is divided into three portions: duodenum, jejunum, and ileum; is related anteriorly to the greater omentum and the abdominal wall; and is connected to the spine by a fold of peritoneum, the **mesentery.** The small bowel is contained in the central and lower part of the abdominal cavity, and is surrounded superiorly and laterally by the large intestine, partly extending below the pelvic brim anterior to the rectum.

The first portion of the duodenum begins at the pylorus and ends at the neck of the gallbladder, posterior to the left lobe of the liver and medial to the gallbladder.

The **duodenal bulb** (first or superior portion) is peritoneal, supported by the hepatoduodenal ligament, and passes anterior to the common bile duct and the gastroduodenal artery, the common hepatic artery, the hepatic portal vein, and the head of the pancreas (Figure 14-6).

The descending duodenum is retroperitoneal and runs posteriorly, parallel and to the right of the spine. It extends from the gallbladder neck, at the level of the first lumbar vertebra, to the body of the fourth lumbar vertebra.

The transverse colon crosses anterior to the middle third of the descending duodenum and is connected by a small amount of connective tissue. The head of the pancreas is medial to this portion; lateral to it is the hepatic flexure of the colon. This portion receives the common

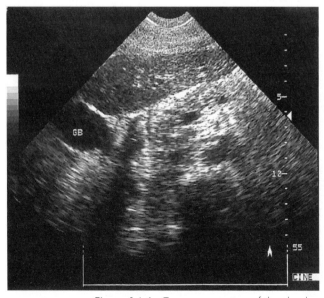

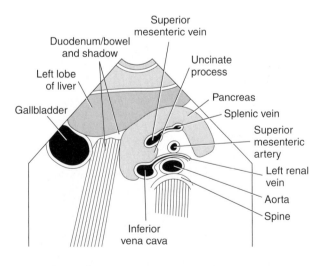

Figure 14-6 Transverse section of the duodenal bulb located between the gallbladder and the head of the pancreas.

bile duct via the ampulla of Vater and secondary pancreatic duct (Santorini's duct) if that is present.

The transverse (third) portion of the duodenum begins at the right of the fourth lumbar vertebra and passes from right to left, anterior to the great vessels and diaphragmatic crura, ending in the fourth portion just to the left of the aorta.

The superior mesenteric vessels course anteriorly to the transverse (third) portion of the inferior duodenum.

The gallbladder, the right lobe of the liver, and the medial portion of the left lobe of the liver are anterior to the C-shaped duodenum.

The fourth portion ascends superiorly on the left side of the spine and aorta as far as the level of the upper border of the second lumbar vertebra, where it bends ventrally and downward to join the proximal jejunum at the duodenojejunal flexure. The ascending portion lies on the left crus of the diaphragm.

The ascending (fourth) portion is held in place by the **suspensory ligament (ligament of Treitz),** a fibromuscular band that courses from the left toward the right crus of the diaphragm. The bowel leaves its retroperitoneal position and becomes intraperitoneal at the level of the suspensory ligament.

At the duodenojejunal flexure, the jejunum is contained within the peritoneum. The jejunum occupies the umbilical and left iliac regions, and the ileum occupies the umbilical, hypogastric, right iliac, and pelvic regions and terminates in the right iliac fossa by opening into the inner side of the origin of the large intestine.

The large intestine begins in the right inguinal region. The cecum is situated below the iliocecal opening as a blind cul-de-sac. The vermiform appendix opens into the cecum approximately 2 to 3 cm below the opening (Figure 14-7). The ascending colon arises from

the right iliac fossa, across the iliac crest, to the visceral surface of the right lobe of the liver. It bends at this point **(hepatic [right] flexure)** and becomes the transverse colon, which crosses the abdomen anterior to the duodenum and just below the transpyloric plane.

The pancreas is posterosuperior to the transverse colon.

Inferior to the spleen, the colon bends **(splenic flexure)** to descend on the left side of the abdomen into the left iliac fossa and over the pelvic brim, where it becomes the sigmoid colon. The pelvic sigmoid colon reaches the midline anterior to the sacrum, where it becomes the rectum, which then descends into the pelvic cavity to the level of the pelvic floor (diaphragm) (Figure 14-8). The rectum penetrates the levator ani muscle to become the anal canal.

At this point the anal canal crosses the pelvic floor, and the GI tract terminates through the opening of the anus.

SIZE

The pharynx is just under 10 cm in length and is broader in the transverse than in the anteroposterior diameter. The largest portion is opposite the cornua of the hyoid bone; its narrowest portion is at the termination in the esophagus.

The esophagus is a muscular tube approximately 23 cm in length. It is the narrowest part of the alimentary canal, and is most contracted at the origin and at the point where it passes through the diaphragm.

The size of the stomach varies considerably. In the adult male its capacity is 2 to 4 L. The greatest length of the stomach is from 25 to 30 cm, from the top of the fundus to the bottom of the greater curvature; its widest diameter is 10 to 12 cm. The distance between the two openings ranges from 7 to 15 cm.

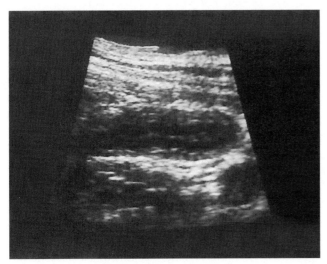
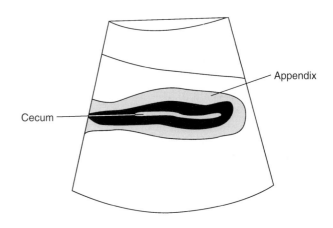

Figure 14-7 Longitudinal section of normal appendix found in the right lower quadrant. The appendix is not usually identified; this was a false positive.

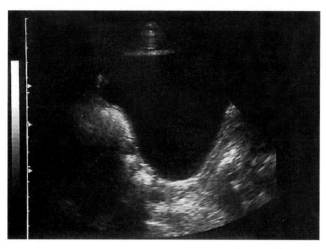
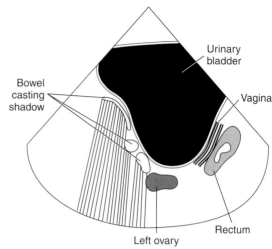

Figure 14-8 Longitudinal section of the rectum in the pelvis.

The pyloric canal is 2 to 3 cm in length.

The small intestine is approximately 6 m in length and 4 cm in diameter. It decreases in size from the origin to the termination.

The duodenum is the smallest, widest, and most fixed portion of the small intestine, measuring some 25 cm in length. It is subdivided into four parts. The superior duodenum (duodenal bulb) is 3 to 5 cm in length, the descending duodenum is approximately 10 cm in length, and the transverse and ascending portions are each 2.5 to 5 cm in length.

The jejunum comprises the upper two fifths of the remaining small intestine or some 2.3 m. Its width is approximately 4 cm. The ileum contains the lower three fifths (3.5 m) of the small bowel and is some 3 cm in diameter.

The large intestine is nearly 2 m in length, largest at the cecum and gradually diminishing in size to the rectum.

GROSS ANATOMY

The gut is a long, hollow tube composed of multiple layers contained within the abdominopelvic cavity and attached by the mesentery.

The esophagus is the most muscular structure of the GI tract. Its outer muscular layer is composed of longitudinal fibers; its inner muscle layer has a circular axis.

The arteries that supply the esophagus derive from the inferior thyroid branch of the subclavian artery, the descending thoracic aorta, the gastric branch of the celiac axis, and the left inferior phrenic artery of the abdominal aorta.

The stomach consists of smooth muscle cells arranged in three layers: an outer longitudinal layer, an inner oblique layer, and a circular middle layer. The two outer layers increase in thickness toward the small bowel.

The stomach has three parts: the fundus superiorly, the body (corpus), which is the major portion of the stomach, and the pylorus. The pylorus is subdivided into three regions: the antrum, the pyloric canal, and the pyloric sphincter.

Five ligamentous structures of the mesentery support the stomach. The **greater omentum,** the **gastrophrenic ligament,** the **gastrosplenic ligament,** and the **lienorenal ligament** support the surface of the greater curvature. The lesser curvature is supported by the **gastrohepatic ligament** of the **lesser omentum.**

Arterial flow to the stomach is supplied by the right gastric branch, the pyloric and right gastroepiploic branches of the hepatic artery, the left gastroepiploic branch and vasa brevia from the splenic artery, and the left gastric artery.

Veins of the stomach are generally parallel to the arterial vessels and drain into the portal system.

The small intestine, like the esophagus and the large intestine, has a two-layered muscular structure, with the outer layer of cells arranged longitudinally and the inner layer of cells following a circular axis.

The duodenum, the jejunum, and the ileum are the parts of the small intestine.

The duodenum is the C-shaped, most proximal portion of the small bowel and contains four segments: superior, descending, transverse, and ascending.

The first portion of the duodenum is not fixed, whereas the remaining portions of the small bowel are bound to the neighboring viscera and the posterior abdominal wall by the extensive peritoneal fold, the mesentery, which allows for freest motion. The fan-shaped mesentery contains blood vessels, nerves, lymphatic glands, and fat between its two layers.

The jejunum is distinguishable from the ileum by the presence of greater vascularity, the presence of **Brunner's (duodenal) glands,** which are similar to the pyloric glands of the stomach, large and thickly set valvulae conniventes, and larger villi. The **valvulae conniventes**

(valves of Kerckring) are large folds of mucous membrane that project into the lumen of the bowel and serve to retard the passage of food and provide a greater absorbing area. They begin to appear about 3 to 5 cm beyond the pylorus and almost entirely disappear in the lower part of the ileum. The ileum connects to the large intestine at the ileocecal orifice.

The large intestine is both shorter and larger than the small gut. This large gut contains the vermiform appendix; the cecum; the ascending, transverse, descending, and sigmoid colons; the right and left colic flexures; the rectum; the anal canal; and the anus.

The colon is divided into segments called **haustra.**

The celiac, superior, and inferior mesenteric arteries supply the small and large intestines. The celiac artery, arising off the anterior abdominal aorta, supplies the duodenum from its right gastric, gastroduodenal, and superior pancreaticoduodenal branches (Figure 14-9).

The superior mesenteric artery (SMA) arises from the anterior surface of the abdominal aorta, passes between the head and neck of the pancreas, and supplies branches to the intestines. The SMA branches to the small bowel include the inferior pancreaticoduodenal, the jejunal, and the ileal arteries (Figure 14-10).

The SMA branches to the large intestine include the ileocolic, the right colic, and the middle colic arteries.

The inferior mesenteric artery (IMA) supplies the large intestine from the left border of the transverse colon to the rectum, arising from the anterior surface of the abdominal aorta at the level of the third lumbar vertebra and descending retroperitoneally.

Branches of the IMA include the left colic, the sigmoid, and the superior rectal arteries.

Venous return from the small and large intestines empties into the portal system via vessels that parallel the SMA branches. These channels may drain directly

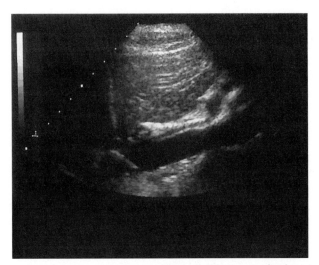
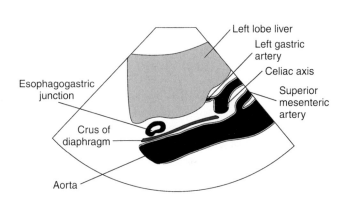

Figure 14-9 Longitudinal section demonstrating the left gastric artery.

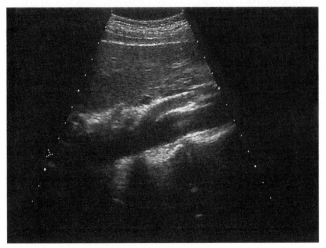
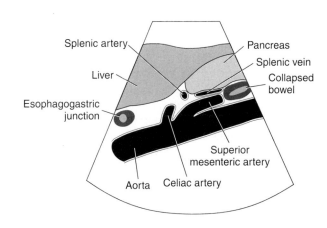

Figure 14-10 Longitudinal section of the superior mesenteric artery (SMA).

into the portal vein, the splenic vein, and the inferior mesenteric vein or the superior mesenteric vein.

The superior mesenteric vein courses to the right of the SMA and joins the splenic vein to form the portal vein, which enters the liver as its major blood supply.

PHYSIOLOGY

The primary functions of the GI tract are the digestion and absorption of nutrients.

The GI tract is the largest endocrine organ in the body. When food is eaten, nervous activity, distention, and chemical stimulation of the GI tract result in the release of hormones from endocrine cells scattered throughout the mucosa from the stomach to the colon. These hormones influence intestinal absorption and act on the secretion of enzymes, water, and electrolytes. The absorption of water, electrolytes, and nutrients influences the motility and growth of the GI tract.

Several GI hormones are well known. **Gastrin** is an endocrine hormone released from the stomach that stimulates the secretion of gastric acid. **Cholecystokinin** is released by the presence of fat in the intestine and serves to regulate gallbladder contraction and gastric emptying. **Secretin** is released from the small bowel and, as "nature's antacid," it stimulates the secretion of bicarbonate, naturally decreasing the acid content of the intestine.

The digestive system breaks down food products—carbohydrates, fats, and proteins—into small, absorbable nutrients.

The GI tract plays a major role in digestion. Food products are reduced to small, absorbable molecules by chemical actions. These actions are initiated by the enzymes present in the juices of the tract.

Food transport and digestion begin in the mouth. The oral cavity, pharynx, and esophagus are coordinated to prepare the food for transport and to transport it to the stomach. The esophagus has two major functions: transport of the food from the mouth to the stomach, and prevention of reflux of the GI contents.

The esophagus transports swallowed material from the pharynx to the stomach, using muscular contractions. The lower esophagus acts as a sphincter, controlling the passage of material entering the stomach. Reflux is prevented by closure of the upper and lower esophageal sphincters between swallows.

The stomach performs important functions related to the storage and digestion of food. It holds a large volume of ingested material, thus providing a storage function.

Digestion involves the breakdown, or hydrolysis, of nutrients to smaller molecules so that they can be absorbed or transported across the intestinal cell. Muscles of the stomach contract and mix the material ingested with gastric juice, thereby facilitating the digestive function of the stomach. The stomach contents are then propelled into the duodenum of the small bowel.

The digestion and absorption of all major food products take place in the small bowel. After the products mix with digestive secretions and enzymes, carbohydrates are reduced to monosaccharides and disaccharides, proteins to peptides and amino acids, and fats to monoglycerides and fatty acids. These nutrients are then absorbed through the intestinal mucosa into the bloodstream. They enter the general circulation via the capillaries into the portal system, or via the lacteals into the intestinal lymphatics. The remaining contents are moved to the large bowel for elimination.

In the large bowel, intestinal material is transformed from a liquid to a semisolid state by the time it reaches the descending and sigmoid colons, as water and electrolytes are absorbed. Most of the absorption process occurs in the cecum. In the sigmoid and rectum, the material is stored and then eliminated.

SONOGRAPHIC APPEARANCE

Visualization of the bowel is impeded by the presence of air or gas within the lumen, which will reflect the sound and thus prevent transmission of the beam (Figure 14-11). The sonographic appearance of bowel depends on the presence or absence of air, gas, feces, or fluid within the lumen, and on the recognition of anatomic landmarks.

The layers of the bowel wall create a characteristic appearance on sonography called a **gut signature,** wherein up to five layers can be visualized. The first, third, and fifth layers are echogenic, and the second and fourth layers are hypoechoic, with an average total thickness of 3 mm if distended and 5 mm if undistended.

Investigators differ as to the histologic structure of the wall layers visible on sonography. Pozniac describes the five principal layers as follows: **mucosa** directly contacts the intraluminal contents and is lined with epithelium having many folds, which increase the absorptive surface and give the mucosal layer its high echogenicity. The **submucosa** beneath it contains blood vessels and lymph channels in connective tissue. The third layer, **muscularis,** contains the circular and longitudinal bands of fiber. The **serosa** is a thin, loose layer of connective tissue, surrounded by the outermost single cell layer of **mesothelium** covering the intraperitoneal bowel loops.

The esophagus is normally recognized at the esophagogastric (EG) junction on a longitudinal scan of the aorta, just to the left of the midline (Figure 14-12). It appears as a target lesion, surrounded by the crura of the diaphragm and anterior to the aorta along the posterior aspect of the left lobe of the liver. The normal esophageal wall measures 5 mm. In the neck, it may be seen posterior to the thyroid gland on the left and is usually recognized by its bull's-eye appearance (Figure 14-13).

Empty loops of bowel also demonstrate the target (bull's-eye) pattern: a thin, hypoechoic sonolucent periphery with an echogenic center of varying size.

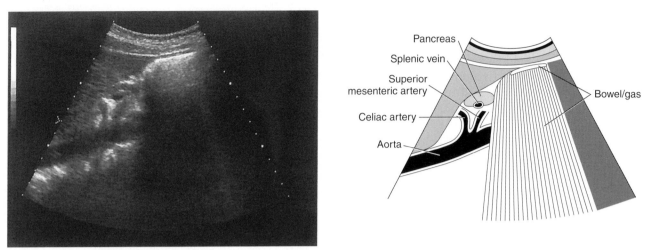

Figure 14-11 Longitudinal section of the abdominal aorta obscured by overlying gas-filled bowel.

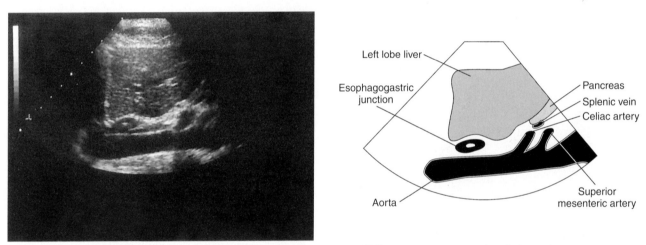

Figure 14-12 Longitudinal section of esophagogastric (EG) junction anterior to the abdominal aorta.

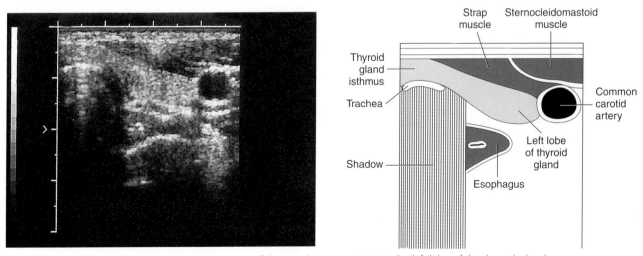

Figure 14-13 Transverse section of the esophagus posterior to the left lobe of the thyroid gland.

The stomach can usually be identified by its characteristic location between the free edge of the left lobe of the liver and the anterior surface of the spleen.

Separation of the fundus of the stomach and the left hemidiaphragm suggests a pathologic process in the subphrenic space, such as an abscess.

The collapsed antrum of the stomach lies anterior to the pancreas (Figure 14-14).

A large mass in the pancreas will displace the stomach anteriorly and perhaps superiorly.

Posterior displacement of the stomach is most probably caused by an enlarged left lobe of the liver, since this lobe is the only structure anterior to the stomach. Splenic enlargement tends to displace the stomach medially.

A fluid-filled stomach may simulate a cystic mass such as a pseudocyst in the left upper quadrant (Figure 14-15).

Sonographic visualization of peristalsis helps to identify bowel and thus differentiate it from cystic masses.

The duodenal bulb is related to the gallbladder and the transverse colon near the hepatic flexure. It is lateral to the head of the pancreas. The duodenum, the gallbladder, and the proper vascular landmarks form a triad that helps to localize the head of the pancreas. Gas in the duodenum, however, may mimic mass lesions or pseudomasses in the pancreas, or a stone-filled gallbladder (Figure 14-16).

A distended gallbladder will indent the superolateral aspect of the duodenal bulb and the descending duodenum.

The proximal portion of the jejunum is inferior to the body and tail of the pancreas and anterior to the left kidney (Figure 14-17).

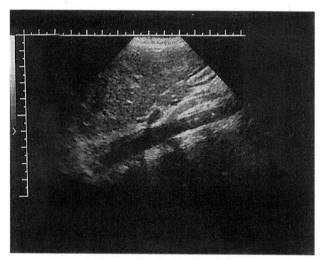
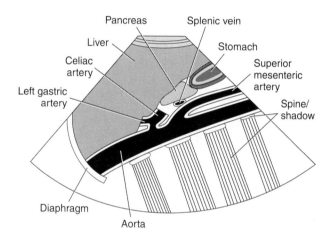

Figure 14-14 Longitudinal section just to the left of the midline, demonstrating the collapsed stomach antrum anteroinferior to the pancreas.

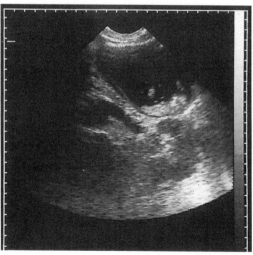
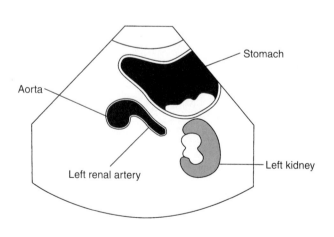

Figure 14-15 Transverse section of a fluid-filled stomach visualized anterior to the left kidney.

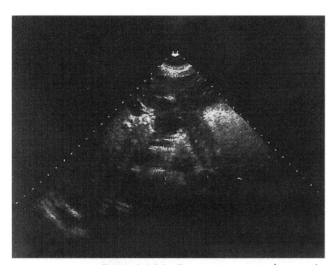
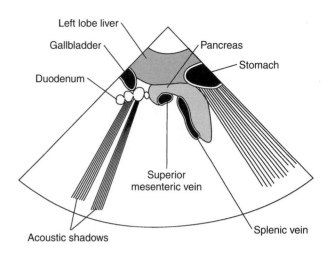

Figure 14-16 Transverse section of gas in the duodenum mimicking stones in the gallbladder or a pseudomass in the head of the pancreas.

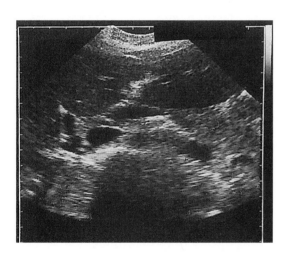
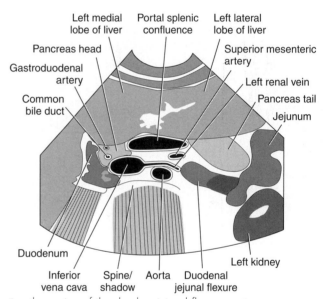

Figure 14-17 Transverse section demonstrating the region of the duodenojejunal flexure posterior to the uncinate process of the pancreas. The jejunum is that portion of small bowel located anterior to the left kidney.

The cecum is medial to the anterior superior iliac spine, and anterior to the iliopsoas muscle.

The vermiform appendix is usually posterior to the cecum, though it may project over the pelvic brim.

The ascending colon is anterolateral to the lower pole of the right kidney. It ascends along the right paracolic gutter to the liver, where it passes anteriorly to the kidney and the descending duodenum as it courses left to form the hepatic flexure.

The collapsed transverse colon may be seen, on longitudinal scans, inferior to the plane of the pancreas and stomach (Figure 14-18). It lies beneath the anterior abdominal wall, throughout its course, and passes anterior to the left kidney as it courses caudally to form the splenic flexure.

The right colic flexure is inferior to the right lobe of the liver and at a lower level than the left colic flexure, which is inferior to the spleen. The right colic (hepatic) flexure may produce artifacts simulating gallbladder disease if it is gas filled, and the left colic (splenic) flexure may mimic the left kidney.

The descending colon is posterior and extends from the splenic flexure to the sigmoid, adjacent to the left flank.

The sigmoid colon is anterior to the external iliac vessels and the sacrum. In females, it is posterior to the

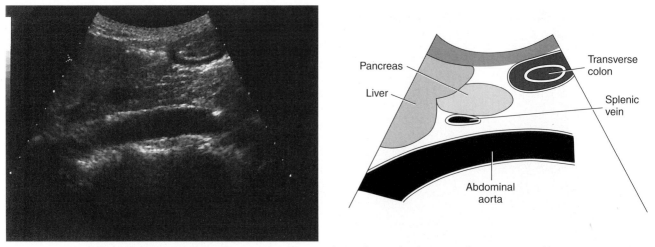

Figure 14-18 Compressed transverse colon noted on a longitudinal section. The transverse colon is seen inferior to the plane of the pancreas and stomach and anterior to the abdominal aorta.

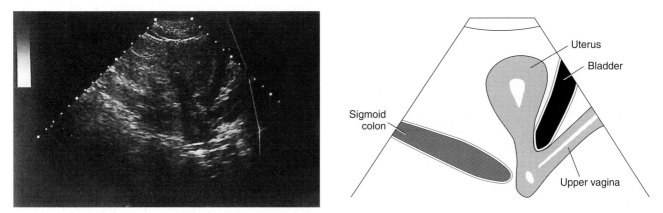

Figure 14-19 Sigmoid colon, superior and posterior to the uterus and vagina.

posterior surface of the uterus and the upper part of the vagina, and in males, posterior to the urinary bladder (Figure 14-19).

The rectum is posterior to the lower uterine segment and the vagina in the female, with the peritoneum over its anterior surface extending to the uterine surface. This forms the **rectouterine pouch,** the pouch of Douglas (posterior cul-de-sac). It is posterior to the prostate gland, the seminal vesicles, and the bladder in the male, and anterior to the levator ani muscles in both the male and female pelvis (Figure 14-20).

SONOGRAPHIC APPLICATIONS

Ultrasound helps to narrow the differential diagnosis of bowel disorders by visualization of the bowel wall and its layers.

Thickening of the bowel wall occurs with infiltration, inflammation, edema, or neoplastic invasion, thus allowing for sonographic recognition of the pathologic

process. Causes of wall thickening include pyloric stenosis, hematoma, intussusception, tumor, appendicitis, and edema.

Inflammation causes ulceration of bowel. Deep or submucosal inflammation such as that found in Crohn's disease causes thickening of the bowel wall.

With serosal inflammation, the inflammatory mass may indent or displace the bowel. Appendicitis is an inflammatory process that exerts such an effect on the cecum.

Normal bowel loops demonstrate peristalsis and are compressible; an inflamed appendix does not exhibit peristalsis and is not compressed. The normal appendix is rarely visualized, except occasionally in a thin patient or when it is surrounded by ascites. Appendicoliths and periappendiceal abscesses can also be visualized.

Bowel becomes dilated when it is obstructed and when ileus occurs. Ileus causes paralysis of bowel loops. Peristalsis is absent in the affected loop or loops of

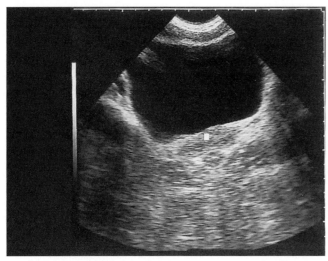
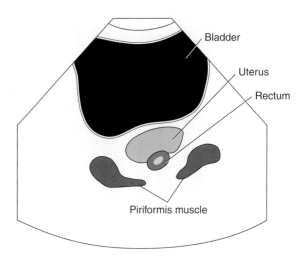

Figure 14-20 Transverse section of rectum posterior to the uterus and anterior to the piriformis muscle.

bowel, which results in gas accumulating in the paralyzed loop. Localized ileus commonly occurs near an inflammatory process.

If bowel becomes obstructed, gas does not pass through the GI tract, and builds up proximal to the obstructed loop. The portion of bowel distal to the obstruction becomes decompressed.

Doppler imaging can be used to assess malrotation of the bowel, which is frequently associated with malposition of the SMA and vein, and the detection of varices as well as the determination of directional flow within them.

Endosonography is useful in evaluating the esophagus, stomach, and rectum. The normal thickness of the esophageal wall is approximately 3 mm as five identifiable layers (Figures 14-21 and 14-22).

Esophageal and gastric lesions assessed with endosonography include varices, typically located in the EG

junction, intramural tumors, and peptic ulcers, which typically demonstrate thickening of all the gut wall layers.

Endoscopic sonography can also depict direct extension of GI malignancies into adjacent soft tissues, and perivisceral adenopathy.

Transrectal endosonography is typically used to identify and stage previously detected cancer. Endorectal ultrasound is considered at least as accurate as computed tomography (CT) for the preoperative staging of rectal carcinoma.

NORMAL VARIANTS

Some 2% to 3% of the population have **Meckel's diverticulum**—the remains of the prenatal yolk stalk (vitelline duct), projecting from the side of the ileum. The diverticulum measures between 5 and 25 cm in length and is attached by a peritoneal fold.

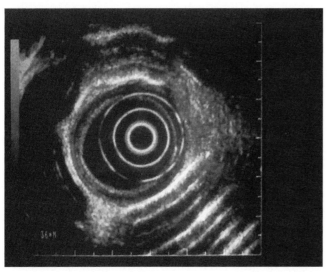
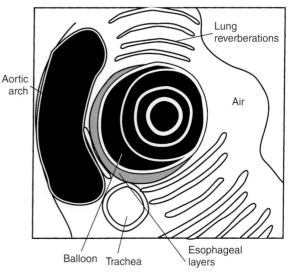

Figure 14-21 Endoscopic section of the upper esophagus, demonstrating wall layer separation. (Photo courtesy Wui Chong, M.D., Vanderbilt Medical Center.)

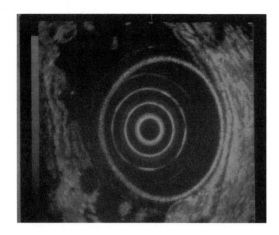

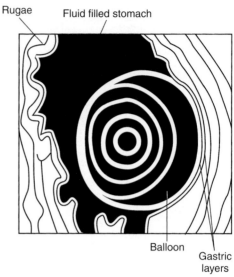

Figure 14-22 Endoscopic section of stomach demonstrating five identifiable wall layers. (Photo courtesy Wui Chong, M.D., Vanderbilt Medical Center.)

REFERENCE CHARTS

■ ■ ■   ASSOCIATED PHYSICIANS

Gastroenterologist: Specializes in treating diseases of the gastrointestinal tract, including the stomach, small and large bowel, gallbladder, and bile ducts.

Internist: Specializes in studying the physiology and pathology of internal organs and diagnosing and treating disorders of those organs.

Oncologist: Specializes in the study and treatment of tumors and malignancies.

Pediatrician: Specializes in guiding the development of children. They are concerned with the prevention and treatment of childhood diseases.

Surgeon: Utilizes operative procedures to treat diseases, trauma, and organ deformity.

Proctologist: Treats disorders of the colon, rectum, and anus.

Otolaryngologist: Specializes in the diagnosis and treatment of diseases and injuries of the ears, nose, and throat.

Radiologist: Specializes in performing and interpreting radiologic diagnostic studies of the gastrointestinal tract.

■ ■ ■   COMMON DIAGNOSTIC TESTS

Examination	Use
ABDOMINAL PLAIN FILM	Bowel gas
	Intestinal obstruction
	Carcinoma
	Appendicolith
	Volvulus

This radiograph is used to evaluate bones and soft tissue densities of the intraabdominal contents. Fluid-filled loops of bowel may be seen as tubular densities. Bowel gas patterns are evaluated and compared with normal gas patterns. Identification of the air-filled stomach, portions of the small intestine, and portions of the colon is possible. The examination is performed by a radiologic technologist and interpreted by a radiologist.

Examination	Use
UPPER GI SERIES (BARIUM SWALLOW)	Hernia
	Strictures
	Obstruction
	Inflammation
	Carcinoma
	Lesions
	Reflux
	Diverticula
	Ulcer disease
	Neoplasms
	Gastritis
	Focal dilatation
	Edema
	Wall thickening

The upper GI series is a set of fluoroscopic and radiographic examinations used to evaluate the GI tract from the esophagus to the small bowel. Fluoroscopy permits observation of real time motion of the tract. Contrast media are used to increase the density of the GI tract so that the anatomy and mucosal detail are visualized. Barium sulfate is most commonly used for these procedures. An iodinated contrast medium is another preparation used to opacify the tract for optimum visualization. Compression and palpation are techniques used by radiologists who perform and interpret the fluoroscopic examinations. Radiologic technologists assist the physician by adjusting the equipment controls, maintaining adequate film supplies, preparing media, and providing patient care and positioning.

These examinations include the following: barium swallow and small-bowel follow-through.

Examination	Use
UPPER GI ENDOSCOPY (EGD)	Biopsy Localized bleeding Dye injection Polyp removal Stent placement Ulcer follow-up Obstruction Hemorrhage control

Upper GI endoscopy is used for diagnostic and therapeutic indications. Following appropriate patient preparation, the endoscope is placed in the throat of the sedated patient. It must be swallowed. The scope is guided through the esophagus and into the stomach and duodenum and provides direct visualization of the upper GI tract. Photography, cytology, and biopsy sampling supplement the procedure, which is usually performed and interpreted by a gastroenterologist.

Examination	Use
BARIUM ENEMA	Obstruction Tumors Inflammation

Similar to the upper GI series, this examination involves the study of the colon. Single or double contrast media are used in the fluoroscopic procedure. Barium sulfate is infused into the cleaned rectum and x-ray studies are performed. The procedure is also used therapeutically in children with non-strangulated intussusception. A radiologist performs and interprets the examination. A radiologic technologist assists the physician.

Examination	Use
COLONOSCOPY **SIGMOIDOSCOPY** **ANOSCOPY**	Polyp removal Bleeding Lesion evaluation Inflammatory bowel

These procedures are done to further evaluate an abnormality previously identified by barium enema. For the colonoscopy, the sedated patient is given a rectal examination, followed by insertion of the colonoscope. Air is infused into the anus and the instrument is moved through the colon to the cecum and terminal ileum. The diagnostic evaluation involves structure visualization, photography, and biopsy or lesion removal. The procedures are similar in sigmoidoscopy, in which the sigmoid colon and rectum are examined, and anoscopy, in which the perianal region and the distal rectum are examined, utilizing smaller probes. The procedures are performed and interpreted by gastroenterologists.

■ ■ ■ **LABORATORY VALUES**

LIVER FUNCTION TESTS

Test	Normal	Increase	Decrease
CO_2	A: 19-24 mM V: 22-26 mM		Severe diarrhea
Carcinoembryonic antigen (CEA) (P)	0-25 mg/ml	Inflammatory bowel disease	
Cholesterol (S)			
Total	150-250 mg/dl		Cancer, fat malabsorption
HDL cholesterol (P)	29-77 mg/dl		
LDL cholesterol (P)	62-185 mg/dl		
VLDL cholesterol (P)	0-40 mg/dl		
Lipids (S)			
Total	400-800 mg/dl		Fat malabsorption
Cholesterol	150-250 mg/dl		
Triglycerides	10-190 mg/dl		
Phospholipids	150-380 mg/dl		
Fatty acids	9.0-15.0 mM/l		
Chloride (CL^-)(U)	110-254 mEq/24 hr		Pyloric obstruction, diarrhea
Potassium (K^+)(U)	25-100 mEq/l		Diarrhea, malabsorption
Sodium (NA^+)(U)	75-200 mg/24 hr		Diarrhea

WB, Whole blood; *P*, plasma; *S*, serum; *U*, urine; *A*, arterial; *V*, venous.

■ ■ ■ **NORMAL MEASUREMENTS**

Nonapplicable.

■ ■ ■ VASCULATURE

ARTERIAL SYSTEM

Vessel	Branch of	Supplies
Esophageal artery	Descending thoracic aorta	Esophagus
Inferior thyroid esophageal branch	Subclavian artery	Esophagus
Left inferior phrenic esophageal branch	Abdominal aorta	Esophagus
Left gastric artery	Celiac artery	Stomach
Esophagus		
Right gastric artery	Hepatic artery	Stomach, duodenum
Short gastric arteries (vasa brevia)	Splenic artery	Stomach
Gastroduodenal artery	Hepatic artery	Stomach, duodenum
Supraduodenal artery	Gastroduodenal artery	Duodenum
Right gastroepiploic artery	Gastroduodenal artery	Stomach, greater omentum
Left gastroepiploic artery	Splenic artery	Stomach, omentum
Superior pancreaticoduodenal artery	Gastroduodenal artery	Pancreas, duodenum
Inferior pancreaticoduodenal artery	Superior mesenteric artery	Pancreas, duodenum
Superior mesenteric artery	Abdominal aorta	Midgut
Inferior mesenteric artery	Abdominal aorta	Hindgut
Right colic artery	Superior mesenteric	Large intestine
Middle colic artery	Superior mesenteric	Transverse colon
Ileocolic artery	Superior mesenteric	Cecum, ascending colon, ileum Appendix
Left colic artery	Inferior mesenteric	Descending colon
Sigmoid artery	Inferior mesenteric	Sigmoid colon
Hemorrhoidal artery	Inferior mesenteric	Rectum, anal canal, anus
Superior rectal artery	Inferior mesenteric	Rectum

VENOUS SYSTEM

Vessel	Tributary to	Drains
Esophageal vein	Azygos	Esophagus
Left gastric vein	Splenic vein	Stomach, esophagus
Right gastric vein	Portal vein	Stomach
Superior mesenteric vein	Portal vein	Midgut
Inferior mesenteric vein	Splenic vein	Hindgut
Portal vein	Liver	GI tract
Left gastroepiploic vein	Splenic vein	Stomach, omentum
Right gastroepiploic vein	Superior mesenteric vein	Stomach, pancreas
Pancreaticoduodenal vein	Splenic vein	Pancreas, duodenum
Ileocolic vein	Superior mesenteric vein	Intestine
Right colic vein	Superior mesenteric vein	Colon
Middle colic vein	Superior mesenteric vein	Colon
Left colic vein	Inferior mesenteric vein	Sigmoid
Superior hemorrhoidal veins	Inferior mesenteric vein	Rectum, anal canal, anus
Superior rectal veins	Inferior mesenteric vein	Rectum

■ ■ ■ AFFECTING CHEMICALS

Nonapplicable

BIBLIOGRAPHY

Agur AMR: *Grant's atlas of anatomy,* ed 9, Baltimore, 1991, Williams & Wilkins.

Applegate EJ: *The sectional anatomy learning system: concepts and applications,* ed 2, Philadelphia, 2001, WB Saunders.

April EW: *Anatomy,* Media, PA, 1984, Harwall.

Basmajian JY, Slonecker CE: *Grant's method of anatomy,* ed 11, Baltimore, 1989, Williams & Wilkins.

Botet JF, Lightdale C: Endoscopic sonography of the upper gastrointestinal tract, *Am J Radiol* 156:63-68, 1991.

Carroll BA: Ultrasonography of the gastrointestinal tract, *Radiology* 172:605-608, 1989.

Fernbach SK, Feinstein KA: Selected topics in pediatric ultrasonography—1992, *Radiol Clin North Am* 30:1011-1031, 1992.

Gooding GAW, Filly RA, Laing FC: Ultrasound of the alimentary tube. In Margulis AR, Burhenne HJ, editors: *Alimentary tract radiology,* vol 1, St Louis, 1989, Mosby.

Gray H: *Anatomy, descriptive and surgical,* ed 15, New York, 1977, Crown Publishers.

Greenberger NJ, Isselbacher KJ: Disorders of absorption. In Braunwald E, Isselbacher KJ, et al, editors: *Harrison's principles of internal medicine,* New York, 1987, McGraw-Hill.

Guyton AC: *Textbook of medical physiology,* ed 10, Philadelphia, 2000, WB Saunders.

Janower ML: The colon: anatomy and examination techniques. In Tavares JM, Ferruchi JT, editors: *Radiology: Diagnosis-Imaging-Intervention,* vol 4, Philadelphia, 1988, JB Lippincott.

Johnson LR, editor: *Gastrointestinal physiology,* St Louis, 1977, Mosby.

Jones B, Braver JM: *Essentials of gastrointestinal radiology,* Philadelphia, 1982, WB Saunders.

Laing FC: Ultrasonography of the acute abdomen, *Radiol Clin North Am* 30:389-404, 1992.

Linder HH: *Clinical anatomy,* Norwalk, CT, 1989, Appleton & Lange.

Monie I: Embryology. In Margulis AR, Burhenne HJ, editors: *Alimentary tract radiology,* vol 1, St Louis, 1989, Mosby.

Moore KL: *The developing human: clinically oriented embryology,* ed 6, Philadelphia, 1998, WB Saunders.

Ngo C, Sarti DA: Simulation of the normal esophagus by a parathyroid adenoma, *J Clin Ultrasound* 15:421-424, 1987.

Pozniac MA, Scanlon K, Yandow D: Ultrasound in the evaluation of bowel disorders, *Semin Ultrasound CT, MR* 8:366-384, 1987.

Rifkin MD: Endorectal ultrasound of the rectal wall, *Semin Ultrasound CT, MR* 8:424-431, 1987.

Rumack CM, Charboneau JW, Wilson SR, editors: *Diagnostic ultrasound,* ed 2, St Louis, 1998, Mosby.

Sarti DA: *Diagnostic ultrasound text and cases,* ed 2, Chicago, 1987, Year Book.

Thomas CL: *Taber's cyclopedic medical dictionary,* ed 19, Philadelphia, 2001, FA Davis.

Torres WE: Radiology of the esophagus. In Gedgaudas-McClees RK, editor: *Handbook of gastrointestinal imaging,* New York, 1987, Churchill Livingstone.

Wilson SR: Ultrasonography of the gastrointestinal tract. In Rifkin MD, editor: *Syllabus: special course ultrasound 1991,* Oak Brook, IL, 1991, Radiological Society of North America, Inc.

Pelvic Sonography

CHAPTER 15

The Male Pelvis

MICHAEL J. KAMMERMEIER

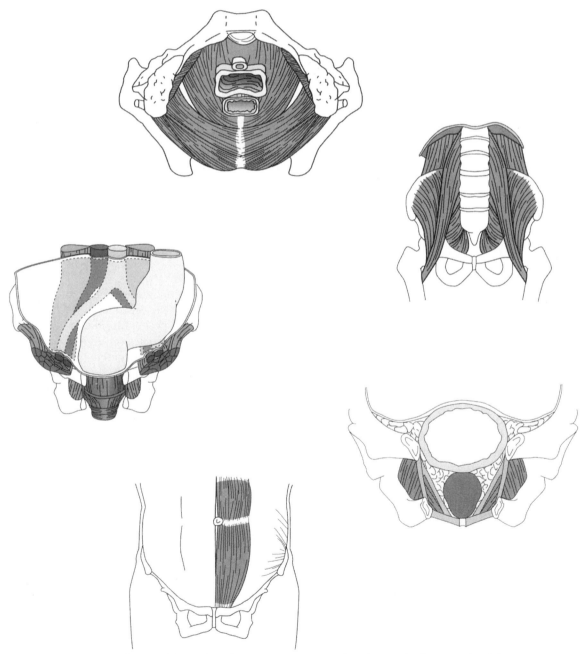

Anatomic layers of the male pelvis. (See Figure 4-4, **A, B, C, E,** and **F** for more details.)

Describe the location of the scrotum, testicles, epididymis, ductus (vas) deferens, seminal vesicles, and prostate.

Describe the size of the testicles and prostate.

Identify the gross anatomy of the scrotum, testicles, ducts, prostate, and penis.

Describe the sonographic appearance of the testicles, seminal vesicles, prostate, and penis.

Identify the associated physicians, related diagnostic tests, and laboratory values.

Define the key words.

■

KEY WORDS ■■■■■■■

Anterior fibromuscular stroma	Pampiniform plexus
Buck's fascia	Penis
Central zone	Peripheral zone
Convoluted seminiferous tubules	Periurethral glandular zone
Corpora cavernosa	Prostate
Corpus spongiosum	Rectum
Cremaster muscle	Rete testis
Denonvillier's fascia	Scrotum
Ductus (vas) deferens	Semen
Ductus epididymis	Seminal vesicles
Efferent ducts	Spermatic cord
Ejaculatory ducts	Spermatogenesis
Epididymis	Testicles/testes
Inguinal canal	Transition zone
Levator ani muscle	Tunica albuginea
Median raphe	Tunica dartos
Mediastinum testis	Tunica vaginalis
Obturator internus muscle	Urethra
	Verumontanum

■

Τhis chapter on the male pelvis/genitourinary system includes the scrotum, testicles, seminal vesicles, prostate, penis, and related structures. Other structures within the male pelvis that are described elsewhere (i.e., the urinary bladder, ureters, muscles, and vasculature) are not included (Figure 15-1).

PRENATAL DEVELOPMENT

Gender is initially determined by the presence (male) or absence (female) of the Y chromosome during conception. Until the seventh or eighth week of gestation, male and female embryos appear identical.

The testicles arise in the fetal upper abdomen near the developing kidneys. In the fourth month, the testes descend to the level of the urinary bladder, where they remain until approximately the seventh month of gestation. The testes descend through the **inguinal canal** and into the scrotum after the seventh month. This de-

scent is hormonally controlled and usually happens during the last month of gestation but occasionally does not occur until the first weeks of neonatal life.

The prostate develops during the third month of gestation. The apex of the urinary bladder (already formed) narrows to form the prostatic urethra. Prostate buds develop as outgrowths of the urethra. These buds develop into tubules, which elongate and multiply to form the lobes of the new prostate gland.

The external genitals of both male and female embryos remain undifferentiated until the eighth week of gestation. Prior to the eighth week, all embryos have a region called the genital tubercle. The genital tubercle is an elevated area between the coccyx and the umbilical cord where the mesonephric and paramesonephric ducts empty. In males, the genital tubercle elongates and develops into the penis.

LOCATION

The **scrotum** is a sac of cutaneous tissue that supports the testicles, or testes, the paired organs of reproduction. The **testicles (testes)** are the male gonads and are classified as both endocrine and exocrine glands. The testes produce sperm, which are transported through a network of ducts (exocrine function) that store and transport the sperm. The accessory organs, the seminal vesicles and the prostate, add secretions called **semen** to the sperm. The penis has two functions: it ejects sperm and semen from the body and excretes urine.

Scrotum and Contents

The scrotum is a pouch of skin that is continuous with the abdomen. It is suspended from the base of the male pelvis between the perineum and the penis. The scrotum contains the testicles, epididymis, and proximal portion of the ductus (vas) deferens.

The epididymis is connected to the superior portion of the testis and runs along the posterior aspect to the base of the testis. The epididymis drains into the ductus deferens at the base of the testis. The ductus deferens courses superiorly and exits the scrotum through the inguinal canal. Once inside the abdominal cavity, each ductus deferens courses along the lateral aspect of the urinary bladder and turns medially and posteriorly to connect with the seminal vesicles.

Seminal Vesicles

The **seminal vesicles** are paired glands that lie posterior to the urinary bladder just superior to the prostate. Each seminal vesicle angles medially toward the apex of the bladder and lies medial to the ureters. Each seminal vesicle joins with its corresponding ductus deferens to form an **ejaculatory duct.** The two ejaculatory ducts course through the prostate gland and empty into the prostatic urethra.

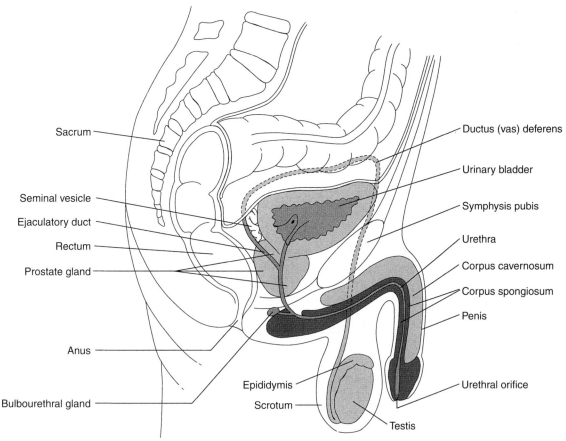

Figure 15-1 Male pelvis. Sagittal cross-section of the male pelvis illustrating the relationships of genital organs to surrounding structures.

Prostate

The **prostate** is a doughnutlike gland that lies inferior to the urinary bladder surrounding the proximal urethra. The prostate lies behind the symphysis pubis and is separated posteriorly from the rectum by the two layers of **Denonvillier's fascia.** Laterally, the prostate is supported by the **obturator internus** and **levator ani muscles.** Prostatic secretions are conveyed through numerous prostatic ducts to the prostatic urethra, located at the central core of the prostate. The fluids are then carried outside the body through the penis via the distal urethra and finally exit through the external urethral orifice.

SIZE

Testis

The normal adult testicle measures approximately 3 to 5 cm (1.5 to 2 inches) in length, 2 to 3 cm (1 inch) in anterior to posterior dimension, and 2 to 3 cm (1 inch) in width. When a male is between the ages of 12 and 17 years, the testicle undergoes rapid growth. Prior to age 12, the average testicular volume is less than 5 ml. After the male reaches maturity, the average testicular volume is approximately 25 ml, with the testicle weighing be-

tween 10 and 15 g. The testicle gradually decreases in size with advancing age.

Epididymis

The epididymis is actually a single, tightly wrapped tube called the ductus epididymis. When unwrapped, the ductus epididymis measures about 6 m (20 feet) in length and about 1 mm in diameter. The epididymis (head, body, and tail combined), as seen grossly, measures only 3.8 cm (1.5 inches) in length. The epididymis empties into the ductus deferens, which measures approximately 45 cm (18 inches) in length.

Seminal Vesicles

The seminal vesicles are convoluted pouchlike structures emptying into the distal portion of the ductus deferens to form the ejaculatory ducts. Each seminal vesicle measures approximately 5 cm (2 inches) in length and less than 1 cm in diameter.

Prostate

The prostate is a single gland weighing about 20 g. It normally measures approximately 4 cm (less than 2 inches) transversely, 3 cm (1.5 inches) in anteroposterior dimension, and 3.8 cm (1.5 inches) in cephalocaudal dimension. Unlike most other organs that atrophy with age, the prostate sometimes enlarges as a result of benign changes in the gland, infection, presence of malignant tumors, or other causes.

GROSS ANATOMY

Figure 15-2 illustrates the scrotum and its contents.

Scrotum

The skin and superficial fascia of the scrotum are continuous with those of the abdomen. Externally, the scrotum is divided into lateral portions by a median ridge called the **median raphe.** Internally, the scrotum is divided into sacs by a septum consisting of the dartos, or **tunica dartos.** The dartos contains superficial fascia and contractile tissue, which is also continuous with the subcutaneous tissue of the abdominal wall and is abundantly supplied by small vessels. Just posterior to the dartos lies the external spermatic fascia, which is a continuation of the external oblique fascia of the abdominal wall. The **cremaster muscle** surrounds each testicle and extends into the abdomen over the spermatic cord. The cremaster muscle is covered by the cremasteric fascia; this is continuous with the internal oblique fascia of the abdomen. Contraction of the cremaster muscle performs the important function of regulating the temperature of the testicles. Deep to the cremaster muscle is the innermost fascial layer of the scrotum, the internal spermatic fascia or infundibuliform fascia. This inner fascia surrounds the covering layers of the testicles, the tunica vaginalis. The **tunica vaginalis** consists of two layers derived from the perineum, an outer parietal layer that is closely attached to the internal spermatic fascia, and an inner visceral layer that is closely attached to the testicle.

Testis

Figure 15-3 illustrates the testis, epididymis, and ductus (vas) deferens.

Each testis is covered by a dense, white fibrous tissue called **tunica albuginea.** The tunica albuginea extends into the posterior wall of the testicle and forms the **mediastinum testis** and interlobar septa. The septa of the mediastinum radiate into the testicle and separate into 200 to 300 lobules. Each lobule contains one to three **convoluted seminiferous tubules,** which produce sperm through a process called **spermatogenesis.** The seminiferous tubules empty the spermatozoa into the straight tubules, which lead to a network of ducts called the rete testis. The **rete testis** is located within the mediastinum testis, and this network connects and exits the testis through the mediastinum testis as a series of coiled **efferent ducts.**

The blood supply to the testicles is via the internal spermatic arteries, which arise from the midabdomen as branches of the aorta just inferior to the renal vessels. The right testicular vein drains into the inferior cava at

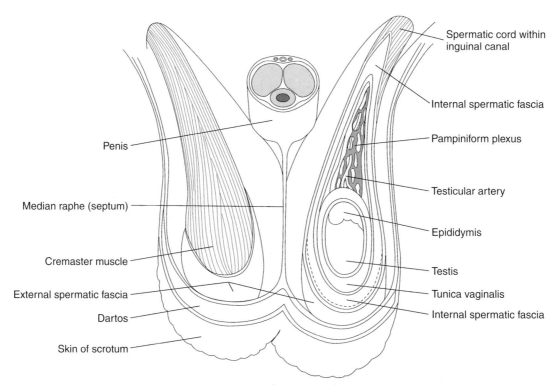

Figure 15-2 Dissected scrotum and its contents.

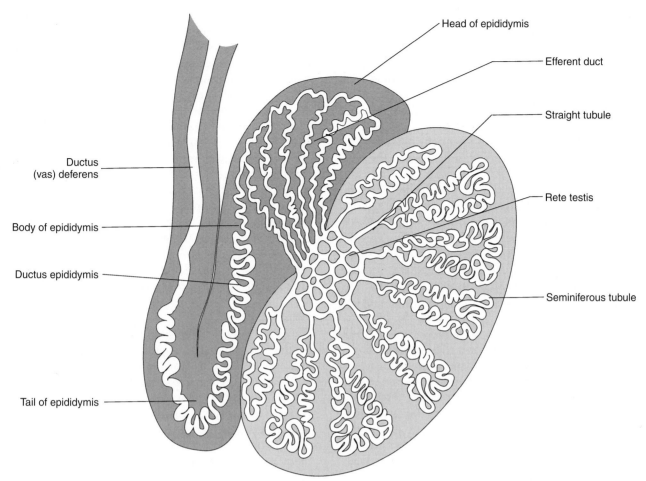

Figure 15-3 Enlarged longitudinal cross-section of testis, epididymis, and ductus (vas) deferens illustrating the complex network of ducts needed to transport sperm.

the level near the renal veins. The left testicular vein drains into the left renal vein.

Epididymis

The epididymis is composed mostly of a single convoluted tube, the **ductus epididymis,** encapsulated by a serosal layer. The ductus epididymis is lined by pseudostratified columnar epithelium, and its walls contain a thin layer of smooth muscle. The ductus epididymis is subdivided into a head (globus major), body, and tail (globus minor). The head of the epididymis is the larger, superior portion consisting mostly of the efferent ducts that empty into the ductus epididymis. The body runs along the posterior aspect of the testis and contains the ductus epididymis. The tail is the smaller, inferior portion, where the ductus epididymis empties into the ductus deferens.

Ductus (vas) Deferens

The **ductus deferens** is a thicker, less convoluted continuation of the ductus epididymis. Three smooth muscle layers contribute to this duct's increased thickness.

At its terminal portion near the seminal vesicles, the ductus deferens dilates; this area is referred to as the ampulla of the deferens.

Spermatic Cord

The two spermatic cords extend from the scrotum through the inguinal canals and internal inguinal rings into the pelvis. Each **spermatic cord** contains the ductus deferens, testicular arteries, venous **pampiniform plexus** (veins that drain the testes and become the spermatic veins superiorly), lymphatics, autonomic nerves, and fibers of the cremaster muscle.

Seminal Vesicles

The seminal vesicles are paired glands, each encapsulated by connective tissue. Beneath the connective tissue is a thin layer of smooth muscle that surrounds the submucosa and mucous membrane. The seminal vesicles join with the ductus deferens to form the ejaculatory ducts, which course through the prostate and empty into the prostatic urethra.

Prostate

The prostate is shaped like a cone with a central core, the prostatic urethra. The tip of the cone, or apex, is the inferior margin of the prostate and provides an exit for the urethra. The base of the gland is the superior aspect, which is in contact with the urinary bladder. The prostate is perforated by the two ejaculatory ducts, which enter the prostate at its posterior margin and course obliquely and anteriorly to join the prostatic urethra near the verumontanum, an area close to the center of the prostate.

The prostate consists of a small anterior fibromuscular region and a much larger posterior glandular region. The **anterior fibromuscular stroma** is located anterior to the prostatic urethra and is generally of less clinical significance because most pathology occurs in the glandular areas. The posterior glandular portion of the prostate has been described as consisting of zones. Dividing the glandular prostate into zones is probably the most useful representation for imaging the prostate. There are four zones within the glandular prostate: the peripheral zone, the central zone, the transition zone, and the periurethral glandular tissue or zone.

The **peripheral zone** is the largest, making up approximately 70% of the glandular prostate. This zone occupies the area lateral and posterior to the distal prostatic urethra. The **central zone** forms about 20% of the glandular prostate and is located at the superior edge bordering the bladder and seminal vesicles. The ejaculatory ducts course through this zone. The **transition zone** comprises only about 5% of the glandular prostate and has two lobes situated on the lateral aspects of the proximal prostatic urethra superior to the verumontanum. The transition zone borders the central zone posteriorly and laterally and the fibromuscular tissue anteriorly. The tissue that lines the proximal prostatic urethra forms the **periurethral glandular zone.** Figure 15-4, *A* depicts the zonal anatomy of the prostate in the coronal plane; Figure 15-4, *B* illustrates the prostatic anatomy in the sagittal plane. The prostate is surrounded by a thin capsule consisting of dense fibrous tissue and smooth muscle. This capsule connects with the muscle layers of the prostatic urethra. The prostatic urethra is divided by the **verumontanum** (area near the center of the prostate) into proximal and distal segments. These proximal and distal segments form an angle of approximately 35 degrees at the verumontanum.

Penis

Figure 15-5, *A* illustrates the gross anatomy of the penis in the coronal plane; Figure 15-5, *B* depicts penile anatomy in the transverse plane.

The **penis** is composed of three cylindrical masses of tissue. There are two **corpora cavernosa** situated dorsolaterally and a single **corpus spongiosum** in the midventral region, which contains the spongy **urethra.** The three corpora are bound and separated by the fibrous tissue called the tunica albuginea. Superficial to the tu-

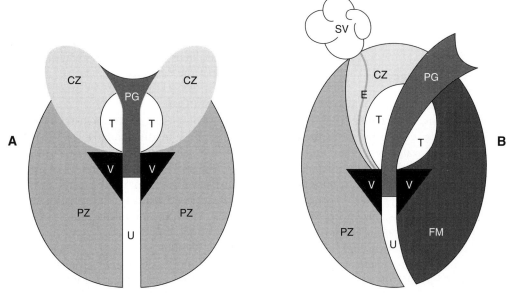

Figure 15-4 A, Zonal anatomy of the prostate in the coronal plane. *PG,* Periurethral glandular tissue (or zone); *CZ,* central zone; *T,* transition zone; *V,* verumontanum; *PZ,* peripheral zone; *U,* prostatic urethra. **B,** Zonal anatomy of prostate in the sagittal plane. *SV,* Seminal vesicles; *CZ,* central zone; *E,* ejaculatory duct; *PG,* periurethral glandular tissue (or zone); *T,* transitional zone; *V,* verumontanum; *PZ,* peripheral zone; *FM,* fibromuscular stroma; *U,* prostatic urethra.

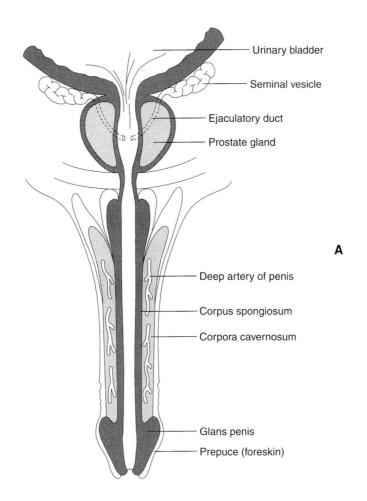

Urinary bladder

Seminal vesicle

Ejaculatory duct

Prostate gland

A

Deep artery of penis

Corpus spongiosum

Corpora cavernosum

Glans penis

Prepuce (foreskin)

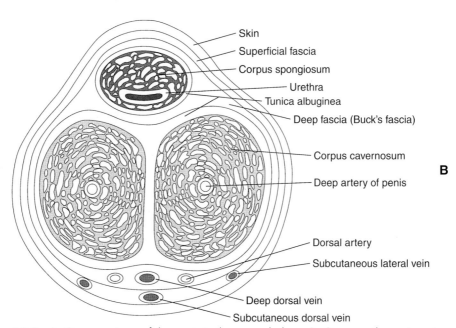

Skin

Superficial fascia

Corpus spongiosum

Urethra

Tunica albuginea

Deep fascia (Buck's fascia)

Corpus cavernosum

B

Deep artery of penis

Dorsal artery

Subcutaneous lateral vein

Deep dorsal vein

Subcutaneous dorsal vein

Figure 15-5   A, Gross anatomy of the penis in the coronal plane. **B,** Gross penile anatomy in short axis for the transverse plane.

nica albuginea is **Buck's fascia,** a thick fibrous envelope, and a loosely applied covering of skin.

The three corpora are composed of smooth muscle and erectile tissue that enclose vascular cavities. The penis becomes enlarged and erect when engorged with venous blood.

The blood supply to the penis and urethra is via the paired internal pudendal arteries, which are branches of the internal iliac arteries. These arteries divide into a deep artery of the penis and the bulbourethral artery. The deep artery of the penis supplies the corpora cavernosa. Branches of the dorsal artery and bulbourethral artery supply the corpus spongiosum, glans penis, and urethra.

The main veins of the penis are the superficial dorsal vein and the deep dorsal vein. The superficial dorsal vein is located outside Buck's fascia, and the deep dorsal vein is beneath Buck's fascia. The superficial and deep dorsal veins connect with the pudendal venous plexus, which drains the penis via the internal pudendal vein.

PHYSIOLOGY

The process by which genetic information is passed from one generation of a species to the next is called reproduction. In human reproduction, 23 chromosomes are passed from the male gamete, or sperm cell, to the female gamete, or ovum, which also contains 23 chromosomes. Through the union of these gametes, a zygote is formed, containing a total of 46 chromosomes. Multiple divisions of the zygote develop into a new organism. The male gametes, or spermatozoa, are produced in the testes by the process of meiosis. The seminiferous tubules within the testicle are lined with spermatogonia. These spermatogonia develop into mature spermatozoa through the process of spermatogenesis. The entire process takes approximately 2 to 3 weeks. Approximately 300 million spermatozoa mature every day. The spermatozoa are transported out of the testes into the ductus epididymis, where the final maturation of the sperm occurs. The spermatozoa can remain viable in storage for up to 4 weeks, after which time they are reabsorbed. The function of the ductal system is to store and help propel the sperm during ejaculation.

The production of sperm might be considered the most important function of the male reproductive system, but without the secretions of the accessory organs, the sperm could not survive to complete the process of reproduction. The seminal vesicles secrete an alkaline, viscous fluid rich in fructose, which contributes to sperm viability. This fluid constitutes about 60% of the volume of semen.

The prostate also produces and secretes an alkaline fluid. Its secretions constitute between 13% and 33% of the volume of semen. This alkaline fluid is believed to neutralize the acid environment of the vagina, uterus,

and fallopian tubes, where fertilization of the ovum takes place.

The reproductive function of the penis is to eject semen into the vagina. Sexual stimulation increases the blood supply to the penis. The penile arteries dilate as the penis is engorged with blood. Expansion of these arteries and blood sinuses within the corpora cavernosa causes compression of the veins that drain the penis; thus most of the blood is retained, resulting in an erection. During ejaculation, increased pressure within the urethra causes the urinary bladder sphincter to close. This mechanism prevents urine from being expelled during ejaculation and semen from entering the bladder.

SONOGRAPHIC APPEARANCE
Scrotal Contents

Sonographically, normal testicular parenchyma is homogeneous, containing medium-level echoes similar in ultrasound appearance to those of the thyroid gland (Figures 15-6 and 15-7). The highly echogenic line running along the long axis of the testis demonstrates the mediastinum testis. This is a normal finding and should not be mistaken for pathology. A few millimeters of anechoic fluid are also normally seen between the two layers of the tunica vaginalis. Excess fluid may indicate pathology (hydrocele).

The head of the epididymis is seen superior and posterior to the testicle. The body and tail of the epididymis are not normally identified. The echogenicity of the epididymis is equal to or slightly greater than that of the normal testicle. However, the texture of the epididymis is generally more coarse in appearance.

The various layers of the scrotum are not normally differentiated on ultrasound. The combination of the scrotal wall layers typically appears as a single, highly echogenic stripe.

The spermatic cord may be visualized as it courses through the inguinal canal. Color flow Doppler is useful in identifying the blood vessels within the cord; however, the ductus deferens is not normally seen.

Seminal Vesicles and Prostate

Ultrasound examination of the seminal vesicles and prostate may be performed either by the transabdominal method through a distended urinary bladder or by the transrectal approach. The transabdominal method is used only to assess the size of the glands, since most pathology is not well demonstrated with this technique. The transrectal approach is superior for scanning the seminal vesicles and prostate because of the close proximity of the transducer to the area of interest.

The transrectal ultrasound appearance of the seminal vesicles and prostate is described below.

Sonographically, the seminal vesicles are demonstrated as structures with low-level echoes superior to

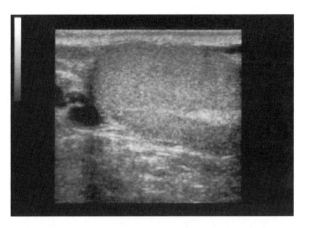
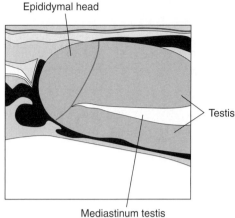

Figure 15-6 Testis in the sagittal plane.

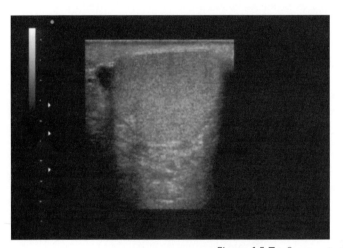
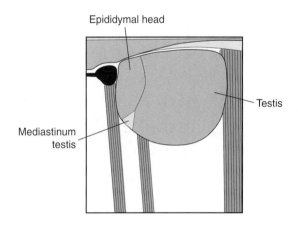

Figure 15-7 Scrotum in the transverse plane.

the prostate. In the transverse plane, the seminal vesicles are seen in their long axis. Figure 15-8 illustrates the seminal vesicles in the transverse plane. Normally they should be symmetric in size, shape, and echogenicity. In the longitudinal or sagittal plane, the seminal vesicles are identified as ovoid structures with low-level echoes superior to the prostate gland. Figure 15-9 demonstrates the prostate and seminal vesicles in the longitudinal plane. The prostate is sonographically heterogeneous, with medium-level echoes. It contains glandular and fibromuscular tissues, which surround the prostatic urethra. The normal prostate should always appear symmetric (Figure 15-9).

Transrectally, in the transverse plane, the prostate will appear semilunar in shape near the base (superiorly) and will become more rounded near the apex (inferiorly). The normal prostate will appear hyperechoic to the normal seminal vesicles. An area of low-level echoes situated anteriorly and in the midline represents the periurethral tissue and fibromuscular stroma. In the normal prostate, the central zone and transition zone cannot be individually distinguished, whereas the peripheral zone may appear more echogenic and homogeneous in comparison. The peripheral zone occupies the posterior and lateral portions of the gland (Figure 15-10).

Longitudinally in the midline, the hypoechoic periurethral tissues will be visualized and may be difficult to differentiate from the anterior fibromuscular stroma, which can also appear hypoechoic. The peripheral zone should normally be homogeneous and slightly more echogenic.

Penis

The most extensive role of penile ultrasonography is in the evaluation of vasculogenic impotence. The advent of duplex ultrasound has made this diagnosis possible. Another use of penile ultrasound is detection of pathologic abnormalities such as fibrosis, tumors, and periurethral diseases.

In the transverse plane, the corpus spongiosum will be seen in the midline, compressed by the transducer,

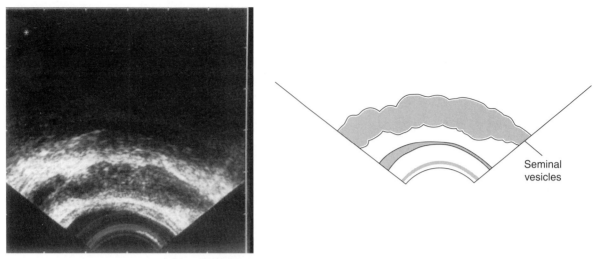

Figure 15-8 Seminal vesicles in the transverse plane.

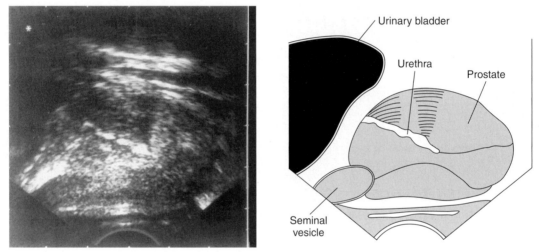

Figure 15-9 Normal sonographic relationship of the prostate and seminal vesicle in the sagittal plane.

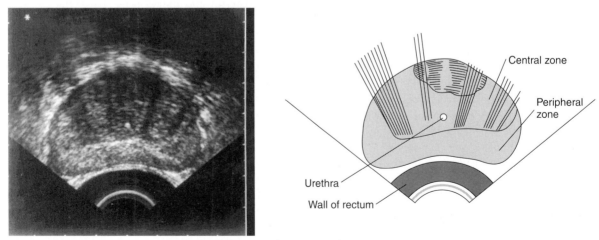

Figure 15-10 Normal prostate in the transverse plane.

and will appear elliptical in shape. Sonographically, the corpus spongiosum should be of homogeneous texture composed of medium-level echoes. The paired corpora cavernosa are posterior to the corpus spongiosum and appear symmetrically round or oval also, with a medium-level homogeneous echo texture. The corpora cavernosa are covered by the highly echogenic tunica albuginea. The echogenic plane dividing the two appears symmetrically round or oval also, with a medium-level homogeneous echo texture. The corpora cavernosa are covered by the highly echogenic tunica albuginea. The echogenic plane dividing the two corpora cavernosa is an extension of the tunica albuginea called the septum penis. Centrally located within the corpora cavernosa are cavernosal arteries, which can be identified by their echogenic walls and pulsations as seen in real time. Figure 15-11 demonstrates the penis in the transverse plane.

In the longitudinal plane, each corpus cavernosum should remain homogeneous with highly echogenic tunica albuginea visualized above and below. The cavernosal arteries will be imaged in their long axis and appear as parallel echogenic lines, representing the walls of the artery, coursing through the middle of the corpora cavernosa. Figure 15-12 illustrates the penis in the longitudinal plane.

SONOGRAPHIC APPLICATIONS
Scrotum
1. Testicular size
2. Inflammatory processes (epididymitis, orchitis)
3. Presence and composition of masses
4. Detection of peritesticular fluid collections (hydrocele)
5. Evaluation of scrotal trauma

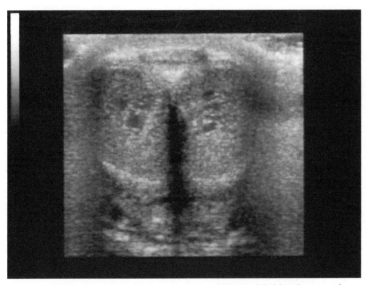
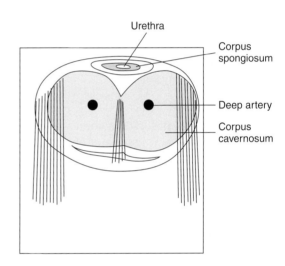

Figure 15-11   Penis in the transverse plane.

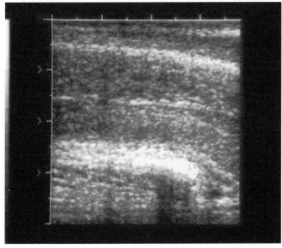
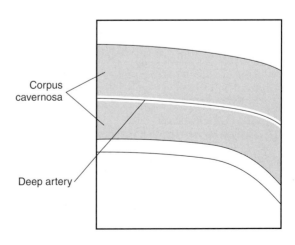

Figure 15-12   Penis in the longitudinal plane.

6. Doppler evaluation to rule out testicular torsion
7. Evaluation of scrotal pain
8. Location of undescended testicles

Prostate

1. Prostatic size and echo texture
2. Evaluation of infection (prostatitis)
3. Detection of masses
4. Evaluation of benign prostatic hypertrophy (BPH)
5. Sonographic correlation of findings on a digital rectal examination
6. Sonographic correlation of evaluated serum prostatic specific antigen (PSA)
7. Evaluation of extracapsular spread of prostatic carcinoma
8. Evaluation of postoperative transurethral resection (TURP)
9. Ultrasound-guided biopsies of prostatic lesions

Seminal Vesicles

1. Evaluate size, symmetry, and echo texture
2. Presence of cysts or calculi
3. Inflammatory processes
4. Congenital anomalies

Penis

1. Detection of fibrosis (Peyronie's disease)
2. Detection of scar tissue and plaques
3. Evaluation of tumors
4. Penile hematoma
5. Evaluation of periurethral disease
6. Doppler evaluation of vasculogenic impotence

NORMAL VARIANTS

Cryptorchidism is a failure of the testicles to descend into the scrotum. Common locations of undescended testes include the abdomen, inguinal canal, and at the external inguinal ring.

REFERENCE CHARTS

■ ■ ■ ASSOCIATED PHYSICIANS

Urologist: Specializes in surgical diseases of the male genitourinary tract and female urinary system.

■ ■ ■ COMMON DIAGNOSTIC TESTS

Magnetic Resonance Imaging (MRI): MRI is a noninvasive imaging modality that is very useful in identifying soft tissue structures. It is performed by a radiologic technologist and interpreted by a radiologist.
Ultrasonography: Second to direct physical palpation by a urologist, it is the method of choice for evaluating the male genitourinary system. It is performed by a radiologic technologist and interpreted by a radiologist.

■ ■ ■ LABORATORY VALUES

Serum Prostatic Specific Antigen (PSA): This is used to evaluate the function of the prostate. Normal serum PSA is less than 4.0. Elevated serum PSA may indicate disease but is not specific for carcinoma.

■ ■ ■ NORMAL MEASUREMENTS

Normal adult testicle: 3 to 5 cm in length; 2 to 3 cm in width; 2 to 3 cm anteroposterior.
Epididymis: 3.8 cm in length; uncoiled, 6 m.
Ductus (vas) deferens: 45 cm.
Seminal vesicles: 5 cm in length, less than 1 cm in diameter.
Prostate: 4 cm transverse, 3 cm anteroposterior; 3.8 cm in length.

■ ■ ■ VASCULATURE

Nonapplicable.

■ ■ ■ AFFECTING CHEMICALS

Nonapplicable.

BIBLIOGRAPHY

Asch MR, Toi A: Seminal vesicles: imaging and intervention using transrectal ultrasound, *J Ultrasound Med* 10:19-23, 1991.

Benson BC, Vickers MA: Sexual impotence caused by vascular disease: diagnosis with duplex sonography, *Am J Radiol* 153:1149-1153,1989.

Coleman BG: *Genitourinary ultrasound: a test/atlas,* New York, 1988, Igaku-Shoin, pp 375-380, 406-412.

Dakin R, Bedigian K, Grube GL: Transrectal ultrasound of the prostate: technique and sonographic findings, *J Diagnostic Med Sonog* 1:1-5, 1989.

DeVere White RW, Plamer JM: *New techniques in urology,* Mt. Kisco, NY, 1987, Futura, pp 235-240, 251-258.

Fornage BD: Normal ultrasound anatomy of the prostate, *J Ultrasound Med Biol* 12:1011-1021, 1986.

Hattery RR, King BF, Lewis RW, et al: Vasculogenic impotence: duplex and color Doppler imaging, *Radiol Clin North Am* 29:629-645, 1991.

Hoddic WK, Hricak H, Jeffrey RB: Scrotal sonography, *Semin Urol* 111(2):146-147, 1985.

Kammermeier MI: Carcinoma of the prostate: what every sonographer should know, *J Diagnostic Med Sonog* 7:139-146, 1991.

Krone KD, Carrol BA: Scrotal ultrasound, *Radiol Clin North Am* 23:121-129, 1985.

Krysiewacz S, Mellinger BC: The role of imaging in the diagnostic evaluation of impotence, *Am J Radiol* 153:1133-1134, 1989.

Littrup PJ, Lee F, McLeary RD, et al: Transrectal ultrasound of seminal vesicles and ejaculatory ducts: clinical correlation, *Radiology* 168:625-628, 1988.

O'Reilly PH, George NJR, Weiss RM: *Diagnostic techniques in radiology,* Philadelphia, 1990, WB Saunders, pp 93-97.

Quam JP, King BF, James EM, et al: Duplex and color Doppler sonographic evaluation and vasculogenic impotence, *Am J Radiol* 153:1141-1147, 1989.

Resnick MI, Ritkin MD, editors: *Ultrasonography of the urinary tract,* ed 3, Baltimore, 1991, Williams & Wilkins, pp 300-309.

Ritkin MD: *Ultrasound of the prostate*, New York, 1988, Raven Press.

Ritkin MD: *Diagnostic imaging of the lower genitourinary tract*, New York, 1985, Raven Press, pp 10-19, 21-26.

Ritkin MD, Kurtz AB, Pasto ME, Goldberg BB: Diagnostic capabilities of high-resolution scrotal ultrasonography: a perspective evaluation, *J Ultrasound Med* 4:13-19, 1985.

Schwartz AN, Lowe M, Berger RE, et al: Assessment of normal and abnormal erectile function: color Doppler flow sonography versus conventional techniques, *Radiology* 180:105-109, 1991.

Schwartz AN, Wang KY, Mack LA, et al: Evaluation of normal erectile function with color flow Doppler sonography, *Am J Radiol* 153:1155-1160, 1989.

Tanagho EA, McAninch JW: *Smith's general urology*, ed 12, Norwalk, CT, 1988, Appleton & Lange, pp 7-13.

Tortora GJ, Anagnostakos NP: *Principles of anatomy and physiology*, ed 5, New York, 1987, Harper and Row, pp 706-708, 713-718,733-735.

Walsh PC, Gittes RF, Perlmutter AD, et al, editors: *Campbell's urology*, ed 5, vol I, Philadelphia, 1986, WB Saunders, pp 47 -69.

CHAPTER 16

The Female Pelvis

BETTY BATES TEMPKIN AND PEGGY MALZI BIZJAK

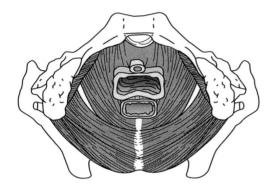
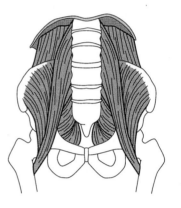
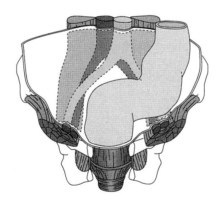
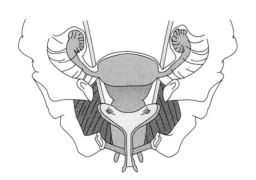
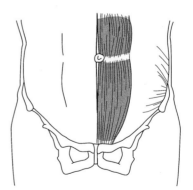

Anatomic layers of the female pelvis. See Figure 4-4, **A, B, C, D,** and **E** for more details.

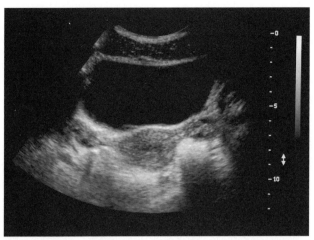

(Courtesy the University of Virginia Health System, Department of Radiology, Division of Ultrasound, Charlottesville, Virginia.)

OBJECTIVES

Describe the anatomy of the female pelvis and its sonographic appearance.

Describe the location of the female pelvic anatomy with relation to immediately adjacent structures.

Describe the sonographic appearance of the muscles and surrounding structures of the true pelvis.

Describe the physiology of the female reproductive organs of the pelvis.

Describe the variable positions of the uterus and their sonographic presentation.

Describe the anatomic layers of the female pelvis.

Define the key words.

KEY WORDS

Adnexa	Internal os
Anteflexed	Isthmus
Anterior cul de sac	Linea terminalis
Anteverted	Menarche
Bicornuate uterus	Multiparous
Broad ligaments	Myometrium
Cervix	Nulliparous
Corpus	Ovulation
Corpus luteum	Parametrium
Endometrial canal	Parity
Endometrium	Posterior cul de sac
External os	Proliferation
False pelvis	Pubic or pubis symphysis
Follicle stimulating hormone (FSH)	Retroflexed
	Retroverted
Fundus	True pelvis
Human chorionic gonadotropin (hCG)	Urinary bladder
	Uterine tubes
Iliac crests	

In most cases, sonography is the imaging method of choice for evaluating the female pelvis. It is a commonly performed examination that requires knowledge of the normal anatomy in the female pelvis and its sonographic (cross-sectional) presentation.

The organs contained within the female pelvis include the genital tract (uterus, vagina, uterine [fallopian] tubes), ovaries, urinary bladder, and pelvic colon. The osseous pelvis forms the outer boundaries of the pelvic cavity. Deep to this bony framework lie the skeletal muscles lining the abdominopelvic cavity.

PRENATAL DEVELOPMENT

The reproductive organs develop with the urinary system from two urogenital folds in the early embryo. Each urogenital fold consists of a gonad and a mesonephros.

Differentiation of the gonads into ovaries or testes depends on the genetic make-up of the embryo. The gonads are initially located in a cephalad position and descend into the true pelvis during fetal development.

The mesonephros is the precursor of the metanephros, the urogenital sinus, the wolffian (mesonephric) ducts, and the müllerian (paramesonephric) ducts. The metanephros and the urogenital sinus form the urinary system. The wolffian and müllerian ducts form the male and female genital tracts, respectively. The müllerian ducts of the female embryo fuse midline to form the vagina, uterus, and fallopian tubes. The wolffian ducts degenerate in the female embryo, leaving only remnants along the broad ligaments and the vaginal walls.

Congenital uterine malformations result in anatomic variations of the uterus, cervix, and vagina resulting from the incomplete fusion or agenesis of the müllerian ducts (Figure 16-1). The **bicornuate uterus** is the most common of the congenital malformations of the female genital tract. It is recognized sonographically by the presence of two endometrial canals that usually communicate at the level of the cervix. Bicornuate uterus is best appreciated in short axis sections as seen in Figure 16-2. Note the gestational sac in the right horn of the uterus and myometrial tissue separating the two endometrial canals.

Congenital ovarian malformations include unilateral müllerian duct anomaly; gonadal dysgenesis; and accessory, lobulated, and supernumerary ovaries. The unilateral müllerian duct anomaly results in a uterus-like parovarian mass, characterized by a central cavity lined by endometrial tissue surrounded by a thick, smooth muscle wall. Gonadal dysgenesis is the absence of both ovaries. It is usually hereditary in nature and associated with an abnormal chromosomal karyotype. In rare cases, unilateral ovarian agenesis may occur. Accessory, lobulated, and supernumerary ovaries are among the rarest of gynecologic malformations.

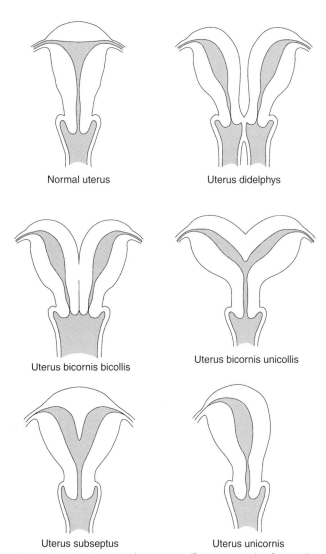

Normal uterus

Uterus didelphys

Uterus bicornis bicollis

Uterus bicornis unicollis

Uterus subseptus

Uterus unicornis

Figure 16-1 Congenital uterine malformations. This figure illustrates some congenital uterine malformations with anatomic variations of the uterus, cervix, and vagina resulting from the incomplete fusion or agenesis of the müllerian ducts. Complete duplication of the vagina, cervix, and uterine horns is seen in *uterus didelphys*. The *bicornuate uterus* has two uterine horns that are fused at one cervix *(uterus bicornis unicollis)* or at two cervices *(uterus bicornis bicollis)*. *Uterus subseptus* is a milder anomaly marked by a midline myometrial septum within the endometrial canal. In some cases, only one müllerian duct develops, forming a single uterine horn and a uterine tube continuous with one cervix and vagina *(uterus unicornis)*.

LOCATION

The location of the pelvis can be defined as that part of the peritoneal cavity extending from the iliac crests superiorly to the pelvic diaphragm inferiorly. The area encompassing the pelvis is described in regions and compartments.

There are three descriptive regions used to describe the area of the pelvis: right iliac, hypogastric, and left iliac (see Figure 4-2). Furthermore, the pelvis is described

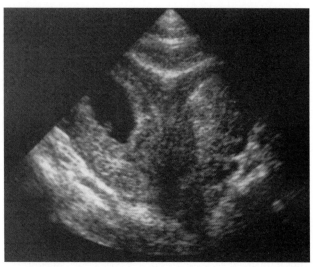

Figure 16-2 This transverse TA image of the pelvis demonstrates a bicornuate uterus containing a gestational sac within the right endometrial cavity. The gestational sac is anechoic and is surrounded by the hyperechoic decidual reaction of the endometrial lining. Myometrial tissue separates the endometrial canals of the left and right uterine horns.

in terms of two structurally continuous compartments that comprise the pelvic cavity area: the true pelvis and the false pelvis.

An arbitrary division defined by the sacral promontory and linea terminalis designates the true and false pelves. The **linea terminalis** is an imaginary arcuate line drawn along the inner surface of the pelvic bone from the pubic or pubis symphysis anteriorly, to the sacral promontory posteriorly that marks the plane separating the false from the true pelvis (Figure 16-3). The **false**

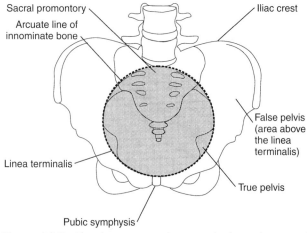

Figure 16-3 The linea terminalis extends from the sacral promontory, along the arcuate lines of the innominate bones, to the pubic symphysis. The true pelvis is the region deep to the linea terminalis. The false pelvis is the region of the abdominopelvic cavity that is superior to the linea terminalis and inferior to the iliac crests.

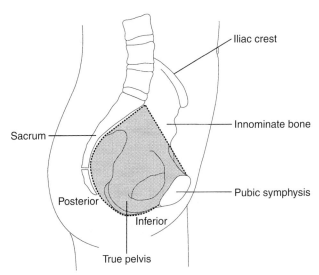

Figure 16-4 The true pelvis is a bowl-shaped cavity that tilts inferoposteriorly.

pelvis (major or greater pelvis) is defined as the more superior aspect of the pelvic cavity, extending from the iliac crests superiorly to the linea terminalis inferiorly. The **true pelvis** (minor or lesser pelvis) extends from the linea terminalis to the pelvic diaphragm inferiorly. It is a

bowl-shaped cavity aligned posteriorly and inferiorly within the skeletal framework (Figure 16-4). The urinary bladder, various loops of small bowel, the genital tract, and the ovaries are situated within the true pelvis.

The nonpregnant *uterus* is located in the hypogastric portion of the peritoneal cavity (or midregion of the true pelvis) between the urinary bladder (anteriorly) and rectum (posteriorly). The *cervical* portion of the uterus enters the vagina and lies at right angles to it.

The *vagina* also sits in the hypogastric portion of the peritoneal cavity between the rectum (posteriorly) and urinary bladder and urethra (anteriorly). It extends superior to inferior, from the uterus to the external genitalia. The external orifice of the vagina is located posterior to the urethral orifice between the labia minora.

The *uterine,* or *fallopian, tubes* extend from the uterus to the ovaries, which are situated more laterally within the true pelvis. The tubes course within the peritoneal folds of the broad ligaments. They are lateral to the uterus, anteromedial to the ovaries, and posterior to the urinary bladder.

The *ovaries* typically lie posterolateral to the uterus within the **adnexa** (peritoneal cavity spaces located posterior to the broad ligaments) (Figure 16-5). Ovaries are quite mobile and influenced by the condition of

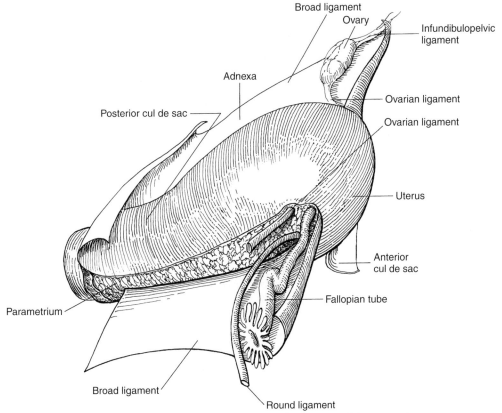

Figure 16-5 The ovaries are situated in the adnexa, the regions of the true pelvis posterior to the broad ligaments. The broad ligaments are double folds of peritoneum extending from the lateral aspects of the uterus to the pelvic wall. The uterine (fallopian) tubes, round ligaments, and ovarian ligaments are all located within the double folds of the broad ligaments.

surrounding structures. Even though their position is variable, the ovaries never move anterior to the uterus or broad ligaments.

During a first pregnancy, it is common for the ovaries to become displaced and never return to their original position. The ovaries in nulliparous (no viable births) women lie in a craniocaudal long axis direction on the iliopsoas muscles of the lateral pelvic walls between the external iliac vessels anteriorly and the internal iliac vessels and ureters posteriorly.

The urinary bladder is fixed inferiorly at its base in the true pelvis, posterior to the pubic symphysis and anterior to the uterus and vagina. It is anchored to the pelvis by pubovesical and lateral ligaments.

Location of the superior portion is variable depending on the amount of urine in the bladder. As the bladder fills with urine, the dome can extend into the false pelvis, displacing movable pelvic organs and loops of small bowel. Only the dome is covered by an extension of peritoneum.

The portions of the *colon* contained within the pelvis include the sigmoid and the rectum. The sigmoid colon lies within the true pelvis and is somewhat variable in length and position. It is continuous with the descending colon in the left lower quadrant of the abdominopelvic cavity and is loosely secured to the posterior pelvic wall by the mesocolon (Figure 16-6). The sigmoid colon descends toward the rectum in the inferoposterior aspect of

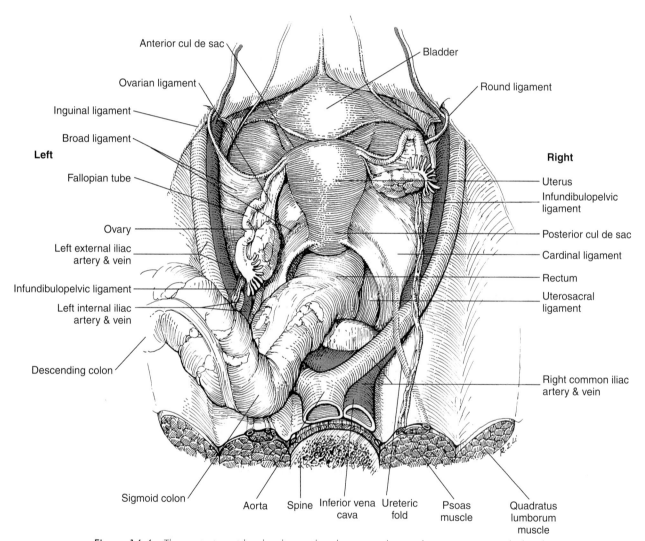

Figure 16-6 The rectosigmoid colon lies within the true pelvis and is continuous with the descending colon in the left lower quadrant of the abdominopelvic cavity. The cardinal ligaments and the uterosacral ligaments provide rigid support for the uterine cervix. The round ligaments extend from the cornua to the anterior wall of the pelvis. These ligaments pass through the inguinal canal and are secured to the external genitalia. The round ligaments maintain the anterior bend of the normal anteverted uterus.

the pelvis at the level of the third sacral vertebra. The rectum is situated posterior to the vagina. It is fixed in its position and is largely retroperitoneal.

SIZE

The size of pertinent female pelvic structures is included with the gross anatomy of female pelvic structures and the Normal Measurements Reference Chart found at the end of this chapter.

GROSS ANATOMY
Skeleton, musculature, ligaments, spaces, organs, colon

Pelvic Skeleton Anatomy
Sacrum, coccyx, innominate bones (ilium, ischium, pubis)
The pelvic skeleton consists of the sacrum, coccyx, and the innominate bones. The *sacrum* and *coccyx* constitute the distal segment of the vertebral spine, and form the posterior border of the pelvic cavity. The *innominate bones* encircle most of the pelvic cavity, forming its lateral and anterior margins. Each innominate bone is comprised of the *ilium, ischium,* and *pubis.* The innominate bones join posteriorly at the sacrum and coccyx and fuse anteriorly at the **pubis** or **pubic symphysis.** The **iliac crests** of the innominate bones define the most superior aspect of the pelvic cavity. The two iliac crests and the pubic symphysis are palpable external landmarks that aid in evaluating the pelvis (Figure 16-7).

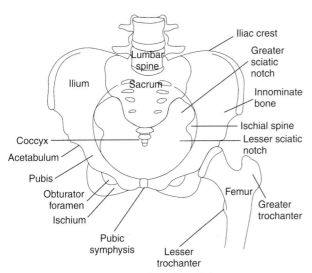

Figure 16-7 The pelvic skeleton.

Pelvic Musculature Anatomy
Psoas, iliopsoas, rectus abdominis, transverse abdominis, obturator internus, piriformis, pelvic diaphragm (pubococcygeus, iliococcygeus, coccygeus)

Psoas Muscles. The psoas major muscles are prominent paired muscles extending across the posterior wall of the abdominopelvic cavity. These muscles originate at the lateral aspects of the lower thoracic vertebrae and course anterolaterally in their descent to the iliac crests.

False Pelvis Musculature
Iliopsoas, rectus abdominis, transverse abdominis
The psoas major muscles join the iliacus muscles at the level of the iliac crests to form the *iliopsoas* bundles of the false pelvis. Each iliopsoas muscle courses anteriorly along the linea terminalis, to travel over the pelvic brim and insert into the lesser trochanter of the femur (Figure 16-8).

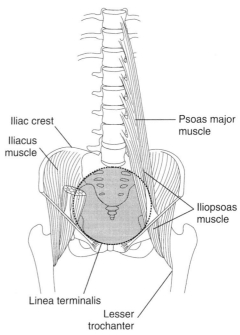

Figure 16-8 In the pelvic musculature, the psoas major muscles and the iliacus muscles join at the level of the iliac crests to form the iliopsoas muscles of the false pelvis. The iliopsoas muscle passes over the pelvic brim, exiting the false pelvis to reach the lesser trochanter of the femur.

Much of the anterior wall of the abdominopelvic cavity is formed by the *rectus abdominis* muscles, which extend from the sixth ribs and the xiphoid process down to the pubic symphysis (Figure 16-9, *A*). These paired muscles are intersected by transverse tendinous bands and are wrapped in a muscular sheath. The rectus sheath fuses with the *transversus abdominis* muscles to form the linea alba at the midline. The transverse abdominis muscles form the anterolateral borders of the abdominopelvic cavity. This muscle group lies deep to the internal and external oblique muscles (Figure 16-9, *B*).

True Pelvis Musculature
Obturator internus, piriformis, pelvic diaphragm (pubococcygeus, iliococcygeus [levator ani], coccygeus)
The *obturator internus muscles* originate along the arcuate line of the innominate bones and course parallel to the

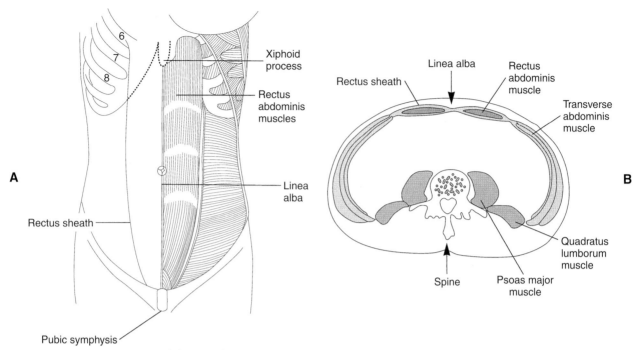

Figure 16-9 Abdominopelvic muscles. **A,** The rectus abdominis muscles extend from the xiphoid process to the pubic symphysis along the anterior abdominal wall. The muscular rectus sheath surrounding the rectus abdominis muscles fuses midline at the linea alba. **B,** Axial section through the midabdomen. The skeletal muscles lining the abdominopelvic cavity include the rectus abdominis muscles anteriorly, the transverse abdominis muscles laterally, and the psoas major and quadratus lumborum muscles posteriorly.

lateral walls of the true pelvis. These triangular muscles narrow inferiorly to pass through the lesser sciatic notch. The obturator internus is secured to the medial aspect of the greater trochanter. The internal surface of this muscle is covered by a tough membranous layer called the obturator fascia (Figure 16-10).

The *piriformis muscles* originate in the most posterior aspect of the true pelvis, along the lower portion of the sacrum, posterior to the uterus. These muscles travel anterolaterally, narrowing to pass through the greater sciatic

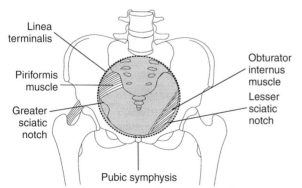

Figure 16-10 The obturator internus muscles line the lateral walls of the true pelvis. The piriformis muscles are situated in the posterior region of the true pelvis and course crossgrain to the obturator internus muscles.

notch. The piriformis muscles are attached to the superior aspect of each greater trochanter (see Figure 16-10).

The *pelvic diaphragm* is a group of skeletal muscles lining the floor of the true pelvis and supporting the pelvic organs (Figure 16-11). This muscular floor is composed of three paired muscles: the pubococcygeus, iliococcygeus, and coccygeus muscles. The *pubococcygeus muscles* are the most medial and anterior muscle pair of the pelvic diaphragm. These muscles extend from the pubic bones to the coccyx, encircling the urethra, vagina, and rectum.

The *iliococcygeus muscles* are located lateral to the pubococcygeus muscles. This pair extends from the obturator fascia and ischial spine anteriorly to the coccyx posteriorly. Together the *pubococcygeus* and *iliococcygeus* muscles form a hammock across the floor of the true pelvis and are termed the *levator ani muscles*. These muscles provide primary support to the pelvic viscera and aid in the contraction of the vagina and rectum. The *coccygeus* muscles are the most posterior muscle pair of the pelvic diaphragm. These muscles extend from the ischial spine to the sacrum and coccyx.

Pelvic Ligaments Anatomy
Broad, round, cardinal, uterosacral, infundibulopelvic, ovarian, pubovesical, lateral

Broad Ligaments Anatomy. The anterior and posterior peritoneal reflections covering the uterus extend

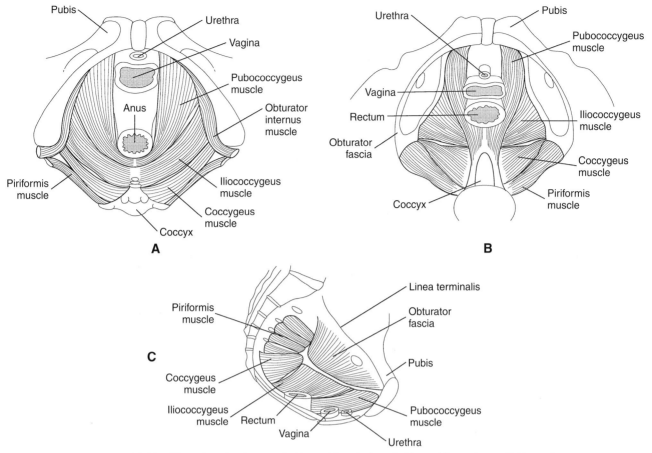

Figure 16-11 The pelvic diaphragm. **A,** Viewed from below. **B,** Viewed from above. **C,** Viewed laterally.

anterolaterally to the walls of the true pelvis. These double folds of peritoneum extend from the uterine cornua to the lateral pelvic walls to form the broad ligaments. The broad ligaments are not true ligaments, and they provide minimal support for the uterus. The fallopian tube, round ligament, ovarian ligament, and vascular structures of the uterus and ovaries are positioned between the two layers of each broad ligament. These structures are surrounded by fat and cellular connective tissue, called the **parametrium.** The spaces within the peritoneal cavity located posterior to the broad ligaments are referred to as the adnexa (see Figure 16-5).

Round Ligaments Anatomy. Three paired ligaments provide structural support to the uterus: the round ligaments, the cardinal ligaments, and the uterosacral ligaments. Each *round ligament* originates at the uterine cornu and courses within the broad ligament to the anterolateral pelvic wall. The round ligament passes over the pelvic brim and through the inguinal canal, and is secured at the labia majora. The round ligaments maintain the forward bend of the uterine fundus.

Cardinal Ligaments, Uterosacral Ligaments Anatomy. The *cardinal* and *uterosacral ligaments* provide more rigid support for the cervix. These ligaments maintain the normal axis of the cervix, roughly perpendicular to the vaginal canal. The cardinal ligaments extend from the upper cervix and isthmus to the obturator fascia at the lateral walls of the pelvis. The uterosacral ligaments extend from the posterior aspect of the cervix around the lateral walls of the rectum to the sacrum (see Figure 16-6).

Infundibulopelvic Ligaments, Ovarian Ligaments Anatomy. There are two paired ligaments supporting the ovaries and maintaining their relative positions in the adnexal regions. The *infundibulopelvic ligament* extends from the infundibulum and the lateral aspect of the ovary to the lateral pelvic wall. The *ovarian ligament* supports the medial aspect of the ovary to the uterine cornu. This ligament lies within the peritoneal folds of the broad ligament. The mesovarium is a short, double fold of peritoneum extending from the posterior aspect of the broad ligament to the ovarian hilum (Figure 16-12).

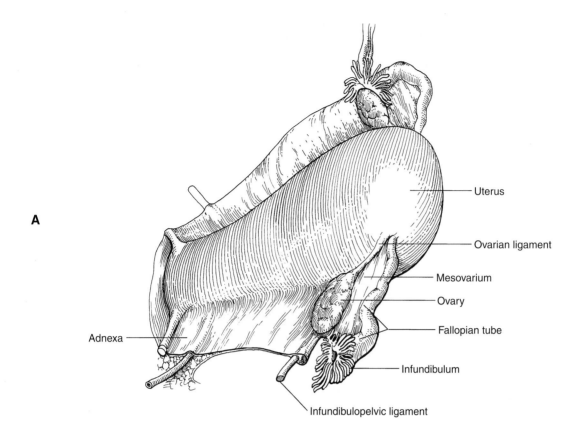

A

Uterus

Ovarian ligament

Mesovarium

Ovary

Fallopian tube

Adnexa

Infundibulum

Infundibulopelvic ligament

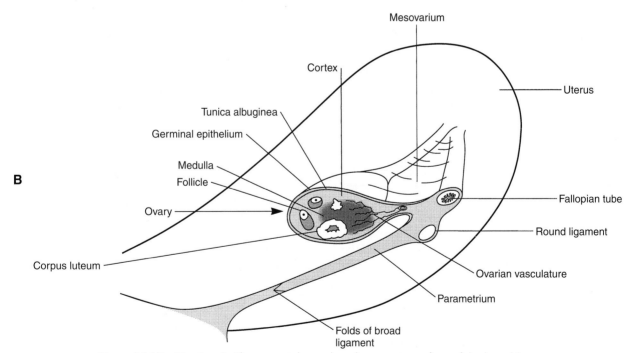

B

Mesovarium

Cortex

Tunica albuginea

Germinal epithelium

Medulla

Follicle

Ovary

Uterus

Fallopian tube

Round ligament

Corpus luteum

Ovarian vasculature

Parametrium

Folds of broad ligament

Figure 16-12 Ovaries. **A,** The ovary is located on the posterior surface of the broad ligament and is anchored in this position by the ovarian and infundibulopelvic ligaments and the mesovarium. The ovaries are the only organs located within the peritoneal cavity that are not covered by peritoneum. **B,** The innermost ovarian tissue is the medulla, composed of ovarian vessels, nerves, and connective tissue. Follicular development takes place in the cortex of the ovary, which surrounds the medulla. The cortex is enclosed by a fibrous capsule called the tunica albuginea. The germinal epithelium is the outermost cellular layer.

Pubovesical Ligaments, Lateral Ligaments Anatomy.
The *pubovesical ligaments* extend anteriorly from the bladder neck and attach to the pubic bones. The *lateral ligaments* extend to fuse with the tendinous arch of the obturator internus muscles.

Pelvic Spaces Anatomy
Anterior cul de sac, posterior cul de sac, space of Retzius

The peritoneal lining of the abdominopelvic cavity covers the anterior and posterior walls of the uterus. The vesicouterine reflection of peritoneum expands over the urinary bladder and covers the anterior wall of the uterus. This reflection creates a shallow space within the peritoneal cavity, known as the **anterior cul de sac** or vesicouterine pouch (Figure 16-13). This space is usually empty but may contain loops of small bowel.

The rectouterine reflection of the peritoneum creates a larger potential space between the posterior wall of the uterus (particularly the cervix) and the anterior wall of the rectum. This space is known as the **posterior cul de sac,** rectouterine pouch, or pouch of Douglas. The posterior cul de sac is the most dependent space in the abdominopelvic cavity. Any fluid collecting within the peritoneal cavity often drains into this space (see Figure 16-13).

The **space of Retzius** separates the anterior bladder wall from the pubic symphysis; it is filled with extraperitoneal fat (see Figure 16-13).

Pelvic Organ Anatomy
Genital tract (vagina, uterus, uterine tubes), ovaries, urinary bladder

Genital Tract Anatomy
Vagina, uterus, uterine tubes

The genital tract (vagina, uterus, and uterine tubes) and ovaries comprise the primary reproductive organs of the female. The vagina, uterus, and uterine tubes all have the same basic structure: cavities enclosed by an inner mucosal lining, a smooth muscle wall, and an outer layer of connective tissue. Together, these communicating cavities are known as the genital tract. Variations in the mucosa and muscular walls of the genital tract are dictated by the location and function of each segment.

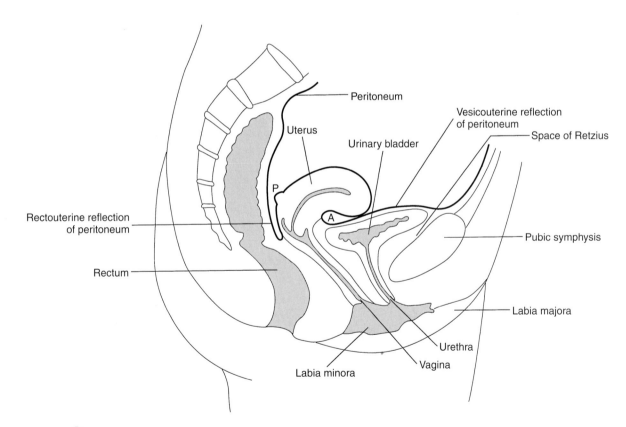

Ⓟ Posterior cul de sac

Ⓐ Anterior cul de sac

Figure 16-13 A midline sagittal plane through the female pelvis. The peritoneal lining of the abdominopelvic cavity is seen covering the superior aspect of the urinary bladder, the uterus, and the anterior region of the rectum. The anterior and posterior cul de sacs are potential peritoneal spaces created by folds in the peritoneum.

Vagina Anatomy

Fornices

The vagina extends from the external genitalia to the uterine cervix. The vaginal canal is approximately 9 cm in length and receives the penis during coitus. The canal also forms the distal portion of the birth canal. The uterine cervix protrudes through the anterior vaginal wall into the upper portion of the vaginal canal. The space within the vaginal canal encircling the cervix forms the *anterior, posterior,* and *lateral* **fornices** of the vagina (Figures 16-14 and 16-15).

The walls of the vagina conform to the general structure of the genital tract. It is composed of a mucosal lining of epithelial cells, a thin smooth muscle wall, and an outer adventitia. The vagina is highly elastic, permitting gross distention during parturition. In the relaxed state, the vaginal walls collapse together, and the epithelial lining folds into transverse ridges, or rugae (see Figure 16-15).

Uterus Anatomy

Fundus, corpus, isthmus, cervix (internal and external os), endometrium, myometrium, serosa

As previously mentioned, the uterus lies in the true pelvis between the bladder and the rectum. Uterine walls are composed of three tissue layers: the endometrium, myometrium, and serosa (see Figure 16-15). The innermost layer of the uterine wall, the **endometrium,** is a mucosal layer that is continuous with vaginal epithelium inferiorly and uterine tube mucosa superolaterally. The endometrium consists of two layers: superficial (functional) and deep (basal). The superficial layer is referred to as the functional layer or functional zone because it increases in size during the menstrual cycle and partially sloughs off at the time of menses. The deep, or basal, layer of the endometrium is composed of dense cellular stroma and mucosal glands; it is not significantly influenced by the menstrual cycle.

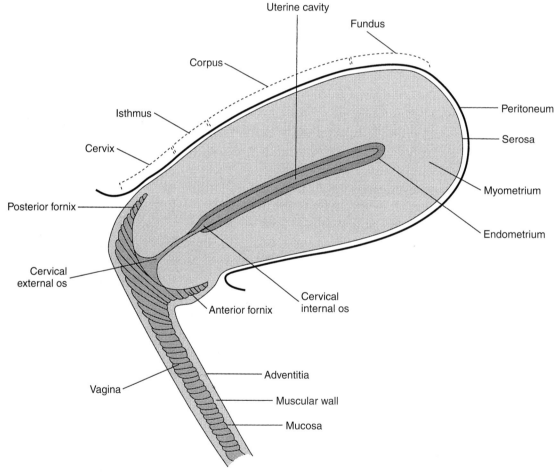

Figure 16-14 The wall of the vagina comprises an inner mucosa, a middle smooth muscle layer, and an outer adventitia. The anterior and posterior fornices of the vagina are seen as spaces between the vaginal walls and the portion of the cervix protruding into the vaginal canal. The uterine wall comprises an inner mucosa, called the endometrium; a thick, smooth muscle wall, called the myometrium; and an outer serosa. The regions of the uterus include the cervix, isthmus, corpus, and fundus. Note the narrow anteroposterior dimension of the uterine cavity.

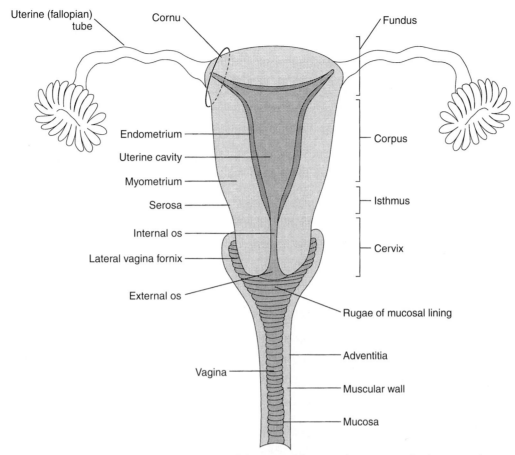

Figure 16-15 Genital tract. In this coronal diagram of the genital tract, notice the three tissue layers that comprise the uterine wall: endometrium, myometrium, and serosa. Note the uterine (fallopian) tubes adjoining the uterus at the cornua. The lateral fornices of the vagina are also evident.

The **myometrium,** or muscle, layer forms the bulk of the uterus. It is composed of three distinct layers of different muscle fibers: outer longitudinal fibers, intermediate spiral bands, and inner circular and longitudinal fibers. This combination of fibers is responsible for the myometrium dramatically enlarging during pregnancy and producing the radial muscle contractions necessary to expel the fetus at parturition.

The **serosa** is the thin membrane that covers the myometrium and forms the outer layer of the uterus.

The uterus is descriptively divided into four parts: fundus, corpus, isthmus, and cervix (see Figure 16-15). The **fundus** is the widest and most superior segment of the uterus situated between the insertion of the uterine tubes at the level of the uterine cornua. It is continuous with the body and largest part of the uterus, called the **corpus.** The corpus is continuous with the uterine cervix at a point marked by a constriction of the uterus called the **isthmus.** During late pregnancy the isthmus is taken up into the corpus to form the lower uterine segment. The **cervix** is the lower cylindrical portion of the uterus that projects into the vagina. The endocervical canal ex-

tends 2 to 4 cm from its **internal os** (or opening), at approximately the same level as the isthmus, where it joins the endometrial canal (uterine canal) to its **external os,** which projects into the vaginal vault. The endometrial, endocervical, and endovaginal canals form a continuous channel through which the fetus passes at birth.

Although the cervix is part of the uterus, the walls of the cervix are structurally unique compared with the rest of the uterus. The smooth muscle fibers are interlaced with collagen fibers, creating a more rigid framework. Furthermore, a histologic difference has been noted between the endometrial and endocervical mucosa in the internal os. The mucosal lining of the vaginal portion of the cervix is identical to the epithelial lining of the vagina.

In childhood, the uterus is approximately 2.5 cm long, 2 cm wide, and 1 cm thick. The mean dimension of the adult **nulliparous** (no births) uterus is approximately 7 cm long and 4 cm wide. **Multiparous** (multiple viable births) uterine mean dimensions are generally 8.5 cm long and 5.5 cm wide. Following menopause, uterine size reduces significantly and the uterus assumes a prepubertal shape. Examples of sonographic measurements of the uterus are shown in Figure 16-16.

Age and **parity** (number of viable offspring) are obviously two important factors influencing uterine size and shape. The corpus and fundus of the uterus show considerably more variation in size than the more rigid cervix. Prior to puberty, the cervix comprises a significantly greater proportion of the organ in the child than in the adult. During puberty, the dimensions of the uterus and endometrial thickness markedly increase. The corpus and fundus portions of the uterus enlarge, changing the uterus from tubular to pear shaped. After **menarche** (menstrual function), the uterus continues to grow for several years. Uterine size is directly related to the number of years postmenarche.

The uterus normally tilts forward, resting on the dome of the bladder. The ligaments and peritoneal connections of this organ allow considerable mobility within the true pelvis. This mobility affords subtle displacements of the uterus with filling of the urinary bladder or the rectum, as well as marked displacement of this organ during pregnancy.

The flexibility of the support structures of the uterus affords considerable variation in normal uterine position (Figure 16-17). When the bladder is empty, the uterus is in an **anteverted** position, in which the cervix and vagina form a 90-degree angle, and the corpus and fundus are tipped or tilted anteriorly. If the corpus and fundus are bent at a greater anterior angle until the fundus is pointing inferiorly and resting on the cervix, the uterine position is described as **anteflexed.**

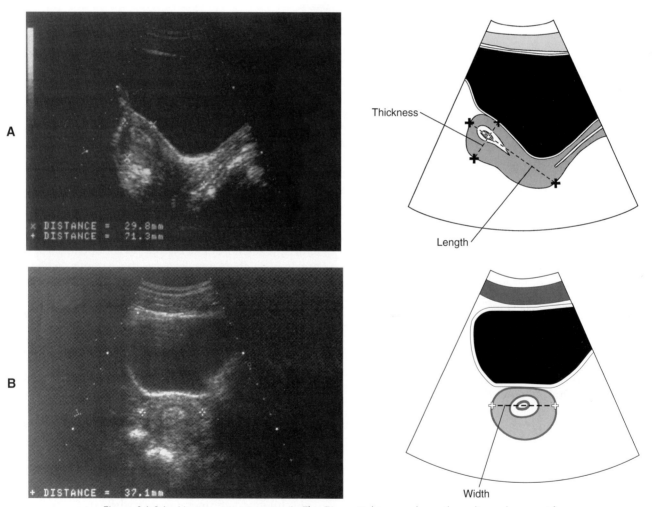

Figure 16-16 Uterine measurements. **A,** This TA sagittal image shows the caliper placement for measuring the longest axis and greatest anteroposterior measurements of the uterus. The length of the uterus is measured from the fundus to the inferior cervical region. The anteroposterior thickness is measured perpendicular to the length at the widest point of the uterine corpus. **B,** This TA transverse image demonstrates the caliper placement for measuring the width of the uterus, which is taken at the widest point of the uterine corpus in a short axis section.

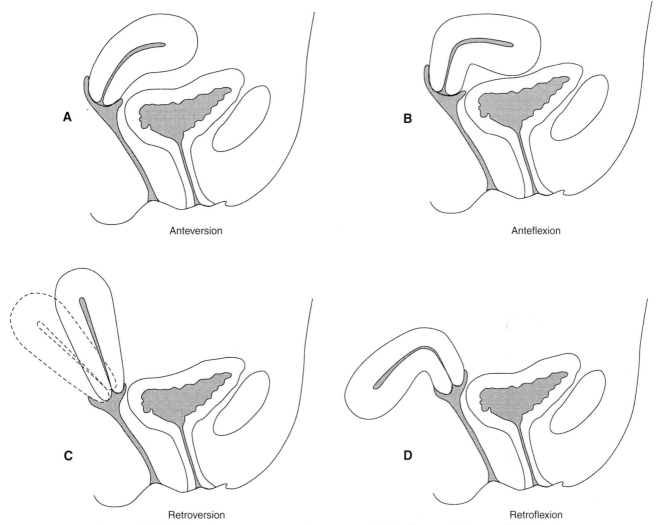

Figure 16-17 Uterine position variations. **A,** Anteversion. **B,** Anteflexion. **C,** Retroversion. **D,** Retroversion with retroflexion.

Inversely, the uterus can also be retroverted and retroflexed. In a **retroverted** position, the corpus and fundus are tipped posteriorly and the angle of the cervix and vagina increases, making them more linearly oriented. If the corpus and fundus are bent at a greater posterior angle until the fundus is pointing inferiorly adjacent to the cervix, the uterine position is described as **retroflexed.**

Uterine Tubes Anatomy
Interstitial segment, isthmus, ampulla, infundibulum

The **uterine tubes** (fallopian tubes, or oviducts) are coiled, muscular tubes emerging from the cone-shaped cornua of the uterus, which are located at the junction of the superior and lateral uterine margins. The uterine tubes vary in length from 7 to 12 cm as they course within the peritoneum along the superior free margin of the broad ligaments until they reach the ovaries.

The uterine tube conducts a mature ovum from the ovary to the uterus through gentle peristalsis of its smooth muscle walls (Figure 16-18, *A*). The mucosal lining of the tube consists of ciliated epithelial cells and secretory cells. The cilia propel a gentle current of fluid, which aids in the transport of ova.

The oviducts may be divided into four segments: interstitial or intramural, isthmus, ampulla, and infundibulum (Figure 16-18, *B*). The **interstitial,** or *intramural,* segment of the uterine tube is the narrowest portion, which is enclosed within the muscular wall of the uterus. The **isthmus** is immediately adjacent to the uterine wall, connected to the interstitial segment. It is a short, straight, narrow portion of the tube. The tube widens laterally, forming the ampullary and infundibular sections.

The longest and most coiled portion of the uterine tube is the **ampulla.** Fertilization most often occurs in

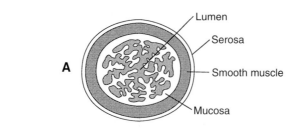

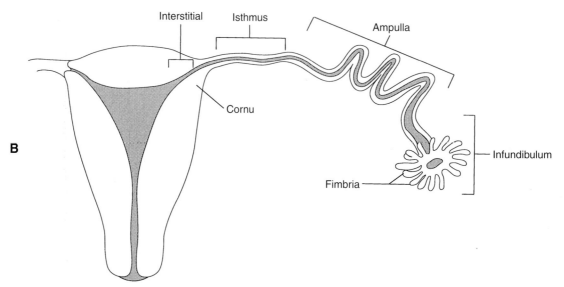

Figure 16-18 Uterine tubes. The uterine (fallopian) tubes or oviducts are continuous with the endometrial cavity at the uterine cornua. The four regions of the oviduct include the interstitial segment, isthmus, ampulla, and infundibulum. **A,** The regions of the uterine tube. **B,** Cross-section through the ampulla of the tube. This section demonstrates the intricate folds of the mucosal lining. The wall of the oviduct comprises the inner mucosa, middle muscular, and outer serosal layers.

the ampulla. The mucosal lining of the ampulla folds into complex matrices, filling much of the tubular lumen.

The *infundibulum* is the funnel-shaped end portion of the oviduct. The tube terminates at the fimbriated end of the infundibulum, and opens into the peritoneal cavity adjacent to the ovary. The peritoneal ostium of the uterine tube is approximately 3 mm in diameter. Specifically, the infundibulum passes through the posterior aspect of the broad ligament to reach the ovary. The oviduct and the ovary are not intimately connected; thus the genital tract creates a channel between the outside and the peritoneal cavity. The fimbriae of the oviduct are fringe-like extensions of the infundibulum, which overlie the ovary and direct the released ovum into the fallopian tube.

Ovarian Anatomy
Tunica albuginea, stroma
The ovaries are paired, almond-shaped organs lying on the posterior surface of the broad ligaments. They are the only organs within the abdominopelvic cavity not lined by visceral peritoneum. The germinal epithelium is a single layer of epithelial cells lining the outer surface of the ovary. (This name arose from the mistaken belief that the germ cells originated from this tissue layer.)

The *tunica albuginea* is a fibrous connective tissue capsule found beneath the epithelial layer. The ovarian *stroma,* or the body of the ovary, consists of the peripheral cortex and the central medulla. The cortex constitutes the bulk of ovarian tissue and is the site of oogenesis, the production of female gametes. The medulla contains the ovarian vasculature, lymphatics, and nerves supported by fibrous connective tissue. This highly vascular core communicates with the parametrium of the broad ligament at the ovarian hilum. The hilum is located along the superoanterior aspect of the ovary.

As previously mentioned, the infundibulopelvic and ovarian ligaments support and maintain the relative position of the ovaries in their adnexal location. In most cases, the ovaries are situated posterolateral to the broad ligaments; however, they are quite mobile and may be located anywhere within the adnexa except anterior to the uterus or anterior to the broad ligaments (see Figure 16-5).

Ovarian size varies during the life span depending on age, menstrual status, pregnancy status, body habitus, and menstrual cycle phase. At birth, the ovaries are relatively large as a result of maternal hormone stimulus. There is little change in ovarian size until age 5 or 6, after which age-related growth is seen, associated with an increase in cystic functional changes. Normal measurements during reproductive years range from 2.5 to 5 cm in length, 0.6 to 2.2 cm in anteroposterior (AP) thickness (or height), and 1.5 to 3 cm in width.

Ovarian volume may also be used as a measure of normal size and is calculated as follows:

$$\text{Volume} = \text{length} \times \text{height (AP thickness)} \times \text{width} \times 0.523$$

In women between 15 and 55 years of age, normal ovarian volume is 6.8 ml. Ovarian volume parameters can be influenced by the presence of a large follicle(s) or pathology. Ovarian volume is only marginally affected by cyclic changes. The lowest volumes can be observed during the luteal phase and highest volumes during the preovulatory phase.

Urinary Bladder Anatomy

The **urinary bladder** is a muscular sac that receives and stores urine produced by the kidneys. It consists of four layers of tissue: an inner mucosa, a submucosa layer, the muscularis, and the outer serosa. The mucosa folds when the bladder is empty, and distends and becomes smooth when the bladder is full. The muscularis layer is comprised of three layers of smooth muscle, called the detrusor muscle. The outermost layer, the serosa, is located at the superior portion of the bladder. It is an extension of pelvic peritoneum (Figure 16-19).

The inferior portion of the urinary bladder is comprised of a posterior base (or trigone area) and the neck, which communicate with the ureters and urethra. The external urethral orifice is located between the labia minora of the external genitalia. The inferolateral surfaces

of the bladder meet anteriorly, and are in contact with the pelvic floor muscles.

The superior and posterior walls of the bladder are lined by visceral peritoneum, which is continuous with the peritoneal lining of the abdominopelvic space. As previously discussed, the peritoneum covering the bladder walls and extending over the uterine fundus creates a potential space between the bladder and the uterus, known as the anterior cul de sac. The space of Retzius, also discussed earlier, separates the anterior bladder wall from the pubic symphysis and is typically filled with extraperitoneal fat (see Figure 16-13).

The urinary bladder is a hollow, symmetric organ, whose size depends on the quantity of contained urine. The wall of a distended bladder normally measures 3 to 6 mm depending on the degree of bladder distension.

Pelvic Colon Anatomy
Sigmoid, rectum

The portions of the large intestine contained within the true pelvis include the **sigmoid colon** and the rectum. The **sigmoid colon** is continuous with the descending colon in the left lower quadrant of the abdominopelvic cavity (see Figure 16-6). The sigmoid colon is loosely secured to the posterior pelvic wall by the mesocolon. The sigmoid colon descends toward the rectum in the inferoposterior aspect of the pelvis. The **rectum** is largely retroperitoneal, and is situated posterior to the vagina.

When the bladder is empty, loops of small bowel rest in the anterior region of the abdominopelvic cavity. A distended urinary bladder pushes the small intestine superiorly, out of the true pelvis.

VASCULATURE

Uterine artery and vein, internal iliac artery and vein, arcuate arteries and veins, radial arteries and veins, straight arteries and veins, spiral arteries and veins, ovarian artery and vein, hypogastric artery, gluteal arteries, vaginal artery, azygos arteries, vascular arch, lymph nodes

Uterine Vasculature

Uterine artery and vein, internal iliac artery and vein, arcuate arteries and veins, radial arteries and veins, straight arteries and veins, spiral arteries and veins

The **uterine artery** is a branch of the **internal iliac artery** and supplies blood to the reproductive organs of the pelvis. The left and right uterine arteries divide into vaginal and uterine branches at the level of the cervix (Figure 16-20, *A*). The uterine branches course along the lateral aspect of the uterus toward the fundus. The arterial and venous uterine branches are located within the peritoneal folds of the broad ligament.

The uterine branches of each uterine artery give rise to the **arcuate arteries.** These arteries loop around the uterus and branch into the radial arteries. The **radial arteries** penetrate the myometrium and give rise to the straight arteries. The **straight arteries** supply the first layer of endometrial tissue, with smaller branches,

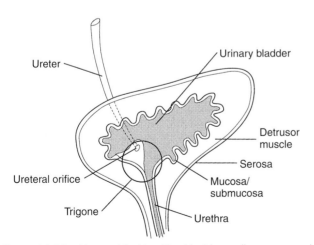

Figure 16-19 Urinary bladder. The bladder wall is composed of an innermost mucosa; followed by a submucosal layer; a thick, middle muscular layer; and an outer serosal lining. The trigone is the region of the urinary bladder at which the ureters enter and the urethra exits this cavity.

Labels: Ureter, Urinary bladder, Detrusor muscle, Serosa, Ureteral orifice, Mucosa/submucosa, Trigone, Urethra

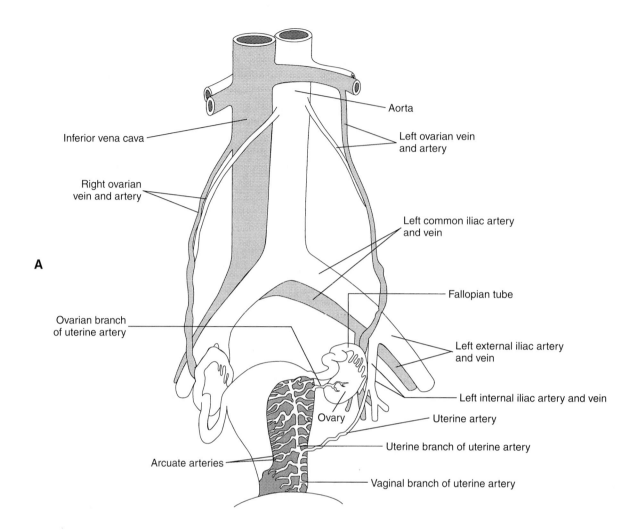

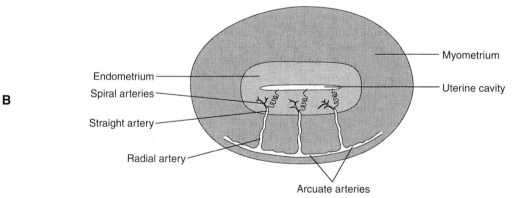

Figure 16-20 Genital tract vasculature. **A,** The uterine artery is a branch of the internal iliac artery. The uterus and vagina receive blood from branches of this artery. **B,** The arcuate arteries encircle the outer tissue of the uterus. The myometrium is penetrated by the radial arteries. The endometrium receives blood from the straight and spiral arteries. The spiral arteries become more dilated during the secretory phase of the menstrual cycle. During menses, the spiral arteries are shed along with much of the endometrial lining. The ovaries receive blood from branches of the uterine artery and from the ovarian arteries arising from the abdominal aorta.

called the *spiral arteries,* perfusing the proliferating endometrium (Figure 16-20, *B*). Flow in the spiral arteries is responsive to hormonal changes of the menstrual cycle. The venous drainage of the uterus is analogous to its arterial supply.

Vaginal Vasculature
Common iliac artery, uterine artery, vaginal artery, azygos arteries
The blood supply to the vagina begins in the pelvis with the **internal iliac artery** and two of its anterior branches, the **uterine and vaginal arteries** (see Figure 16-20, *A*). Among other things, the uterine artery provides blood for the cervix. Branches of the cervical branch of the uterine artery anastomose with branches of the vaginal artery to form the anterior and posterior *azygos arteries* of the vagina.

Uterine Tubes Vasculature
Vascular arch
The uterine tubes' vascular supply comes from the **vascular arch** formed by the anastomosed ovarian and uterine arteries. Vascular arch branches pass through the mesosalpinx of the broad ligament, to meet the uterine tubes.

Ovarian Vasculature
Uterine artery and vein, ovarian artery and vein
The blood supply to the ovary is maintained by two separate vascular pathways. First, the uterine branches of the **uterine artery** and **vein** give rise to ovarian branches at the level of the cornu. The ovarian branches travel laterally within the broad ligament to reach the ovarian hilum.

Second, the left and right **ovarian arteries** branch off the abdominal aorta inferior to the renal arteries. The ovarian arteries course anterior to the psoas and iliopsoas muscles within the retroperitoneum. They travel medially along the infundibulopelvic ligaments to reach the ovarian hilum. The **ovarian veins** follow a similar ascent to the inferior vena cava, with slight variation in that the left ovarian vein drains into the left renal vein (see Figure 16-20, *A*).

Urinary Bladder Vasculature
Hypogastric artery, gluteal arteries, uterine and vaginal arteries
Blood is supplied to the urinary bladder by the superior, middle, and inferior vesicles, derived from the anterior trunk of the **hypogastric artery.** Small visceral branches of the obturator and inferior **gluteal arteries** along with branches derived from the **uterine** and **vaginal arteries** also supply blood to the bladder.

Pelvic Lymph Nodes
External iliac, internal iliac, common iliac
The main groups of pelvic lymph nodes include the external and internal iliac lymph nodes and the common iliac lymph nodes. The **external iliac nodes** accompany the external iliac artery and vein and are situated in the false pelvis and pelvic sidewalls. **Internal iliac nodes** surround the internal iliac vessels, and the **common iliac nodes** are associated with the common iliac artery.

PHYSIOLOGY
Between puberty and menopause, the female reproductive system normally undergoes monthly cyclical changes. The menstrual cycle usually follows a 28-day course, during which a single ovum reaches maturity and is released into the genital tract. Hormones secreted by the anterior pituitary gland and by the ovary itself control changes in the ovary and the endometrium throughout this cycle.

The Ovarian Cycle
At menarche the ovaries contain thousands of primordial follicles, each composed of a single primary oocyte and surrounding follicular cells. During the follicular phase of the ovarian cycle (days 1 to 14), 10 to 20 primordial follicles begin to mature. **Follicle stimulating hormone (FSH)** is a gonadotropin produced by the anterior pituitary gland, which initiates follicular development. This initial maturation process results in the development of several follicles, each composed of multiple cellular layers.

The primary follicle contains the primary oocyte surrounded by a membranous protein layer, called the zona pellucida. Proliferating follicular cells, collectively called the zona granulosa, encircle this layer. Outer connective tissue layers of the primary follicle include the theca interna and the theca externa (Figure 16-21).

As each primary follicle grows, the oocyte reaches a mature size. The follicular antrum is a fluid-filled cavity that forms between the cellular layers of the zona granulosa. The developing oocyte rests along the wall of the follicular antrum and is surrounded by the cumulus oophorus, a layer of follicular cells continuous with the zona granulosa. At this stage of development, the oocyte and its surrounding structures are called the secondary follicle. The theca interna cells of multiple secondary follicles fulfill an endocrine function as they differentiate into estrogen-secreting cells. The hormone estrogen promotes proliferation of the endometrium.

Although many follicles develop in the ovaries in response to FSH, only one primary follicle matures completely to be released at ovulation (see Figure 16-21). Most of the follicles undergo follicular atresia beyond the stage of the secondary follicle. One secondary follicle continues to mature to become a graafian or dominant follicle prior to ovulation (see Figure 16-21). The ovum continues to mature through meiotic division, forming the secondary oocyte. Now the oocyte floats freely within the enlarged follicular antrum of the graafian follicle. The follicular cells of the cumulus oophorus now

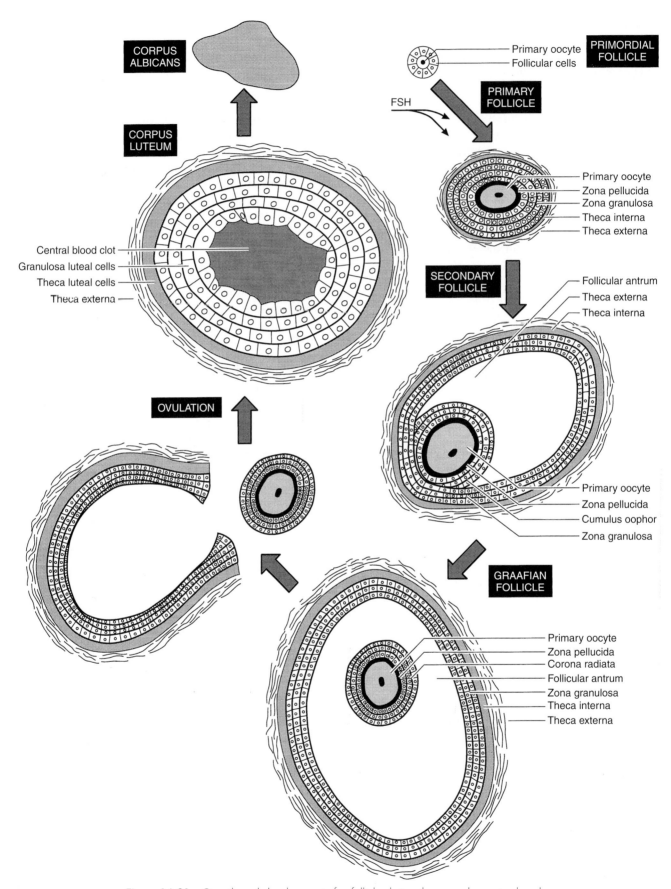

Figure 16-21 Growth and development of a follicle during the normal menstrual cycle.

completely surround the zona pellucida and the secondary oocyte, and are called the corona radiata.

The theca interna cells of the graafian follicle continue to produce estrogen. The graafian follicle migrates to the surface of the ovary, while the remaining secondary follicles undergo atresia. At approximately day 14 of the ovarian cycle, **ovulation** occurs when the mature ovum is expelled into the peritoneal cavity. The fimbria of the oviduct draw the released egg into the infundibulum.

At ovulation, 5 to 10 ml of follicular fluid are released into the peritoneal cavity, settling into the posterior cul de sac between the uterus and rectum. The ruptured graafian follicle collapses, fills with blood, and is transformed into a temporary endocrine gland. This begins the luteal phase of the ovarian cycle (days 15 to 28). The remaining follicular structure is now called the **corpus luteum** and contains a central blood clot surrounded by granulosa luteal cells, theca luteal cells, and the theca externa.

The granulosa luteal cells enlarge and secrete progesterone, which promotes glandular secretions of the endometrium. The theca luteal cells continue the estrogen secretion of their precursors (theca interna), maintaining the proliferated endometrial lining of the uterus. The outer theca externa cells support the rich vascular network characteristic of an endocrine gland.

Luteinizing hormone (LH) is produced throughout the ovarian cycle by the anterior pituitary gland. This hormone promotes secretion of estrogen and progesterone by the ovary. Both estrogen and LH peak immediately prior to ovulation. While the corpus luteum depends on LH, progesterone negatively inhibits the production of LH. Consequently, the corpus luteum eventually regresses due to lack of LH stimulation, and only a fibrous tissue mass, called the corpus albicans, remains in the ovary (see Figure 16-21). When the levels of estrogen and progesterone diminish, the thickened endometrial lining of the uterus is shed through menstruation (Figure 16-22).

Pregnancy interrupts the normal menstrual cycle. The developing placenta secretes **human chorionic gonadotropin (hCG)** following implantation of the fertilized ovum. This hormone has an analogous function to LH, maintaining the corpus luteum. Thus, during pregnancy, the corpus luteum continues to secrete estrogen and progesterone throughout the first trimester. The placenta ultimately takes over this endocrine function and the corpus luteum regresses, forming the corpus albicans.

The Endometrial Cycle
The days of the menstrual cycle are numbered according to changes in the endometrial lining of the uterus. Days 1 through 5 generally correspond to menses, when the thickened superficial layer of the endometrium is shed.

Proliferation is the next phase of the endometrial cycle, occurring between menses and ovulation. The endometrium thickens under the influence of estrogen, preparing the uterine cavity to receive the fertilized egg.

Ovulation usually occurs near the fourteenth day of the menstrual cycle, marking the beginning of the secretory phase. The continued production of estrogen and now progesterone by the corpus luteum promotes continued thickening and swelling of the endometrium. Exocrine glands of the endometrial lining secrete a glycogen-rich mucus, preparing a suitable environment for implantation.

In the absence of fertilization, the production of LH, estrogen, and progesterone diminishes, and a new cycle begins on day 1 with menses. The timing of menses and proliferation in the endometrial cycle correspond to the follicular phase of the ovarian cycle (days 1 to 14). The secretory phase of the endometrial cycle corresponds to the luteal phase of the ovarian cycle (days 15 to 28).

SONOGRAPHIC APPEARANCE
Skeleton, musculature, ligaments, spaces, organs, colon, vasculature
Standard examination of the female pelvis is composed of transabdominal sonography (TAS) combined with transvaginal sonography (TVS) (Figures 16-23 to 16-27). In some cases, standard TAS and TVS studies may be supplemented by TA (transabdominal) and TV (transvaginal) color flow Doppler and by hysterosonography (HS).

TAS of the female pelvis is performed through the full urinary bladder, which provides a wide sonic window and larger field of view than a TV approach. TVS provides better anatomic detail than TAS because the high-frequency transducer can be placed closer to an area of interest. Ideally, TAS may show the size and location of a mass, which can then be better characterized with TVS.

Sonographic Appearance of the Pelvic Skeleton
Sacrum, coccyx, innominate bones (ilium, ischium, pubis)
Sonography is *not* the modality of choice for evaluating osseous structures because sound waves cannot penetrate their density; thus, bones cast shadows. On the other hand, the distinctive sonographic appearance of the pelvic skeleton creates useful landmarks. The highly echogenic vertebrae of the lower spine form the posterior boundary of the true pelvis (Figure 16-28). The iliac crests of the innominate bones can be identified as hyperechoic linear structures casting posterior shadows. These crests can be visualized extending from the near field to the far field on a TA image when the approach is along the superolateral aspect of the pelvis (Figure 16-29).

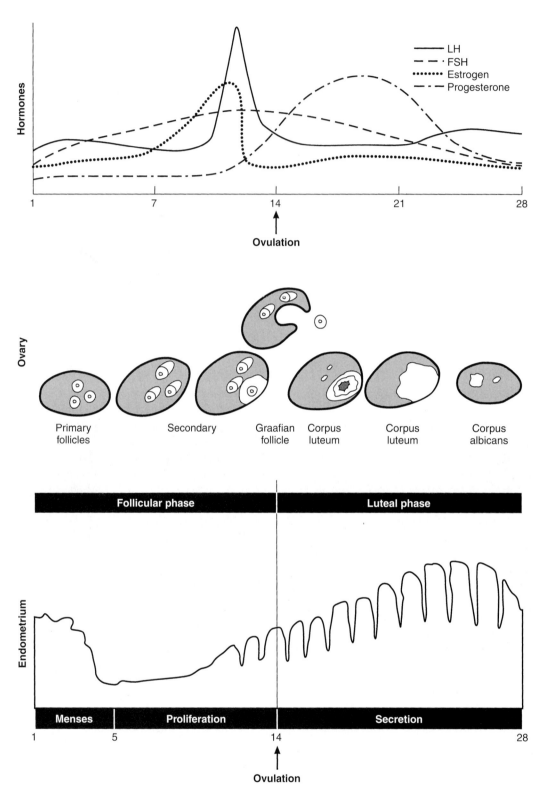

Figure 16-22 Menstrual cycle. The first day of bleeding corresponds to the first day of the female menstrual cycle. The thickened endometrial lining of the uterus is shed during menses. At this point, the production of follicle stimulating hormone (FSH) promotes the follicular phase of the ovarian cycle. Developing follicles within the ovaries begin to produce estrogen, which in turn causes proliferation of the endometrial lining. At approximately day 14 of the menstrual cycle, luteinizing hormone (LH) peaks; at this point, ovulation occurs, and the graafian follicle releases a mature ovum. The latter half of the menstrual cycle corresponds to the luteal phase of the ovary, during which the corpus luteum produces estrogen and progesterone. These hormones promote the secretory phase of the endometrial cycle, during which the endometrium continues to thicken. Inhibited production of LH at the end of the menstrual cycle leads to a breakdown of the corpus luteum and the shedding of the endometrium with the onset of menses.

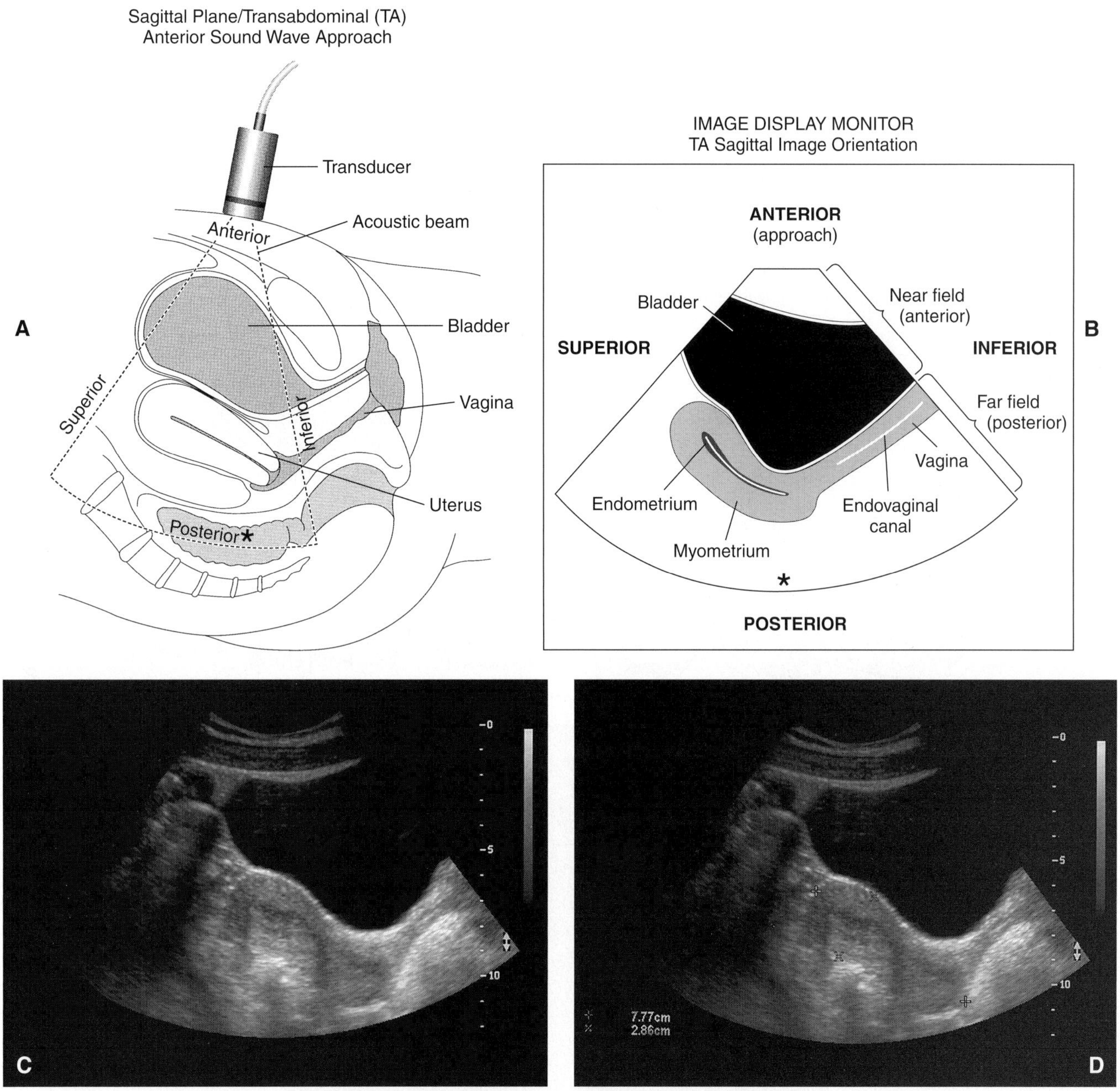

Sagittal Plane/Transabdominal (TA)
Anterior Sound Wave Approach

A

Transducer

Acoustic beam

Anterior

Bladder

Vagina

Uterus

Posterior*

Superior

Inferior

IMAGE DISPLAY MONITOR
TA Sagittal Image Orientation

B

ANTERIOR
(approach)

Bladder

Near field
(anterior)

SUPERIOR

INFERIOR

Far field
(posterior)

Endometrium

Vagina

Myometrium

Endovaginal
canal

*

POSTERIOR

C

D

7.77cm
2.86cm

Figure 16-23 Sagittal plane transabdominal (TA) pelvic imaging. **A,** Illustrates how TA pelvic sonography is performed from an anterior approach using the fully distended urinary bladder as an acoustic window. **B,** Image orientation of the sagittal plane on the image display monitor. The anterior portion of the pelvis is displayed in the near field of the image, and the posterior region of the pelvis is displayed in the far field of the image. In a sagittal plane, the left and right sides of the image correspond to the superior and inferior regions of the pelvis, respectively. **C,** Sonogram from a midsagittal plane in TA pelvic imaging. The fully distended urinary bladder is the large anechoic structure with bright walls in the near field of the image, anterior to the uterus. Notice the smooth contour and medium gray echo texture of the uterine myometrium and vaginal walls. Note how the uterus is pushed superoposteriorly by the distended bladder, and is roughly perpendicular to the ultrasound beam. **D,** Represents the caliper placement for measuring the long axis section of the uterus from a TA sagittal plane. *Denotes corresponding location. (C and D, Half-tone images courtesy the University of Virginia Health System, Department of Radiology, Division of Ultrasound, Charlottesville, Virginia.)

Transverse Plane/Transabdominal (TA)
Anterior Sound Wave Approach

A

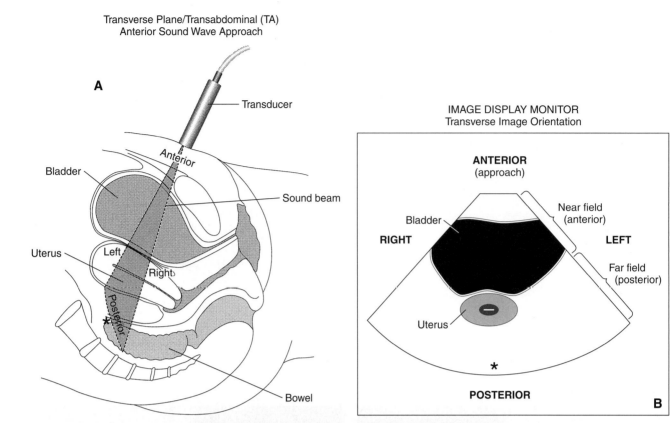

Transducer

Anterior

Bladder

Sound beam

Uterus

Left

Right

Posterior

*

Bowel

IMAGE DISPLAY MONITOR
Transverse Image Orientation

ANTERIOR
(approach)

Bladder

RIGHT

Near field
(anterior)

LEFT

Far field
(posterior)

Uterus

*

POSTERIOR

B

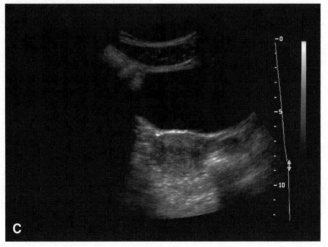

C

Figure 16-24 Transverse plane TA pelvic imaging. **A,** Illustrates the anterior transducer position for TA imaging of the pelvis in the transverse plane. **B,** Image orientation of the transverse plane on the image display monitor. The near and far fields of the transverse image correspond to the anterior and posterior regions of the pelvis, respectively. The left and right sides of the image correspond to the right and left sides of the pelvis, respectively. **C,** TA, transverse sonogram of a short axis section of the uterus. Note the anechoic urinary bladder in the near field of the image, anterior to the medium gray uterus. *Denotes corresponding location.

Sagittal Plane/Transvaginal (TV)

A

Anterior

Uterine
myometrium

Superior

Uterine
endometrium

*

Collapsed urinary
bladder

Transducer in
vaginal canal

Inferior

Posterior

Sound beam

Rectum

Bowel

TV Sagittal Image Orientation

B

Superior

Anterior

Inferior

Posterior

Inferior

**ROTATE
IMAGE**

Anterior

Posterior

Superior

IMAGE DISPLAY MONITOR

INFERIOR
(approach)

Near field
(inferior)

Uterine
endometrium

ANTERIOR

POSTERIOR

Far field
(superior)

*

Uterine
myometrium

SUPERIOR

Bowel

C

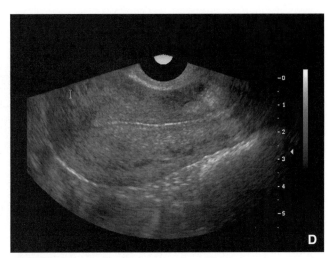

D

Figure 16-25 Sagittal Plane/Transvaginal (TV) pelvic imaging. **A,** The endovaginal transducer position for TV imaging of the pelvis; **B** and **C,** The TV sagittal image orientation and the rotation of the image on the display monitor. The apex of the TV image corresponds to anatomic structures that are closest to the face of the transducer. In the sagittal plane, the near field of the TV image generally corresponds to the inferior region of the true pelvis. The far field of the TV image generally corresponds to the superior region of the true pelvis. The left and right sides of the display monitor correspond to anterior and posterior regions of the pelvis, respectively. **D,** Longitudinal section of the uterus from a midsagittal plane in TV pelvic imaging. Note the limited field of view (compared with TA imaging) but the increase in anatomic detail. *Denotes corresponding location.

Coronal Plane/Transvaginal (TV)
Inferior Sound Wave Approach

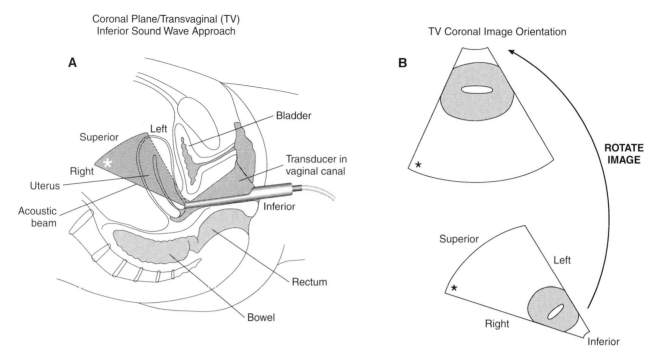

TV Coronal Image Orientation

ROTATE IMAGE

IMAGE DISPLAY MONITOR

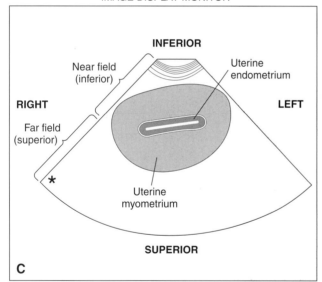

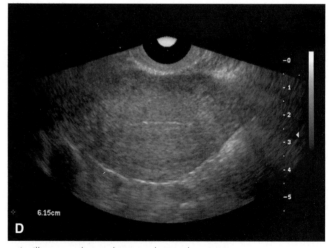

Figure 16-26 Coronal plane TV pelvic imaging. **A,** Illustrates the endovaginal transducer position for TV imaging of the pelvis. With an empty urinary bladder, the fundus of the anteverted uterus is tilted forward toward the anterior abdominal wall. Consequently, the coronal TV imaging plane demonstrates a short axis section of the anteverted or anteflexed uterus. **B** and **C,** Illustrate the TV coronal image orientation and the rotation of the image on the display monitor. The near and far fields of the coronal TV image correspond to inferior and superior regions of the pelvis, respectively. The left and right sides of the display monitor correspond to the right and left sides of the pelvis, respectively. **D,** Short axis section of the uterus from a coronal plane in TV pelvic imaging. As mentioned previously, note the limited field of view (compared with TA imaging) but the increase in anatomic detail. *Denotes corresponding location. (D, Half-tone image courtesy the University of Virginia Health System, Department of Radiology, Division of Ultrasound, Charlottesville, Virginia.)

IMAGE DISPLAY MONITOR

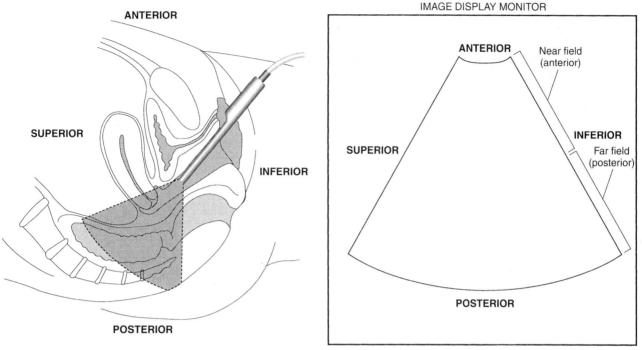

Figure 16-27 TV imaging: anteroinferior approach. Most TV imaging is performed from a standard inferior approach as demonstrated in Figures 16-25 and 16-26. However, manipulation of the TV transducer causes variation from the standard TV image orientation previously described. For example, when the transducer is lifted anteriorly (toward the pubic symphysis), the acoustic beam is directed more posteriorly. In this case, the near and far fields of the sagittal image correspond to anterior and posterior regions of the pelvis, respectively. Similarly, from a more anterior TV approach, the left and right sides of the image display monitor more closely correspond to superior and inferior regions of the pelvis. A posterior TV approach would also cause significant variation in image orientation. Thus, image orientation for TVS may vary between authors and ultrasound texts.

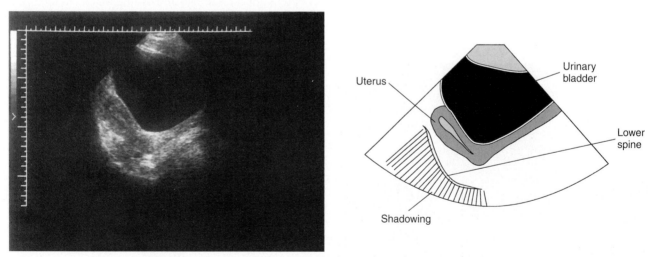

Figure 16-28 Pelvic skeleton. The lower vertebral spine forms the posterior boundary of the true pelvis. The vertebral bodies appear highly echogenic and cast posterior shadows.

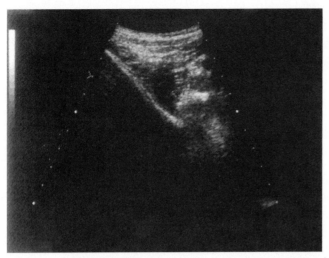

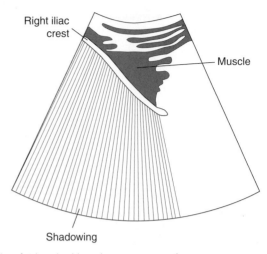

Figure 16-29 Pelvic skeleton. The iliac crest is easily identified as highly echogenic, extending superiorly on this longitudinal view. As with the spine, the iliac crest is reflective and casts shadows so that structures behind the crest cannot be visualized.

Sonographic Appearance of Pelvic Musculature

Iliopsoas, obturator internus, pelvic diaphragm, (pubococcygeus, iliococcygeus, coccygeus), pirifprmis, rectus abdominis

The muscles most commonly visualized in TA pelvic sonography include the iliopsoas muscle bundles, obturator internus muscles, pelvic diaphragm muscles, piriformis muscles, and rectus abdominis muscles. The skeletal muscles of the pelvis exhibit the same characteristic low-gray sonographic muscular pattern seen from other muscles throughout the rest of the body. The pelvic muscles typically appear hypoechoic to the pelvic organs. Linear striations in the muscles can be visualized when imaged in a plane longitudinal to the muscle fibers. The

skeletal muscles define the external borders of the abdominopelvic cavity.

The *iliopsoas muscle bundle* formed by the psoas major and iliacus muscles exhibits low-gray echoes with a distinct, fairly central, hyperechoic focus from the iliopsoas fascia that lies between the psoas major and iliacus muscle. The paired iliopsoas muscles can be identified on each side of the reflective lateral walls of the urinary bladder, in the anterior portion of the pelvis. The anechoic external iliac vessels and homogeneous rectus abdominis muscle can be identified anterior to the iliopsoas. In short axis, the iliopsoas appear rounded and distinctive due to their contrasting hyperechoic centers (Figure 16-30). In longitudi-

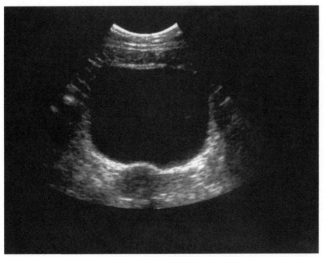

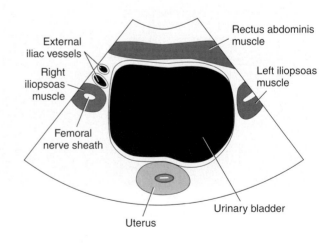

Figure 16-30 Pelvic musculature. This TA transverse section shows how the iliopsoas muscles are lateral to the urinary bladder. These skeletal muscles have low-level echoes and appear hypoechoic to their echogenic foci, the femoral nerve sheath.

nal sections the low-gray iliopsoas muscle bundle is ovoid and divided by the femoral nerve sheath, which appears thick, horizontal, and hyperechoic compared with the muscle (Figure 16-31).

The *obturator internus muscles* appear posterior and medial to the iliopsoas muscles. They present sonographically as thin, bilateral, linear, low-level echoes abutting the lateral walls of the urinary bladder (Figure 16-32). The obturator internus muscles are best seen in TA transverse images of the true pelvis.

The muscles of the *pelvic diaphragm (pubococcygeus, iliococcygeus [levator ani muscles], coccygeus)* are easiest to visualize in TA transverse views of the most inferior portions of the true pelvis. These bilateral muscles are seen medial to the obturator internus muscles adjacent and posterior to the cervix and vagina (see Fig-

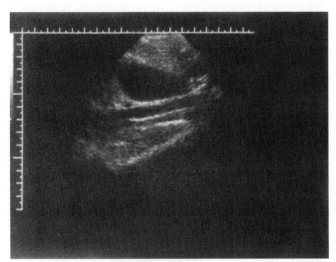

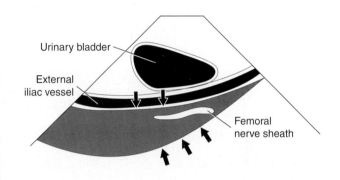

Figure 16-31 Pelvic musculature. This TA longitudinal section is a right parasagittal view of the pelvis, just lateral to the right ovary. This view demonstrates the low-level echoes of the iliopsoas muscle (shown by arrows), and the central hyperechoic femoral nerve sheath. The anechoic external iliac vein is seen anterior to the muscle.

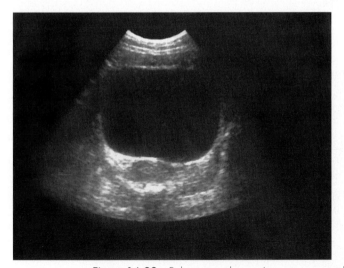

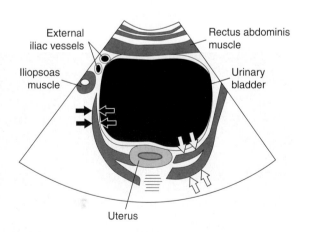

Figure 16-32 Pelvic musculature. In a transverse plane, the obturator internus muscles are seen transversely as thin structures with low-level echoes, paralleling the lateral walls of the urinary bladder *(black arrows)*. The levator ani muscles of the pelvic diaphragm are seen hammocking across the pelvic floor, posterior to the cervix *(white arrows)*. The right iliopsoas muscle is seen anterolaterally. The right external iliac artery and vein can be identified as circular, anechoic structures anterior to the iliopsoas muscle. The rectus abdominis muscle is seen lining the anterior abdominal wall, anterior to the urinary bladder.

ures 16-32 and 16-33). Sonographically, they present as low-level, mildly curved, linear echoes.

The bilateral hypoechoic *piriformis muscles* can be visualized posterior to the uterus and anterior to the sacrum (Figure 16-34).

The paired, paramedian *rectus abdominis muscles* are easiest to identify in a transverse or short axis section of the pelvis. They appear low gray in the most anterior portion of the abdominopelvic wall. Thin, bright lines representing the rectus sheath delineate the anterior and posterior borders (see Figure 16-31).

Sonographic Appearance of Pelvic Ligaments

Unless they are outlined by free intraperitoneal fluid, the ligaments of the female pelvis, with the exception of the broad ligaments (Figure 16-35), are not routinely identified sonographically.

Sonographic Appearance of Pelvic Spaces
Anterior cul de sac, posterior cul de sac, space of Retzius

It is not uncommon or abnormal to visualize a small amount of free fluid between the cervix and the rectum, in the *posterior cul de sac.* Identification of a large amount of fluid in the posterior cul de sac, between the uterus and urinary bladder in the *anterior cul de sac,* in the lateral pelvic recesses, or in Morison's pouch suggests an abnormal intraperitoneal fluid collection.

The *space of Retzius* may be sonographically significant when the urinary bladder appears to be displaced posteriorly. This is a characteristic feature of masses in

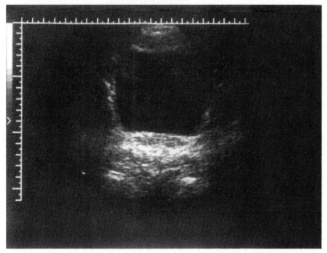

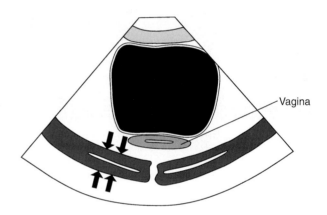

Figure 16-33   Pelvic musculature. This TA image from a transverse plane demonstrates the low-gray, mildly curved levator ani muscles posterior and lateral to the vagina *(between arrows).*

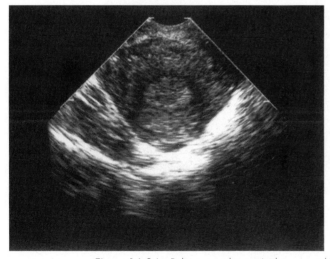

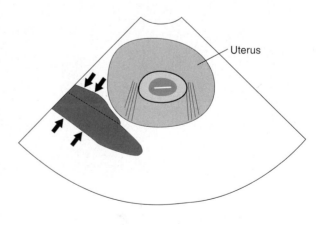

Figure 16-34   Pelvic musculature. In this coronal TV image, the bilateral, low-gray piriformis muscle is visualized in the right posterior region of the pelvis *(black arrows).* The corresponding piriformis muscle on the left side is obscured by overlying bowel gas in the left region of the pelvis.

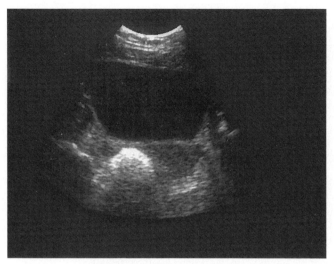

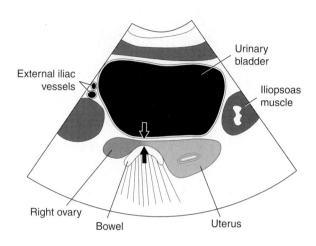

Figure 16-35 Broad ligament. This transverse TA image shows a longitudinal section of the broad ligament *(between arrows)*, which appears as the region of medium- to low-level echoes extending between the uterine cornu and the ovary. The uterine tube is not sonographically distinguished.

the space of Retzius, as other pelvic masses typically displace the bladder anteriorly or inferiorly.

Sonographic Appearance of Pelvic Organs
Genital tract (vagina, uterus, uterine tubes), ovaries, urinary bladder

Genital Tract Appearance
Vagina, uterus, uterine tubes

The sonographic presentations of the vagina, uterus, and uterine tubes are very similar because they share the same basic structure: cavities enclosed by an inner mucosal lining, a smooth muscle wall, and an outer layer of connective tissue. Variations in the sonographic ap-

pearance of the mucosa and muscular walls of the genital tract are dictated by size, location, and function of each segment.

Vagina Appearance. The vagina can be identified in the inferior portion of the pelvis between the urinary bladder (anteriorly) and rectum (posteriorly). Longitudinally, the vagina appears as a tubular extension of the uterus. In short axis, the vagina has a flattened, oval shape. The muscular vaginal walls appear low gray and homogeneous with smooth contours. The central mucosal lining of the normally collapsed vaginal canal walls appears thin, linear, and bright (Figures 16-36 and 16-37). The muscles of the pelvic diaphragm and any

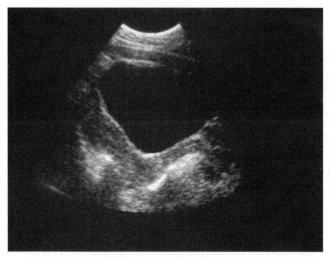

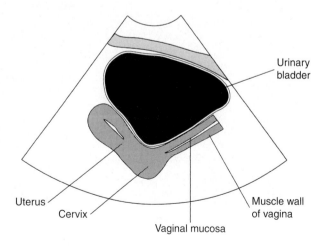

Figure 16-36 The vagina. In this TA image from a sagittal plane, the vagina is seen posterior and inferior to the distended, anechoic urinary bladder. Notice how the muscular walls of the vagina exhibit low- to mid-level echoes and surround the thin, hyperechoic central mucosal lining.

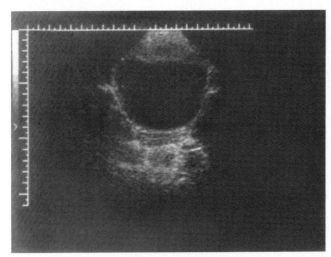

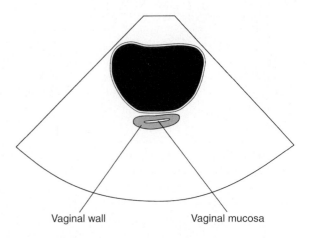

Vaginal wall   Vaginal mucosa

Figure 16-37 The vagina. In this TA image from a transverse plane, the vagina is visualized posterior to the anechoic urinary bladder. The central vaginal mucosa appears hyperechoic compared with the low-gray appearance of the muscular vaginal walls. Note the smooth contour of the vaginal walls.

fluid in the posterior cul de sac can be visualized posterior to the vagina.

Uterus Appearance. The uterus is well-visualized sonographically, using either TAS or TVS. Size and sonographic pattern of the uterus are described according to corresponding cyclical changes.

As mentioned earlier, the endometrial layer of the uterus is composed of a deep basal layer and superficial layer (or functional zone). Sonographically, the basal layer appears highly echogenic due to the reflective mucosal glands that compose the layer. The superficial layer generally appears hypoechoic compared with the bright basal layer. The central, linear, opposing surfaces of the endometrium that form the endometrial canal present sonographically as a bright, reflective, thin, midline strip, called the endometrial stripe.

The width of the endometrium is greatest near the uterine fundus and narrows toward the cervix (Figure 16-38). Measurement of endometrial thickness is most accurate on a longitudinal section of the uterus taken in the sagittal plane and should include the endometrial layers anterior and posterior to the reflective endometrial canal

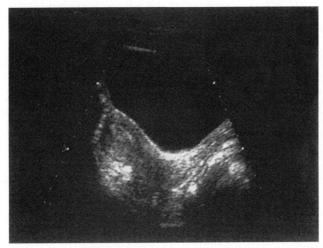

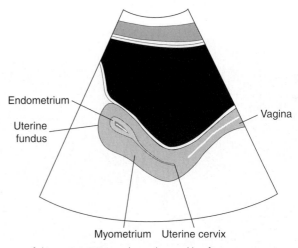

Endometrium

Uterine fundus

Vagina

Myometrium   Uterine cervix

Figure 16-38 The uterus. This is a midsagittal TA image of the uterus. Notice how the width of the endometrium is greatest near the fundus and narrows toward the cervix. In longitudinal sections of the uterus, like this one, the endometrial canal appears as a very thin, centrally located, bright stripe that is hyperechoic compared with the myometrium. The walls of the uterus are normally compressed together, collapsing the uterine cavity, which gives it a single stripe appearance. In some cases, the continuous endometrial, cervical, and vaginal canals can be imaged together in the same longitudinal section.

(Figure 16-39). Some refer to this as the "double-layer" thickness. The darker hypoechoic halo from the inner myometrial layer should not be part of the measurement.

As the thickness of the endometrium changes cyclically with the menstrual cycle, so does its sonographic appearance. During the menstrual phase, the endometrium appears thin and bright as the superficial layer is shed. In the early proliferative phase (days 5 to 9), the endometrium measures 4 to 8 mm thick and appears linear and hyperechoic to surrounding structures. Later in the proliferative phase (days 10 to 14), the functional zone of the endometrium thickens under the influence of estrogen and is hypoechoic compared with the bright, echogenic basal layer. Just prior to ovulation near the 14th day of the menstrual cycle, the endometrium measures from 6 to 10 mm and takes on a multilayered appearance (Figure 16-40). The bright endometrial stripe is surrounded by the thickened, hypoechoic, functional zone. The functional zone is separated from the inner layer of the myometrium by the fairly thin hyperechoic basal layer. This layered appearance continues during the early secretory phase when the endometrium achieves its maximum echogenicity and thickness from 7 to 14 mm (Figure 16-41). During the secretory phase (days 15 to 28), the functional zone is even thicker and edematous from the influence of progesterone and becomes isoechoic to the basal layer (see Figure 16-41). The endometrium normally measures less than 8 mm in postmenopausal women.

The myometrium is isoechoic to and continuous with the muscular walls of the vagina. As mentioned earlier, the uterine myometrium comprises the bulk of uterine tissue and consists of three sonographically distinguishable muscle fiber layers. The outer longitudinal fiber layer appears hypoechoic to the intermediate layer and is separated from the intermediate layer by anechoic arcuate vessels. The spiral fiber bands of the intermediate layer comprise the thickest and most echo-dense layer

that exhibits a mid- to low-gray, homogeneous echo texture. The inner circular and longitudinal fibers are significantly less echogenic than the intermediate layer and give the appearance of a thin hypoechoic halo surrounding the endometrium (Figure 16-42).

During periovulatory and menstrual phases, myometrial contractions have been identified sonographically as a rippling effect along the endometrium, extending from the cervix to the fundus. These muscular contractions are thought to play a role in sperm transport.

The only notable sonographic characteristic of the outer serosa layer of the uterus is its smooth contour. It is otherwise indistinguishable.

The sonographic pattern of the cervix is similar to that of the rest of the uterus (Figure 16-43). The muscular walls are homogeneous, with mid- to low-gray echoes surrounding the thin, hyperechoic endocervical mucosal lining (Figure 16-44). The endocervical canal is a continuation of the endometrial canal and appears as a fairly thin, bright echogenic stripe. It is normal to occasionally see anechoic fluid in the endocervical canal, particularly during the preovulatory phase. In some cases, shadows are cast by air visualized in the vaginal fornices surrounding the external os of the cervix (Figure 16-45; see Figure 16-44, *B*).

The internal os of the cervix is difficult to visualize except during pregnancy, when it is identified as the point where the cervical canal and the amniotic membrane or presenting parts meet. The external os is recognized as the point where the anterior and posterior lips of the cervix meet. In most cases, TVS provides a clear image of the cervix. In situations where TVS is contraindicated and TAS does not provide enough detailed information of the cervix, translabial (transperineal) sonography provides another scanning option. In translabial imaging, the cervical canal is generally oriented at a right angle from the distal vagina.

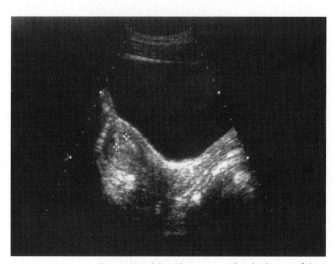

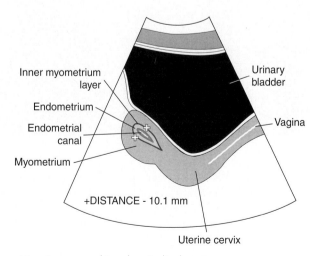

Figure 16-39 The uterus. The thickness of the endometrium is measured in a longitudinal section of the uterus from a sagittal plane, at its greatest dimension.

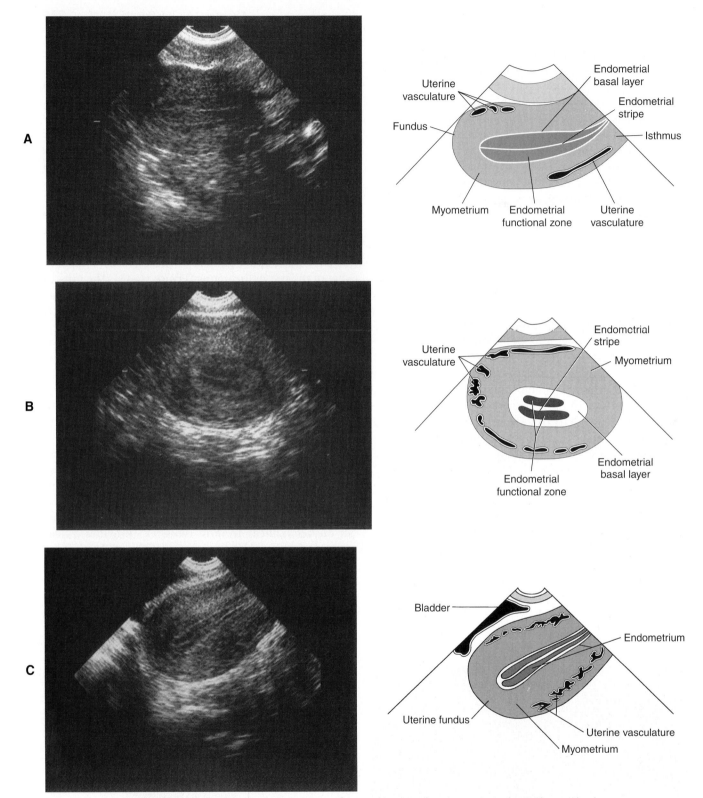

Figure 16-40 Multilayered appearance of preovulatory endometrium. **A,** In this TV longitudinal section of the uterus, notice how thick the endometrium is. The bright hyperechoic stripe of the endometrial canal is surrounded by the low-gray functional zone, the thickest portion of the endometrium. The functional zone is separated from the hypoechoic inner myometrial layer by the thin, bright basal layer of the endometrium. **B,** This TV coronal plane demonstrates a short axis section through the anteverted uterus. The myometrium exhibits low- to mid-level gray echoes, and the endometrium presents with a multilayered preovulatory appearance. **C,** This TV sagittal view shows a longitudinal section of an anteverted uterus prior to ovulation. The multilayered appearance of the endometrium presents as a central hyperechoic line surrounded by a thicker, hypoechoic layer, surrounded by a thin, hyperechoic border. A small quantity of anechoic urine is seen in the urinary bladder. The uterine vessels can be identified as anechoic areas along the periphery of the myometrium.

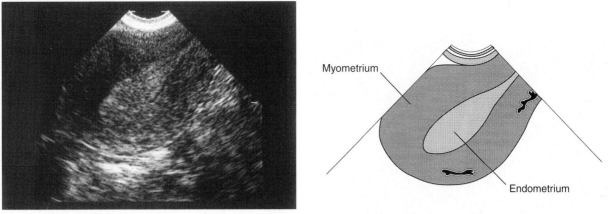

Figure 16-41 Secretory phase endometrial appearance. In this TV sagittal image showing a longitudinal section of the uterus, the appearance of the endometrium during the secretory phase is demonstrated. In addition to an increased overall thickness, the endometrial basal layer, functional zone, and canal become isoechoic.

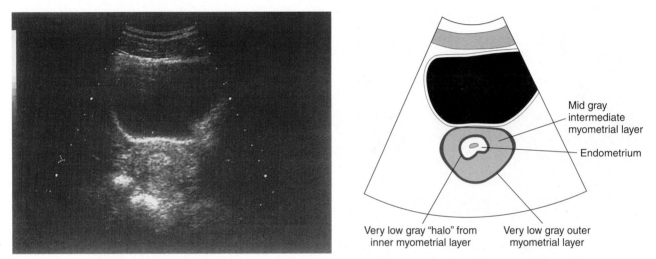

Figure 16-42 Myometrium. This TA transverse image and short axis section of the uterus clearly distinguishes the muscle fiber layers of the myometrium. The inner and outer layers appear hypoechoic compared with the mid-gray intermediate layer. In transverse views like this of the pelvis, short axis sections of the uterus can be identified posterior to the bladder as round or oval low-level echo textures distinguished by the bright, horizontal, centrally located stripe representing the endometrial canal. It is fairly easy to recognize the uterus because of the sharp contrast in appearance between the anechoic distended bladder and low-gray echo texture of the uterus.

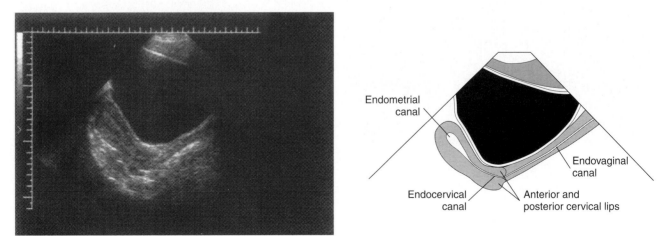

Figure 16-43 The cervix. This sagittal TA image shows a longitudinal section of the cervix at the most inferior aspect of the uterus, closest to the vagina. Notice how the anterior and posterior lips of the cervix can be outlined as the cervix protrudes into the vagina, which lies at right angles to the cervix.

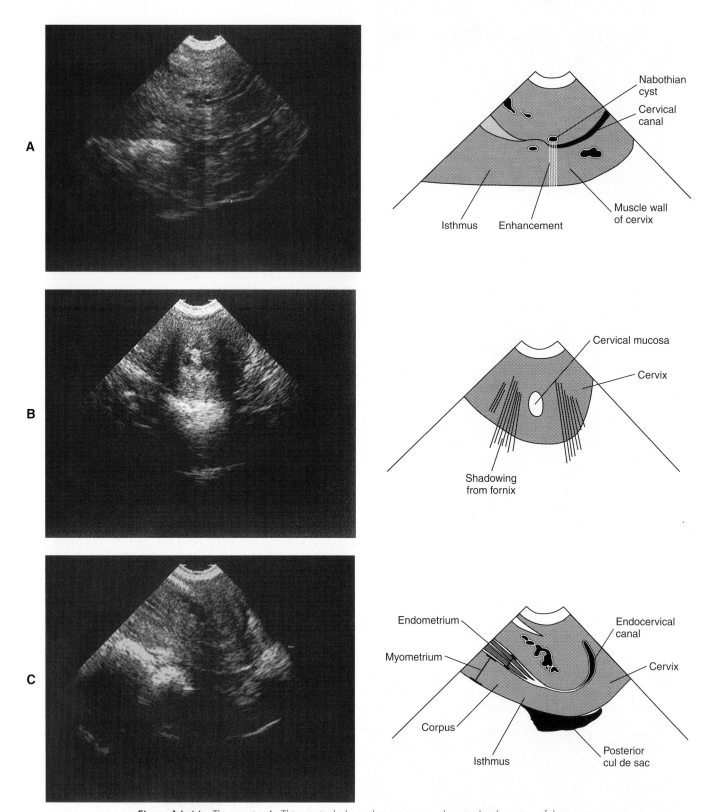

Figure 16-44 The cervix. **A,** This sagittal plane demonstrates a longitudinal section of the cervix. The uterus is in the normal anteverted position. A slight quantity of anechoic fluid is seen within the cervical canal. A small nabothian cyst is seen within the wall of the cervix exhibiting posterior enhancement. **B,** In the coronal TV plane of the true pelvis, the anteverted uterus is demonstrated in short axis sections. Shadowing from the vaginal fornices is identified at the level of the cervix. Notice how TVS provides more detailed visualization of the cervical canal than TAS provides. **C,** This sagittal TV image shows a longitudinal section of the cervix in an anteflexed uterus. A small quantity of anechoic fluid is seen in the endocervical canal and the posterior cul de sac.

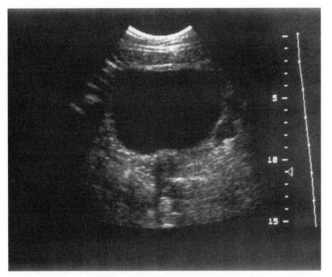
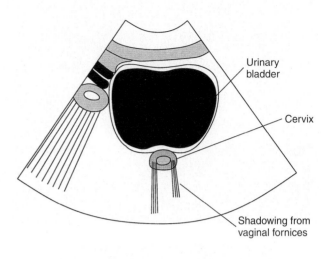

Figure 16-45 The cervix. In this TA transverse image, shadowing from the vaginal fornices clearly denotes the level of the cervix seen in short axis.

On TAS when the urinary bladder is full, the uterus appears "straightened out" rather than anteflexed. If the uterus is retroverted, with the fundus pointing posteriorly, it can be difficult to image the fundus with TAS as a result of attenuation of sound by the anterior portion of the uterus. This echo-poor appearance is referred to as the "dropout" phenomenon. Usually, the dropout in the fundus of a retroverted uterus is not a problem for TVS.

Uterine Tubes Appearance. Unless there is free fluid in the lateral pelvic recesses or tubal pathology, the infundibulum, ampulla, and isthmus cannot be identified sonographically. The interstitial portion of the oviduct, however, can be imaged with TVS. It appears as a 1-cm long, tenuous, echogenic line arising from the endometrial canal and extending through the uterine wall.

Ovarian Appearance. The bilateral, almond-shaped ovaries are most commonly identified lateral to the uterine fundus, usually with the long axis vertically orientated (Figure 16-46). Normal ovarian echo texture is homogeneous unless otherwise interrupted by anechoic ovarian follicles, a common finding during reproductive years. Generally the ovary presents sonographically with a hypoechoic periphery representing the tunica and a low-gray echogenic center representing the stroma. The ovaries usually appear hypoechoic to the uterine myometrium. Sonographic landmarks include the hypoechoic iliopsoas

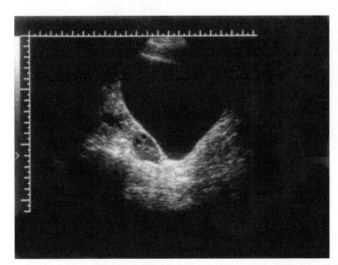
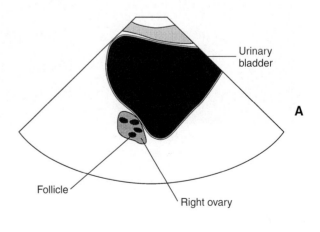

Figure 16-46 Ovaries. **A,** The almond shape of the ovary is apparent in this sagittal TA image. The ovaries appear low gray and hypoechoic compared with the uterine myometrium, and several small anechoic follicles are seen within the ovary.

continued

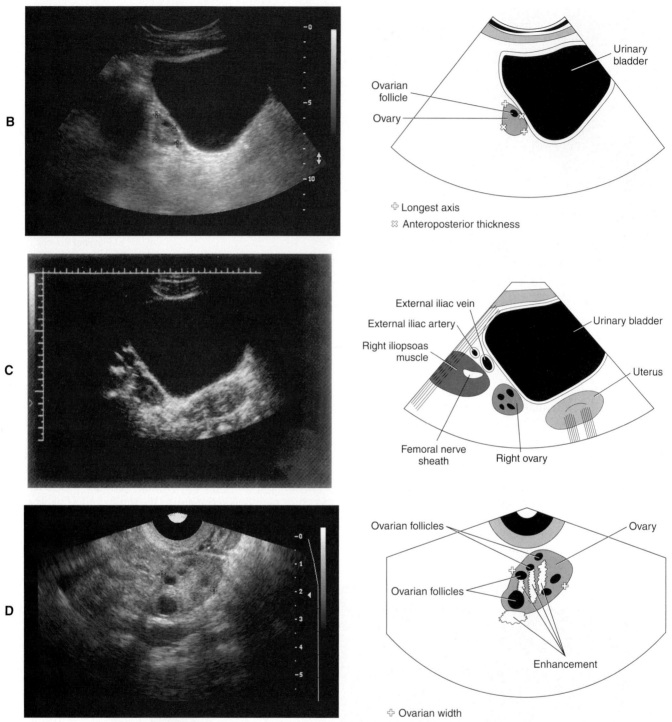

B
C
D

Longest axis
⊗ Anteroposterior thickness

Urinary bladder
Ovarian follicle
Ovary

External iliac vein
External iliac artery
Right iliopsoas muscle
Urinary bladder
Uterus
Femoral nerve sheath
Right ovary

Ovarian follicles
Ovary
Ovarian follicles
Enhancement

Ovarian width

Figure 16-46, cont'd   B, The length and thickness of the ovary are measured on a longitudinal view, and depending on the lay of the ovary, that may be viewed in either a sagittal or transverse plane. The length is calculated from the longest dimension of the ovary. The anteroposterior thickness is measured perpendicular to the length. C, The transverse transabdominal image demonstrates the anatomic position of the ovary relative to its surrounding structures. The very low-gray iliopsoas muscle and anechoic external iliac vessels are seen right lateral to the right ovary. The cervix is visualized medial to this right ovary. More often, the ovary will be identified lateral to the uterine corpus or fundus. D, The width of the ovary is measured on a short axis section. The anteroposterior thickness would be measured perpendicular to the width. (B and D, Half-tone images courtesy the University of Virginia Health System, Department of Radiology, Division of Ultrasound, Charlottesville, Virginia.)

muscles and anechoic external iliac vessels anterolateral to the ovaries and the anechoic internal iliac vessels posterior to the ovaries. TAS and especially TVS provide excellent definition of the ovaries and follicular structures.

As mentioned earlier, ovarian volume is marginally affected by cyclical changes. The lowest volumes are seen during the luteal phase and highest volumes during the preovulatory phase. Developing follicles within the ovary vary in both size and number. The anechoic appearance of a follicle accompanied by bright, hyperechoic posterior enhancement is due to the fluid-filled follicular antrum (Figure 16-47).

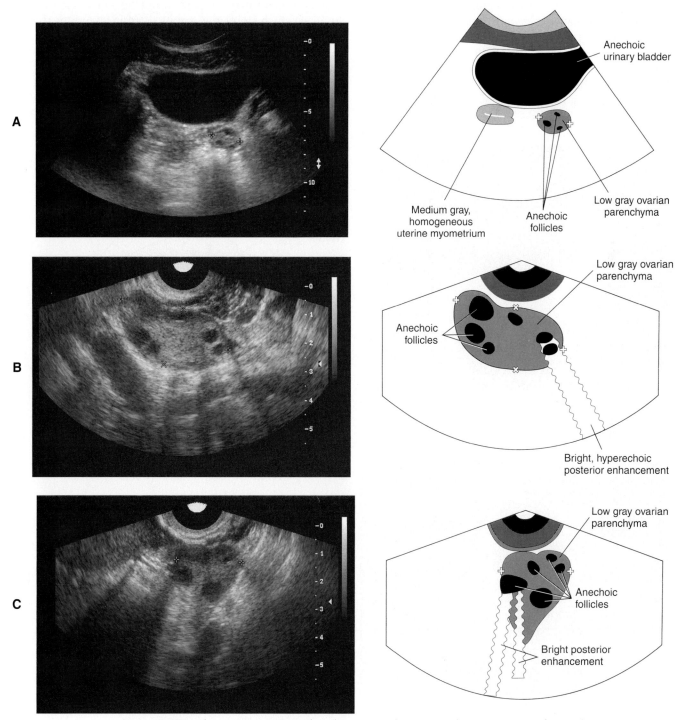

Figure 16-47 The ovaries. A, B, and C demonstrate the sonographic appearance of normal ovarian parenchyma and developing follicles. In A, notice how the ovary is hypoechoic compared with uterine myometrium. (Half-tone images courtesy the University of Virginia Health System, Department of Radiology, Division of Ultrasound, Charlottesville, Virginia.)

The oocyte and cellular layers of the developing follicle cannot be identified sonographically. However, just prior to ovulation, the granulosa layer separates from the theca layer, resulting in a low-gray, hypoechoic ring. Also at this time, the cumulus oophorus of the secondary follicle can occasionally be seen as a thin hyperechoic crescent along the wall of the anechoic follicular antrum (Figure 16-48). A mature graafian or dominant follicle presents as anechoic, with smooth hyperechoic walls, and measures approximately 20 mm (within a range of 16 to 28 mm) (Figure 16-49).

Following ovulation, the anechoic fluid of the ruptured graafian follicle can be identified in the posterior cul de sac, molding to the shape of surrounding structures. Usually, bright acoustic enhancement through the fluid can be identified behind the posterior cul de sac (Figure 16-50). Also following ovulation, the corpus luteum appears irregular in shape and contains internal echoes due to hemorrhage and blood clot. The internal echoes vary in appearance from multiple, fine, bright septations, to diffuse, low-level echoes (Figure 16-51). This blood clot may become completely anechoic over time, at which point the corpus luteum resembles the sonographic appearance of a mature follicle. Eventually, the corpus luteum regresses, leaving a small amount of scar tissue in the ovary, called the corpus albicans, which appears as a hyperechoic focus within the ovarian stroma (Figure 16-52).

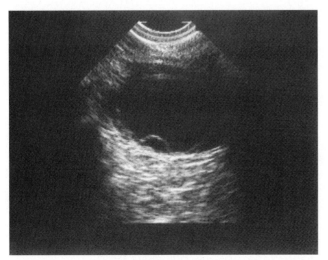

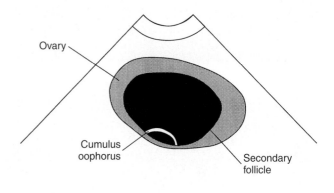

Figure 16-48 Cumulus oophorus. The cumulus oophorus appears as a thin, bright crescent along the wall of the mature follicle. The secondary oocyte is contained within the cumulus oophorus.

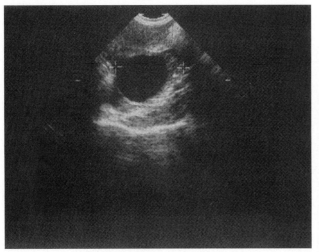

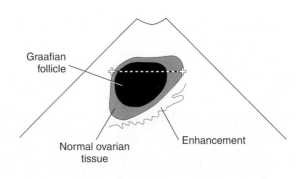

Figure 16-49 Graffian follicle. This coronal TV image demonstrates a mature graafian follicle within the ovary. Sonographically, dominant follicles appear anechoic with smooth walls, and are round or oval in shape. Mature follicles are usually 18 to 22 mm in size and exhibit posterior enhancement.

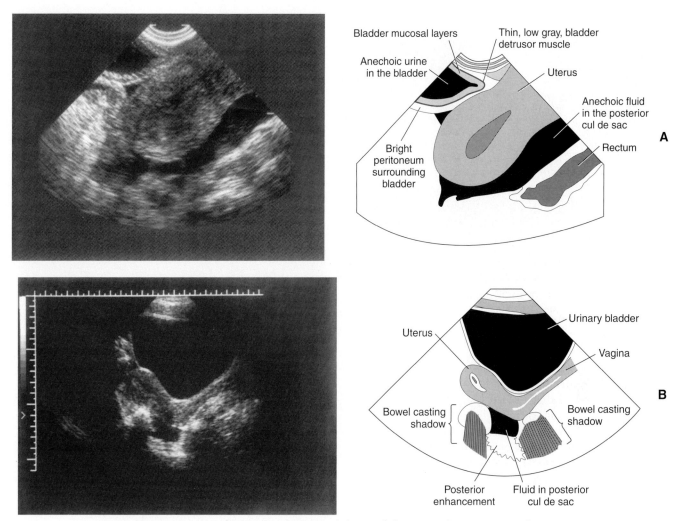

Figure 16-50 Anechoic fluid in the posterior cul de sac, following ovulation. **A,** Note the partially filled urinary bladder in the upper left corner, which correlates to an anteroinferior orientation in this TV sagittal image. Notice how the inner mucosa of the bladder wall is less visible, and the relaxed detrusor muscle and the peritoneal lining surrounding the bladder are clearly visualized. **B,** The rectum and sigmoid colon of the pelvic bowel are often visualized in sagittal TA images. The rectum usually appears bright and reflective, posterior to the vagina. The sigmoid colon has a similar appearance and lies posterior to the uterus.

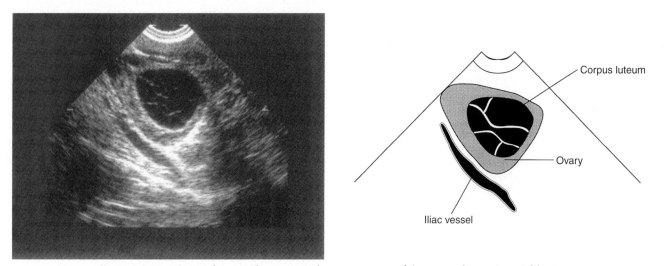

Figure 16-51 Corpus luteum. The sonographic appearance of the corpus luteum is variable. In this TV coronal section, the corpus luteum is visualized with multiple fine septations.

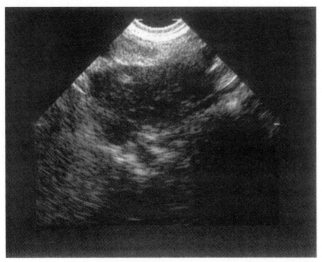
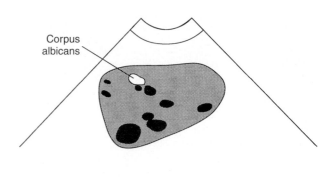

Corpus
albicans

Figure 16-52 Corpus albicans. The corpus albicans is the remaining scar tissue in the ovary following regression of the corpus luteum. This TV image shows the corpus albicans, which appears as a highly echogenic foci within the ovary.

Urinary Bladder Appearance. It is important to note that the size and shape of the bladder can vary depending on the quantity of urine being stored at any given time. Nevertheless, the distended bladder should appear symmetric on ultrasound. The fully distended urinary bladder presents as a large, anterior, anechoic structure in the midregion of the true pelvis surrounded by smooth, hyperechoic, uniformly thick walls.

On superior short axis sections the distended bladder has a rounded appearance. Inferiorly, the short axis bladder sections appear square, shaped by the pelvic musculature and bones. In longitudinal sections, the contour of the posterior surface of the bladder can normally appear somewhat indented by an anteverted uterus. The bladder lumen is not visible when it is collapsed.

As mentioned earlier, the bladder is composed of four layers of tissue: an inner mucosa, a submucosa layer, the muscularis, and the outer serosa. The thin inner layers of mucosa appear as narrow bright lines along the circumference of the bladder (Figure 16-53). The middle muscularis, or muscular, layer of the bladder wall stretches thin with bladder distention and is not well-visualized sonographically. When the bladder is only slightly distended, the relaxed detrusor muscle can be visualized as a hypoechoic layer surrounding the mucosa (Figure 16-54; in 16-50, *A*, notice how the detrusor muscle is better appreciated with TVS). The thin outer serosal layer of the bladder is sonographically indistinct.

Normally the ureters are not sonographically appreciated as they enter the bladder. However, the effect of the ureters ejecting urine into the bladder can be routinely observed on real-time examination. As discussed

in Chapter 12, hyperechoic ureteral jets, or squirts of urine, can be visualized in the trigone portion of the bladder (see Figure 12-28).

Sonographic Appearance of the Pelvic Colon

Loops of bowel within the pelvic cavity appear heterogeneous due to content. Bowel can present as bright and reflective, anechoic, or a combination of both.

Small bowel is displaced superiorly when the urinary bladder is full for TAS. During TVS, peristalsis can be observed in the loops of small bowel around the uterus and ovaries. In some cases, gas in the small intestine can obscure visualization of the ovaries.

Like the small bowel, the sonographic appearance of the rectosigmoid colon is variable, depending largely on content. Typically, the sigmoid colon and the rectum contain gas and fecal material that cast a posterior acoustic shadow (Figure 16-55).

Sonographic Appearance of Pelvic Vasculature

Uterine Vasculature Appearance. The high resolution of TVS provides visualization of much of the uterine vasculature. Vessels coursing within the peripheral myometrium appear as anechoic tubular structures (see Figure 16-40).

As a rule, the uterine arteries and veins can be identified with color flow Doppler (TAS or TVS) lateral to the cervix and ascending lateral to the uterus in the broad ligament to the junction of the uterine tubes and uterus.

During the periovulatory period the spiral arteries can be identified in the functional zone of the endometrium with TV color flow Doppler. In cases of infertility, the spiral arteries cannot be imaged.

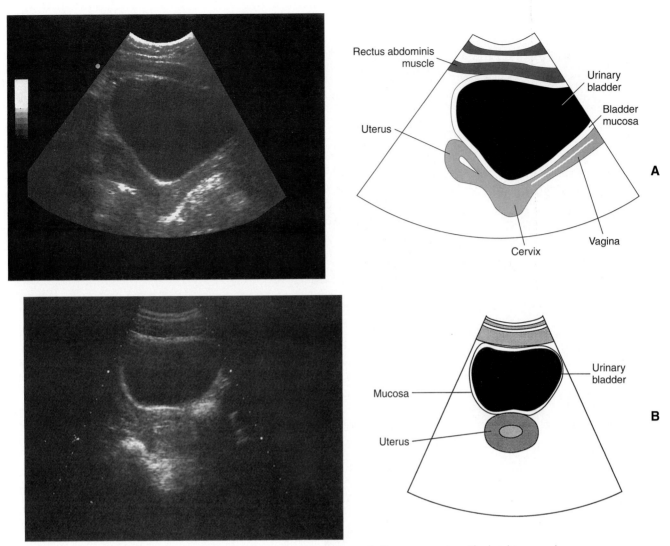

A

B

Figure 16-53 Urinary bladder. **A,** Longitudinal section. **B,** Short axis section. The bright mucosal lining of the distended anechoic bladder is seen along its circumference. The muscular wall of the bladder is stretched thin due to distention; thus the detrusor muscle is not visible. Notice how the bladder appears square in short axis. The low-gray appearing uterus can be identified in both images, posterior to the bladder.

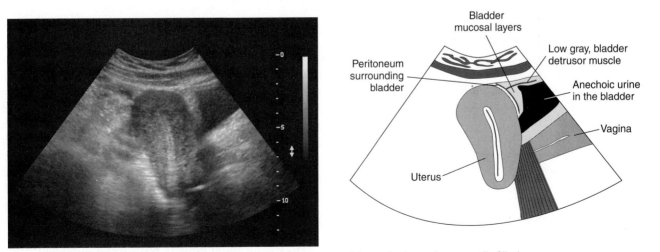

Figure 16-54 Urinary bladder. Sagittal TA image of the midpelvis with a partially filled urinary bladder. In this case the detrusor muscle is relaxed and is seen as a low-gray layer of the bladder wall. Note how the entire uterus is difficult to visualize without the acoustic window of a fully distended urinary bladder.

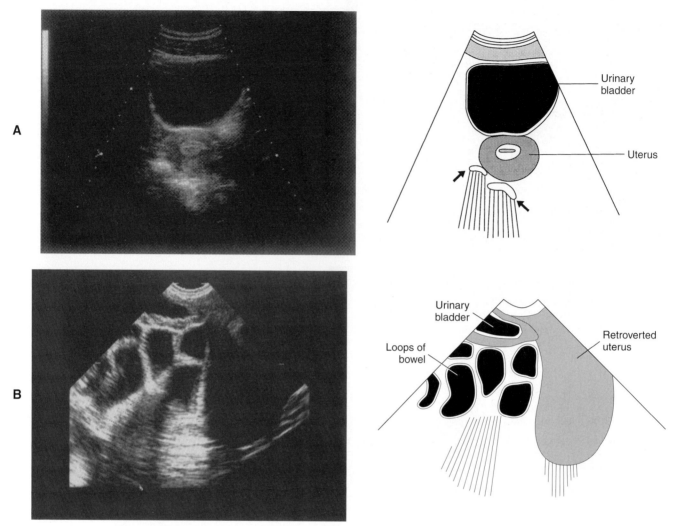

Figure 16-55 Pelvic colon. **A,** This transverse TA image shows a reflective portion of the sigmoid colon *(arrows)* posterior to the uterus. **B,** Peristaltic loops of small bowel are often visualized transvaginally. Anechoic, fluid-filled loops of bowel are seen resting in the anterior cul de sac. In this sagittal image, notice that the uterus is moderately retroverted. Note also the thickness of the partially distended bladder wall. (Half-tone images courtesy the University of Virginia Health System, Department of Radiology, Division of Ultrasound, Charlottesville, Virginia.)

Ovarian Vasculature Appearance. Color flow and spectral Doppler are valuable tools in assessing blood flow to the ovaries and to ovarian masses. During the normal ovulatory cycle, the functional ovary receives greater vascular perfusion between days 9 and 28 of the menstrual cycle. This is reflected in a lower resistance Doppler waveform in the ovary producing the dominant follicle. A low resistance waveform has a high amount of diastolic flow. The luteal phase is the best time to observe blood flow within the ovary using power Doppler and TV color flow Doppler. In postmenopausal women, ovarian flow cannot be detected.

Pelvic Lymph Node Appearance. Normal pelvic lymph nodes are not appreciated sonographically. Abnormally large nodes appear hypoechoic to surrounding structures or even anechoic with indistinct hyperechoic walls. Typically, they appear in multiples and are closely related in groups. Pathologically enlarged lymph nodes in the pelvis would be visualized in the areas surrounding the common iliac artery, external iliac artery and vein, pelvic sidewalls, and in the area of the false pelvis.

SONOGRAPHIC APPLICATIONS

Sonographic imaging of the female pelvis has multiple applications but is generally used to rule out the presence of a mass. If a mass is found, sonography can provide the site of origin, size, and composition. This modality is more limited, however, in providing definitive diagnoses of the benignity or malignancy of such

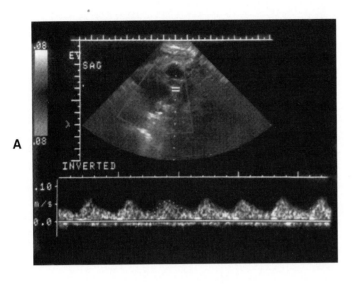

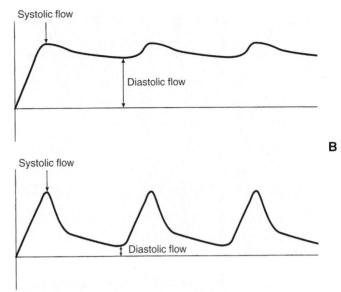

Figure 16-56 Ovarian Doppler. **A,** A low resistance waveform, obtained in the ovarian artery. Low resistance vessels exhibit a high amount of flow during diastole. **B,** An ovarian artery with higher resistance. **C,** Doppler signal obtained from a malignant ovarian tumor. The low resistance of this vessel is reflected in the low pulsatility index of 0.79.

masses. Clinical studies utilizing TV color flow Doppler and spectral Doppler suggest great potential for differentiating benign from malignant tumors using these techniques (Figure 16-56).

Gynecologic sonography can also be used to diagnose congenital uterine anomalies, pelvic inflammatory processes, and suspected ectopic pregnancy. In addition, ultrasound plays a significant role in diagnosing and managing infertility. Pelvic sonography is used in assessing contributing causes of infertility such as endometriosis, congenital anomalies, myomas, and pelvic inflammatory disease. Sonography is routinely utilized for follicle monitoring in infertility cases, particularly in patients undergoing hormone therapy. Ultrasound guidance is also important for ovum retrieval prior to in vitro fertilization.

Another application of pelvic sonography is detecting intrauterine contraceptive devices (IUDs, IUCDs). Figure 16-57 demonstrates four common types of IUDs. These devices generally appear highly reflective with varying degrees of posterior acoustic shadowing. Figures 16-58 and 16-59 demonstrate the typical sonographic patterns of IUDs.

Further use of pelvic sonography includes the evaluation of ovaries in posthysterectomy patients. In the absence of the uterus, the ovaries typically rest within the posterior cul de sac. Figure 16-60 illustrates a TA midsagittal plane posthysterectomy.

Hysterosonography (HS) is an imaging technique developed to better evaluate the endometrium. HS has provided a more accurate distinction between endome-

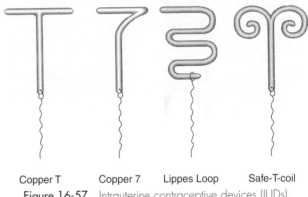

| Copper T | Copper 7 | Lippes Loop | Safe-T-coil |

Figure 16-57 Intrauterine contraceptive devices (IUDs).

trial abnormalities such as hyperplasia, polyp, fibroid, or carcinoma.

NORMAL VARIANTS

Normal variations of the uterus identifiable on ultrasound consist of specific uterine positions that include tilting of the uterus to the right or left, tilting of the uterine fundus and body posteriorly (retroversion) (Figure 16-61), and bending of the uterine fundus and body posteroinferiorly (retroflexion). It should be noted that these position variations are considered to be normal standard deviations unless the uterus is displaced by pathology.

A congenital ovarian malformation identifiable with ultrasound alters the normal shape of the ovary, giving it a distinctive L-shape. The ovary appears normal in all other respects.

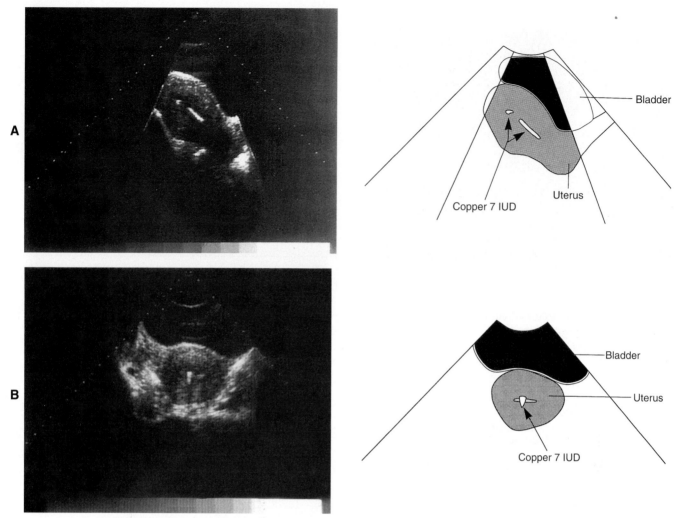

Figure 16-58 Copper Seven IUD. **A,** The Copper Seven IUD is easily visualized in a sagittal view and longitudinal section of the uterus. This contraceptive device is highly echogenic and rests within the endometrial cavity. **B,** This transverse TA image demonstrates the appearance of the Copper Seven IUD within the endometrial canal in a short axis section of the uterus.

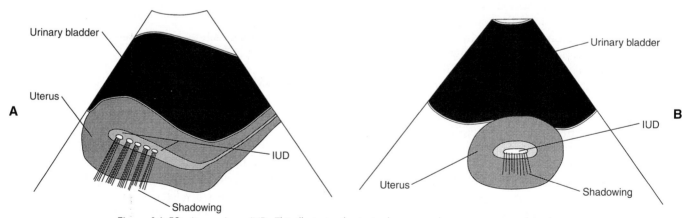

Figure 16-59 Lippes Loop IUD. This illustrates the typical sonographic appearance of the Lippes Loop IUD in short **(A)** and long **(B)** axis within the endometrial canal. Posterior shadowing is frequently associated with IUDs.

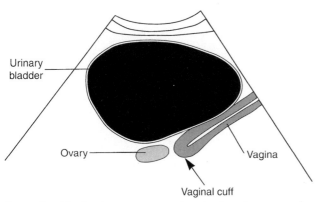

Figure 16-60 Posthysterectomy pelvis. In this illustration of a sagittal TA image of the pelvis posthysterectomy, the vaginal cuff is identified and the uterus is absent. The ovaries can often be identified in the region of the posterior cul de sac.

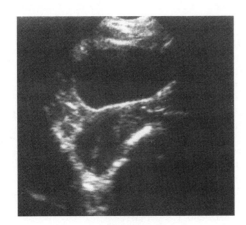

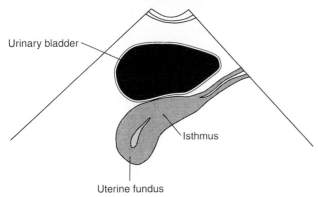

Figure 16-61 Normal variant. In a TA sagittal plane, a longitudinal section of a retroverted uterus shows the fundus tilted posteriorly.

REFERENCE CHARTS

■ ■ ■   ASSOCIATED PHYSICIANS

Gynecologist: A physician specializing in female reproduction, including physiology, endocrinology, and diseases of the genital tract.

Endocrinologist: A physician specializing in the physiologic and pathologic association of hormonal secretions of the body.

Obstetrician: A physician specializing in the medical care of pregnant women.

Radiologist: A physician specializing in the administration and interpretation of diagnostic medical imaging.

■ ■ ■   COMMON DIAGNOSTIC TESTS

Computed Tomography and Magnetic Resonance Imaging: CT and MRI are both extremely important diagnostic tools in evaluating the female pelvis. Improvements in contrast agents continue to enhance the superior tissue characterization of these modalities. These tests are performed by trained technologists and interpreted by radiologists.

Laparoscopy: An endoscopic procedure performed under local or general anesthesia in which a telescopic instrument is inserted into the abdominal cavity from the area of the navel. The laparoscope can be manipulated in order to visualize the abdominal or pelvic organs. This test is performed and interpreted by a gynecologist.

Hysteroscopy/Salpingoscopy: An endoscopic procedure in which a telescopic instrument is inserted through the vagina and into the uterus. This test allows visualization of the interior uterine walls. This technique can also be used to visualize the fallopian tubes. These tests are performed and interpreted by a gynecologist or a similarly trained physician.

Hysterosalpingography: A radiologic examination of the uterus and fallopian tubes following dye (contrast agent) administration. Tubal blockage and structural abnormalities of the uterus can be diagnosed. This procedure is performed and interpreted by a radiologist.

Hysterosonography: A sonographic procedure used to examine the endometrium and uterine cavity. The procedure provides enough detail to differentiate endometrial pathologies that are otherwise not distinguishable with standard TAS or TVS. Radiologists perform the procedure and interpret the results.

■ ■ ■   LABORATORY VALUES

Human Chorionic Gonadotropin (hCG): A highly accurate blood pregnancy test. This hormone is produced by the placental trophoblastic cells and plays an important role during the first trimester of pregnancy.

Leukocytosis: An abnormally high serum white blood cell count (exceeding 10,000 per mm³). This condition is indicative of an infectious process (such as pelvic inflammatory disease).

Hysterosonography: A sonograph used to examine the endometrium and uterine cavity.

Estrogen/Progesterone: These hormones are produced by the ovary during the normal menstrual cycle. Serum concentrations of these hormones can be useful in evaluating ovulatory function.

■ ■ ■   NORMAL MEASUREMENTS

	Length	Width	Thickness
Vaginal canal	9 cm		
Cervical canal	2-4 cm		
Premenarchal uterus	2.5 cm	2 cm	1 cm
Nulliparous uterus	7 cm	4 cm	3 cm
Multiparous uterus	8.5 cm	5.5 cm	4.5 cm
Uterine tubes	7-12 cm		
Adult ovary	2.5-5 cm	1.5-3 cm	0.6-2.2 cm
Ovarian volumes*	Mean (ml)		
Premenarche (3-15 years)	3.0±2.3		
Menstruating	9.8±5.8		
Premenopausal	6.8		
Postmenopausal (1-5 years after)	6.2±2.7 to 4.0±1.8		
Postmenopausal (10-15 years after)	2.8±2.1 to 2.2±1.4		

*Length × width × thickness (height) × 0.523

■ ■ ■   VASCULATURE

Uterine Vasculature:
Aorta—common iliac artery—uterine—internal iliac artery—uterine artery—arcuate arteries—radial arteries—straight arteries—spiral arteries—spiral veins—straight veins—radial veins—arcuate veins—uterine vein—internal iliac vein—common iliac vein—inferior vena cava.

Ovarian Vasculature:
PATHWAY ONE. Aorta—common iliac artery—internal iliac artery—uterine artery—ovarian branch of uterine artery—ovarian branch of uterine vein—uterine vein—internal iliac vein—common iliac vein—inferior vena cava.

PATHWAY TWO. Aorta—right ovarian artery—right ovarian vein—inferior vena cava or aorta—left ovarian artery—left ovarian vein—left renal vein—inferior vena cava.

■ ■ ■   AFFECTING CHEMICALS

Birth Control Pills: Estrogen and progestin provide a highly effective form of birth control. These medications mimic the hormonal conditions of pregnancy, resulting in an anovulatory state.

Diethylstilbestrol (DES): A synthetic estrogen commonly administered to pregnant women from the late 1940s to the early 1970s. This medication was thought to reduce the risks of spontaneous abortion. DES was taken off the market after it was discovered to cause multiple problems involving the reproductive organs of offspring exposed to the drug in utero. A small, irregular, T-shaped uterus is a common malformation associated with DES exposure.

Menotropins (Pergonal), Urofollitropin (Metrodin), Clomiphene Citrate (Clomid): Medications commonly prescribed in infertility to stimulate follicular maturation and induce ovulation.

BIBLIOGRAPHY

Cooperberg P, Richenberg J: Ultrasound of the uterus. In Callen PW, editor: *Ultrasonography in obstetrics and gynecology*, ed 4, Philadelphia, 2000, WB Saunders, pp 819-821, 824, 829.

Dill-Macky MJ, Atri M: Ovarian sonography. In Callen PW, editor: *Ultrasonography in obstetrics and gynecology*, ed 4, Philadelphia, 2000, WB Saunders, pp 859, 861.

Levi CS, Holt SC, Lyons EA, et al: Normal anatomy of the female pelvis. In Callen PW, editor: *Ultrasonography in obstetrics and gynecology*, ed 4, Philadelphia, 2000, WB Saunders, pp 781, 785, 790, 796, 799, 801-809.

Scheerer LJ, Bartolucci L: Ultrasound evaluation of the cervix. In Callen PW, editor: *Ultrasonography in obstetrics and gynecology*, ed 4, Philadelphia, 2000, WB Saunders, pp 577, 580.

SECTION V

Obstetrics

CHAPTER 17

First Trimester Obstetrics (0 to 12 Weeks)

BETTY BATES TEMPKIN AND PEGGY MALZI BIZJAK

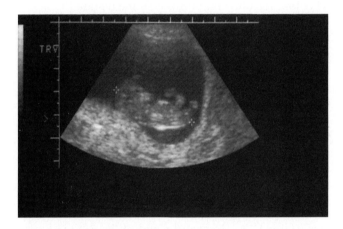

OBJECTIVES

Describe the role of the female reproductive system in creating and supporting a developing embryo.

Describe the sonographic appearance of the gestational sac and early embryo.

Describe the sonographic appearance of embryologic development.

Describe the sonographic appearance of the placenta during the first trimester.

Describe how gestational age is determined sonographically during the first trimester.

Be familiar with related tests performed during the first trimester.

Define the key words.

KEY WORDS

Alimentary canal	Anteflexion
Amnion	Anteverted position
Amniotic cavity	Basal layer
Amniotic fluid	Blastocyst
Amniotic fluid volume (AFV)	Chorion
	Chorion frondosum

Chorion laeve	Implantation
Chorionic plate	Lacunae
Chorionic sac	Luteinizing hormone (LH)
Chorionic villi	Mean sac diameter (MSD)
Corpus luteum	Mesencephalon
Cotyledons	Morula
Crown-rump length (CRL)	Neuroplate
Decidua	Oligohydramnios
Decidua basalis	Omphalomesenteric duct
Decidua capsularis	Placenta
Decidua parietalis (vera)	Placental substance
Decidual reaction	Polyhydramnios
Double bleb sign	Primary yolk sac
Double sac sign	Progesterone
Embryonic disk	Prosencephalon
Endometrium	Retroflexion
Estrogen	Retroversion
Follicle stimulating hormone (FSH)	Rhombencephalon
Gestational age (GA)	Syncytiotrophoblastic tissues
Gestational sac	Trophoblastic cells
Human chorionic gonadotropin (HCG)	Vitelline duct
	Zygote

Chapters 17 and 18 describe the anatomy, physiology, embryology, and ultrasound appearance of the embryo/fetus and its support structures at various stages of pregnancy. Chapter 19 describes high-risk pregnancies and associated ultrasound studies and ultrasound-guided procedures.

The first trimester of pregnancy is a remarkable sequence of events. The period of time for the first trimester is based on a 28-day menstrual cycle. It can be defined as 12 weeks after the first day of the last menstrual period. Typically, the term **gestational age (GA)** is synonymous with menstrual age and is used to date the age of a pregnancy. The first trimester includes ovarian, embryonic, and fetal phases of development; therefore understanding normal development and the rapid changes that occur in early pregnancy is important for obtaining accurate, interpretable sonographic images.

MATERNAL PHYSIOLOGY AND EMBRYO DEVELOPMENT

As discussed in Chapter 16, preparation of the female reproductive organs for support of a pregnancy begins 14 days prior to conception. The first and second weeks of the first trimester are days 1 to 14 of the menstrual cycle. During the first 2 weeks, an ovarian follicle matures, and usually on the 14th day, ovulation occurs (Figure 17-1). The ovarian phase, or cycle, depends on **follicle stimulating hormone (FSH)** to promote the follicular growth and a rise in **luteinizing hormone (LH)** resulting in ovulation (rupture of follicle and release of ovum). Following ovulation, the follicle transforms into the **corpus luteum,** which produces **progesterone** and a small amount of **estrogen** to prepare the uterus for **implantation.** During pregnancy, the corpus luteum may become enlarged and cystic (fluid filled) (Figure 17-2). The corpus luteum can reach greater than 6 cm in diameter by 7 weeks. Thereafter, it gradually diminishes without complication.

Fertilization usually takes place within 1 day of ovulation, day 15, at the ampulla of the fallopian tube and is considered complete when the egg and sperm fuse to form a **zygote.** The zygote, or cell mass, repeatedly divides and eventually forms a cluster of 16 or more cells, the **morula.** The morula exits the fallopian tube on the 18th or 19th day and enters the uterine cavity. Endometrial fluid penetrates the cell mass, creating a blastocyst cavity that converts the cell mass into an outer trophoblast layer and inner embryoblast layer (or **embryonic disk**). A **primary yolk sac** forms adjacent to the embryonic disk. The outer cell layer eventually creates the chorionic membranes of the fetal portion of the **placenta.** The inner embryoblast layer eventually develops into the embryo, amnion, umbilical cord, and the primary and secondary yolk sac. By the 20th or 21st day, the **blastocyst** begins to implant into the decidualized **endometrium,** a term applied to the functional layer of the gravid endometrium (Figure 17-3). By the 28th day, the blastocyst has become fully embedded within the myometrium of the uterus and implantation is complete.

During week 4, there is a rapid proliferation of the **syncytiotrophoblastic tissues** (**trophoblastic cells** that contact the endometrium), resulting in a primitive uteroplacental circulation. Primary **chorionic villi** are finger-like projections of the outer trophoblast layer that extend into deciduate endometrium. Chorionic villi are formed, surrounded by pools of maternal blood called **lacunae.** The primary yolk sac regresses as the secondary yolk sac

forms between the **amnion** (innermost membrane of the embryo) and the **chorion** (outermost tissues of the embryo). A bilaminar embryo disk distinguishes itself from the embryoblast layer. It lies between the secondary yolk sac and developing amnion (Figure 17-4).

Also during the 4th week as the embryo grows and elongates, a long, hollow tube is formed on the anterior surface of the embryo that develops into the **alimentary canal.** The canal is the rudimentary gastrointestinal system and divides into the foregut (the most superior end), midgut, and hindgut (the most inferior end). The foregut will eventually give rise to the pharynx, esophagus, stomach, and proximal duodenum. It will also give rise through outpouching to the liver and pancreas. The midgut gives rise to the small intestine and a portion of the colon. The hindgut eventually develops into the distal colon, rectum, and portions of the bladder.

The **neuroplate,** the most primitive component of the neurologic axis, develops after 4 to 5 weeks. This plate forms the neurocrest and neurotube. The neurotube eventually forms the brain and spinal cord.

The fetal lungs begin development as small-paired buds arising from the anterior surface of the most superior portion of the tube that becomes the alimentary canal. The fetal lung buds are present at about 5 weeks of GA and form numerous branching buds, which grow and increase in number until 17 weeks of gestation.

During week 5, a woman's normal menstrual flow is usually absent and suspect of pregnancy. The chorionic cavity (**gestational sac**) expands to a diameter of 5 mm (see Figure 17-4). Toward the end of the 5th week, the bilaminar embryonic disk changes into a trilaminar structure (three layers: endoderm, mesoderm, ectoderm).

The embryonic phase is weeks 6 to 10 and is considered a critical phase of human development. Major structures begin to form and although organ function is minimal, the primitive heart starts to beat at the beginning of the 6th week.

The embryonic heart begins as two tubes that eventually fuse along their midlines to form a very primitive tubular heart. Later in the first trimester, the four-chambered heart is formed by a series of folds and fusions of tissues in the tubular pump. Initially, the heart is required only to move blood across the circulatory system of the yolk sac. Following development of the four chambers, the heart pumps fetal blood throughout the growing embryo/fetus and its attendant placenta (see Chapter 23).

By week 6, the neurotube has developed into the primitive embryonic brain that consists of three segments: forebrain (the **prosencephalon**), midbrain (the **mesencephalon**), and hindbrain (the **rhombencephalon**). The forebrain develops into the cerebrum, lateral ventricle, and thalamus. The midbrain becomes the adult midbrain

NORMAL EVENTS IN THE FIRST FOUR WEEKS OF GESTATION

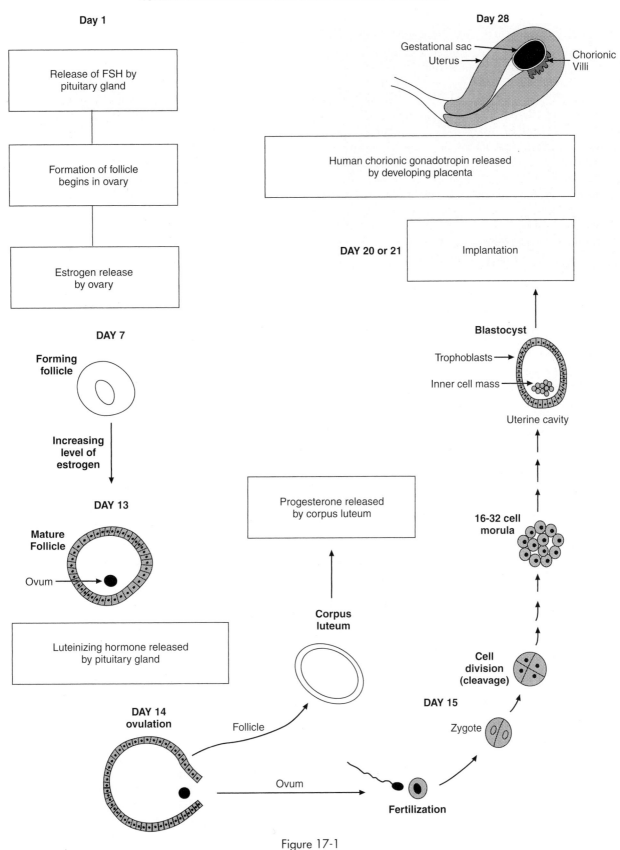

Figure 17-1

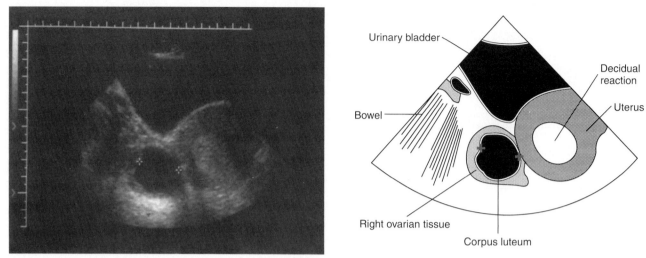

Figure 17-2 Transverse pelvis section. Anechoic corpus luteum cyst is adjacent to the homogeneous myometrium of the uterus. Note the hyperechoic appearance of the early decidual reaction of the endometrium. A corpus luteum usually has thick hyperechoic walls surrounding echogenic content. Its appearance can, however, range from a hyperechoic slit encircled by hypoechoic walls to a large solid or cystic mass.

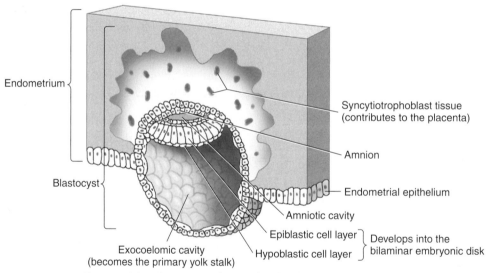

Figure 17-3 Blastocyst implanting the decidualized endometrium.

and forms the aqueduct of Sylvius. The hindbrain grows into the adult pons, medulla, and cerebellum and forms the fourth ventricle.

While it is growing, the embryo folds on itself along its different surfaces to differentiate anatomy. Two lateral folds lead to the formation of the anterior and lateral abdominal walls. At the same time, the midgut forms from the roof of the yolk sac, thereby reducing the connection between them to a narrow yolk stalk. At approximately 7 or 8 weeks, the yolk stalk fuses with the **omphalomesenteric duct (vitelline duct)** to become the umbilical cord. The umbilical cord is the connection between the embryo/fetus and placenta. It contains the vessels (two arteries, one vein) through which

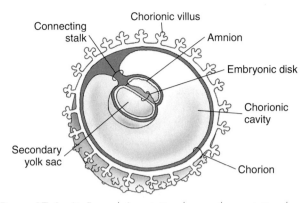

Figure 17-4 At 5 weeks' gestational age, the gestational sac (chorionic cavity) measures 5 mm in diameter and is well-visualized sonographically. The bilaminar embryo is situated between the newly formed amniotic cavity and secondary yolk sac. This anatomic relationship is described in sonography as the "double bleb" sign.

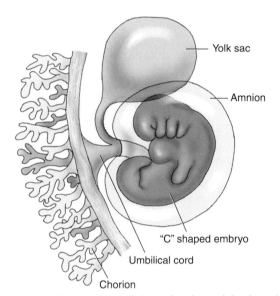

Figure 17-5 Between 7 and 8 weeks, the umbilical cord resolves and the embryo changes from flat to C shaped.

embryonic/fetal blood passes to and from the placenta. As the amnion continues to expand, it will form an external covering for the umbilical cord and embryo. At this point, the appearance of the embryo changes from flat and trilaminar to a C-shaped embryo with limb buds (Figure 17-5). The heart comes to lie ventrally and the brain cranially.

Mineralization of the fetal skeleton begins at 8 weeks. The skull and femur are adequately mineralized by 11.5 to 12 weeks. During the 8th to 11th weeks the small bowel usually herniates out of the embryo at the base of the umbilical cord. This is a normal event, and the bowel retracts into the embryo by 12 weeks of development.

Functional fetal kidney tissue appears at approximately 10 weeks. The production of fetal urine does not occur until early in the second trimester. (The fetal kidneys and bladder are discussed in Chapter 18.) By the end of the 10th week, major organ systems are established, and the embryo demonstrates human features.

Weeks 11 and 12, the final 2 weeks of the first trimester, begin the fetal phase. Growth is rapid and organ development continues. Fetal intestinal activity begins the 11th week of development and fetal swallowing usually the 12th week. As mentioned, the skull and femur are adequately mineralized by 11.5 to 12 weeks. The fetal head is disproportionately large compared with the body and constitutes one half of the length. As development continues, the head and body subsequently become more proportional.

DEVELOPMENT OF THE PLACENTA

Placentation is the sequence of events that follows implantation of the embryo, leading to the development of the placenta. The mother and embryo/fetus are joined together through adjacent uterine (maternal) and trophoblastic (embryonic/fetal) vascular structures. The maternal portion of the placenta is the section of decidualized endometrial lining of the uterus where implantation occurs **(decidua basalis).** The fetal portions of the placenta are the chorionic villi that form from the trophoblast layer (outer cell layer of the blastocyst) (Figure 17-6).

Decidua is the term applied to the gravid endometrium. It is the functional reaction of the endometrial lining to pregnancy. The endometrium becomes thick and edematous from vascular and structural changes to accommodate embryo implantation and development. During these changes, the decidua differentiates into three distinct areas, the decidua basalis, capsularis, and parietalis, all of which, except the deepest, is shed at parturition. The decidua basalis is the portion of thick decidua at the implantation site, which makes it the maternal portion and deepest layer of the placenta. The **decidua capsularis** is a thin portion of endometrium that overlies the section of gestational sac facing the uterine cavity. The **decidua parietalis** (or **decidua vera**) is the remaining endometrium, or peripheral portion, that is unoccupied by the implanted ovum (Figure 17-7).

As previously discussed, the fetal components of the placenta are the chorionic villi. Part of these villi degenerate to form a membranelike structure, the smooth

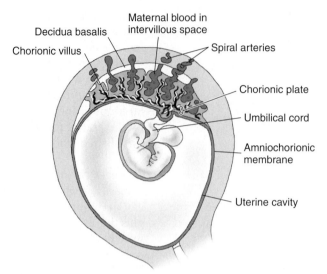

Figure 17-6 Chorionic villi invade the decidua basalis, forming embryo-maternal circulation. Resulting intervillous spaces receive maternal blood from the spiral arteries that surround and perfuse villi containing fetal blood.

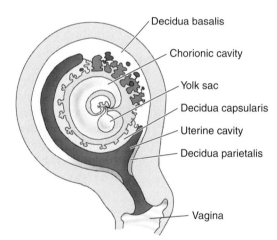

Figure 17-7 Differentiation of the gravid endometrium into decidua basalis (implantation site), capsularis (overlies sac facing uterine cavity), and parietalis (remainder of endometrium).

chorion (**chorion laeve,** or "chorionic membrane"). The rest of the villi compose the **chorion frondosum,** the portion of chorion at the implantation site that actively invades the decidua basalis to establish nutrition for the embryo. The chorion frondosum villi are surrounded by maternal tissue called the lacunar network. The lacunar network is a tissue extremely rich in small blood vessels and which, after contact with the villi, breaks down and forms small pools of maternal blood, or lacunae. It is the contact of the villi of the embryonic circulatory system with the maternal lacunae that facilitates the transfer of oxygen and metabolites and the transfer of carbon dioxide and waste products (see Figure 17-6).

Each chorionic villus branches to form groups of villi. Large groups of villi are known as **cotyledons,** and groups of cotyledons form between one and five lobules. As the gestation increases in size, so do its requirements for nutrition and waste product removal. The placenta also increases in size to keep up with this increasing demand. At 12 weeks, the placenta is between 1 and 2 cm in thickness. By 40 weeks of gestation, the placenta may be between 2.5 and 4 cm in thickness. The diameter of a term placenta can be as much as 20 cm.

The placenta may be divided into three basic areas: (1) The **chorionic plate** is the portion toward the inside of the sac (touching the amniotic membrane); (2) the **basal layer** (base plate) is that portion on the outside (touching the uterus); and (3) the **placental substance** is the placental material between the basal layer and the chorionic plate. Functional circulatory groups separate the lobes of the placenta. Small venules course through the substance of the placenta, becoming progressively larger as they converge, eventually forming a single umbilical vein. Conversely, two umbilical arteries enter the substance of the placenta and progressively divide with the villi to form even smaller vessels. As previously discussed, the single umbilical vein and the two umbilical arteries comprise the umbilical cord that connects the fetus to the placenta.

The placenta also functions as an endocrine gland. It produces **human chorionic gonadotropin (HCG),** which communicates to the rest of the body that a gestation is present within the uterus. The maternal blood, which supplies the oxygen and nutrients and removes waste products and carbon dioxide, arrives at the placenta via the spiral arterioles. These blood vessels coil their way up to the base of the placenta from the endometrial layer of the uterus.

DEVELOPMENT OF FETAL MEMBRANES

Prior discussion included that two fetal membranes surround the embryo, the amnion and the chorion. The amniotic membrane develops from the inner blastocyst layer and enlarges to enclose the **amniotic cavity,** which is separated from the secondary yolk sac by the small bilaminar embryonic disk (see Figure 17-4). The following illustrations show how the amnion and cavity enlarge to accommodate the developing embryo. The amniotic membrane remains attached to the embryo at the cord insertion site and ultimately covers the umbilical cord. The yolk sac, within the shrinking chorionic cavity, moves away from the embryo. The amnion and its cavity grow rapidly, containing the developing embryo and the **amniotic fluid** that "bathes" it throughout its course of development. The amnion consists of four connective layers and one epithelial layer; it is not a vascular membrane.

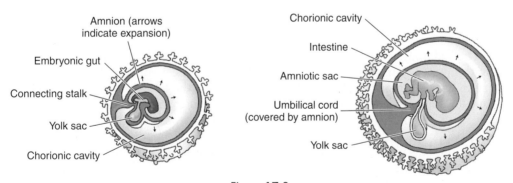

Figure 17-8

As mentioned, the chorionic membrane (smooth chorion, or chorion laeve) develops from the outer blastocyst layer. This vascular structure encloses the chorionic cavity, which surrounds the amnion, yolk sac, and embryo. The following illustration shows that as development continues, the chorionic membrane and cavity shrink; the amniotic membrane and cavity enlarge. Eventually, the membranes fuse, usually after 16 weeks. Complete fusion of the amniotic and chorionic membranes occurs with obliteration of the chorionic cavity.

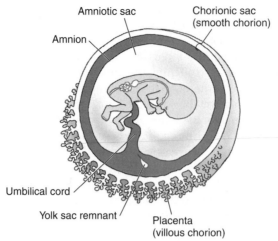

Figure 17-9

DEVELOPMENT OF AMNIOTIC FLUID

Amniotic fluid is the liquid enclosed by the amnion. It surrounds and bathes the embryo/fetus. Amniotic fluid has several important functions: (1) it permits symmetric growth of the embryo/fetus, (2) it prevents adhesions from forming in the fetal membranes, (3) it cushions the embryo/fetus and acts as a shock absorber, (4) it helps to maintain proper temperature of the embryo, (5) it allows normal development of the respiratory, gastrointestinal, and musculoskeletal systems, (6) it helps to prevent infection, and (7) it may be a source of nutrients for the developing embryo.

Amniotic fluid volume (AFV) depends on the balance between its production and its removal or absorption. During pregnancy, the structures responsible for production and passage of fluid into the amniotic cavity are the chorion frondosum, chorionic and amniotic membranes, skin, and respiratory and urinary tracts. Structures involved in the reduction of amniotic fluid are the gastrointestinal system and the amniotic-chorionic interface. Intramembranous and transmembranous pathways are also involved with the exchange, across membranes, of amniotic fluid and fetal blood (intramembranous) and amniotic fluid and maternal blood (transmembranous).

The first trimester contributes very little in the production of amniotic fluid. Electrolytes, water, urea, and creatinine pass freely through the membranes and into the cavity. Later, amniotic fluid is produced primarily by the lungs and kidneys. Fetal lung fluid leaves the trachea during breathing, becoming part of the amniotic fluid. The exact amount is unknown. Urine production also becomes part of amniotic fluid. Urine contribution is estimated at about 30% of fetal body weight daily.

The quantity of amniotic fluid increases until about 30 weeks of gestation. At that point, the volume of fluid begins to decrease considerably until delivery. The reduction of amniotic fluid is due primarily to the gastrointestinal system (swallowing amniotic fluid) and absorption of amniotic fluid into fetal blood perfusing the surface of the placenta. Fetal swallowing removes about half of the daily urine produced. At term, the fetus may swallow up to 50% of the AFV. It should be noted that at one time the respiratory system was considered part of AFV reduction; however, the current theory is that the lungs do not provide a pathway for the absorption of fluid in the normal fetus.

The volume of amniotic fluid reflects the state of gestational well-being. In fact, many abnormalities are associated with marked increases **(polyhydramnios)** or decreases **(oligohydramnios)** in the AFV. (Various methods of calculating AFV are discussed in Chapter 18.)

SONOGRAPHIC APPEARANCE OF FIRST TRIMESTER ANATOMY

Transvaginal sonography has made it possible to routinely image early structures. A sonographer needs to be familiar with embryology and how it presents sonographically to be able to distinguish normal and abnormal development. Early identification of anomalies influences decisions about pregnancy termination or fetal therapy.

Uterine Position Appearance

It is important to recall, from Chapter 16, the variable positions of the uterus (Figure 17-10). These positions may affect the sonographic appearance of the uterus and ultimately the appearance of an early gestation.

The uterus is normally located in the midline of the true pelvis in an **anteverted position.** In this position, the uterine body is bent at the isthmus slightly anterior toward the anterior abdominal wall so that the corpus and fundus rest on the dome of the bladder. A common variation in position is **anteflexion,** which is defined by a marked anterior flexion of the uterus at the isthmus. Filling of the bladder usually straightens out the uterus so it does not appear anteflexed on transabdominal imaging. **Retroflexion** is easy to identify sonographically because of the backward bend of the uterine fundus, which is angled posteriorly toward the posterior cul de sac. Another variation of uterine position is **retroversion.** In this instance, the cervix is tilted posteriorly, causing the uterine fundus to extend as far posteriorly as the rectum. A retroverted uterus can be difficult to image transabdominally, particularly the fundus, which may appear "echo poor." Alternatively, the retroverted fundus is not a problem in transvaginal scanning.

Gestational Sac Appearance

An intrauterine gestational sac is the term used by sonologists to describe the fluid-filled **chorionic sac,** which is the first fundamental sonographic finding in early pregnancy. Transvaginal transducers can visualize the gestational sac as early as 3 to 5 weeks. Normally it is located within the fundus or midportion of the uterus and appears as a small, round or oval, anechoic, fluid-filled collection enclosed by hyperechoic "walls" (the bright choriodecidual reaction).

As the normal gestational sac enlarges, it has a distinct sonographic appearance known as the **double sac sign.** This sign distinguishes a "pseudo sac" associated

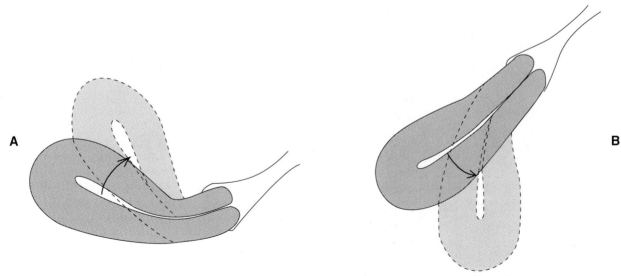

Figure 17-10 Variations in uterine position. **A,** Anteverted uterine position. Dotted lines show anteflexed position. **B,** Retroverted uterine position. Dotted lines indicate retroflexed position. In some cases the uterus may in fact be anteverted and retroflexed, anteverted and anteflexed, retroverted and anteflexed, or retroverted and retroflexed.

with ectopic pregnancies from a gestational sac. The following image demonstrates the double sac sign. Two hyperechoic concentric lines are seen surrounding a portion of the gestational sac. The line closest to the sac is the decidua capsularis (DC)—smooth chorion. The peripheral line is the decidua parietalis (DP). The uterine cavity is the anechoic, fluid-filled space between these two lines. The uterine cavity is always a potential hypoechoic space or anechoic space containing a small amount of fluid visualized between the DC and DP. The decidua basalis (DB) combines with the chorion frondosum at the gestational sac–endometrium interface; it appears hyperechoic and thick due to developing placental tissue. Note how the posterior portion of the image is enhanced by the bright through transmission.

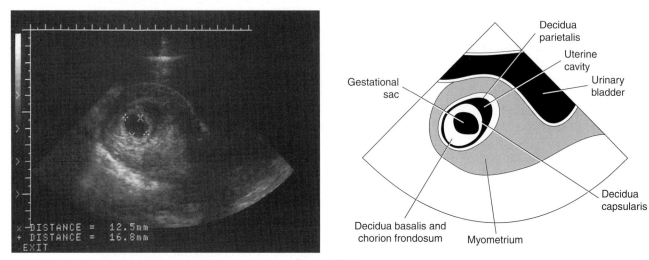

Figure 17-11

Yolk Sac Appearance

The secondary yolk sac is the first structure identified within the gestational sac. As seen in the image below, the yolk sac appears small and round with bright walls and an anechoic fluid-filled center. Normally, it measures less than 6 mm. Transvaginally, the yolk sac can be identified as early as the 5th week. Using a transabdominal approach, the yolk sac should be visible by the 7th week.

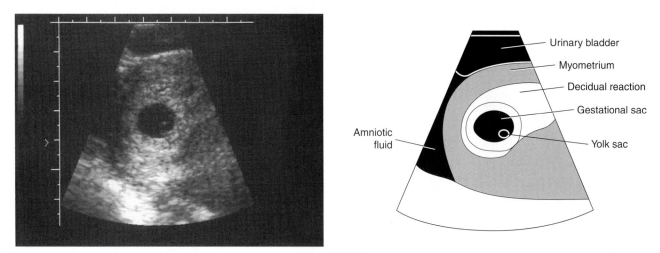

Figure 17-12

Sonographic visualization of the yolk sac confirms pregnancy and rules out a pseudo sac. The yolk sac also serves as a landmark for locating the embryonic disk and cardiac activity. A faint flickering motion visualized adjacent to the yolk sac represents neurologically active heart tissue. It is often seen before the embryo can be sonographically distinguished. As previously discussed, the yolk sac and embryo retreat from one another as the amnion and its cavity enlarge and the chorionic cavity obliterates. The yolk sac comes to lie outside of the amniotic cavity, remaining attached to the embryo by the vitelline (omphalomesenteric) duct. Although small, the duct can be sonographically identified as the bright, hyperechoic, linear connection between the embryo and yolk sac, surrounded by anechoic fluid.

Embryo Appearance

At 5 to 6 gestational weeks the embryo is evident with transvaginal scanning. At this point, it is about 1 to 2 mm in length, ovoid or shapeless, and hugs the wall of the gestational sac.

As seen in the following image, the embryo appears as a small, highly echogenic, focal thickening along the bright outside edge of the yolk sac, surrounded by anechoic chorionic fluid.

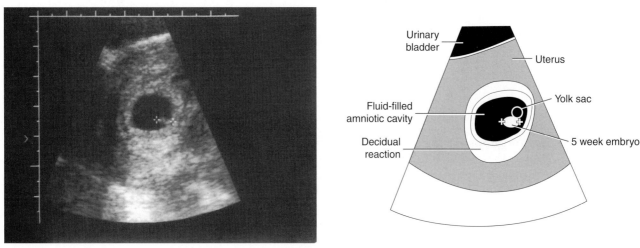

Figure 17-13

At 6 weeks' GA, it is not possible to distinguish the embryo crown ("cephalic end"/"cephalic pole") from the rump ("caudal end"/"caudal pole"), but by the 7th week, as seen in the next image, the embryo begins to assume a shape that reveals the head at one end and rump at the other.

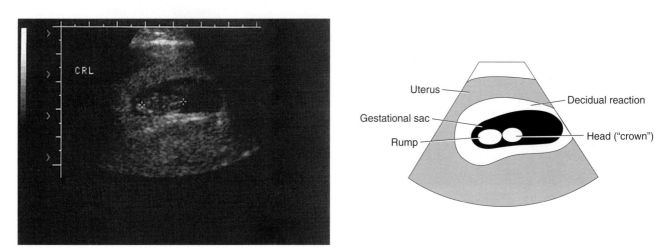

Figure 17-14

Fetal limb buds should start to be visible by 8 weeks as the embryo develops a C-shaped configuration (see Figure 17-5). The crown becomes prominent and contains the anechoic developing rhombencephalon (cystic hindbrain). In some cases, a tail-like appendage is identifiable at the rump. Because of embryonic curvature, length measurements, as discussed earlier, are often neck-rump rather than crown-rump lengths. The umbilical cord is well-visualized at 8 weeks. It appears thick and about as long as the embryo (Figure 17-15).

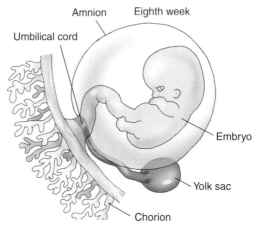

Figure 17-15 The 8th week of development.

The cord grows at a rate similar to that of the embryo. As it increases in length, it develops multiple spiral turns thought to be caused by helic arterial muscle layers. As mentioned, the cord is composed of two umbilical arteries and one umbilical vein that appear anechoic with walls that are thick and bright. The normal diameter of the cord is less than 2 cm. The next two images are the cord viewed in short axis. It presents as one large anechoic circle with thick hyperechoic walls, flanked by two small anechoic circles with thick hyperechoic walls.

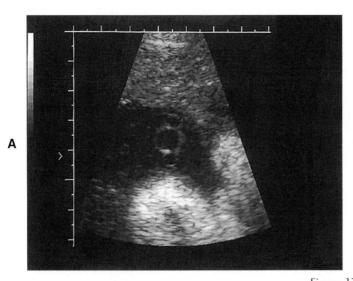

A

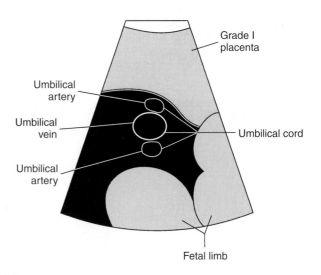

Figure 17-16

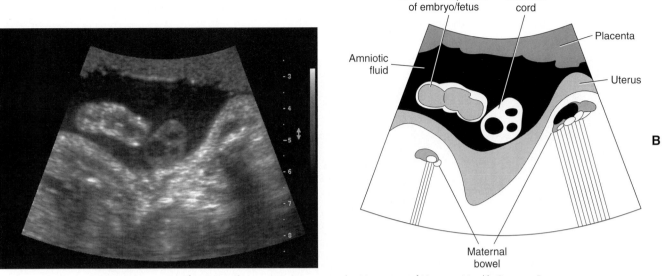

Figure 17-16, cont'd (B, Half-tone image courtesy the University of Virginia Health System, Department of Radiology, Division of Ultrasound, Charlottesville, Virginia.)

Umbilical cord blood vessels enter the embryo/fetus at the umbilicus and immediately diverge there. The umbilical vein runs superiorly to join embryo/fetal portal circulation. The umbilical arteries course inferiorly along both sides of the urinary bladder and can be differentiated from dilated ureters with color Doppler ultrasound as seen in the following image, a black-and-white version of color flow.

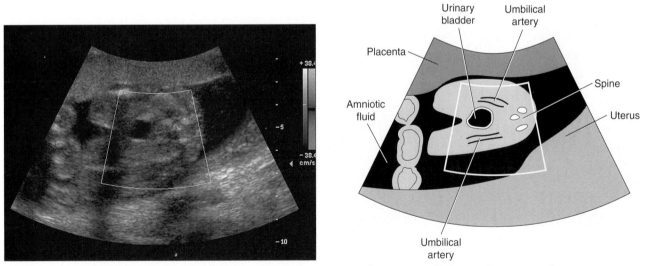

Figure 17-17 (Half-tone images courtesy the University of Virginia Health System, Department of Radiology, Division of Ultrasound, Charlottesville, Virginia.)

The image below shows a 9.5-week-old embryo. All four developing limbs can be seen, as well as the normal protruding caudate pole referred to as the embryonic tail that resolves with further development.

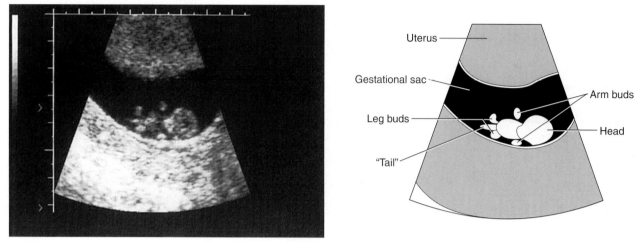

Figure 17-18

This next image shows a 10.6-week gestation with normal gut herniation into the base of the umbilical cord. Also, at this point, the head becomes disproportionately large compared with the body and constitutes one half of the length. As development continues, the head and body subsequently become more proportional.

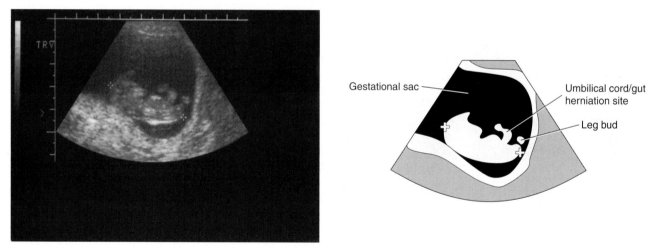

Figure 17-19

During week 10, the fluid-filled anechoic stomach and homogeneous embryonic liver can be seen, and the brain may appear hypoechoic or anechoic. By 12 weeks, however, two bright structures can be visualized within the fetal skull. These structures, as seen in the following image, represent the choroid plexus, which produces cerebrospinal fluid in the embryo.

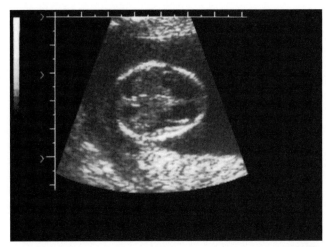
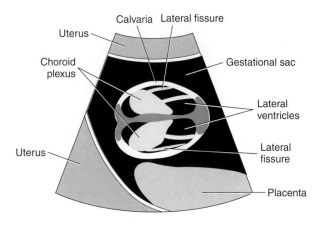

Figure 17-20

Individual fingers and toes are usually identified by the 11th week, and the anechoic, urine-filled bladder might be seen but should always be visualized by week 13. This femur measurement image includes the anechoic, urine-filled bladder.

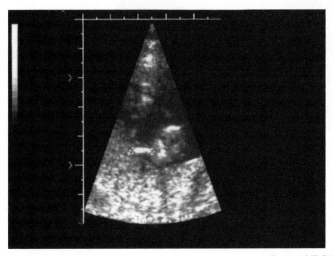
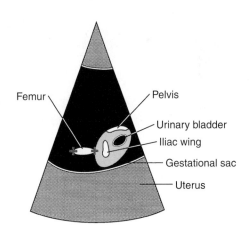

Figure 17-21

As mentioned earlier, the skull and femur are adequately mineralized by 11.5 to 12 weeks. The next two images demonstrate how bone attenuates the sound waves and is therefore highly reflective and hyperechoic compared with surrounding structures. As bones increase in size, they demonstrate posterior acoustic shadowing.

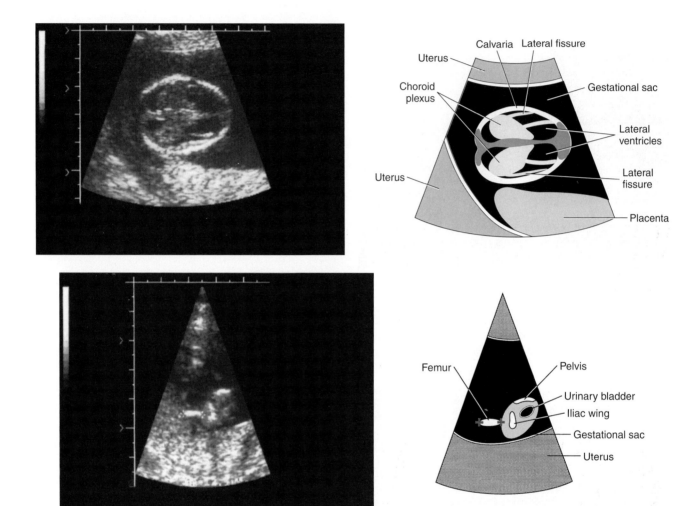

Figure 17-22

Placenta Appearance

What begins as a diffusely thick hyperechoic ring surrounding the early gestational sac changes to a hyperechoic focal area of thickening, the chorionic frondosum, which eventually becomes the placenta. This image clearly shows the differentiated deciduas, including the decidua basalis that combines with the chorionic frondosum to become the placenta.

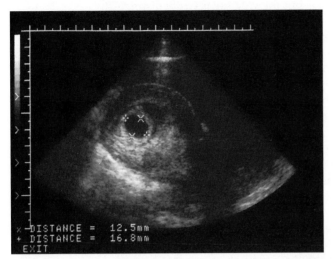
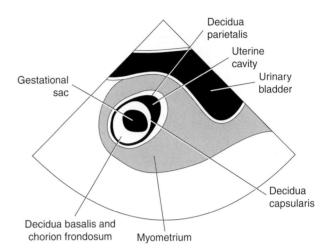

Figure 17-23

The placenta appears homogeneous to heterogeneous. It is primarily medium-level, homogeneous echoes that are interrupted by the retroplacental complex early in the second trimester of pregnancy and later by retroplacental and intraplacental arteries. The homogeneous substance of the placenta is further interrupted by "insertion" of the umbilical cord shown in the color flow image below. Ultrasound identification of the cord insertion into the placenta is important for certain invasive obstetric procedures such as fetal blood sampling. The area is considered optimal because the cord is fixed at this location, making the needle approach more accurate.

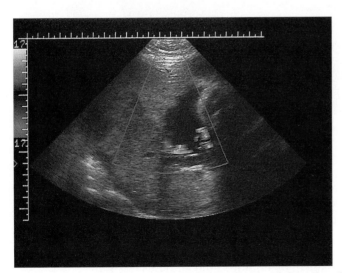
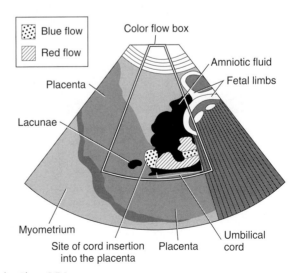

Figure 17-24   (See Color Plate 25.)

Membrane Appearance

Sonographic identification of the amnion and its cavity confirms the presence of an intrauterine gestational sac. Its size and appearance determine whether an early pregnancy is progressing normally. The amniotic membrane is very thin, and as a rule, is not visualized prior to 7 weeks' GA. Once in a while, however, it is identifiable as a small, round, echogenic ring containing anechoic fluid; it is contiguous with the embryo but on the opposite side of the yolk sac. The amniotic membrane and yolk sac are approximately the same size, but the yolk sac is easily distinguishable because it is the thicker and the most echogenic of the two. **Double bleb sign** has been used to describe the sonographic appearance of this early anatomic relationship.

By 7 weeks' GA or when the embryo is 7 mm long **(crown-rump length [CRL])**, the amniotic membrane has developed beyond the double bleb sign. It is best visualized with transvaginal transducers and high gain settings and appears as a thin, bright, hyperechoic membrane outlining the anechoic, fluid-filled amniotic cavity (or sac) containing the echogenic embryo. As development continues in the first trimester, the CRL and amniotic sac diameter increase 1 mm per day; interestingly, these measurements are equal throughout the first trimester. Occasionally, when the amnion is not visualized, it does not indicate an abnormality. When the amnion completely fuses with the chorion, between 12 and 16 weeks' GA, the amniotic membrane is no longer visible.

Prior to fusion of the amnion and chorion, the chorionic cavity can only be appreciated sonographically when the amniotic membrane is visible. Another sonographic marker of the chorionic cavity is the distinctive chorionic fluid, which is more echogenic than the anechoic amniotic fluid. This image shows the low-level echoes in chorionic fluid that are probably from increased concentrations of protein and albumin within the chorionic cavity.

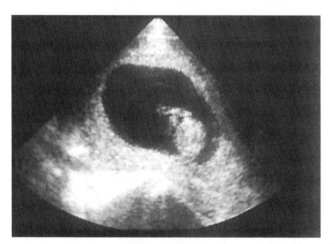 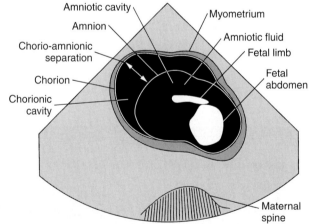

Figure 17-25

Amniotic Fluid Appearance

Amniotic fluid appears anechoic; however, it is not unusual to view free-floating particles in the fluid. In most cases this occurs in the early to mid second trimester of pregnancy. The particles are believed to be fetal vernix (flakes of skin) with no pathologic significance.

As mentioned, the amount of amniotic fluid is a sonographic marker for fetal well-being. In the past, sonographic assessment of amniotic fluid amounts was subjective. Extremes of too little fluid (oligohydramnios) or too much fluid (polyhydramnios) were fairly easy for experienced sonologists and sonographers to recognize; however, there were no criteria for use by less experienced examiners. The importance of amniotic fluid in fetal development brought about the development of methods to accurately assess the AFV throughout pregnancy. (Because these assessments are more applicable to second and third trimester gestations, they will be discussed in Chapter 18.)

SONOGRAPHIC DETERMINATION OF GESTATIONAL AGE

Every gestation begins as a single cell, but eventually individual differences in growth rate give rise to a range of sizes and biologic variations, all of which are normal for a given GA. Early in the pregnancy these individual differences are much less pronounced than they are later. Therefore the most accurate time to date a pregnancy is during the first trimester when variations are relatively minimal.

Measurement guidelines for dating pregnancy during the first trimester are gestational sac (no yolk sac, embryo, or heartbeat) at 5 weeks' GA, gestational sac with yolk sac (no embryo, no heartbeat) at 5.5 weeks' GA, gestational sac with yolk sac (living embryo too small to measure) at 6 weeks' GA, and CRL of the embryo from 6 weeks + days to 12 weeks' GA. Several methods such as sac volumes and mean diameters have been developed to determine gestational sac size to calculate gestational/ menstrual age. Many institutions use the **mean sac diameter (MSD)** method. Three measurements of the chorionic/gestational sac—length, depth, and width—are obtained, summed, and then divided by 3 to determine the MSD. Length and depth are measured on a longitudinal image section and width on a transverse section.

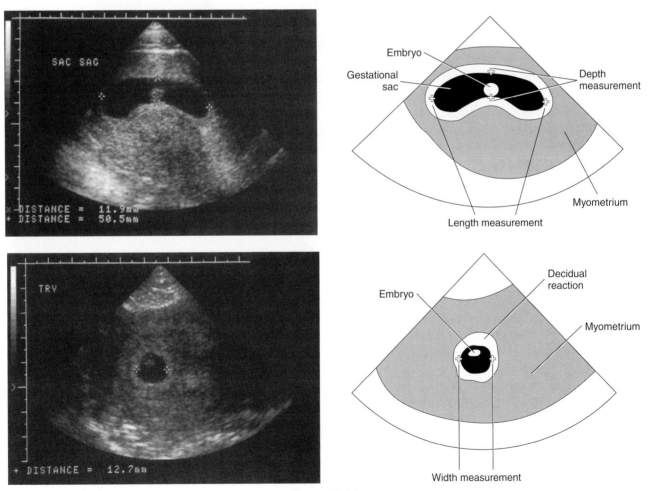

Figure 17-26

To accurately obtain the mean internal diameter of the chorionic sac, measurement calipers are placed at the fluid-tissue interface; the wall (the bright choriodecidual reaction) is not included in the measurement. Gestational age (in days) is calculated by adding 30 to the MSD (in millimeters):

Mean Sac Diameter + 30 = Gestational Age (in days)

The CRL is commonly accepted as the most accurate assessment of GA. Measurement guidelines for CRL are embryonic disk length (not possible to distinguish the crown from the rump) at 6 weeks + days' GA, neck-rump measurement (prominent head flexion makes longest axis from neck to rump) at 6+ weeks to 8 weeks' GA, and CRL (head extends, making true crown-rump long axis) at 8+ weeks to 12 weeks' GA.

The CRL measurement is reported to be accurate to within ± 4.7 days for dating pregnancies. The following image demonstrates correct caliper placement for CRL measurement. The CRL measured 36.9 mm, which correlates to a 10.7 week GA. Several methodology tables are available that convert CRL (in millimeters) to GA.

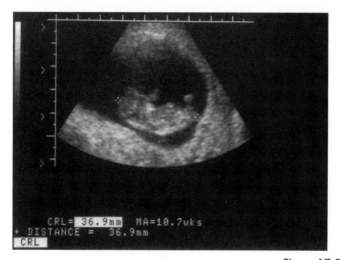
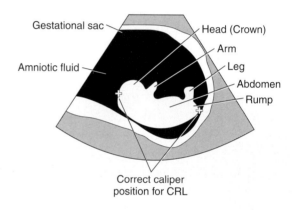

Figure 17-27

As development continues into the second trimester, CRL measurements are replaced by biparietal measurements of the fetal head and femur length measurements to determine GA.

SONOGRAPHIC APPLICATIONS

Ultrasound can be used to confirm or rule out a variety of things during the first trimester. The most common indications for a first trimester ultrasound are:

- Gestational age (GA): Confirmation of GA for patients who require invasive studies such as chorionic villi sampling, elective repeat cesarean delivery, or elective termination of pregnancy.
- Vaginal spotting or bleeding: Rule out ectopic pregnancy, threatened abortion, abortion in progress, or incomplete or complete abortion.
- Large for dates: Rule out a mass, a multiple gestation, a fetal anomaly, or an incorrect menstrual history.
- Small for dates: Rule out embryonic/fetal death, blighted ovum, ectopic pregnancy, fetal anomaly, or incorrect menstrual history.
- Pelvic pain: Rule out a mass, a placental abruption, or an ectopic pregnancy.
- Fetal growth: Determine cases of severe preeclampsia, diabetes mellitus, renal disease, chronic hypertension, or fetal malnutrition.

- Substance abuse or prescription drugs early in pregnancy: Rule out embryonic/fetal anomalies and determine fetal growth rate.
- Fetal presentation: Determine when presenting part cannot be established in labor.
- Trauma: Determine embryonic/fetal well-being.
- History of miscarriage: Determine the status and well-being of an early gestation.
- History of multiple gestations or fertility drug treatment: Determine the number of gestations.

In 1984, a fact-finding panel of the National Institutes of Health issued guidelines for ultrasound examinations during pregnancy. Although the panel recommended diagnostic ultrasound for multiple obstetric indications, it did not endorse routine ultrasound screening in pregnant women. This was based on the fact that there is not enough evidence to demonstrate that the clinical benefits of such screening would outweigh the economic, legal, and psychological costs involved. The panel stated that there is no evidence to indicate that either the woman or the fetus is harmed during these studies.

NORMAL VARIATIONS

Uterine Synechia (Amniotic Sheets)

Synechias are membranes formed from scarring or adhesions secondary to surgery or infection. They extend from the uterus with amnion and chorion growing around them. The membrane is four layers thick (two layers of amnion and two of chorion) and highly echogenic. Synechia do not attach to the embryo/fetus and are not associated with gestational abnormalities. They should not be confused with amniotic bands. This image shows the hyperechoic, membranous appearance of synechia.

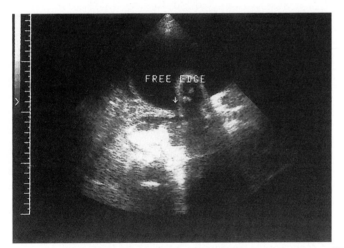
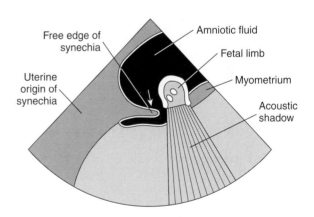

Figure 17-28

Myometrial Contraction(s)

Contractions of the myometrium of the uterus are frequently seen on sonograms and should not be confused with a myoma (uterine mass). Contractions are distinguishable by their inward bulge without disturbing uterine contour and their temporary nature.

REFERENCE CHARTS

■ ■ ■   ASSOCIATED PHYSICIANS

Obstetrician/Gynecologist: Manages preterm obstetric care and delivers the fetus. This physician is also responsible for the care of the infant immediately following delivery.

High-Risk Obstetrician: Specializes in the preterm management of women whose pregnancies are at risk due to various medical conditions, and delivers the fetus. This physician is also responsible for the care of the infant immediately following delivery.

Fertility Specialist: Typically, this physician is an obstetrician/gynecologist who specializes in treating disorders of the female reproductive system associated with fertility and pregnancy.

Radiologist/Sonologist: Specializes in the administration and diagnostic interpretation of ultrasound and other imaging modalities.

■ ■ ■   COMMON DIAGNOSTIC TESTS

Pregnancy Test: Detects human chorionic gonadotropin (hCG) levels in urine or blood when pregnancy exists. A lab technician usually runs the test, which is interpreted by a pathologist or obstetrician/gynecologist.

Beta-hCG Test: Blood is tested to quantitate the serum level of hCG to estimate gestational age. A lab technician usually runs the test, which is interpreted by a pathologist or obstetrician/gynecologist.

Maternal/Paternal Blood Typing: Determines blood type and whether Rh factor is positive or negative. The Rh factor is a group of autoantibodies that react with a person's own immunoglobulin.

Chorionic Villus Sampling (CVS): Transabdominal or transcervical penetration of the uterus and amniotic sac for a sample of the chorion covered by villi, which is used for obtaining pertinent genetic information regarding the embryo/fetus.

Computed Tomography (CT): Evaluation of fetal and maternal anatomy when sonographic evaluation is indeterminate. CT is generally used as a "last resort" because of the radiation exposure and in most cases is limited to assessment of the acute maternal abdomen.

Magnetic Resonance Imaging (MRI): Traditionally used to evaluate maternal anatomy during pregnancy and abnormalities such as adnexal masses, which require further characterization beyond the ultrasound findings. Typically, MRI evaluation of the fetus is hindered by fetal motion.

■ ■ ■   LABORATORY VALUES

hCG: An hCG of 2000 is the level at which a sac will be seen in most normal early pregnancies.

Alpha-Fetoprotein (AFP): Found in maternal blood and amniotic fluid. Elevated levels indicate fetal abnormalities or defects.

Triple Marker Screening (AFP, uE3, hCG): Abnormal levels of alpha-fetoprotein (AFP), unconjugated estriol (uE3), and human chorionic gonadotropin (hCG) are indicators of certain embryonic/fetal abnormalities, possible multifetal gestations, and combined with maternal age, screening markers for Down syndrome.

■ ■ ■   NORMAL MEASUREMENTS

Mean Sac Diameter (MSD): Length + Depth + Width / 3

Gestational Sac: Visible with transvaginal sonography when MSD is 2 to 3 mm. This corresponds to 4 weeks' GA. Visible transabdominally when MSD is 5 mm, which corresponds to 5 weeks' GA.

Gestational Age (GA) (in days):
MSD (in millimeters) + 30 = GA (in days)
MSD of 6 mm corresponds to 36 gestational days.

Crown-Rump Length (CRL): Long axis measurement of the embryo. CRL increases by approximately 1 mm/day.

Yolk Sac: Maximum diameter is 5 to 6 mm, which corresponds to a CRL of 30 to 45 mm.

■ ■ ■   VASCULATURE

Internal iliac artery—Paired uterine arteries—Multiple arcuate arteries—Arcuate branches enter the endometrium—Spiral arteries—Located within decidua basalis—Invading trophoblastic chorionic villi plug the spiral arteries and erode small portions of the decidua, which enlarges to form—Intervillous spaces—Receive maternal blood from spiral arteries

■ ■ ■   AFFECTING CHEMICALS

Menotropins (Pergonal), Urofollitropin (Metrodin), Clomiphene Citrate (Clomid): Medications prescribed for infertility to stimulate follicular maturation and induce ovulation. In some cases, these medications have been associated with multifetal gestations.

BIBLIOGRAPHY

Barth RA, Crowe HC: Ultrasound evaluation of multifetal gestations. In Callen PW, editor: *Ultrasonography in obstetrics and gynecology*, ed 4, Philadelphia, 2000, WB Saunders, pp 171-191.

Callen PW: Amniotic fluid: its role in fetal health and disease. In Callen PW, editor: *Ultrasonography in obstetrics and gynecology*, ed 4, Philadelphia, 2000, WB Saunders, pp 638-656.

Filly RA, Hadlock FP: Sonographic determination of menstrual age. In Callen PW, editor: *Ultrasonography in obstetrics and gynecology*, ed 4, Philadelphia, 2000, WB Saunders, pp 146-153.

Grannum PA: The genitourinary tract. In Nyberg DA, Mahoney BS, Pretorius DH, editors: *Diagnostic ultrasound of fetal anomalies*, St Louis, 1990, Mosby.

Laing FC, Frates MC: Ultrasound evaluation during the first trimester of pregnancy. In Callen PW, editor: *Ultrasonography in obstetrics and gynecology*, ed 4, Philadelphia, 2000, WB Saunders, pp 105-110.

Levine D: Ectopic pregnancy. In Callen PW, editor: *Ultrasonography in obstetrics and gynecology*, ed 4, Philadelphia, 2000, WB Saunders, pp 912-914.

Lyons EA, Levi CS: Ultrasound in the first trimester of pregnancy. In Callen PW, editor: *Ultrasonography in obstetrics and gynecology*, Philadelphia, 1982, WB Saunders.

National Institutes of Health Consensus Development Conference, Washington, DC, 1984, US Government Printing Office.

Queenan JT, Gadow EC: Polyhydramnios: chronic versus acute, *Am J Obstet Gynecol* 108:349-355, 1970.

Rempen A: Diagnosis of viability in early pregnancy with vaginal sonography, *J Ultrasound Med* 9:711-716, 1990.

Robinson HP, Fleming JEE: A critical evaluation of sonar crown-rump length measurements, *Brit J Obstet Gynecol* 82:703-708, 1975.

Sohaey R, Woodard P: The spectrum of first-trimester ultrasound findings, *Diag Radiol* 25(2):53-76, 1996.

CHAPTER 18

Second and Third Trimester Obstetrics (13 to 42 Weeks)

BETTY BATES TEMPKIN AND PEGGY MALZI BIZJAK

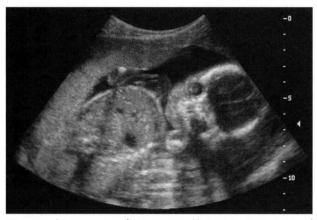

(Courtesy the University of Virginia Health System, Department of Radiology, Division of Ultrasound, Charlottesville, Virginia.)

OBJECTIVES

Describe the sonographic appearance of and the role of the placenta in supporting gestation.

Describe the significance of the location of the placenta in relation to the internal cervical os.

Describe the sonographic appearance of the fetus and surrounding structures.

Describe the sonographic presentation of the development of fetal anatomy.

Describe the sonographic markers used to properly orient the transducer planes for the BPD, HC, and AC.

Define the key words.

KEY WORDS

Abdominal circumference (AC)	Aqueduct of Sylvius
Amniotic fluid index (AFI)	Arachnoid layer
Amniotic fluid volume (AFV)	Biparietal diameter (BPD)
	Brachiocephalic

Brain stem	Foramina of Luschka
Cavum septum pellucidum	Fronto-occipital diameter (FOD)
Cephalic index (CI)	
Cerebellar vermis	Head circumference (HC)
Cerebellum	Lacunae
Cerebrospinal fluid (CSF)	Lateral ventricles
Cerebrum	Ligamentum teres
Choroid plexus	Ligamentum venosum
Cisterna magna	Meconium
Cisterns	Meninges
Dolichocephalic	Midbrain
Ductus arteriosus	Neurotube
Ductus venosus	Ossify
Dura mater	Pia mater
Dural sinuses	Placenta previa
Falciform ligament	Subarachnoid spaces
Falx cerebri	Thalamus
Femur length (FL)	Umbilical arteries
Foramen of Magendie	Umbilical vein
Foramen of Monro	Ventricles
Foramen ovale	Vernix

The second and third trimesters of a pregnancy are a progressive period when the organs and organ systems formed during the first trimester become fully developed. By the twelfth week the majority of organs formed during the first trimester are located in their final anatomic positions. Thus the first trimester can be termed "a trimester of differentiation and development," and the second and third trimesters may be referred to collectively as "trimesters of growth and maturation."

This chapter addresses the organs, organ systems, and associated structures that can be examined with sonography during the second and third trimesters of pregnancy and the measurements used to determine gestational age during this time.

THE PLACENTA

The tremendous amount of growth that occurs during the second and third trimesters is highly dependent on the ability of the fetus to acquire nutrients and oxygen. It is also dependent on fetal ability to remove the waste products of metabolism. The organ that accomplishes these tasks is the placenta.

The enormous circulatory surface provided by the many fetal and maternal blood vessels allows nutrients and metabolic waste products to be exchanged in the placenta. Carbon dioxide is at a much higher concentration in the fetal blood and thus tends to move into the maternal blood. Oxygen is at a much higher level in the maternal bloodstream and thus moves into the fetal blood. The placenta thus functions as an organ of respiration for the fetus.

The placenta may be sonographically visible by 10 weeks. As discussed in Chapter 17, it appears as the thick-ened, hyperechoic portion of the rim of tissue surrounding the gestational sac. At 12 to 13 weeks, the early placenta appears homogeneous and hyperechoic. Intervillous blood flow can be demonstrated with color or power Doppler sonography. During the second and third trimesters the placenta's appearance becomes slightly darker. In some cases, small anechoic areas representing maternal venous lakes, or **lacunae,** may interrupt the otherwise homogeneous appearance. It is often possible to see a swirl-like motion within these lakes. This presumably represents very slow circulation of maternal blood. A prominent venous lake is shown in Figure 18-1. Anechoic tubular structures on the uterine surface of the placenta representing maternal marginal veins may also be visualized (Figure 18-2). Between 14 and 15 weeks the placenta is well-established, and the retroplacental complex can be observed. It presents as a hypoechoic area, composed of the decidua, myometrium, and anechoic

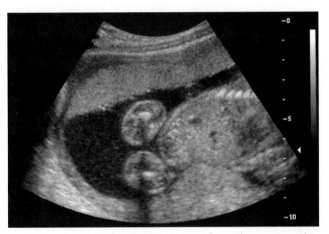
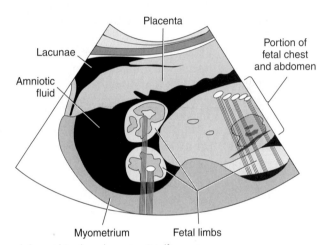

Figure 18-1 A normal anechoic maternal venous lake within the placenta. (Half-tone image courtesy the University of Virginia Health System, Department of Radiology, Division of Ultrasound, Charlottesville, Virginia.)

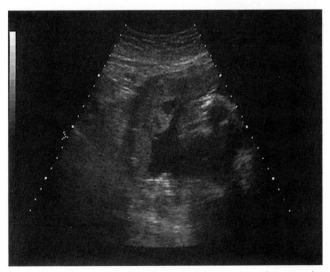
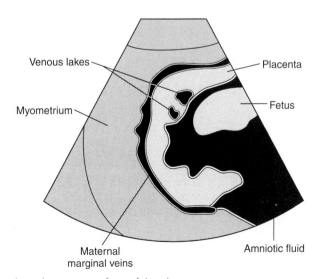

Figure 18-2 Anechoic maternal marginal veins along the uterine surface of the placenta.

uterine vessels. At 16 to 18 weeks, color power Doppler may be able to demonstrate small intraplacental arteries. By the third trimester the mature placenta becomes extremely vascular. Both retroplacental and intraplacental arteries are readily identified as widespread, anechoic structures with hyperechoic walls.

Some experts believe that placental volume in the second trimester can be used as an accurate predictor for abnormal fetal outcome. In most cases, the placenta should be approximately equal in thickness (in millimeters) to the gestational age in weeks ±10 mm. Measuring the placenta is not standard practice; however, in most cases, it should not exceed 4.0 cm. With experience, a sonographer can generally recognize a placenta that appears too thick or too thin secondary to a primary pathology.

Throughout pregnancy, the placenta matures and calcifies (the sonographic sign of "aging") at a fairly reproducible rate. During the 1970's, Grannum et al developed placental grading. This method classifies placental maturation according to sonographic appearance (Figure 18-3).

The categories of placental classification are:

1. Grade 0: Represents the normal placenta throughout pregnancy. A Grade 0 placenta has a smooth chorionic plate (sac border), a substance that is devoid of focal hyperechoic areas, and a basal layer (uterine border) that is free of hyperechoic densities as well. The placental substance (between borders) appears homogeneous, with medium-level to low-level echoes; it may be interrupted by anechoic lacunae.

2. Grade I: The chorionic plate shows some subtle indentation. The homogeneous placental substance exhibits a few scattered, hyperechoic, punctate densities (calcifications). The basal layer of a Grade I placenta appears hypoechoic to anechoic. These placental findings are considered as normal changes at any time after 34 weeks of development.

3. Grade II: This category of placenta exhibits mild or medium-sized indentations in the chorionic plate. The homogeneous substance of the placenta contains scattered, hyperechoic, "comma-like" densities (calcifications). The basal plate in a Grade II placenta contains a few small, linear, hyperechoic densities. Grade II placental findings are considered normal at any time after 36 weeks of development.

4. Grade III: A Grade III placenta contains indentations in the chorionic plate that extend as far as the basal layer, dividing the placenta into segments. The otherwise homogeneous substance of the placenta may contain both highly echogenic and anechoic areas. The hyperechoic echoes will be significantly larger than the small, scattered calcifications seen in the Grade I placenta, and may exhibit acoustic shadowing. The basal layer of a Grade III placenta has very long, hyperechoic, linear echoes and may, in advanced stages, appear as an unbroken line. Grade III placental findings are considered normal at any time after 38 weeks of development.

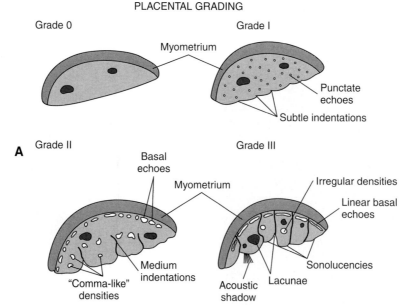

Figure 18-3 Placental grading. **A,** The aging process of the placenta. Note the increase in densities (calcifications) and how the contour of the placenta changes from smooth to markedly irregular.

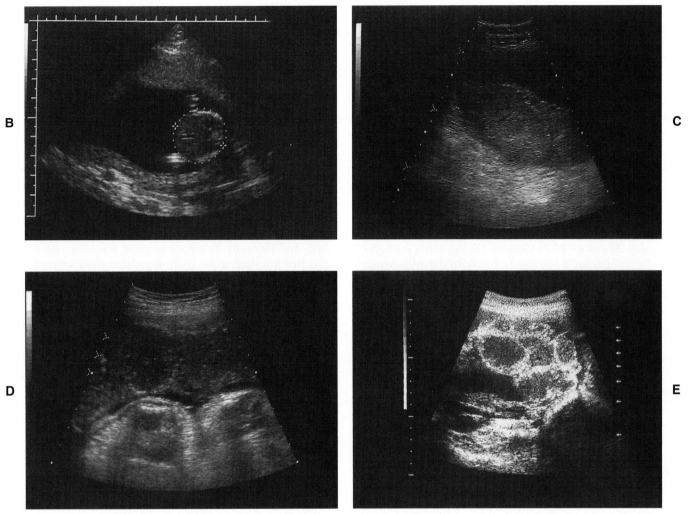

Figure 18-3, cont'd B to E, Placenta images. B, Grade 0. C, Grade I. D, Grade II. E, Grade III.

Initially it was believed that the placental grading system, which essentially measures amounts of calcification within the aging placenta, could be used as a means to date a gestation. Experts attempted to correlate placental maturity with lung maturity. It is now known that dating the gestation by placental grading techniques is highly inaccurate. However, there is a distinct relationship between the age of the gestation and the grade of the placenta. The appearance of a Grade I placenta (if it occurs at all) should occur after 34 weeks. A Grade II should appear after 36 weeks, and a Grade III placenta should appear after 38 weeks. Appearance of these grades before the stated times may indicate an abnormality. When the placenta exhibits premature aging or accelerated calcification, it is usually due to maternal cigarette smoking or to thrombotic disorders or the medicines used to treat them.

Sonographic evaluation of the placenta also includes its position within the uterus relative to the internal os of the cervix to rule out placenta previa. **Placenta previa** occurs when any portion of the internal cervical os is covered by part of the placenta. There are three types of placenta previa: total, partial, and marginal. Total (or complete) placenta previa occurs when the entire cervical os is obstructed by an overlying placenta. Generally, vaginal bleeding during the second or third trimesters indicates it. Patients usually require cesarean deliveries rather than vaginal deliveries that would be dangerous for the fetus and mother. Partial (or incomplete) previa occurs when the overlying placenta blocks a portion of the cervical os. This condition is associated with vaginal bleeding and necessitates cesarean section. Marginal previa exists when the placenta extends up to but not above the internal cervical os. These patients have follow-up examinations during the final weeks of the pregnancy to see if the position of the placenta has changed as the uterus enlarges to accommodate the growing fetus.

Occasionally, the term *low-lying placenta* or *potential placenta* is used to describe a placenta that stops within a few millimeters of the internal cervical os. In follow-up examinations, the placenta frequently appears to move upward and away from the internal os, when in fact it is the stretched lower uterine segment that has moved due to the growing fetus pushing the uterus upward.

There are three causes of placenta previa: a low-lying placenta in a normal uterus, a low-lying placenta due to the presence of a benign fibroid tumor, and a vascular malformation that causes placental formation only in the lower portion of the uterus.

AMNIOTIC FLUID

The fetal effect on amniotic fluid volume increases with the pregnancy. During the third trimester, fetal kidneys may produce between 600 and 800 ml of fluid per day; near term, the fetus may swallow up to 450 ml of fluid per day. As discussed in Chapter 17, the volume of amniotic fluid reflects the state of gestational well-being. For that reason, various methods of calculating **amniotic fluid volumes (AFV)** have been developed. One method assesses the AFV by totaling the individual pockets of amniotic fluid. The maximum vertical pocket (MVP) method to assess the AFV was developed to determine oligohydramnios (deficiency in the amount of amniotic fluid). It uses the greatest vertical dimension of the single deepest pocket of amniotic fluid free of cord and extremities. Most institutions use 2 cm as the minimum normal amount; less than 2 cm usually indicates oligohydramnios. An alternative method, the four-quadrant analysis, assesses AFV by finding the **amniotic fluid index (AFI).** The following illustration shows how this measurement is based on the division of the gravid uterus into four equal quadrants using the umbilicus and linea nigra.

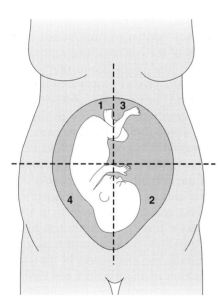

The anteroposterior diameter of the deepest amniotic fluid pocket free of cord and extremities in each quad-

rant is measured. These four measurements are added together to total the AFI. The sum should equal 8 cm to be considered normal.

In the early to mid second trimester of pregnancy, it is not unusual to view free-floating hyperechoic particles in the otherwise anechoic amniotic fluid. The particles are believed to be fetal **vernix** (flakes of skin and hair) with no pathologic significance.

FETAL ORGAN SYSTEMS
Musculoskeletal System

The fetal skeleton is seen earlier and more consistently than any other organ system. The axial skeleton begins to form between the sixth and eighth menstrual weeks, beginning with the vertebrae and ribs, followed by the skull and sternum. The appendicular skeleton also begins to form during the sixth menstrual week when the upper and lower limbs first appear as small buds on the lateral body wall. This is followed by formation of the pectoral and pelvic girdles. The soft tissues of the skeleton develop in a similar sequence to that of the skeletal structures. The bones continue to grow and accumulate minerals **(ossify)** throughout the second and third trimesters.

Sonographic Appearance

Bone and Cartilage. As early as the latter half of the first trimester, ultrasound is able to demonstrate how ossified portions of the fetal skeleton appear highly echogenic compared with the mid-gray, hypoechoic appearance of adjacent cartilaginous structures.

The bright reflection of the fetal skeleton is an indication of the degree of mineralization that has taken place within the developing bones. The density of bone attenuates the sound waves, preventing through transmission. The sound waves are reflected from the surface of the bones, causing a highly echogenic appearance with a shadow cast behind it. As discussed in Chapters 1 and 4, the degree of echogenicity depends on the density of the bone, its distance from the sound beam, and the angle at which the beam strikes the bone. The brightest reflections occur at normal (perpendicular) incidence.

Axial Skeleton. During the second and third trimesters the majority of bones or components of bones of the axial skeleton can routinely be visualized. This includes the fetal spine, and even though it matures at varying degrees and levels, the vertebrae have a highly reflective appearance, making them easy to recognize. Three primary ossification centers of each vertebra are sonographically distinguishable. They are the anterior centrum of the body and one on each side of the posterior neural arch. As ossification continues, the transverse processes, pedicles, and laminae can be differentiated (Figure 18-4).

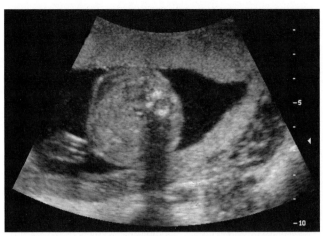
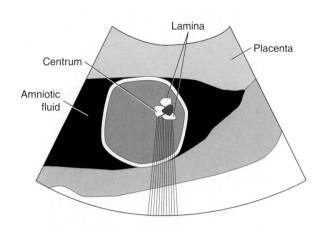

Figure 18-4 Transverse axial section of the lumbar spine. Note the reflective centrum and defined echogenic ossification of the laminae. (Half-tone image courtesy the University of Virginia Health System, Department of Radiology, Division of Ultrasound, Charlottesville, Virginia.)

The anterior ossification center of the vertebrae is equidistant from the two posterior ossification centers. In short axis, these bright echoes are parallel, or actually converge toward each other (Figure 18-5). Normal vertebral laminae angle inward, the opposite of the outward splaying of the laminae observed with spina bifida, a bony anomaly.

Several vertebrae imaged at once in a longitudinal section appear as two rows of closely spaced reflectors on each side of the hypoechoic spinal cord. These two rows are roughly parallel, but they are wider in the cervical and lumbar regions and narrower in the sacral region (Figure 18-6).

In the region of the thorax, the echogenic rib cage is easily identified and serves as an excellent anatomic landmark. The reflective ribs found between the spine and the sternum stand out against the mid-gray background of the lungs and heart muscle.

In the skull region a number of vivid, echogenic bones can be visualized. The calvaria, composed of the frontal, temporal, parietal, and occipital bones, is easily distinguishable. Similarly, the cartilaginous portions of these bones, the cranial sutures, are commonly seen (Figure 18-7) as well as the fontanelles or "bone free windows" to the fetal brain. The petrous ridge and greater wing of the sphenoid bone are visualized without difficulty as they delineate the anechoic anterior, middle, and posterior cranial fossae. In almost all normal cases, the mandible, bony nasal

ridge, and orbits can be identified. Usually, in older fetuses, the orbital contents can be assessed. The globe and lens appear very low gray and hypoechoic to adjacent structures. The bright retrobulbar fat and bony orbital walls appear hyperechoic compared with the mid-gray appearance of the rectus muscles, optic nerve, and eyelid.

Appendicular Skeleton. During the early to mid second trimester the majority of bones of the appendicular skeleton can be visualized. In most cases, the upper extremity phalanges, metacarpals, radius, ulna, humerus, clavicle, and scapula can be identified. Because the metacarpals and metatarsals are ossified at 16 weeks, they are easier to distinguish than the carpals and tarsals (except for the tarsal talus and calcaneus), which remain cartilaginous throughout pregnancy. Figure 18-8 shows all five digits of a 33-week fetal hand. The lower extremity phalanges, metatarsals, tibia, fibula, and femur can also be imaged in the first half of the second trimester as well as the hip and knee joints.

In short axis, the long bones of the forearms and lower legs appear as two bright, echogenic foci surrounded by hypoechoic soft tissue. Normally these bones end at the same level distally. Proximally the ulna is longer than the radius. In the lower leg, the tibia is the medial bone; the fibula, the lateral. In long axis and longitudinal sections, the long bones appear "long" and highly echogenic with posterior acoustic shadowing (Figure 18-9). *Text continued on p. 330*

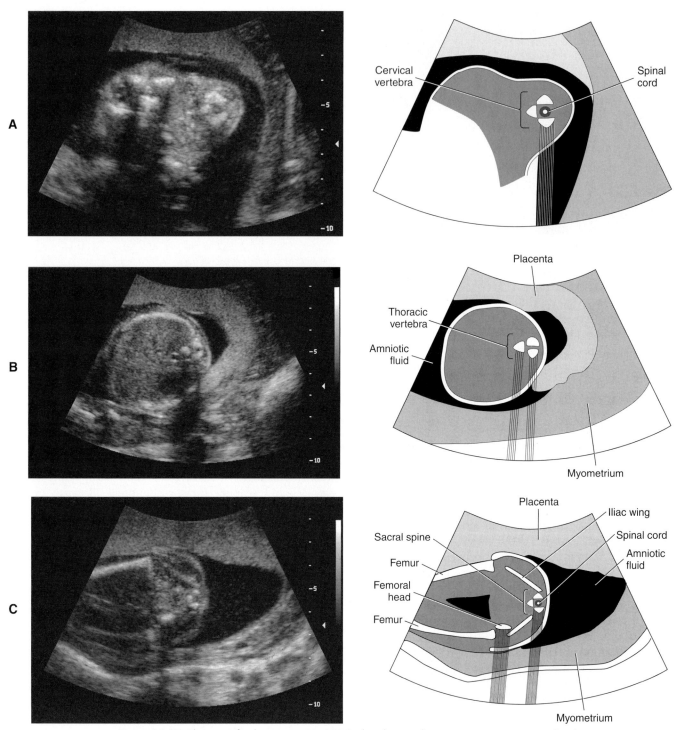

Figure 18-5 Short axis fetal spine sections. Note their hyperechoic appearance compared with adjacent structures. **A,** Cervical vertebra. **B,** Thoracic vertebra. **C,** Sacral spine. The bright, reflective pelvic iliac bones serve as excellent landmarks for confirming the caudal portion of the fetal spine in short axis. (Half-tone images courtesy the University of Virginia Health System, Department of Radiology, Division of Ultrasound, Charlottesville, Virginia.)

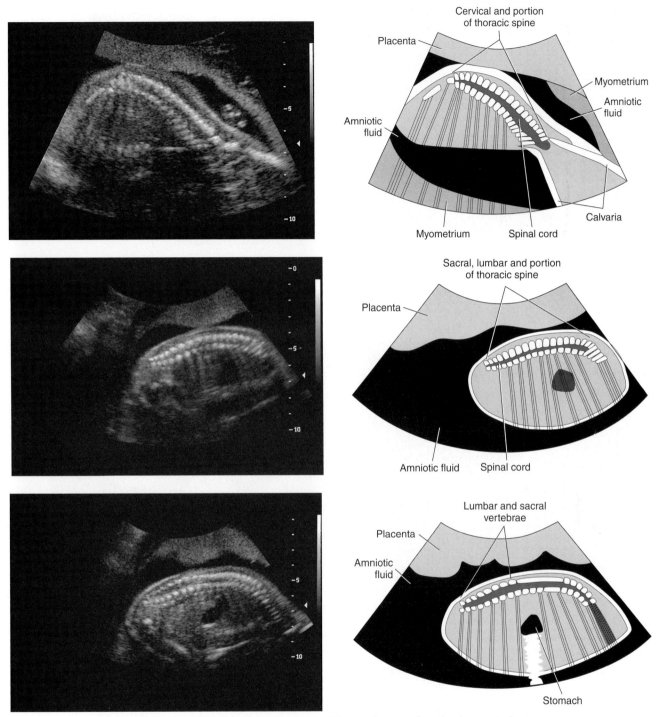

Figure 18-6 Longitudinal fetal spine sections. Observe how much wider the cervical spine section is compared with the normal tapering of the vertebrae in the sacral area. Gaps between vertebral bodies are composed of the nonossified margins of adjoining vertebral bodies and the intervertebral disks. Spinal cord neural tissue appears echogenic and hypoechoic compared with the bright meninges and vertebral bodies. (Half-tone images courtesy the University of Virginia Health System, Department of Radiology, Division of Ultrasound, Charlottesville, Virginia.)

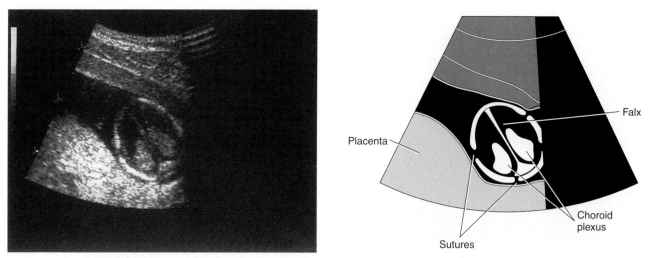

Figure 18-7 Skull sutures. Observe the hypoechoic appearance of the cartilaginous sutures compared with the bright reflection from the bones that make up the calvarium or skull. These sutures, sagittal, coronal, and lambdoid, along with the fontanelles act as the windows for sonographic brain imaging. These "gaps" between the skull bones allow the sound waves to pass through.

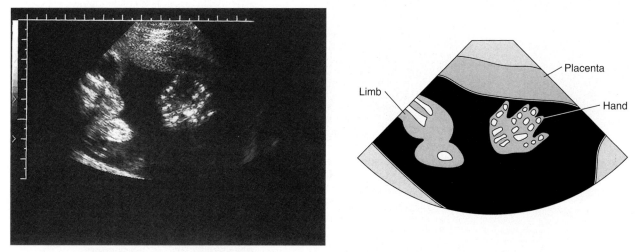

Figure 18-8 Hand. All five highly echogenic digits of this 33-week fetal hand can be identified. The hypoechoic areas between the pieces of bone are cartilages that assist hand movement. Ossified carpal bones cannot be visualized. Note their conglomerated hypoechoic bands between the distal radius and ulna to the proximal metacarpal ossification centers.

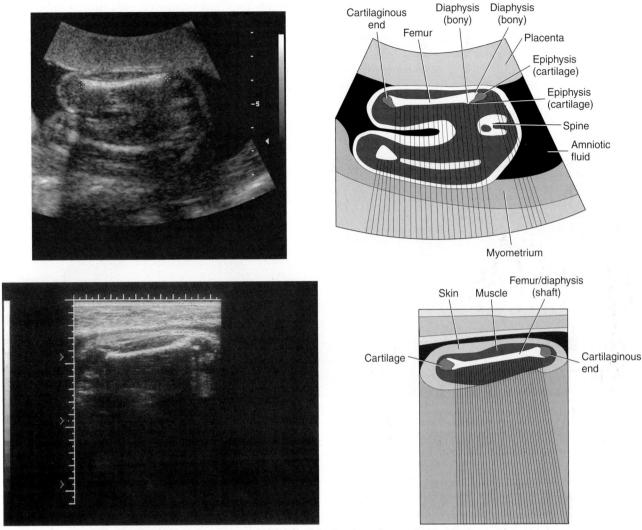

Figure 18-9 Femur. Longitudinal sections of the bright, reflective femur. The hypoechoic areas immediately adjacent to each bony end of the femur are the cartilaginous ends of the bone. Shadowing prevents the full thickness of the ossified diaphysis of long bones from being visualized. Therefore the width of the cartilaginous epiphysis can appear greater than the width of the bony diaphysis. When both femurs are visualized, the shadowing can also give the appearance that the femur in the far field of the image is bowed. The posterior shadow cast by the femur becomes more apparent with advancing gestational age. (Half-tone image at top courtesy the University of Virginia Health System, Department of Radiology, Division of Ultrasound, Charlottesville, Virginia.)

Muscles. Generally, normal fetal muscles appear hypoechoic compared with adjacent structures. However, in some cases, as seen in the following image, muscles may appear so hypoechoic that they are mistaken for anechoic fluid, especially in the abdominal wall where they can mimic the appearance of ascites (abnormal fluid). Current high-resolution ultrasound equipment makes it possible to differentiate the individual layers of the transversus abdominus, and internal and external oblique muscles. These muscles can be identified as the hypoechoic area between the bright subcutaneous and peritoneal fat.

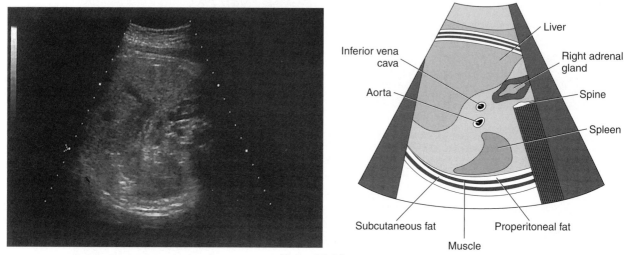

Figure 18-10

Cardiovascular System

This discussion will concentrate on the sonographic presentation of uterine and fetal blood vessels as well as the fetal heart. Given that the anatomy of the heart and great vessels is the focus of Chapter 23, this discussion will concentrate on the features unique to the fetal heart and their sonographic presentation.

The fetal vascular system has some unique features that do not exist after birth. As discussed in Chapter 17, the umbilical cord contains one vein and two arteries. The **umbilical vein** carries oxygenated blood from the placenta to the fetus, where it connects with the left portal vein in the liver. Following birth, the umbilical vein closes off, and eventually becomes the **ligamentum teres.** Specifically, the umbilical vein courses from the midline of the fetal abdominal wall posteriorly and slightly cephalad into the liver along the free margin of the **falciform ligament.** It joins the umbilical segment of the left portal vein, which courses superiorly and to the right, forming the transverse portion, or pars transversa, of the left portal vein, where it joins the right portal vein.

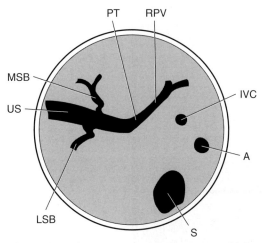

Figure 18-11 Fetal/left portal circulation. *US,* Umbilical segment of left portal vein; *LSB,* lateral segment branch; *MSB,* medial segment branch; *PT,* pars transversa of left portal vein; *RPV,* right portal vein; *S,* stomach; *A,* aorta; *IVC,* inferior vena cava.

The **ductus venosus,** which shunts oxygenated blood into the inferior vena cava, originates from the pars transversa, or in some cases more rightward. It courses unbranched to join the left, or middle, hepatic vein and ultimately the inferior vena cava. Shortly before birth, the ductus venosum closes and becomes the fibrous **ligamentum venosum,** marking the left anterolateral border of the caudate lobe of the liver.

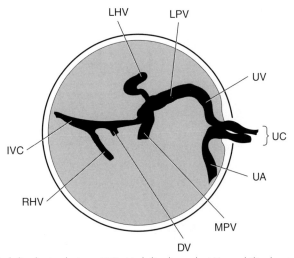

Figure 18-12 Umbilical circulation. *UC,* Umbilical cord; *UA,* umbilical artery; *UV,* umbilical vein; *LPV,* umbilical segment of left portal vein; *DV,* ductus venosus; *RHV,* right hepatic vein; *IVC,* inferior vena cava.

These next figures show the umbilical cord insertion into the placenta and into the fetus. As discussed in Chapter 17, ultrasound identification of the cord insertion into the placenta is important for invasive obstetric procedures such as fetal blood sampling. The area is considered optimal because this is the only location where the cord is fixed, making needle approach more accurate. At the cord insertion site into the fetus, the umbilical vein courses superiorly and to the right to enter the liver and become part of portal circulation; the **umbilical arteries** run inferiorly along the margin of the urinary bladder and ultimately carry blood from the fetus back to the placenta. Some of the blood, however, does bypass the umbilical arteries at the internal iliac arteries to oxygenate and nourish the lower extremities of the fetus.

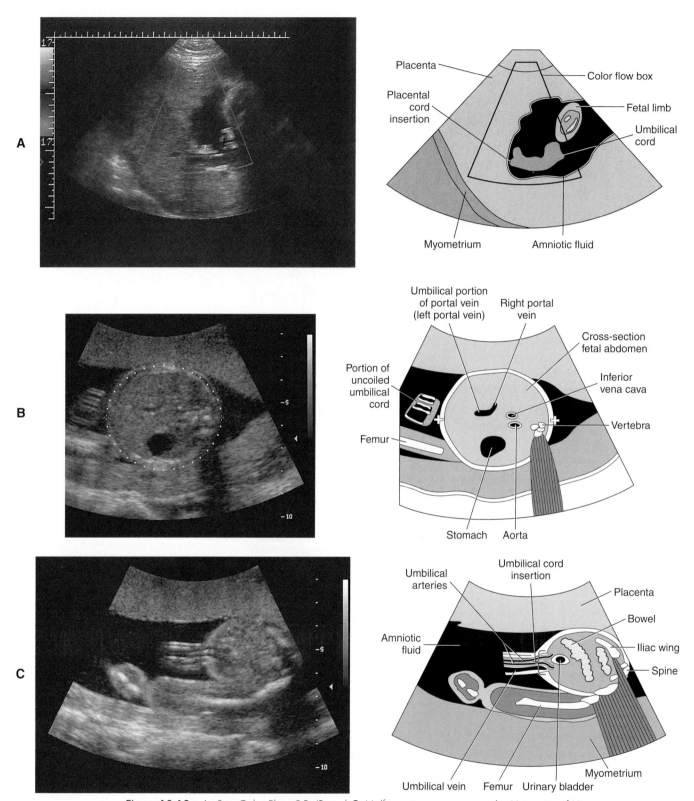

Figure 18-13 **A,** See Color Plate 25. (**B** and **C,** Half-tone images courtesy the University of Virginia Health System, Department of Radiology, Division of Ultrasound, Charlottesville, Virginia.)

Prior to birth, the anatomy of the heart and great vessels is the same as that discussed in Chapters 23 and 24, such as four chambers comprised by two atria and two ventricles, atrioventricular connections (valves), and inflows and outflows (great vessels). However, the fetal heart also includes two unique features, the foramen ovale and ductus arteriosus. As illustrated below, the fetal heart allows blood to move from right to left in the atrial chambers via the **foramen ovale.** This opening between the atria may remain patent after birth, but is held closed by the normal pressure gradient between left and right atria. The pulmonary artery and the aorta are connected by the **ductus arteriosus.** This duct allows blood to move from the pulmonary artery to the aorta. Because the fetal lungs do not have a respiratory function, they do not require large quantities of blood. The ductus arteriosus closes at (or shortly after) birth.

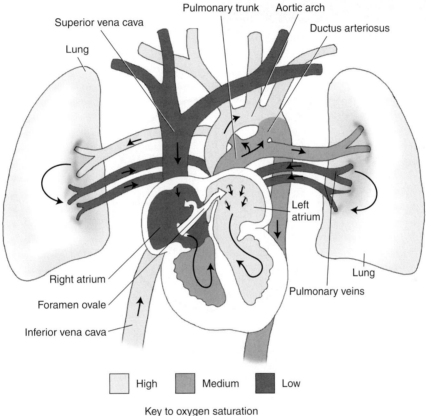

Figure 18-14

Sonographic Appearance

Heart Chambers and Septa. The fetal heart can be visualized as a four-chambered structure as early as 15 weeks and certainly by 20 weeks (Figure 18-15). Chamber walls appear hyperechoic compared with the anechoic blood within them. They should appear relatively symmetric, divided by the bright atrioventricular septa, which should be "broken" only at the foramen ovale. Normally the heart should be visualized on the left side of the thorax. The axis of the heart should be tilted approximately 45 degrees to the anteroposterior axis of the fetal thorax and pointed to the left (Figure 18-16). Sometimes it is necessary to image the ventricles and atria separately because of fetal position (Figure 18-17).

Cava, Aorta, and Pulmonary Artery. As seen in the following images, sonography also provides information regarding the position and size of the great vessels. Blood vessels in the fetus appear as they do after birth, bright walls and anechoic,

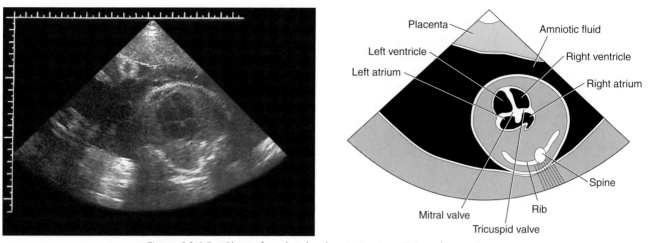

Figure 18-15 Classic four-chamber heart view in a 34-week gestation.

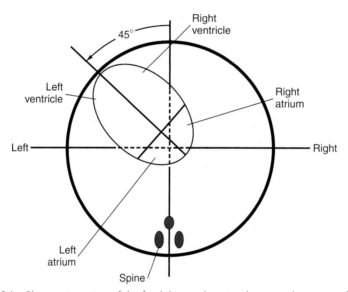

Figure 18-16 Short axis section of the fetal thorax showing the normal position of the heart.

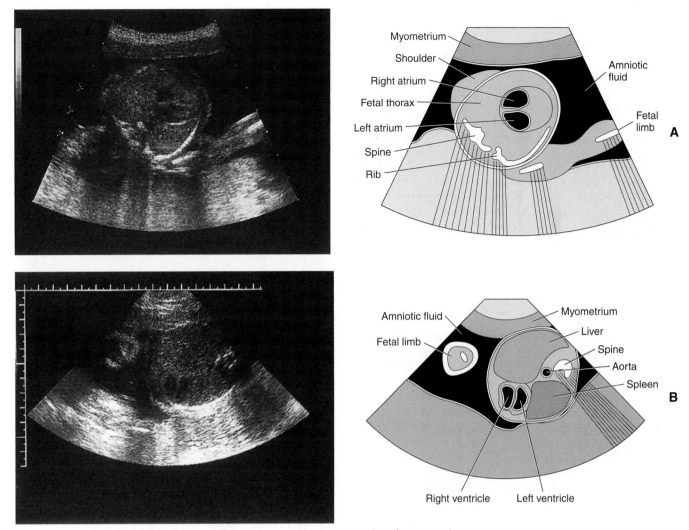

Figure 18-17 Heart. **A,** Atria. **B,** Ventricles of a 27-week gestation.

blood-filled lumens. Identification of the great arteries and outflow tracts in their usual positions confirms normal ventriculoarterial connections. Notice how the left atrium lies closest to the spine and the right ventricle lies closest to the anterior chest wall. Both atria and both ventricles are approximately the same size.

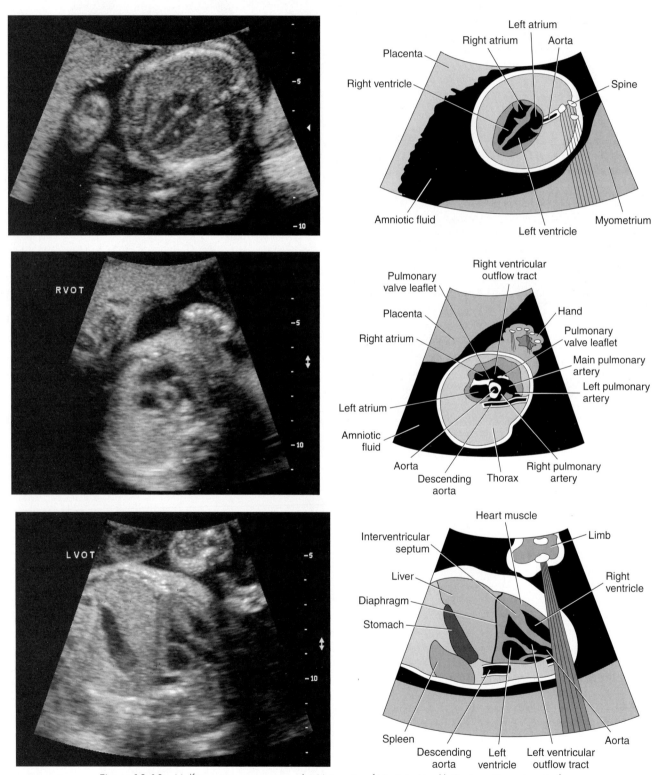

Figure 18-18   Half-tone images courtesy the University of Virginia Health System, Department of Radiology, Division of Ultrasound, Charlottesville, Virginia.

During the second trimester the superior vena cava, thoracic aorta, and pulmonary artery appear in the upper mediastinum, just superior to the heart. In older fetuses, the transverse aorta branches (brachiocephalic, left common carotid, left subclavian), right common carotid, and jugular veins are frequently seen. The posterior position of the abdominal aorta and inferior vena cava in the abdomen makes them easy to identify. The iliac arteries and veins are also frequently observed. Color Doppler is useful for identifying smaller branches of the abdominal aorta, such as the celiac axis, superior mesenteric artery, and renal arteries and veins.

Respiratory System

The lungs begin development as small-paired buds branching off the primitive alimentary canal during the fifth menstrual week. These buds increase in size, and multiple diverticula (outpouchings) form until about 17 weeks of gestation. The surfaces for gas exchange are not developed during this period. Therefore respiration is not possible, and fetuses born during this period are unable to survive. The primitive lungs mature and become capable of functioning sometime after 25 weeks' gestation. Some fetuses born at this stage will survive if given intensive care. During the last weeks of gestation, the final stage of development of the lungs begins. The lungs grow until they nearly fill the thoracic cavity. Lung growth continues into early childhood. The ability of the lungs to function can be measured in utero by monitoring the lecithin to sphingomyelin ratio (LS ratio), described in Chapter 19.

Sonographic Appearance

Upper Respiratory Tract. The portions of the fetal upper respiratory tract visible with sonography include the nose, nasal cavity and septum, and the palate. The presence of anechoic amniotic fluid in portions of the tract makes structures such as the pharynx, hypopharynx, piriform sinuses, and the epiglottis (in older fetuses) commonly visible. When the hypopharynx is fluid filled, the larynx is usually detectable. Generally, the fluid-filled trachea can be traced from its distal end, passing posterior to the aortic arch.

Lungs, Ribs, and Diaphragm. Early in pregnancy, identification of the lungs is derived more from the structures adjacent to them such as the heart (medially), ribs (superolaterally), diaphragm (inferiorly), and liver (inferiorly). The homogeneous lung tissue contrasts with the anechoic heart chambers. The ribs are easily recognized by their highly reflective, hyperechoic appearance. In a longitudinal section, the diaphragm is seen as a hypoechoic line separating the lungs from the abdomen (Figure 18-19). It should appear slightly concave, with the cuplike portion opening toward the abdomen and the arched position pointing toward the thorax. It is not unusual to see

the diaphragm move with fetal respiration, especially during the latter half of the third trimester. During part of the second trimester, the homogeneous, mid-gray appearance of the liver and lungs is the same. The lungs become more echogenic as the pregnancy progresses.

Gastrointestinal System

As discussed in Chapter 17, during the fourth gestational week, the foregut and hindgut develop from embryonic folds. The midgut is connected to the yolk sac. The foregut divides into the esophagus, stomach, and duodenum in the fifth week. The liver, gallbladder, pancreas, and spleen arise as diverticula from the primitive alimentary tube. The midgut splits into the remainder of small bowel, ascending colon, and a portion of transverse colon. The hindgut differentiates into the remainder of transverse colon, descending colon, and rectum. In the second trimester, bidirectional bowel peristalsis occurs. By the third trimester, peristalsis is unidirectional from the esophagus to the anus.

During the mid-to-late second trimester, fetal **meconium** ("waste") will accumulate in the bowel. It consists of swallowed amniotic fluid, glandular secretions, vernix, and bile. The cecum acts as an accumulation point for this fetal waste material.

Sonographic Appearance. As early as the end of the first trimester, several components of the fetal gastrointestinal system, such as the tongue, along with the stomach, gallbladder, liver, and bowel can be identified sonographically.

Oral Cavity and Esophagus. The oral cavity including hard and soft palates and the tongue are visualized fairly consistently with sonography. On the other hand, the proximal portion of the esophagus is nearly impossible to see; however, the mid and distal portions may occasionally be visualized anterior to the descending thoracic aorta as five parallel lines. The lines are created by the hypoechoic muscular wall and hyperechoic serosa and lumen.

Stomach and Gallbladder. Because they are the only subdiaphragmatic fetal gastrointestinal system structures normally filled with fluid, the stomach and gallbladder are consistently easy to identify. The fluid-filled stomach appears as an anechoic structure on the left side of the fetal abdomen (Figure 18-20). The size of the stomach is variable and depends on the amount of amniotic fluid swallowed by the fetus. The bile-filled gallbladder appears as an anechoic structure on the right side of the fetal abdomen (Figure 18-21). The gallbladder may be difficult to visualize after 32 weeks' gestation. It is thought that it contracts, releasing bile, due to initiation of gallbladder function.

Liver. By the second trimester, the homogeneous, mid-gray liver is routinely visualized occupying the right

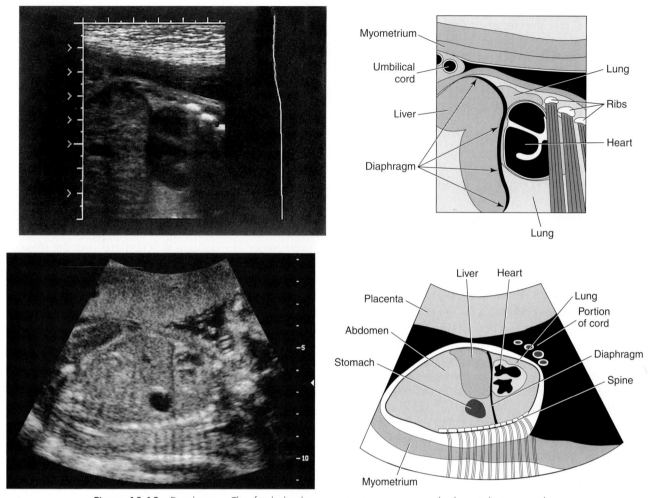

Figure 18-19 Diaphragm. The fetal diaphragm appears as a smooth, hypoechoic muscular boundary between the thorax and the abdomen. (*Bottom*, Half-tone image courtesy the University of Virginia Health System, Department of Radiology, Division of Ultrasound, Charlottesville, Virginia.)

side and much of the rest of the fetal abdomen (see Figure 18-21). In the early phases of pregnancy the liver margins may appear ill defined. The fetal liver is the largest parenchymal organ of the gastrointestinal system and of the abdomen. It is the site of production of red blood cells and is proportionately much greater in size in the fetus than in the adult; the left lobe extends as far as the left abdominal wall. It is the large size of the fetal liver that forces the diaphragm upward into the thorax and causes the fetal heart to be in a nearly horizontal plane.

The anechoic umbilical vein coursing through it interrupts the smooth parenchyma of the fetal liver. The vein's course is nearly perpendicular to the axis of the fetus as it nears its bifurcation point within the liver. Because of this, it is possible to see a fairly lengthy segment of the vein in a perpendicular transverse section taken at a level of the fetal stomach (Figure 18-22). The umbilical vein, stomach, spine, and liver are important landmarks for measurement of the fetal abdominal di-

ameter or abdominal circumference (described later in this chapter). The cord insertion into the fetal abdomen is shown in Figure 18-23.

Pancreas. The pancreas is the other major parenchymal organ of the gastrointestinal system; it is rarely seen. In some instances, the fetal pancreas may appear hyperechoic to adjacent structures and is visualized lying between the anechoic fluid-filled stomach (posterior wall) and anechoic splenic vein.

Spleen. Even though the spleen is not a gastrointestinal organ, it is associated with the liver by virtue of portal-splenic circulation (see Chapter 7). It arises from mesenchymal cells of the dorsal mesogastrium. Between 12 and 24 weeks' gestation, the spleen functions as a hematopoietic organ; lymphocyte and monocyte production continue throughout adult life. Like the fetal liver, the fetal spleen is routinely visualized from the second trimester onward. It occupies the left upper quadrant of the fetal abdomen; it is bounded laterally by the

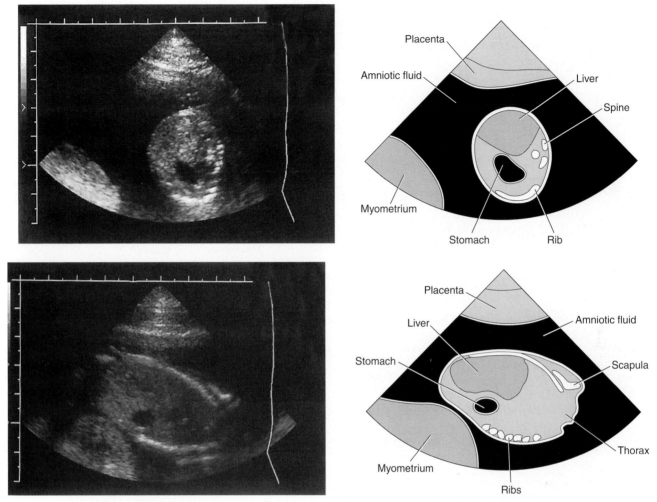

Figure 18-20 Stomach. The fluid-filled fetal stomach is routinely visualized on the left side of the abdominal cavity. It appears anechoic with relatively smooth walls. Stomach size and shape are determined by the amount of fluid it contains.

ribs, posteromedially by the spine, anteromedially by the stomach, posteriorly by the kidney, superiorly by the diaphragm, and inferiorly its margin is variable. As seen in Figure 18-21, the sonographic appearance of the fetal spleen is comparable to the fetal liver, that is, mid-gray and homogeneous with indistinct margins during early development. Comparatively, the adult spleen appears slightly hypoechoic to the liver.

Small and Large Bowel. Through the second and third trimesters, the small bowel gradually becomes more noticeable. Depending on how modern the ultrasound equipment is, small bowel loops and the bowel wall can be well-distinguished. The muscle layers of the bowel wall appear hypoechoic compared with the remarkably echogenic serosa and subserosa.

When the pregnancy nears term, the small bowel is readily imaged in virtually all fetuses. It is thought that mesenteric fat deposits delineate individual bowel loops, which facilitate identification. By late pregnancy

it is normal to see a small amount of anechoic fluid within the small bowel and hyperechoic areas of meconium (fetal waste).

The fetal colon is in the same anatomic position as in the adult. The colon ascends from the right flank to the liver, where it bends (at the "hepatic flexure") and traverses the abdomen inferior to the stomach to the spleen where it bends ("splenic flexure") and then descends toward the left flank, meeting the sigmoid colon and rectum. Figure 18-24 shows amniotic, fluid-filled portions of the ascending and transverse colon. Collapsed, the fetal colon typically appears hypoechoic compared with adjacent structures.

Genitourinary System

The fetal genitourinary system consists of the kidneys, ureters, urinary bladder, urethra, and genitalia. The kidneys, which form in association with urethral buds, develop between 7 and 9 weeks of gestation and become

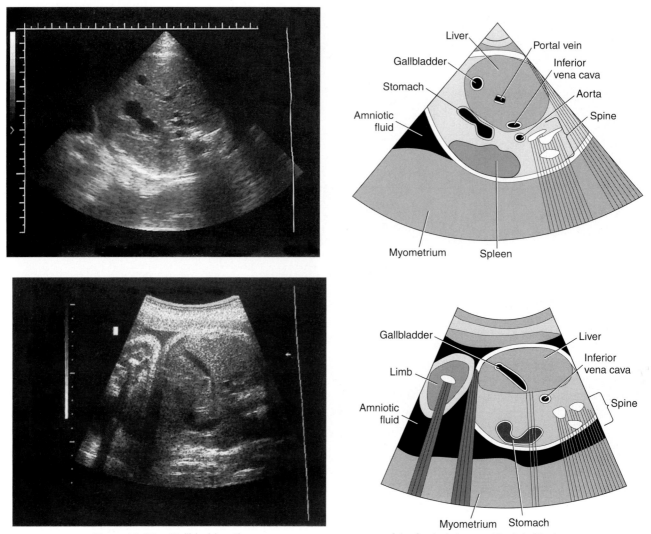

Figure 18-21 *Gallbladder. Short axis or transverse sections of the fetal abdomen. The bile-filled fetal gallbladder is typically visualized on the right side of the abdominal cavity. It appears anechoic with smooth walls. Gallbladder lie is variable; therefore, the long axis can be identified in any scanning plane. The size and shape of the gallbladder depend on the amount of fluid (prior to bile production) or bile it contains.*

functional at approximately 10 weeks of menstrual age. The bladder and ureters are formed at approximately 6 menstrual weeks of development.

Following the sixteenth week of gestation, the majority of amniotic fluid arises from fetal urination. Assessment of the quantity of amniotic fluid, therefore, constitutes the initial step in the evaluation of the fetal genitourinary system. A normal amount of amniotic fluid implies the presence of at least one functioning kidney.

Sonographic Appearance

Kidneys. Even though fetal kidney position is variable and the sonographic appearance of the kidneys is difficult to differentiate from adjacent structures, they may, in some cases, be identified sonographically as early as 15 to 16 weeks. Typically, consistent recognition of fetal kidneys begins during the twentieth week. Later in pregnancy, the bright, hyperechoic, retroperitoneal fat surrounding the kidneys makes them easier to visualize.

The fetal kidneys grow at a rate that keeps them proportionately equal to the other developing fetal structures. In general, the length of the fetal kidneys may be represented by the length of four to five vertebrae of the fetus. The ratio of kidney diameter to the diameter of the fetal abdomen should remain between 0.27 and 0.23 throughout the gestation.

Cortex, Medulla, and Sinus. The normal fetal renal cortex usually appears slightly hypoechoic relative to surrounding structures. It appears interrupted by the anechoic medullary pyramids typically separated by

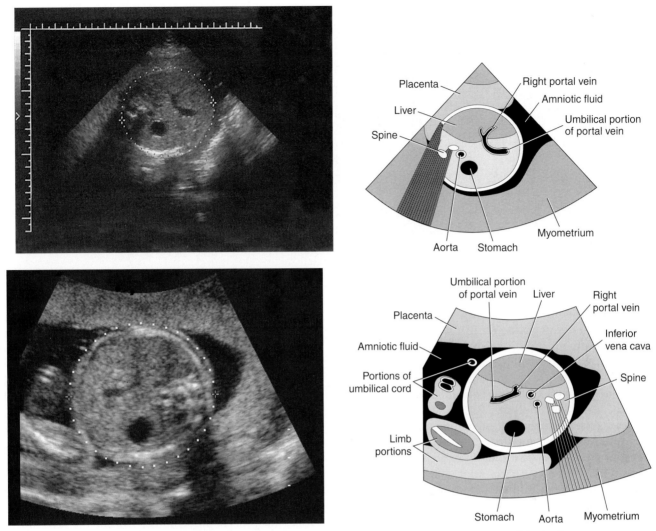

Figure 18-22 Umbilical portion of the portal vein. Short axis or transverse sections of the fetal abdomen. Notice how the umbilical portion of the portal vein lies in the midline of the abdomen, then curves toward the liver as the right branch of the portal vein becomes visible. (Half-tone image at bottom courtesy the University of Virginia Health System, Department of Radiology, Division of Ultrasound, Charlottesville, Virginia.)

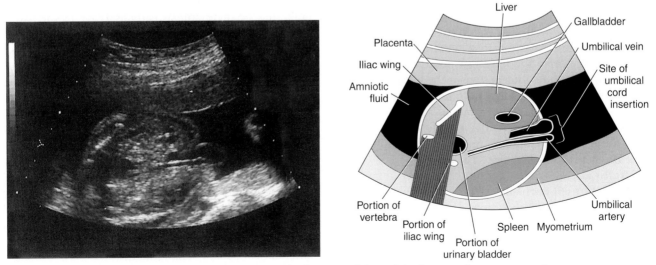

Figure 18-23 Cord insertion. Longitudinal section of the umbilical vein and one artery as they enter the fetal abdominopelvic cavity.

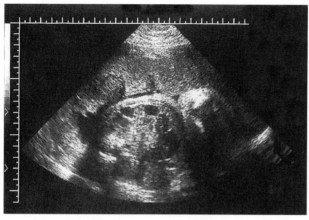
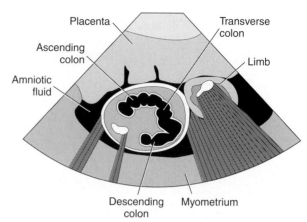

Figure 18-24   Colon. The anechoic fluid it contains distinctly delineates portions of the ascending, transverse, and descending colon.

columns of Bertin (cortical extensions). Unlike adult kidneys, there is very little fat in the fetal renal sinus, making it virtually indistinguishable or very slightly hyperechoic compared with the cortex. Because of this, it is common to visualize normal, urine-filled, intrarenal collecting structures; the urine-filled infundibula and renal pelvis appear anechoic.

Normal fetal kidneys can be identified in their paraspinous location; longitudinal sections appear elliptical; transverse sections appear round (Figure 18-25).

Ureters. As a rule, normal fetal ureters are not visualized sonographically. In almost all cases, identification of a fetal ureter is an indication of pathologic dilation.

Urinary Bladder. By 15 weeks' menstrual age, over 90% of all normal fetal urinary bladders can be visualized. Figure 18-26 demonstrates the ultrasound appearance of the fluid-filled fetal urinary bladder. Note how the bladder is located at the midline of the fetal pelvis. Also notice the thin, hyperechoic bladder wall surrounding the anechoic fluid. With normal fetal renal function, the size of the fetal bladder will often be seen to increase and decrease in size during an ultrasound examination. Identification of the urine-filled fetal urinary bladder is necessary to establish renal function. If the bladder is not seen, the fetus can be examined in 30-minute to 45-minute intervals when the fetus normally fills and empties its bladder. If the bladder still cannot be visualized, follow-up studies are usually mandatory. The fetal bladder grows in proportion to the rest of the fetus during the remainder of pregnancy, and its visualized size depends on the degree of filling.

Urethra. Occasionally the urethra may be identified in male fetuses. If the penis is erect, the urethra presents as a bright, reflective line running along the length; otherwise it is not identifiable.

Genitalia. From the early second trimester, fetal gender can be established sonographically. Determination of fetal gender depends on the visualization of either the male scrotum or the female labia. Assignment of gender should not be made on the basis of the presence or absence of a fetal penis. The penis may be quite small and not visualized, suggesting the presence of a female fetus, or a female clitoris may suggest the presence of a small penis. Thus if the gender of the fetus is to be determined, the labia must be distinguished from the scrotum. Figure 18-27 demonstrates the ultrasound appearance of male and female external genitalia in utero.

Fetal male genitalia are easier to identify than female genitalia. The mid-gray to low-gray, homogeneous penis and scrotum are most apparent. In some cases, the testes have been differentiated within the scrotum as early as the third trimester. It is not unusual for small, anechoic testicular hydroceles (fluid collections) to be visualized bilaterally. Details of the penis, including the glans, urethra, and corpora cavernosa, may also be identified; in some cases, even the foreskin is visible. The prostate cannot be distinguished.

In the fetal female, the bilateral major and minor labia may be detectable as early as 17 or 18 menstrual weeks. The major labia flank the minor labia; they appear more echogenic than the hypoechoic minor labia. The bright, linear, vaginal cleft lies at the midline, between the minor labia. Typically, the fetal uterus and ovaries cannot be visualized.

Adrenal Glands. While the fetal adrenal glands are not part of the genitourinary system, their close proximity to the kidneys and relatively conspicuous appearance make them a significant sonographic marker. The triangular shaped adrenals appear to "cap" the upper renal poles. High-resolution scanning reveals a low-gray organ, predominantly hypoechoic to the liver and renal cortex on the right and the spleen and renal cortex on the left. Figure 18-28 shows the relationship of the adrenal gland to the fetal kidney.

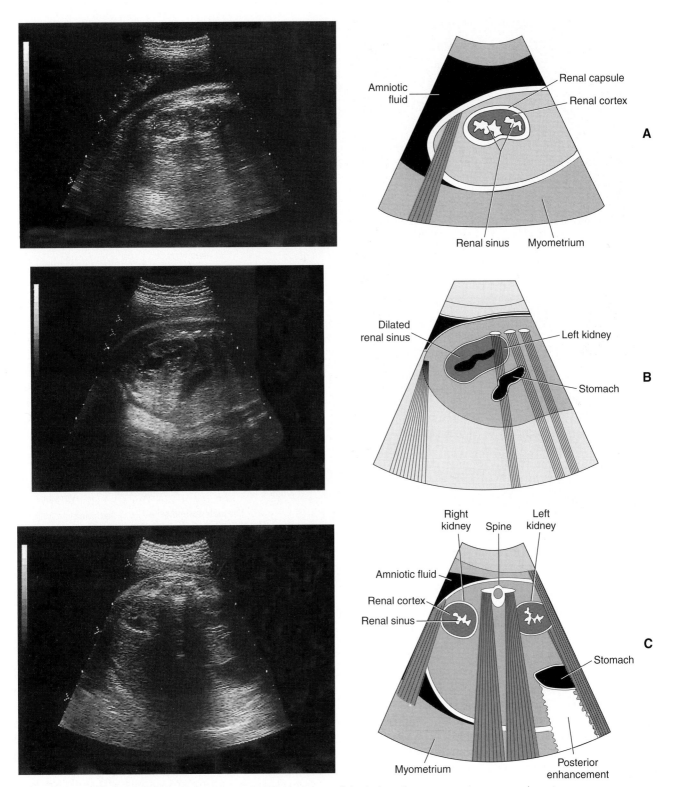

Figure 18-25 Kidneys. **A,** Longitudinal section of the kidney (between measurement calipers). The distinctive elliptical shape and bright renal capsule assist sonographic identification of the kidneys. Later in the trimester, the reflective retroperitoneal fat visualized surrounding the kidneys also makes visualization easier. Notice the classic contrast in appearance between the vivid renal sinus and low-gray appearance of the renal cortex. **B,** In this longitudinal section the area of the renal sinus appears anechoic because the collecting system is marginally dilated with urine/fluid. **C,** In a transverse or short axis section the kidneys appear round or circular. Notice how close they lie to the lumbar spinal ossification centers bilaterally.

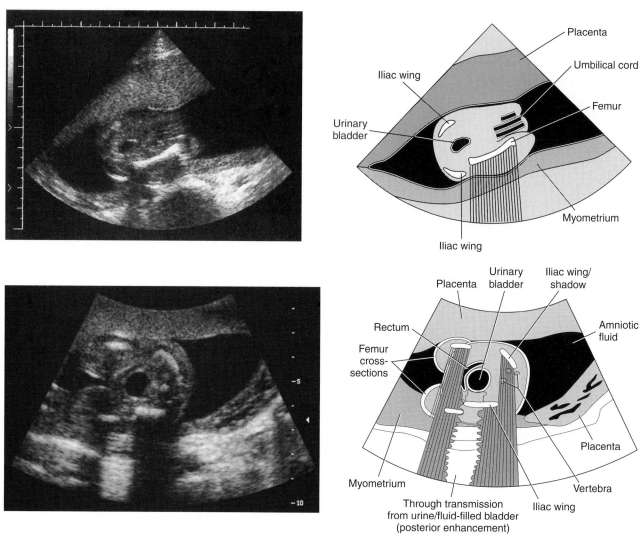

Figure 18-26 Urinary bladder. The urine-filled fetal bladder is easily recognized in the fetal pelvis because of its characteristic anechoic appearance and midline position. Another distinction is the thin, hyperechoic bladder wall that virtually disappears when the bladder is fully distended. Notice the difference in size between these bladders. Changes in the volume of the urinary bladder not only confirm fetal urine production but also, with time, differentiate the bladder from pathologic structures in the pelvis, such as cysts, that have the same sonographic appearance. (Half-tone image on bottom courtesy the University of Virginia Health System, Department of Radiology, Division of Ultrasound, Charlottesville, Virginia.)

Central Nervous System

The central nervous system consists of the brain and the spinal cord. It arises from the posterior surface of the embryo (ectoderm). A linear depression is formed along the midline of the early embryo. The borders of the depression fold over to form the **neurotube** that gives rise to the spinal cord and the brain. Closure of this tube begins in midembryo and continues in both cephalad and caudad directions, completing the cephalad first. The brain is composed of three elements: the brain stem, the cerebrum, and the cerebellum. Membranes known as the meninges, which also surround the spinal cord, surround these elements. The brain and spinal cord have an elaborate system of circulation composed of ventricles, cisterns, and sinuses.

The **brain stem** is composed of the medulla, pons, midbrain, thalamus, and hypothalamus. It is a continuation of the spinal cord and is the base of the brain. The medulla oblongata is closest to the spinal cord and is responsible for control of respiration, heart rate, blood pressure, and certain involuntary reflexes (sneezing, coughing, and so on). The *pons* is located between the medulla and the cerebellum and helps to regulate respiration. The pons also transmits signals from the spinal cord to the cerebellum and cerebrum. The **midbrain** sits between the pons and the thalamus. It relays

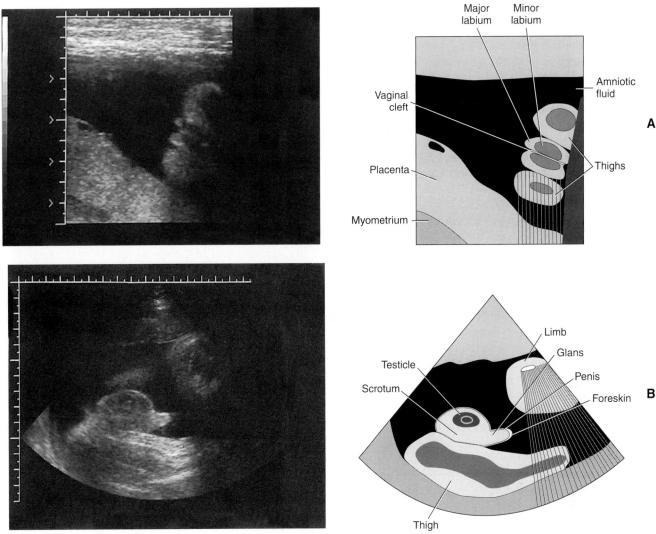

Figure 18-27 Genitalia. **A,** Female genitalia in a 32-week gestation. Female gender is confirmed only when the major and minor labia have been identified. **B,** Male genitalia in a 30-week gestation.

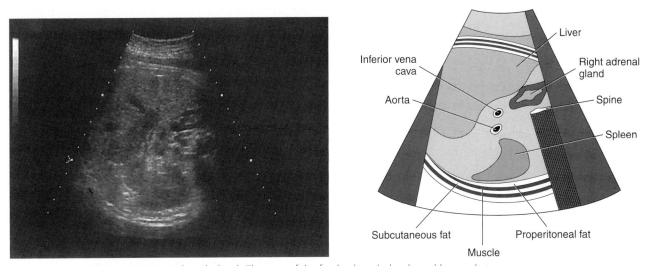

Figure 18-28 Adrenal gland. The size of the fetal adrenal glands and hypoechoic appearance of the cortex make it distinguishable from surrounding structures. The right adrenal is immediately posterior to the inferior vena cava.

signals from one part of the brain to another and controls head and eye movements. The thalamus and hypothalamus are superior to the midbrain. The thalamus is a relay system for cerebral impulses. The hypothalamus is the communication relay between the nervous system and the endocrine system.

The **cerebrum** is the center of higher mental faculties. It is concerned with the interpretation of impulses and voluntary muscular activities; it is the largest component of the brain and is composed of five lobes: parietal, temporal, occipital, frontal, and insula (or isle of Reil), the only lobe not named for an overlying bone. The cerebral (or callosal) fissure that extends anteriorly to posteriorly almost completely divides the cerebrum into two lateral hemispheres; the corpus callosum keeps them connected. The sylvian fissure separates the parietal and temporal lobes. The insula lies in a central location deep in the cerebrum between the sylvian fissures.

The **cerebellum** helps to coordinate movements, balance, and posture; it is located just below the cerebrum and superoposterior to most of the brain stem. The cerebellum is composed of two lateral hemispheres. A small central lobe, the vermis, relays information between the two hemispheres.

The **meninges** are composed of three layers. The **dura mater** is the outermost layer and functions as a tough protective cover. The **arachnoid layer** is a fibrous cobweblike structure and is the thin middle layer. The **pia mater** is a delicate and highly vascularized inner layer that closely follows the contours of the brain and spinal cord. The meninges not only provide protection for the central nervous system, but also facilitate cerebrospinal fluid movement from the subarachnoid space to the dural sinuses. The dura mater is actually two layers. The thicker outer layer firmly adheres to the bones of the skull. The thin inner layer follows the basic curvature of the brain, and together with the arachnoid and pia mater layers, serves to separate the structures of the brain. At the area where the outer and inner layers first separate, there are small spaces. Collectively these spaces are known as the **dural sinuses.**

Cerebrospinal fluid (CSF) is similar to plasma in chemical composition except for the concentration of sodium ions, which is much higher in CSF. CSF fills the central canal of the spinal cord, the ventricles of the brain, and the subarachnoid space. It also is present within the cisterns of the brain (discussed later in this chapter). CSF acts as a protective cushion encasing the brain and spinal cord, and regulates the pressure within the spaces that it fills. CSF may also have a metabolic role; however, this role is not clearly defined.

Ventricles of the brain are part of a system that helps manufacture and distribute CSF. Four ventricles constitute this system. There are two **lateral ventricles,** one in each cerebral hemisphere. The lateral ventricles are the

first and second ventricles. They contain five regions: the frontal horns (most anterior), the lateral bodies (most superior), the occipital horns (most posterior), the temporal (most lateral), and the atria (the juncture of the temporal and occipital horns with the body of the lateral ventricle). The lateral ventricles are connected to the third ventricle by the **foramen of Monro,** which runs from the juncture of the frontal horn and body of the lateral ventricle to the roof of the third ventricle. The third ventricle is found in the midline of the brain and is located centrally in the thalamus. The fourth ventricle is also found in the midline in a more posterior location. The third and fourth ventricles are connected by a long tubular structure known as the **aqueduct of Sylvius,** and the fourth ventricle is also connected to the central canal of the spinal cord by two lateral ducts, the **foramina of Luschka,** and a single medial duct, the **foramen of Magendie.**

The **choroid plexus** is found in the lateral ventricles (with the exception of the frontal and occipital horns) and the third and fourth ventricles. Choroid plexus is a highly vascularized tissue that develops from the pia mater that secretes CSF. CSF flows from the lateral ventricles to the third and fourth ventricles; to the subarachnoid space; then to the dural sinuses, where it is absorbed in the venous bloodstream. The subarachnoid space (the space between the pia mater and the arachnoid layer) is very small in most areas, but in certain areas it is enlarged, and CSF will pool. These areas are called **cisterns.** The lumbar cistern is the largest of these spaces and is found in the distal end of the spine. Other such cisterns are found in various locations within the brain. The largest of these cisterns is the **cisterna magna,** which is located at the base of the cerebellum in a posterior location within the skull (Figure 18-29).

Two internal carotid arteries and two vertebral arteries supply the circulatory system of the brain. The vertebral arteries join in the inferior and posterior portion of the brain to form basilar arteries, which enter the circle of Willis. The internal carotid arteries enter the circle laterally and inferiorly. The middle cerebral arteries arise laterally from the circle of Willis and course medially to the sylvian fissures. Paired anterior and posterior cerebral arteries also arise from this circle. The veins draining the brain are all tributaries of the dural sinuses and drain into the internal jugular veins.

The spine is a continuation of the brain stem. It contains a nerve bundle floating in CSF and covered by meninges. The CSF in the spinal column freely communicates with the CSF in the cranium.

Sonographic Appearance

Intracranial Anatomy. By the eleventh gestational week, the ovoid appearance of the large lateral ventricles filled with highly echogenic choroid plexus is easily

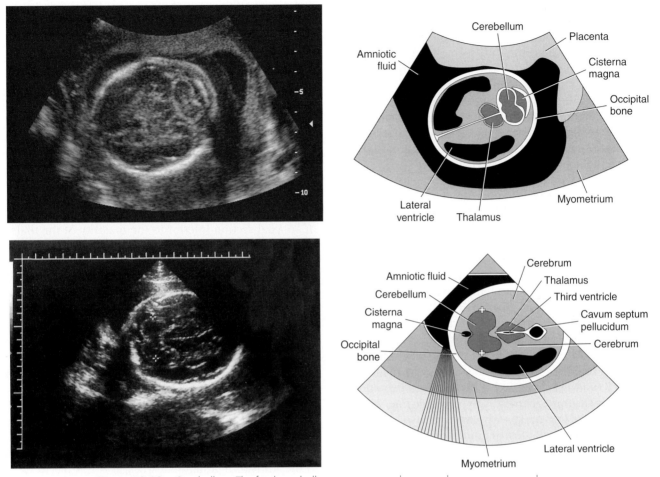

Figure 18-29 Cerebellum. The fetal cerebellum appears very low gray, homogeneous, and symmetric. (Half-tone image at top courtesy the University of Virginia Health System, Department of Radiology, Division of Ultrasound, Charlottesville, Virginia.)

identified. The choroid plexus are the most prominent intracranial structures seen at this time. They are bright, drumstick-shaped structures on either side of the falx cerebri in the posterior portion of the brain. The falx is the bright, reflective fold of dura mater in the cerebral fissure that separates the cerebral hemispheres. The anechoic frontal horns are free of the choroids, yet are easily identified because they are filled with CSF. Except for the areas containing choroid plexus, the remaining portions of the lateral ventricles are clearly delineated by anechoic CSF. Ventricle walls appear vivid and hyperechoic to the CSF and mid-gray to low-gray brain matter. At this point of development only the rudiments of the occipital and temporal horns are present. Also at this time, the homogeneous, medium-level to low-level gray appearance of the cerebrum, cerebellum, brain stem, and highly reflective third ventricle is established and will remain fairly consistent, other than developmental enlargement, throughout the gestation. The brain linings (dura-arachnoid and pia) are also established and have the distinction of appearing very bright or hypere-

choic compared with adjacent structures. The **falx cerebri** is a significant sonographic marker because it is an extremely bright reflection. The falx is seen at right angles to the sound beam in the axial plane as a reflective line dividing the homogeneous, mid-gray to low-gray cerebrum into equal right and left halves. The **cerebellar vermis** often appears strikingly echogenic due to its intertwined meninges covering; it is the reflective line dividing the homogeneous, low-gray cerebellum.

Peripheral to the edges of the brain are **subarachnoid spaces** that range in appearance from anechoic to varying levels of echogenicity; some are filled with anechoic CSF and some with echogenic mater, and some with areas of both.

As development continues, specific portions of brain matter are identifiable as they differentiate sonographically. Nuclei such as the caudate and lentiform appear as low-level, gray echoes, hypoechoic to surrounding structures with the exception of anechoic CSF. The tegmentum portion of the brain stem is also hypoechoic as opposed to the ventral area of the pons that presents as an area of mid-gray or moderate echogenicity, a little brighter than the nuclei and tegmentum.

Highly reflective brain fissures can be identified prior to 20 weeks. Two are commonly seen, the small and less important parieto-occipital fissure and the larger lateral fissure that is often mistaken for the lateral wall of the lateral ventricles, an error that can present as hydrocephalus (overenlargement of the lateral ventricles). By 38 to 42 weeks (term), the lateral fissure closes with progressive growth of the parietal and temporal lobes and eventually becomes the sylvian cistern.

The occipital and temporal horns of the lateral ventricles can be identified by the eighteenth or twentieth gestational week. Like the frontal horns, the occipital horns do not contain any choroid plexus. At this stage all of the components of the lateral ventricles have developed. Nevertheless, their shape and proportion will change as they and adjacent neural tissue continue to grow. Between 24 weeks and term, the increase in brain volume causes the slow-growing lateral ventricles and choroid plexus to gradually become less prominent.

The **thalamus** is a diamond-shaped area visualized in the center of an axial section taken through the temporal lobe of the brain; it appears homogeneous with medium-level to low-level echoes and is divided into two equal sections by the third ventricle, a hyperechoic line, which extends upward into the space between the two halves. At times a very small quantity of fluid, which appears anechoic, can be seen giving the third ventricle a slitlike appearance. The **cavum septum pellucidum** is another anechoic, fluid-containing structure seen in the midline of the brain. It appears as two small, bright lines separated by CSF, parallel to the falx. This structure contains more fluid than the third ventricle. It is located superoanterior to the thalamus and third ventricle and lies between the frontal horns and bodies of the two lateral ventricles.

An axial section just above the level of the thalamus should show three hyperechoic lines parallel with the long axis of the head. The middle of these three lines is the falx cerebri. It should be seen to bisect the head left to right. Lateral to the falx are two bright lines. These represent the lateral borders of the lateral ventricles. The distance from the falx to either of the lines should be approximately one-third the distance from the falx to one side of the calvarium (skull) or less. Figure 18-30 is an image of normal lateral ventricles in an 18-week gestation. Prior to 18 weeks, the ventricles fill most of the skull, and this rule does not apply, but should hold, beyond 18 weeks of gestation.

The posterior portion of the brain can be visualized in an axial section inferior to the majority of the thalamus. The cerebellum should appear symmetric, homogeneous, and of medium-level to low-level echogenicity. The cerebellum in a 22-week fetus is shown in Figure 18-29. The cisterna magna is a subarachnoid space seen in a posteroinferior position with respect to the cerebellum. It appears anechoic because it is filled with CSF.

Spinal Cord. The hypoechoic spinal cord is clearly visible by the fifteenth or sixteenth week. It can best be seen in a longitudinal section, lying between the highly reflective, echogenic vertebrae.

Familiarity with the development of fetal intracranial anatomy and its sonographic presentation assists the sonographer in recognizing normal versus abnormal anatomy at different growth stages. For instance, prior to the thirteenth gestational week, it is normal to view the choroid plexus filling the lateral ventricle. It assumes a more posterior location between 13 and 15 weeks, and the anterior horns of the lateral ventricles become quite prominent. In some cases, the prominent anterior horns have been mistaken for abnormally large ventricles (ventriculomegaly). Similarly, development of the

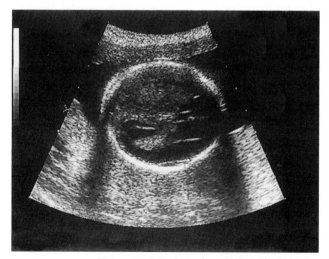

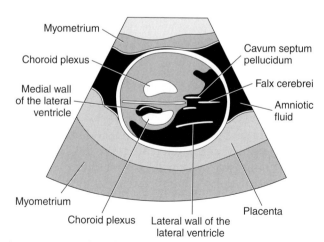

Figure 18-30 Lateral ventricles. The lateral ventricles appear anechoic because they are filled with cerebrospinal fluid; their walls appear hyperechoic and bright. This image shows a lateral ventricle in an 18-week gestation.

corpus callosum is not complete until the eighteenth or twentieth gestational week. Scans prior to this time have, in some instances, wrongly suggested agenesis of the corpus callosum. In the same way, before 18 to 22 weeks, the undeveloped cerebellar vermis leaves the inferior portion of the fourth ventricle only covered by the thin ventricular roof, giving the appearance of abnormal communication between the fourth ventricle and cisterna magna. Later in gestation, this finding suggests the presence of brain malformation.

DETERMINATION OF GESTATIONAL AGE DURING THE SECOND AND THIRD TRIMESTERS

The transition between first and second trimesters (12 to 13 weeks) is the accepted time to make the transition from crown-rump length (CRL) measurements to **biparietal diameter (BPD), head circumference (HC) and abdominal circumference (AC),** and **femur length (FL)** measurements to predict gestational age.

Biparietal Diameter

The BPD can be appropriately measured through any plane of section that traverses the third ventricle and thalami. The transducer must be perpendicular to the parietal bones and positioned to intersect the third ventricle and thalami (Figure 18-31). (Refer to the Central Nervous System section to review the sonographic appearance of these brain structures.)

To accurately measure the BPD, the calvaria (cranium) must be symmetric and smooth, and measurement cursors may be positioned in one of three ways: inner edge of near calvarial wall to outer edge of far calvarial wall, outer edge of near calvarial wall to inner edge of far calvarial wall, and middle of near calvarial wall to middle of far calvarial wall. Many institutions utilize the second method (Figure 18-32, *A*).

The recognizable symmetry of the calvaria and thalami (on either side of the third ventricle) makes it easy to recognize the correct plane of section to obtain accurate and consistent measurements of the BPD. Charts are available that correlate the BPD measurement with gestational age, and most modern ultrasound equipment computes an age while the measurement is obtained.

Cephalic Index

At times a number of conditions such as multiple gestations and breech presentations can alter the shape of the fetal head; therefore, the **cephalic index (CI)** should always be determined to assess head shape. The BPD along with a **fronto-occipital diameter (FOD)** is utilized to calculate the CI :

$$BPD/FOD \times 100 = \text{Cephalic Index}$$

The FOD is measured from the outer edge to the outer edge of the calvaria (Figure 18-32, *B*). Today, most ultrasound machines compute the CI using the long and short axes from the HC. The CI should be between 0.72 and 0.86. If the CI is above 0.86, the head is wider than average, or **brachiocephalic.** If the CI is under 0.72, the head is narrower than average, or **dolichocephalic.** The HC is usually used for dating the pregnancy when the CI is abnormal.

Head Circumference

Unlike the BPD, HC is best obtained through a single plane of section that must be perpendicular to the thalami, the third ventricle (like the BPD), *and* the cavum septum pellucidum and tentorium.

To accurately measure the HC, the calvaria should appear symmetric and smooth. In cases where the entire perimeter of the calvaria is not demonstrated, the ellip-

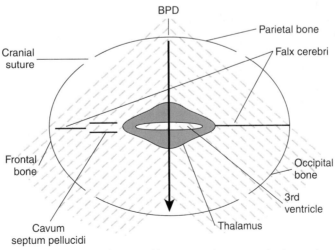

Figure 18-31 This illustrates how the sound beam must be perpendicular to the parietal bones *and* intersect the third ventricle and thalami to obtain an accurate plane for a biparietal diameter measurement (BPD).

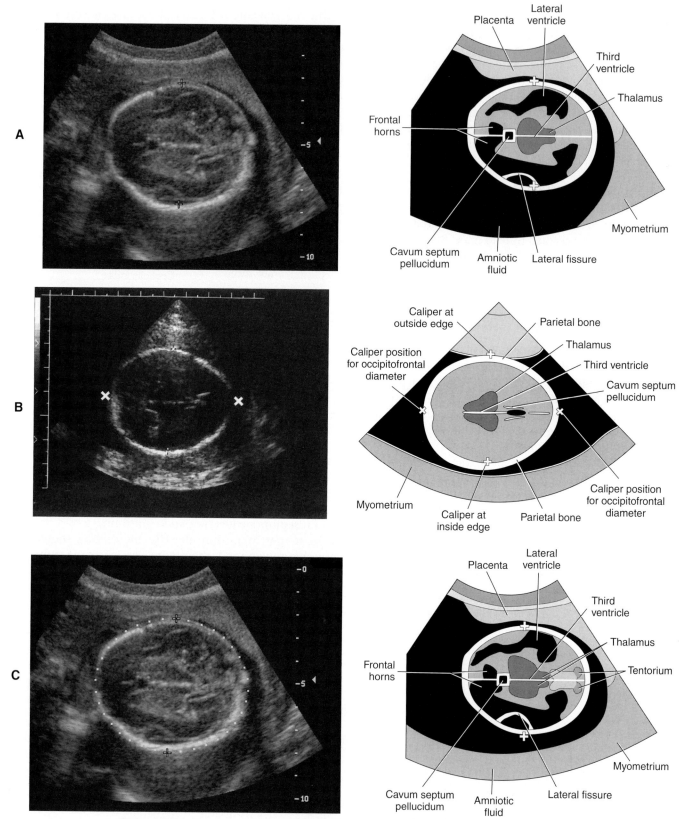

Figure 18-32 Head measurement levels. **A,** Demonstrates caliper placement (outer to inner) and anatomic level for a BPD measurement. **B,** Position of calipers (outer to inner and outer to outer/horizontal) for BPD and fronto-occipital diameter (FOD) measurements. **C,** Demonstrates caliper placement (outer to outer/vertical) and anatomic level for a head circumference (HC) measurement. (**A,** and **C,** Half-tone images courtesy the University of Virginia Health System, Department of Radiology, Division of Ultrasound, Charlottesville, Virginia.)

tical measurement cursor on most machines will adequately estimate the portions not imaged. Cursors should be placed at the outer edge of the near calvarial wall to the outer edge of the far calvarial wall (Figure 18-32, *C*). Care should be taken not to fit the ellipse to the surrounding skin edge. Charts are available that correlate the HC measurement with gestational age, and most modern ultrasound equipment computes an age while the measurement is obtained.

As mentioned, the BPD can be obtained through multiple planes, the HC through a single plane of section. Therefore the HC image can be used to obtain the BPD. On the other hand, a BPD image cannot necessarily be used to obtain the HC unless it is at the single level that includes the cavum septum pellucidum and tentorium along with the thalamus and third ventricle.

Abdominal Circumference

As seen in Figure 18-33, the AC is measured through a single plane of section where the umbilical vein branches, and the right and left portal veins are continuous with one another. At this level, the shortest length of the umbilical vein is visualized. Other sonographic markers for the correct AC level include the fetal spine that appears as three bright, echogenic reflectors, and the anechoic fluid-filled stomach may be seen on the fetus' left.

The fetal abdomen should appear round or nearly round for an accurate AC measurement. The elliptical measurement cursor is fit to the skin edge (Figure 18-34). Charts are available that correlate the AC measurement with gestational age and, as previously mentioned, most modern ultrasound equipment computes an age while the measurement is obtained.

The AC is considered the most difficult measurement to consistently obtain due to the times when the AC landmarks can be less than optimal to image. In these cases, the "roundest" appearance of the abdomen is utilized. At this level, the anteroposterior and transverse diameters of the abdomen should be equal or nearly equal. Because not all ultrasound instruments have the ability to trace or draw ellipses, the AC can be determined by adding the anteroposterior and transverse diameters of the abdomen (measured from skin edge to skin edge) and multiplying the total sum by 1.57:

$$(D1 + D2) \times 1.57 = AC$$

Standard reference tables are used to correlate the AC with predicted age. Other charts use the AC and HC to estimate fetal weight.

Femur Length

The fetal femur can be measured as early as 12 weeks of development to predict gestational age. The proper plane of section is simply the long axis of the bone. This can be confirmed by showing the highly reflective femoral head and femoral condyle in the same plane. Measurement cursors are placed at the bone-cartilage interface, which are the ossified portions of the metaphysis and diaphysis. The hypoechoic cartilaginous ends of the femur are not included in the measurement.

Figure 18-35, *A* demonstrates the measurement of a fetal femur. Both femurs should always be measured. If the femur lengths do not agree with head or abdominal measurements, the humeri should also be measured (Figure 18-35, *B*). Charts (often part of ultrasound machine software as mentioned) are available that correlate estimated gestational age with femur and humerus lengths.

In relatively rare cases, when the BPD, HC, or FL is not obtainable, additional measurement parameters (and correlating charts) to estimate fetal age can be utilized. They include long axis measurements of the fetal tibia, fibula, radius, ulna, clavicle, or foot. Furthermore, interorbital and intraorbital diameters and transverse diameter of the cerebellum are preferred by some experts as supplementary methods for estimating fetal age.

Following the first trimester, fetal age estimates should be based on the multiple measurement parameters discussed in this chapter, preferably before 20 weeks' gestation. Most experts agree that the optimal combination of parameters is based on HC and FL.

Inaccurate measurements can lead to misdiagnoses and serious potential errors in the clinical management of the patient and gestation. Learning the guidelines for obtaining fetal measurements and using them consistently and accurately provide the essential information for correct interpretation.

NORMAL VARIANTS
Lemon Sign

Appears as bilateral, frontal, concave scalloping of the calvaria.

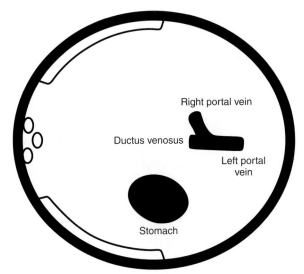

Figure 18-33 Anatomic level for abdominal circumference (AC) measurement.

Right portal vein

Ductus venosus

Left portal vein

Stomach

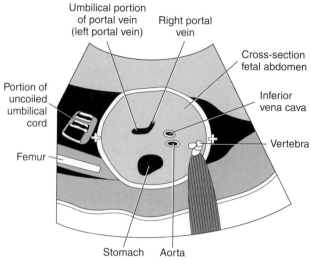

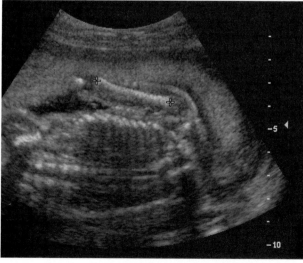

Figure 18-34 Abdominal measurement level. Demonstrates caliper placement (outer skin edge to outer skin edge) and plane of section to obtain the AC measurement. The AC is measured at the position where the short axis diameter of the liver is the greatest. Sonographically, this is identified as the short axis section where the anechoic right and left portal veins are continuous with one another. Some refer to this appearance as the "hockey stick." Note that this is also where the shortest length of the umbilical portion of the left portal vein is visualized. (Half-tone image courtesy the University of Virginia Health System, Department of Radiology, Division of Ultrasound, Charlottesville, Virginia.)

A
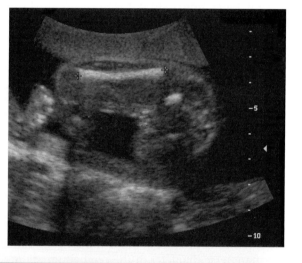

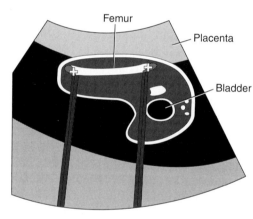

B
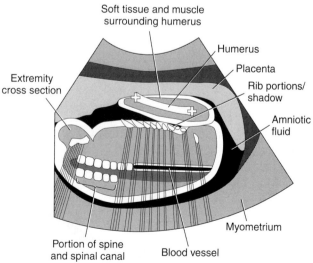

Figure 18-35 Long bone measurements. The long axis of the femur and humerus are used for measurements to determine gestational age. If both cartilaginous ends of the long bones are visualized, this guarantees that the plane of section is the long axis. Measurement is confined to the ossified portions. A, Femur measurement. B, Humerus measurement. (Half-tone images courtesy the University of Virginia Health System, Department of Radiology, Division of Ultrasound, Charlottesville, Virginia.)

Prominent Cisterna Magna

If no other malformation(s) is identified, this is a normal finding.

Choroid Plexus Cyst

If no other malformation(s) is identified, this is a normal finding that usually resolves by 24 to 26 gestational weeks.

Cavum Vergae

Normal prominent posterior continuation of the cavum septum pellucidi, which may simulate a dilated third ventricle or arachnoid cyst.

Fetal Hair

Commonly seen in the third trimester and should not be mistaken for a calvarial mass or scalp edema.

Prominent Cardiac Moderator Band

Normal enlargement or prominence of the moderator band can simulate a ventricular thrombus or neoplasm.

REFERENCE CHARTS

■ ■ ■ ASSOCIATED PHYSICIANS

Obstetrician/Gynecologist: Manages preterm obstetric care and delivers the fetus. This physician is also responsible for the care of the infant immediately following delivery.

High-Risk Obstetrician: Specializes in the preterm management of women whose pregnancies are at risk due to various medical conditions, and delivers the fetus. This physician is also responsible for the care of the infant immediately following delivery.

Fertility Specialist: Typically, this physician is an obstetrician/gynecologist who specializes in treating disorders of the female reproductive system associated with fertility and pregnancy.

Radiologist/Sonologist: Specializes in the administration and diagnostic interpretation of ultrasound and other imaging modalities.

■ ■ ■ COMMON DIAGNOSTIC TESTS

Pregnancy Test: Detects human chorionic gonadotropin (hCG) levels in urine or blood when pregnancy exists. A lab technician usually runs the test, which is interpreted by a pathologist or obstetrician/gynecologist.

Beta-hCG Test: Blood is tested to quantitate the serum level of hCG to estimate gestational age. A lab technician usually runs the test, which is interpreted by a pathologist or obstetrician/gynecologist.

Maternal/Paternal Blood Typing: Determines blood type and whether Rh factor is positive or negative.

Antibody Screen: Blood test for Rh factor, which is a group of autoantibodies that react with a person's own immunoglobulin.

Glucose Screen: Blood test for diabetes between 24 and 28 weeks' gestation.

Doppler Ultrasound: Various Doppler ultrasound applications to evaluate maternal and fetal blood flow, including the blood vessels of the placenta.

Amniocentesis: Transabdominal or transcervical penetration of the uterus and amniotic sac for aspiration of a sample of amniotic fluid used for obtaining pertinent genetic information regarding the fetus.

Computed Tomography (CT): Evaluation of fetal and maternal anatomy when sonographic evaluation is indeterminate. CT is generally used as a "last resort" because of the radiation exposure, and in most cases is limited to assessment of the acute maternal abdomen.

Magnetic Resonance Imaging (MRI): Traditionally used to evaluate maternal anatomy during pregnancy and abnormalities such as adnexal masses, which require further characterization beyond the ultrasound findings. Typically, MRI evaluation of the fetus is hindered by fetal motion.

■ ■ ■ LABORATORY VALUES

Alpha-Fetoprotein (AFP): Found in maternal blood and amniotic fluid. Elevated levels indicate fetal abnormalities or defects.

Triple Marker Screening (AFP, uE3, hCG): Abnormal levels of alpha-fetoprotein (AFP), unconjugated estriol (uE3), and human chorionic gonadotropin (hCG) are indicators of certain embryonic/fetal abnormalities, possible multifetal gestations, and combined with maternal age, screening markers for Down syndrome.

■ ■ ■ ROUTINE MEASUREMENTS

Biparietal Diameter (BPD): Easily obtained, reproducible measurement of the fetal head used to calculate an estimated age. An accurate BPD can be obtained through any plane of section that intersects the thalami and third ventricle. Generally, measurement cursors are placed from the outer edge of the near calvarial wall to the inner edge of the far calvarial wall. Experts believe the BPD to be most accurate prior to 20 menstrual weeks.

Standard reference tables are used to correlate the BPD with predicted age.

Head Circumference (HC): Elliptical measurement along the calvarial margins that is used to calculate an estimated age. The HC is best obtained through a single plane of section that must be perpendicular to the thalami, third ventricle, cavum septum pellucidum, and tentorium. Measurement cursors should be placed at the outer edge of the near calvarial wall to the outer edge of the far calvarial wall.

Standard reference tables are used to correlate the HC with predicted age.

Abdominal Circumference (AC): Elliptical measurement along the abdominal skin margin used to calculate an estimated age. The AC is best obtained at the short axis level of the abdomen where the right and left portal veins are continuous with one another. Elliptical measurement cursors should be placed at the skin edge.

Standard reference tables are used to correlate the AC with predicted age. Additional charts use the AC and HC to estimate fetal weight.

Femur Length (FL): Long axis measurement of the ossified portions of the fetal femur used to calculate an estimated age. An accurate FL is when the cartilaginous femoral condyle and femoral head are visualized simultaneously. They are not included in the femoral measurement; cursors are placed at the ossified ends of the metaphysis and diaphysis.

Standard reference tables are used to correlate the HC with predicted age.

Cephalic Index (CI): Calculated measurement to assess fetal head shape. The BPD along with the FOD (fronto-occipital

diameter measured from the outer edge to the outer edge of the calvaria) is utilized to calculate the CI as follows:

$$BPD/FOD \times 100 = Cephalic\ Index$$

A normal CI is between 0.72 and 0.86.

Amniotic Fluid Index (AFI): Calculated measurement to determine the amniotic fluid volume (AFV). Anteroposterior fluid measurements from four equal, gravid uterine quadrants are added together to total the AFI. An 8-cm AFI is considered normal.

■ ■ ■ AFFECTING CHEMICALS

Menotropins (Pergonal), Urifollitropin (Metrodin), Clomiphene Citrate (Clomid): Medications prescribed for infertility to stimulate follicular maturation and induce ovulation. In some cases, these medications have been associated with multifetal gestations.

■ ■ ■ VASCULATURE

Fetal Circulation

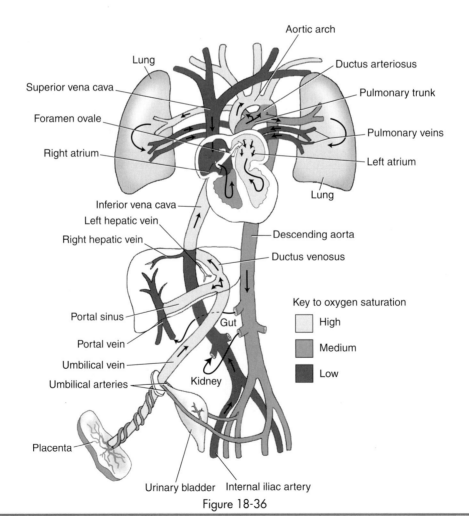

Figure 18-36

REFERENCES

Blecker OP, Kloostennan GJ, Breur W, et al: The volumetric growth of the human placenta: a longitudinal ultrasonic study, *Am J Obstet Gynecol* 149:512-517, 1977.

Budorick NE: The fetal musculoskeletal system. In Callen PW, editor: *Ultrasonography in obstetrics and gynecology*, ed 4, Philadelphia, 2000, WB Saunders, p 331.

Chervenak FA, Jeanty P, Cantraine F, et al: The diagnosis of fetal microcephaly, *Am J Obstet Gynecol* 149:512-517, 1984.

Clautice-Engle T, Pretorius DH, Budorick NE: Significance of nonvisualization of the fetal urinary bladder, *J Ultrasound Med* 10:615-618, 1991.

Cooper C, Mahoney BS, Bowie JD, et al: Prenatal ultrasound diagnosis of ambiguous genitalia, *J Ultrasound Med* 4:4433-4436, 1989.

Filly RA, Feldstein VA: Fetal genitourinary tract. In Callen PW, editor: *Ultrasonography in obstetrics and gynecology*, ed 4, Philadelphia, 2000, WB Saunders, p 517.

Filly RA, Feldstein VA: Ultrasound evaluation of normal fetal anatomy. In Callen PW, editor: *Ultrasonography in obstetrics and gynecology*, ed 4, Philadelphia, 2000, WB Saunders, pp 254, 262-263, 273.

Filly RA, Hadlock FP: Sonographic determination of menstrual age. In Callen PW, editor: *Ultrasonography in obstetrics and gynecology*, ed 4, Philadelphia, 2000, WB Saunders, pp 153, 154, 158.

Grannum PT, Bracke M, Silverman R, et al: Assessment of fetal kidney size in normal gestation by comparison of ratio of kidney circumference to abdominal circumference, *Am J Obstet Gynecol* 136:249-254, 1980.

Hadlock FP, Vincoff NS: Sonographic evaluation of fetal lung maturity. In Callen PW, editor: *Ultrasonography in obstetrics and gynecology*, ed 4, Philadelphia, 2000, WB Saunders, p 632.

Hadlock FP, Harrist RB, Carpenter RJ, et al: Sonographic estimation of fetal weight, *Radiology* 150:535-540, 1984.

Harris RD, Alexander RD: Ultrasound of the placenta and umbilical cord. In Callen PW, editor: *Ultrasonography in obstetrics and gynecology*, ed 4, Philadelphia, 2000, WB Saunders, p 598.

Hill LM: Ultrasound of the fetal gastrointestinal tract. In Callen PW, editor: *Ultrasonography in obstetrics and gynecology*, ed 4, Philadelphia, 2000, WB Saunders, p 457, 480.

Hoddick WK, Mahoney BS, Callen PW, et al: Placental thickness, *J Ultrasound Med* 4:479-482, 1985.

Hopper KD, Komppa GH, Williams BP, et al: A reevaluation of placental grading and its clinical significance, *J Ultrasound Med* 3:161-266, 1984.

Mahoney B: The genitourinary system. In Callen PW, editor: *Ultrasonography in obstetrics and gynecology*, ed 2, Philadelphia, 1988, WB Saunders, p 256.

Merz E, Mi-Sook KK, PeW S: Ultrasonic mensuration of fetal limb bones in the second and third trimesters, *J Clin Ultrasound* 15: 175-183, 1987.

Moore KL: *The developing human: clinically oriented embryology*, ed 6, Philadelphia, 1998, WB Saunders.

Nyberg DA, Mack LA, Pattern RM, et al: Fetal bowel: normal sonographic findings, *J Ultrasound Med* 6:3-8, 1987.

Petrucha RA, Platt LD: Relationship of placental grade to gestational age, *Am J Obstet Gynecol* 144:733, 1982.

Pilu G, Falco P, et al: Ultrasound evaluation of the fetal neural axis. In Callen PW, editor: *Ultrasonography in obstetrics and gynecology*, ed 4, Philadelphia, 2000, WB Saunders, 277.

Robinson HP, Hood VD, Adam AH, et al: Diagnostic ultrasound: early detection of fetal neural tube defects, *Obstet Gynecol* 56:705-710, 1980.

Warda AH, Deter RL, Rossavik IK, et al: Fetal femur length: a critical re-evaluation of the relationship to menstrual age, *Obstet Gynecol* 66:69, 1985.

Zafaranloo S, Gerard PS, Wise G: Sonographic assessment of fetal male genitalia, *J Diag Med Sonog* 7:205-207, 1991.

CHAPTER 19

High-Risk Obstetric Sonography

BETTY BATES TEMPKIN AND PEGGY MALZI BIZJAK

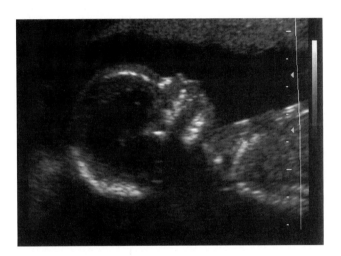

OBJECTIVES

Describe the indications for a biophysical profile.
Describe how biophysical profiles are scored.
Describe the benefits of fetal Doppler velocimetry studies. Give examples.
Define amniocentesis and its purpose.
Describe chorionic villus sampling (CVS) and its purpose.
Describe the indications for fetal blood sampling.
Describe the difference between dizygotic and monozygotic twin gestations.
Define the key words.

KEY WORDS

Alpha-fetoprotein (AFP)	Fraternal twins
Amniocentesis	L-S ratio
Biophysical profile	Monochorionic-diamniotic
Chorionic villus sampling (CVS)	twins
	Monochorionic-monoamniotic twins
Dichorionic-diamniotic twins	Monozygotic twins
Dizygotic twins	Umbilical cord Doppler

High-risk pregnancies are those in which there was a previous child with an abnormality such as a neural tube defect, there is a preexisting or existing maternal condition that may jeopardize the pregnancy, or there is a suspected or detected abnormality. In most high-risk cases, additional ultrasound evaluation or ultrasound-guided procedures are required. This chapter addresses the ultrasound studies utilized for those higher-risk pregnancies.

Indications for prenatal ultrasound evaluations in high-risk pregnancies include conditions such as postdates, multiple pregnancy, advanced maternal age, intrauterine growth retardation, and maternal diabetes mellitus. Having an abnormal biochemical screening or previous child with a chromosomal disorder, neural tube defect as mentioned, developmental defect, or malformation syndrome are also considered high-risk indicators for ultrasound assessment.

FETAL SONOGRAPHIC BIOPHYSICAL PROFILE

There are times when it is necessary to determine whether or not a fetus is in distress. In order to assess the status of the fetus, a **biophysical profile** may be performed. It is a test that measures fetal well-being. Biophysical profiles are usually reserved for ultrasound cases with abnormal or ambiguous findings. Several fetal biophysical variables are observed to predict perinatal outcome; they are fetal heart rate, fetal body movements, fetal tone, fetal breathing movements, amniotic fluid volume, and placental grading. Evaluations begin with a nonstress, electronic fetal heart rate monitoring followed by real-time ultrasound assessment of the other biophysical components. The examination ends when each of the biophysical components meets normal criteria or 30 minutes of real-time ultrasonography have elapsed. A scoring system is utilized in which each biophysical activity or component is scored as 0 (when abnormal) or 2 (when normal). Scores of 8 or higher are associated with good perinatal outcome. Scores lower than 8 are generally followed up with additional testing or induced delivery.

The criteria for scoring biophysical profiles may vary among institutions but generally, the normal fetal biophysical profiles are based on the following observations within 30 minutes: the presence of two or more fetal heart rate accelerations of at least 15 beats per minute in amplitude and at least 15 seconds' duration associated with fetal movement in a 20-minute period, and fetal body movement consisting of three or more gross body movements that may include arching of the back or neck or twisting of the trunk. Simultaneous limb and trunk movements are counted as a single movement. Fetal tone consists of at least one incident of limb motion from a position of flexion to extension and rapid return to flexion. Fetal breathing movements are noted as at least one, 60-second episode. Amniotic fluid volume consists of the presence of fluid throughout the uterus and a pocket measuring at least 2 cm or more in vertical diameter. Placental grading (discussed in Chapter 18) is noted as 0, 1, or 2.

An alternative method for assessing the amount of amniotic fluid or determining the amniotic fluid index (AFI) is the four-quadrant analysis. This measurement is based on the division of the gravid uterus into four equal quadrants using the umbilicus and linea nigra. The anteroposterior diameter of the deepest amniotic fluid pocket in each quadrant is measured. These four measurements are added together to total the AFI. The sum should equal 8 cm to be considered normal. In most cases, sonographers only include the pockets that are free of extremities and the umbilical cord.

Biophysical profiling is recognized as a reliable method of assessing fetal well-being to predict perinatal outcome in high-risk pregnancies.

DOPPLER ULTRASOUND EVALUATION

Doppler studies of placental and fetal circulation can provide significant data concerning fetal well-being, making it possible to improve fetal outcome.

Umbilical cord Doppler is an examination technique that measures the resistance of blood flow within the placenta. The Doppler signal from the two umbilical arteries is obtained with continuous-wave, or in some cases, pulse-wave, Doppler. The spectrum of the signal is analyzed to determine the diastolic flow. The extent of diastolic flow is directly related to the flow resistance of the placenta. There is good correlation between the absence of effective diastolic flow and a poor outcome. In some institutions a poor high-resistance flow pattern will increase the likelihood of an induced delivery. The thought is that the damage to the fetus may be minimized by its removal from an inadequate environment.

Doppler measurements may also be used to assess maternal circulation to the uterus. During pregnancy the uterine arteries have very low pulsatility and may appear almost as venous signals when the Doppler waveform is examined. However, a modest cardiac pattern should be obtained. Examples of umbilical artery and maternal uterine artery Doppler waveforms are presented in Figures 19-1 and 19-2.

Fetal responses and adaptation to changes in the intrauterine environment can be evaluated by observing fetal blood circulation. This discussion will focus on applicable blood circulation excluding the fetal heart, since it was discussed in Chapter 18.

Absence of the end-diastolic fetal aortic velocity can easily be determined and is a good predictor of fetal well-being. In fetuses with absent end-diastolic velocity of the thoracic or abdominal aorta, perinatal outcome is poor. Furthermore, abnormal fetal aortic flow velocity

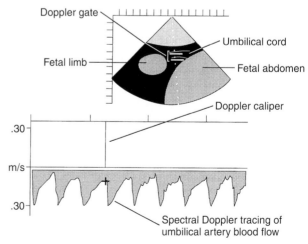

Doppler gate
Fetal limb
Umbilical cord
Fetal abdomen
Doppler caliper
.30
m/s
.30
Spectral Doppler tracing of umbilical artery blood flow

Figure 19-1 Ultrasound pulsed Doppler interrogation of the umbilical artery. This is a normal low-resistance waveform.

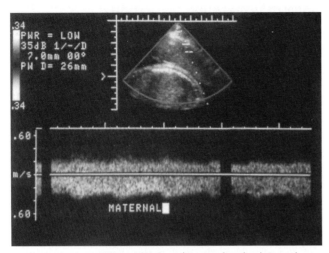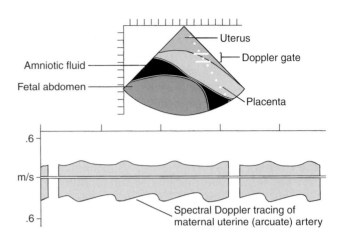

Figure 19-2 Ultrasound pulsed Doppler interrogation of uterine circulation during the third trimester. The waveform on top of the line is a venous signal. The waveform under the line is that of a uterine artery. Note their similarity. The artery has a very low pulsatility.

waveforms have been associated with neurologic dysfunctions such as lower verbal and global IQ.

Doppler velocity of the renal arteries is clinically applicable for assessing the fetal behavioral state. High renal vascular impedance is an indicator of a fetus that is too small for its gestational age. This becomes more obvious with the presence of oligohydramnios. Additionally, there seems to be a significant correlation between the AFI and the renal artery systolic/diastolic ratio.

Normally the fetal splenic artery has a lower pulsatility than the renal artery. Abnormal splenic artery velocity may be utilized in predicting fetal hypoxia. In addition, some fetuses that are small for their gestational age demonstrate a decrease in resistance in the splenic artery.

In severe cases of intrauterine growth retardation, the fetal hepatic artery can usually be detected. The flow velocity waveform displays a low-impedance, high-velocity blood flow, suggesting redistribution of the hepatic artery as well as the cerebral, adrenal, and coronary arteries.

Doppler investigation of the umbilical vein is another gauge of fetal well-being. Extraabdominal umbilical venous flow displays regular pulsations up to 15 weeks of gestation; beyond that, the venous pulsations gradually disappear. Occurrence of venous pulsations later in pregnancy is an ominous sign that indicates congestive heart failure in compromised fetuses.

Doppler velocimetry of the ductus venosus plays a valuable role in prenatal fetal assessment. It is easy to distinguish from surrounding vessels and has an acceptable reproducibility with little variation. Abnormal ductus venosus velocity may be useful in determining fetal cardiac disease, severe growth retardation, fetal anemia, and various chromosomal abnormalities.

Abnormal flow velocity waveform of the inferior vena cava (IVC) is another key sign of fetal compromise. In fetal hypoxia the pulsatility of blood flow in the IVC increases.

With high-risk pregnancies, the improvement in outcome of the compromised fetus depends on early identification. Doppler velocimetry studies can provide early data that are critical in the detection and management of fetal abnormalities.

ULTRASOUND-GUIDED PROCEDURES
Amniocentesis

Certain invasive obstetric procedures are routinely assisted by ultrasound for a safer and more accurate study. One of these is transabdominal **amniocentesis,** the penetration of the uterus and amniotic sac for aspiration of a sample of amniotic fluid. The fluid contains desquamated fetal cells that can be grown in tissue culture and used for a variety of metabolic assays or DNA extraction. Ideally, amniocentesis is performed at approximately 16 weeks' gestation. Any earlier increases the risk of possible complications.

Amniotic fluid markers of fetal lung maturity often influence perinatal management. The amniotic fluid is tested to detect two chemicals: lecithin and sphingomyelin. The ratio of lecithin to sphingomyelin, the **L-S ratio,** measures the degree of fetal lung development. Depending on the L-S ratio, elective delivery may be delayed to allow time for the lungs to develop, and in mandated preterm deliveries, prenatal medications are administered to prevent or decrease the severity of respiratory distress.

When the amniotic fluid is analyzed to determine its biochemical components, one component, **alpha-fetoprotein (AFP)** is a protein whose concentration increases beyond normal limits when certain defects are present. Of particular interest is the karyotype (a chromosomal map) to detect Down's syndrome. Many other genetic abnormalities can be detected by this procedure, and the list is growing as research continues. Also, through research in molecular biology, molecular probes have been devised that can detect a great number of genetic disorders, which will give test results in a shorter period of time than other conventional cell culture and chromosomal banding techniques.

Ultrasound plays several roles during the amniocentesis procedure. First, ultrasound is used to assess gestational age, viability, anatomy, number of gestations, and placenta location. Second, the position of the desired pocket of amniotic fluid is determined. The abdomen is then prepped with sterile washes, and the physician anesthetizes the skin and subcutaneous tissues. A sterile cover is positioned over the transducer, and sterile gel is used as the scanning couplant. Next, the position of the amniotic fluid pocket is reconfirmed. In some institutions a sterile needle will be affixed to the ultrasound transducer. In others, the transducer is positioned to visualize the amniocentesis needle as it is inserted "freehand" into the amniotic sac. During the procedure, ultrasound provides confirmation that the fetus is not in the needle's path and that the needle is in the correct position for fluid aspiration. Following the procedure, ultrasound assesses fetal viability.

As a rule, amniocentesis performed with ultrasound guidance is a safe procedure, but it has the potential to cause serious complications such as premature rupture of membranes, premature labor, and premature separation of the placenta. Additional complications may include injury to the fetus from the needle, fetal or maternal bleeding, placental hemorrhage (if a transplacental approach is used), and even fetal death. Considering the possible complications, each case is evaluated individually, weighing the benefits of the information provided from an amniocentesis against the risks.

Chorionic Villus Sampling

Chorionic villus sampling (CVS) was developed as an early first trimester means of collecting tissue for genetic analysis, using placental tissue buds or chorionic villi. Because this test can be performed as early as 10 to 12 menstrual weeks, it offers a greater advantage to a woman who is at high risk for giving birth to an abnormal infant. If an affected fetus is diagnosed, and the decision is made to terminate the pregnancy, the medical and psychological risks are fewer with a first trimester termination compared with a second trimester termination.

As in amniocentesis, ultrasound is used prior to the procedure to determine viability, number, trophoblast location, and sampling path. There are two commonly used approaches to CVS, transcervical and transabdom-

inal. The placental implantation site and the position of the uterus dictate the choice of method. Either the abdomen or cervix is prepped with sterile washes, and the physician anesthetizes the site. A sterile cover is positioned over the transducer, and sterile gel is used as the scanning couplant. In both cases, ultrasound guidance informs the clinician when an area rich in chorionic villi has been reached and the collecting device is in place for sampling.

CVS does carry certain risks. Following the procedure, spontaneous bleeding or even spontaneous abortion can occur. Generally, procedure-related fetal loss rate due to CVS is extremely low; however, spontaneous abortion has been estimated to occur in approximately 1% of cases.

Fetal Blood Sampling and Fetal Intravascular Transfusion

Ultrasound is essential for safe and reliable access to fetal circulation. The most common indications for the sampling of fetal blood are the confirmation of abnormal findings found on amniocentesis or CVS and the need for rapid chromosomal diagnosis. Analysis of fetal blood requires 48 to 72 hours as compared with 2 to 3 weeks with amniocentesis. Additional indications that require the sampling of fetal blood include diagnosis of a structural anomaly on ultrasound, assessment of fetal anemia, hemophilia and other clotting disorders, and immunodeficiencies and other white cell disorders.

Therapy by intrauterine transfusion of red cells into the umbilical vein is recommended in fetuses with severe hydrops and anemia. Red cells or platelets are routinely transfused for fetal isoimmunization. A transfusion of thrombocytes may be considered in fetuses with severe thrombocytopenia.

The method of choice for fetal blood sampling and fetal intravascular transfusion is as follows. Prior to the procedure, the area of the umbilical cord insertion into the placenta is established with ultrasound. This area is considered optimal because the cord is fixed at this location. In some cases, a free loop of cord may be used; however, the approach is more difficult due to cord movement. The mother is sedated for her own comfort and to reduce movement of the fetus. The abdomen is prepped with sterile washes, and a sterile cover is positioned over the transducer. Sterile gel is used as the scanning couplant. While the physician anesthetizes the skin and subcutaneous tissues, ultrasound is used to check the angle of the needle insertion. Next, under ultrasound guidance, a spinal or transfusion needle is advanced into the umbilical circulation.

The complication rate following fetal blood sampling and fetal intravascular transfusion procedures depends on the indication for the procedure. Fetuses with intrauterine growth retardation and/or structural anomalies are at the highest risk for fetal distress.

Clearly, ultrasound is essential for establishing accuracy during invasive obstetric procedures, making it a valuable asset for prenatal diagnosis and therapy.

MULTIFETAL GESTATIONS

The increase in multiple births since 1980 has been attributed to increased fertility treatments and older maternal populations. Multifetal gestations are considered high-risk pregnancies, both for the fetus and the mother. Complications in multifetal gestations parallel those of single gestations but occur with higher frequency, including preterm birth, intrauterine growth retardation, and fetal anomalies. Complications unique to multifetal gestations include conjoined twins, acardiac twins, twin embolization with co-twin demise, and twin-to-twin transfusion syndrome. Maternal complications associated with multifetal gestations compared with single gestations include a higher incidence of preeclampsia, hypertension, placenta abruption, placenta previa, and prepartum and postpartum hemorrhage. The complications and anomalies described for twins are generally applicable to each additional gestation; the risk and severity are usually accentuated.

Sonography is of great value in determining the type of twinning and in accurately identifying fetal complications and anomalies associated with multiple gestations, thus significantly contributing to perinatal management.

Embyology of Multifetal Gestations

Twin gestations result from fertilization of either two separate ova (**dizygotic,** or **fraternal**) or a single ovum (monozygotic, or identical). Each dizygotic twin develops embryologically similarly to a single gestation. All dizygotic twins form their own blastocyst, resulting in separate amnions (diamniotic) and separate placentas (dichorionic).

Monozygotic, or identical, **twins** occur after fertilization of a single ovum. The number of chorions (placentas) and amnions is variable and depends on when the zygote (fertilized ovum) divides relative to differentiation of the chorion and amnion. There are three types of monozygotic twins: dichorionic-diamniotic, monochorionic-diamniotic, and monochorionic-monoamniotic (Figure 19-3).

Division of the zygote prior to day 4 (before blastocyst formation) results in a **dichorionic-diamniotic** gestation. Each embryo will have an individual placenta and amniotic sac. Division between 4 and 8 days (after blastocyst formation but before amnion differentiation) results in a **monochorionic-diamniotic** gestation. This is the most common type of monozygotic twin gestation. The embryos will share a common placenta but have their own amniotic sac. Division beyond 8 days postfertilization (after amnion formation) results in a **monochorionic-monoamniotic** gestation. The embryos will share a common placenta and share a single amniotic sac. In rare cases, division can occur to the embryonic disk more than 13 days postfertilization, resulting in conjoined, or "Siamese," twins. The later the division, the greater the number of shared organs. All conjoined twins are monozygotic, monochorionic-monoamniotic gestations.

Understanding the embryologic sequence for chorion and amnion formation is essential to the sonographic assessment of multifetal gestations. With twin gestations, all dichorionic twins are diamniotic, and all monoamniotic twins are monochorionic. Monochorionic gestations can be either diamniotic or monoamniotic because the amnion forms after the chorion.

Sonographic Assessment of Multifetal Gestations

There are special considerations in the ultrasound examination of multifetal gestations.

All twins should be carefully evaluated with ultrasound to verify the number of chorions and amnions. It should be determined whether the developing embryos, or fetuses, reside in a single amniotic sac or are separated by a membrane(s), or reside in multiple amniotic sacs; whether the chorion/placenta is single and shared or individual and multiple. This determination can be challenging, particularly beyond the first trimester when it may not be possible. For example, a monozygotic dichorionic-diamniotic gestation is identical in appearance to that of a dizygotic gestation. Both involve two complete embryos, two complete sacs, and two separate placentas. Quite often, later in pregnancy, the borders of the placentas will move close to each other and may finally fuse, making differentiation between a monochorionic or dichorionic pregnancy difficult if not impossible.

From the 6th through 10th gestational weeks, sonographic identification of the number of gestational sacs is an accurate method for predicting chorionicity. An early gestational sac appears as a 2- to 5-mm round, fluid-filled structure surrounded by a rim of high-amplitude echoes, which corresponds to the chorion. Early in development, the amniotic membrane is closely applied to the forming embryo, and the fluid-filled gestational sac, as identified on ultrasound, is predominantly chorionic fluid and representative of the chorionic cavity. Therefore counting the number of gestational sacs (chorionic cavities) accurately predicts chorionicity (number of placentas). Two sacs imply dichorionicity, three sacs trichorionicity, and so on. At approximately 10 weeks of gestation, the amniotic cavity enlarges until it obliterates the chorionic cavity, and in twin gestations, the amnions become opposed and form an intertwin or interfetal membrane.

During the second and third trimesters, the sonographic criteria for determining chorionicity shift to fetal gender, appearance of the interfetal membrane, and number of placentas. If twin fetuses are of opposite gender (dizygotic/fraternal), they are always dichorionic and diamniotic. If, however, the twins are the same gen-

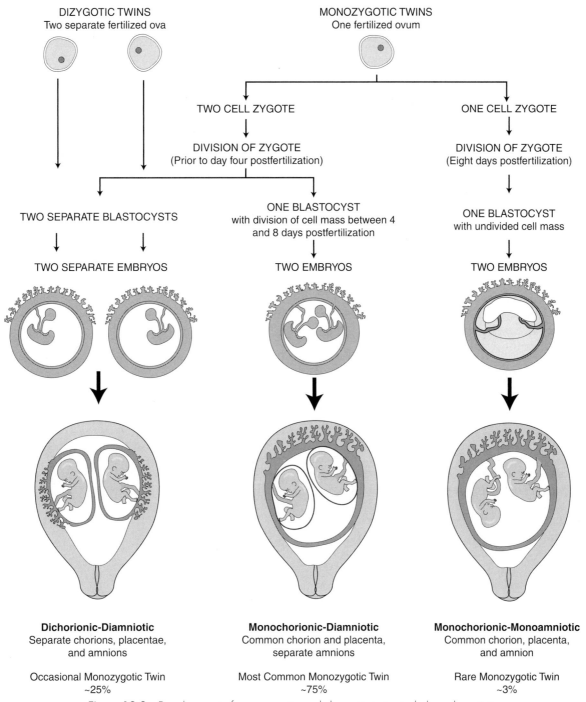

DIZYGOTIC TWINS
Two separate fertilized ova

MONOZYGOTIC TWINS
One fertilized ovum

TWO CELL ZYGOTE

ONE CELL ZYGOTE

DIVISION OF ZYGOTE
(Prior to day four postfertilization)

DIVISION OF ZYGOTE
(Eight days postfertilization)

TWO SEPARATE BLASTOCYSTS

ONE BLASTOCYST
with division of cell mass between 4
and 8 days postfertilization

ONE BLASTOCYST
with undivided cell mass

TWO SEPARATE EMBRYOS

TWO EMBRYOS

TWO EMBRYOS

Dichorionic-Diamniotic
Separate chorions, placentae,
and amnions

Occasional Monozygotic Twin
~25%

Monochorionic-Diamniotic
Common chorion and placenta,
separate amnions

Most Common Monozygotic Twin
~75%

Monochorionic-Monoamniotic
Common chorion, placenta,
and amnion

Rare Monozygotic Twin
~3%

Figure 19-3 Development of monozygotic and dizygotic twins including placentation

der (identical or fraternal) or the gender is not identified, chorionicity cannot be established and only genetic analysis can determine the type prior to delivery.

In a diamniotic twin gestation, whether placentas are shared or not, a membrane should be seen sonographically, separating the fetuses. The thickness of this interfetal membrane can predict chorionicity, whether the pregnancy is monochorionic or dichorionic. The membrane in a diamniotic-monochorionic twin gestation is two layers thick, consisting of two amnions only, one from each fetus. The membrane in a diamniotic-dichorionic twin gestation is the thickest: four layers thick, with two amnions plus two chorions.

Sonographic identification of separate placentas in multifetal gestations depends on the proximity of implantation of the blastocysts. The further apart the implantation, the less likely the placentas are to become fused along their borders, making differentiation easier and the number count accurate. Identification of a single placenta with sonography does not differentiate between a monochorionic gestation and a dichorionic gestation with two continuous fused placentas. However, sonographic identification of two separate placentas in a twin pregnancy does determine dichorionicity.

Utilizing transvaginal sonography, the amnion is visible by the 7th or 8th week of gestation, when the crown-rump length is 8 to 12 mm. Diamnionicity is recognizable as two separate gestational sacs. Monoamnionicity is confirmed when a single amniotic sac containing two embryos is identified.

Amnionicity can also be established by identifying the number of yolk sacs. Sonographically, the yolk sac is identified approximately 2 weeks earlier than the amnion. Therefore, in a monochorionic twin gestation, identification of two yolk sacs is an accurate method for confirming diamnionicity in the first trimester before visualization of the amniotic membrane. Monochorionic-monoamniotic gestations are associated with a single yolk sac or, in rare cases, a partially divided yolk sac, depending on when the zygote divides.

THE EXPANDING ROLE OF ULTRASOUND IN HIGH-RISK OBSTETRICS

This chapter presented the role of ultrasound in high-risk pregnancies. In most cases, high-risk pregnancies utilize the ultrasound examinations and ultrasound-guided procedures discussed in this chapter. As new clinical management procedures evolve for handling high-risk pregnancies, ultrasound will continue to play a critical role in the development of new approaches to fetal prenatal diagnosis and therapy.

Recently, fetal surgical procedures have been carried out with a high degree of success. These procedures require the use of ultrasound for, first, detecting the anomaly, and second, locating an incision point within the uterus for extracting the fetus for surgery. The post-surgical period also requires ultrasound examination of the surgical site.

The appeal of ultrasound in managing high-risk pregnancies is that it is a safe procedure that offers an abundance of information that directly impacts maternal and fetal management and ultimately reduces adverse perinatal outcome.

REFERENCE CHARTS

■ ■ ■ ASSOCIATED PHYSICIANS

High-Risk Obstetrician: Specializes in the preterm management of women whose pregnancies are at risk due to various medical conditions, and delivers the fetus. This physician is also responsible for the care of the infant immediately following delivery.

Obstetrician/Gynecologist: Manages preterm obstetric care and delivers the fetus. This physician is also responsible for the care of the infant immediately following delivery.

Fertility Specialist: Typically, this physician is an obstetrician/gynecologist who specializes in treating disorders of the female reproductive system associated with fertility and pregnancy.

Radiologist/Sonologist: Specializes in the administration and diagnostic interpretation of ultrasound and other imaging modalities.

■ ■ ■ COMMON DIAGNOSTIC TESTS

Fetal Biophysical Profile: Ultrasound evaluation to assess fetal well-being by evaluating multiple fetal biophysical activities.

Doppler Ultrasound: Various Doppler ultrasound applications to evaluate maternal and fetal blood flow, including the blood vessels of the placenta.

Amniocentesis: Transabdominal or transcervical penetration of the uterus and amniotic sac for aspiration of a sample of amniotic fluid used for obtaining pertinent genetic information regarding the fetus.

Chorionic Villus Sampling (CVS): Transabdominal or transcervical penetration of the uterus and amniotic sac for a sample of the chorion covered by villi, which is used for obtaining pertinent genetic information regarding the embryo/fetus.

Fetal Blood Sampling: Generally follows confirmation of abnormal findings on amniocentesis or CVS or the need for rapid chromosomal diagnosis. Analysis only requires 48 to 72 hours, much shorter than the time required for amniocentesis or CVS.

Fetal Blood Transfusion: Fetal therapy involving fetal intravascular transfusion of red cells or platelets for isoimmunization.

Computed Tomography (CT): Evaluation of fetal and maternal anatomy when sonographic evaluation is indeterminate. CT is generally used as a "last resort" because of the radiation exposure and in most cases is limited to assessment of the acute maternal abdomen.

Magnetic Resonance Imaging (MRI): Traditionally used to evaluate maternal anatomy during pregnancy and abnormalities such as adnexal masses, which require further characterization beyond the ultrasound findings. Typically, MRI evaluation of the fetus is hindered by fetal motion.

■ ■ ■ LABORATORY VALUES

Alpha-Fetoprotein (AFP): Found in maternal blood and amniotic fluid. Elevated levels indicate fetal abnormalities or defects.

Triple Marker Screening (AFP, uE3, hCG): Abnormal levels of alpha-fetoprotein (AFP), unconjugated estriol (uE3), and human chorionic gonadotropin (hCG) are indicators of certain fetal abnormalities, possible multifetal gestations, and combined with maternal age, screening markers for Down syndrome.

■ ■ ■ NORMAL MEASUREMENTS

Refer to Chapter 18.

■ ■ ■ VASCULATURE

Refer to Chapter 18.

■ ■ ■ AFFECTING CHEMICALS

Menotropins (Pergonal), Urofollitropin (Metrodin), Clomiphene Citrate (Clomid): Medications prescribed for infertility to stimulate follicular maturation and induce ovulation. In some cases, these medications have been associated with multifetal gestations.

BIBLIOGRAPHY

Arduini D, Rizzo G: Fetal renal artery velocity waveforms and amniotic fluid volume in growth-retarded and post-term fetuses, *Obstet Gynecol* 77:370, 1991.

Barth RA, Crowe HC: Ultrasound evaluation of multifetal gestations. In Callen PW, editor: *Ultrasonography in obstetrics and gynecology,* ed 4, Philadelphia, 2000, WB Saunders, pp 171-181.

Callen PW: Amniotic fluid: its role in fetal health and disease. In Callen PW, editor: *Ultrasonography in obstetrics and gynecology,* ed 4, Philadelphia, 2000, WB Saunders, pp 642-644.

Coleman BG, Grumbach K, Arger PH, et al: Twin gestations, *Radiology* 165(2):449, 1987.

Copperberg PL, Carpenter CW: Ultrasound as an aid to intrauterine transfusion, *Am J Obstet Gynecol* 128:239-241, 1977.

Crane IP, Beaver HA, Cheung SW: First trimester chorionic villus sampling versus mid-trimester genetic amniocentesis: preliminary results of a controlled prospective trial, *Prenatal Diag* 8:355-356, 1988.

Gall SA, editor: *Multiple pregnancy and delivery,* St Louis, MO, 1996, Mosby.

Goldberg JD, Norton ME: Genetics and prenatal diagnosis. In Callen PW, editor: *Ultrasonography in obstetrics and gynecology,* ed 4, Philadelphia, 2000, WB Saunders, pp 31-34.

Grannum PT, Copel IA, Plaxe SC, et al: In utero exchange transfusion by direct intravascular injection in severe erythroblastosis fetalis, *N Engl J Med* 314:1431-1434, 1986.

Hadlock FP, Vincoff NS: Sonographic evaluation of fetal lung maturity. In Callen PW, editor: *Ultrasonography in obstetrics and gynecology,* ed 4, Philadelphia, 2000, WB Saunders, pp 627-628.

Hecher K, Snijders R, Campbell S, et al: Fetal venous, intracardial, and arterial blood flow measurements in intrauterine growth retardation, *Am J Obstet Gynecol* 173:10, 1995.

Mahony BS, Filly RA, Callen PW: Amnionicity and chorionicity in twin pregnancies, *Obstet Gynecol* 84(1):107, 1994.

Manning EA, Platt LD, Sipos L: Antenatal fetal evaluation: development of a fetal biophysical profile, *Am J Obstet Gynecol* 136:787-795, 1980.

Mari G, Abuhamad AZ, Uerpairojkit B, et al: Blood flow velocity waveforms of the abdominal arteries in appropriate- and small-for-gestational-age fetuses, *Ultrasound Obstet Gynecol* 6:15, 1995.

Maxwell DJ, Johnson P, Hurley P, et al: Fetal blood sampling and pregnancy loss in relation to indication, *Br J Obstet Gynecol* 98:982, 1991.

Spellacy WN, Handler A, Ferre CD: A case-control study of 1253 twin pregnancies from a 1982-1987 perinatal database, *Obstet Gynecol* 75(2):168, 1990.

Tekay A, Campbell S: Doppler ultrasonography in obstetrics. In Callen PW, editor: *Ultrasonography in obstetrics and gynecology,* ed 4, Philadelphia, 2000, WB Saunders, pp 692-694, 699-706.

Veille J-C, Penry M, Muller-Haubach E: Fetal renal pulsed Doppler waveform in prolonged pregnancies, *Am J Obstet Gynecol* 169:882, 1993.

Vintzileos AM, Hanley ML: Antepartum fetal assessment by ultrasonography. In Callen PW, editor: *Ultrasonography in obstetrics and gynecology,* ed 4, Philadelphia, 2000, WB Saunders, pp 660-668.

Vyas S, Nicolaides KH, Campbell S: Renal artery flow-velocity waveforms in normal and hypoxemic fetuses, *Am J Obstet Gynecol* 161:168, 1989.

Warren WB, Timor-Tritsch I, Peisner DB, et al: Dating the early pregnancy by sequential appearance of embryonic structures, *Am J Obstet Gynecol* 161(3):747, 1989.

Small Parts Sonography

CHAPTER 20

The Thyroid and Parathyroid Glands

WAYNE C. LEONHARDT

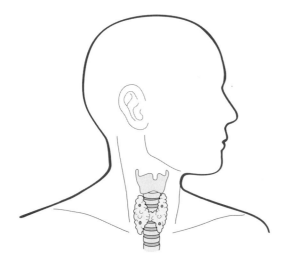

Longus colli muscle (LCM)	Sternohyoid muscle (SH)
Major neurovascular bundle (MAJNB)	Sternothyroid muscle (ST)
Minor neurovascular bundle (MINB)	Strap muscles
	Superior thyroid artery
Omohyoid muscle (OH)	Superior thyroid vein
Parathormone	Thymus
Parathyroid hormone (PTH)	Thyroid stimulating hormone (TSH)
Pituitary gland	
Pyramidal lobe	Thyrotropin
Recurrent laryngeal nerve	Thyroxine (T$_4$)
Sternocleidomastoid muscle	Triiodothyronine (T$_3$)
	Vagus nerve

OBJECTIVES

Describe the sonographic appearance of the normal thyroid, parathyroid glands, and relevant adjacent anatomic structures in the neck on sectional sonograms.
Describe the physiology of the thyroid and parathyroid glands.
Describe various shapes of normal parathyroid glands.
Describe clinical laboratory tests, related diagnostic tests, normal laboratory values, and associated physicians in the work-up of thyroid and parathyroid glands.
Describe the sonographic indications for thyroid and parathyroid gland studies.
Define the key words.

KEY WORDS

Calcitonin	Hypothalamus
Ectopic parathyroid glands	Inferior thyroid artery
Extrathyroidal veins and arteries	Inferior thyroid vein
	Infrahyoid muscle
Hyperparathyroidism	Isthmus

THYROID GLAND

The thyroid gland is an endocrine gland (one of the ductless glands, which release their secretion into the blood) consisting of two lateral lobes and a connecting portion called the **isthmus** (Figure 20-1). The thyroid gland secretes three significant hormones: thyroxine (T$_4$), triiodothyronine (T$_3$), and calcitonin, which affect body metabolism, growth, and development.

PRENATAL DEVELOPMENT

The thyroid gland arises from a median, saclike entodermal diverticulum (the thyroid sac), which begins to thicken during the third week of embryologic development. It arises at the level of the first and second pharyngeal pouches (epithelial entodermal-lined cavities that give rise to a number of vital organs within the embryo) of the ventral wall of the pharynx. The stalk between the thyroid and the tongue is called the thyroglossal duct. It opens in the embryo at the foramen cecum, located at the base of the tongue. The thyroglossal duct atrophies by the sixth week of embryonic development, and by the eighth week, thyroid follicles begin to form. They acquire colloid by the third month of development. The thyroglossal duct normally closes after

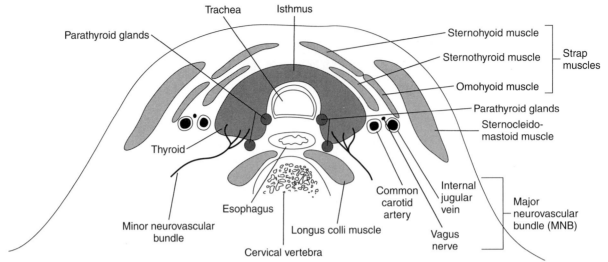

Figure 20-1 Transverse thyroid anatomy, parathyroid glands, and relevant adjacent structures. Shaded circles represent normal location of parathyroid glands.

birth. If it persists, cysts, fistulas, or an accessory pyramidal lobe may develop.

Aberrant thyroid tissue may be found anywhere along the path of the thyroid gland. The descent begins at the level of the foramen cecum to the first tracheal ring (Figure 20-2). The lingual type accounts for 90% of ectopic thyroids.

LOCATION

The thyroid is composed of right and left lobes connected across the midline by the isthmus. It is located in

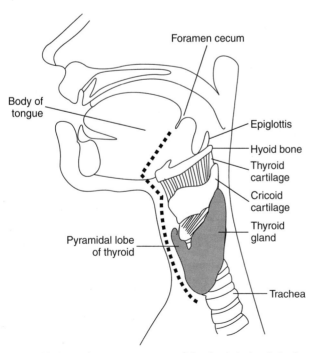

Figure 20-2 Embryonic migration of the thyroid gland. Broken line indicates path of migration.

the anteroinferior part of the neck below the larynx and anterior to the trachea. The isthmus unites the lower third of the lobes at the level of the second, third, and fourth tracheal rings (see Figure 20-1). The thyroid gland is generally shaped like a U or a low-slung H (Figure 20-3, A). In the latter, the cross bar represents the isthmus, and the vertical bars represent two conical lateral (right and left) lobes, rounded below and tapered above. In the transverse plane, the thyroid gland has a horseshoe appearance (see Figure 20-1).

In cross-section, the thyroid is outlined posterolaterally by the common carotid artery (CCA) and the internal jugular vein (IJV), medially by the trachea (T), and anterolaterally by the infrahyoid or **strap muscles** and **sternocleidomastoid muscles. Infrahyoid muscles** are double-layered muscle planes located anterior to the neck and superficial to the larynx, trachea, and thyroid gland. They include the **sternohyoid (SH), sternothyroid (ST), omohyoid (OH),** and thyrohyoid (TH). The **longus colli muscle (LCM),** esophagus (E), and **minor neurovascular bundle (MINB),** consisting of the inferior thyroid artery and recurrent laryngeal nerve, mark the posterior border of the thyroid. The **major neurovascular bundle (MAJNB)** located posterolateral to the thyroid gland consists of the CCA, IJV, and the **vagus nerve.** It is encased by the carotid sheath, which consists of areolar tissue. The vagus nerve is visualized posterolateral to the thyroid lobes between the CCA and IJV (see Figure 20-1).

SIZE

The size and shape of the thyroid gland vary in normal patients. In general, tall, thin individuals have elongated lateral lobes that can measure up to 7 to 8 cm in the longitudinal plane. Shorter, obese patients tend to exhibit oval lateral lobes measuring less than 5 cm. As a

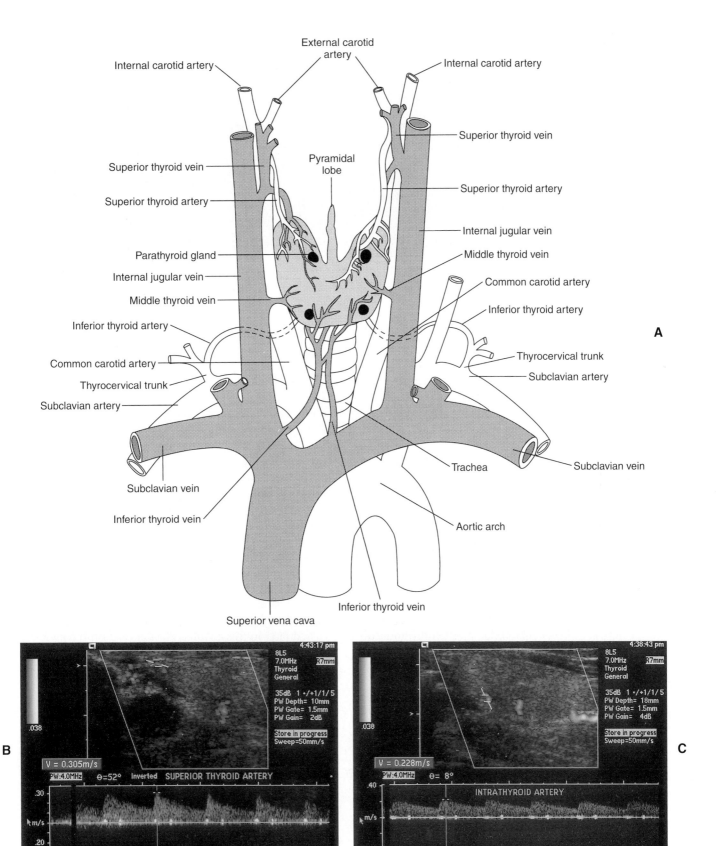

Figure 20-3 A, Frontal view of the thyroid and parathyroid regions. Dark circles, normal parathyroid locations. B, Color Doppler axial section of the thyroid gland and superior thyroid artery demonstrating arterial flow with a peak systolic velocity of 0.305 m/s. (See Color Plate 26.) C, Color Doppler imaging of an intrathyroidal artery demonstrating a peak systolic velocity of 0.228 m/s. (See Color Plate 27.)

continued

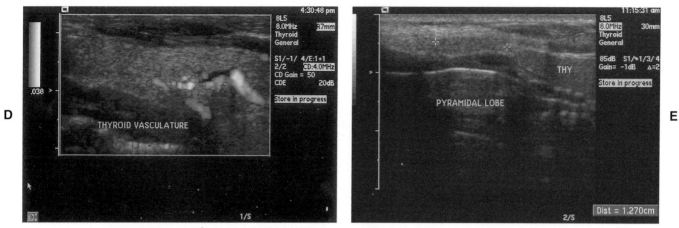

Figure 20-3, cont'd D, Color imaging axial section of the thyroid gland demonstrating intrathyroid and extrathyroid vasculature. (See Color Plate 28.) E, Sagittal view, axial section of the upper pole of the thyroid and pyramidal lobe (calipers).

result, normal thyroid gland measurements have a wide range of variability. The adult thyroid gland measures approximately 4 to 6 cm in length, 1.3 to 1.8 cm in anteroposterior (AP) diameter, and 1.5 to 2 cm in width (Figures 20-4 and 20-5). The isthmus measures approximately 2 to 6 mm in AP diameter (Figure 20-6). In newborns and children, the gland measures approximately 2 to 3 cm in length, 0.2 to 1.2 cm in AP diameter, and 1 to 1.5 cm in width. The right lobe is usually larger than the left. Average weight of the thyroid is approximately 25 g.

GROSS ANATOMY

The thyroid gland is composed of right and left lobes connected by an isthmus. It is covered by two thin layers of connective tissue. The first layer is the pretracheal fascia, or false thyroid capsule, which surrounds the gland. The second layer is the true thyroid capsule, adherent to the gland surface. Thyroid parenchyma is composed of follicles (glandular epithelium and col-loid), connective tissue, stroma, blood vessels, nerves, and lymphatics.

PHYSIOLOGY

The thyroid plays a major role in growth and development, and regulates basal metabolism by the synthesis, storage, and secretion of thyroid hormones. It produces and secretes three hormones: **triiodothyronine (T_3)**, **thyroxine (T_4)**, and **calcitonin.** The secretion of these hormones is regulated by the **hypothalamus** and the **pituitary gland.** Thyroid secretion is primarily controlled by **thyroid stimulating hormone (TSH)** secreted by the anterior pituitary gland. Thyroxine is the primary hormone (90%) secreted by the thyroid. Triiodothyronine represents a small portion (approximately 10%).

Calcitonin is secreted by the parafollicular cells (C cells) of the normal thyroid. Its primary function is to decrease blood calcium levels, preventing hypercalcemia. This hormone works the opposite of parathormone, discussed later in this chapter. Plasma calcitonin concentra-

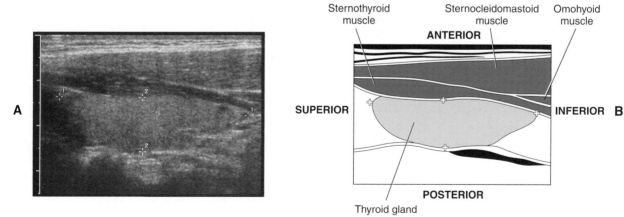

Figure 20-4 A, Longitudinal sagittal view, axial section of thyroid gland. B, Caliper placement measuring the length and anterior/posterior (AP) diameter. Note position of calipers, Dist 1 and Dist 2.

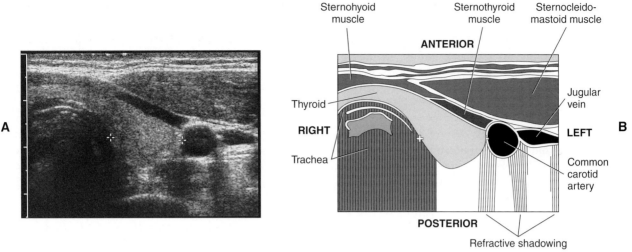

Figure 20-5 **A,** Transverse view, longitudinal section. **B,** Measurement of left lobe of thyroid gland. Note placement of calipers.

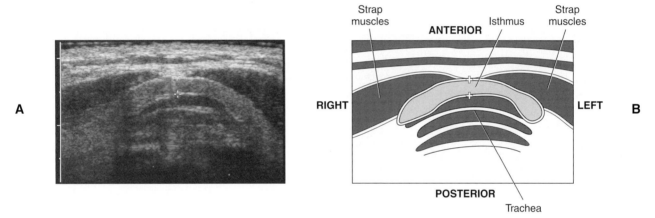

Figure 20-6 **A,** AP measurement of isthmus. **B,** Transverse view, longitudinal section.

tion level is elevated in a number of conditions; more importantly, it is elevated in the majority of patients with medullary thyroid carcinoma. The thyroid is composed of follicles filled with colloid, which is secreted by cuboidal epithelioid cells lining the periphery of the follicle. Colloid consists mainly of a glycoprotein, thyroglobulin, which contains thyroid hormones within its molecule. When thyroid hormone is needed, TSH, or **thyrotropin,** secreted by the anterior pituitary gland, triggers the release of hormones into the bloodstream. The secretion of TSH is regulated by the thyrotropin-releasing factor, produced by the hypothalamus. The level of thyrotropin-releasing factor is controlled by the basal metabolic rate (BMR). A decrease in BMR results from a low concentration of thyroid hormones, causing an increase in thyrotropin-releasing factor. This causes an increase in TSH secretion and an increase in the release of these hormones. Once the blood level of hormones is returned to normal, the BMR stabilizes and TSH secretion ceases.

BLOOD SUPPLY

The thyroid is a highly vascular gland. Its blood supply consists of paired superior and inferior thyroid arteries and veins, and often middle thyroid veins. The **superior thyroid artery** is the first branch of the external carotid artery. It runs downward and forward to the apex of the lateral lobe. The **inferior thyroid artery** is the largest branch of the thyrocervical trunk of the subclavian artery. It ascends to the inferior pole of the gland. Superior thyroid veins accompany the superior thyroid arteries (see Figure 20-3, *A*). The mean diameter of major thyroid arteries is between 1 and 2 mm. Normal peak systolic velocities range between 20 and 40 cm/sec. Intraparenchymal arteries exhibit peak systolic velocities between 15 and 30 cm/sec (see Figure 20-3, *B* and *C*). **Superior thyroid veins** arise above the anterolateral surface of the gland, cross the CCA, and empty into the IJVs above the thyroid cartilage. **Inferior thyroid veins** arise in the venous plexus of the thyroid gland, communicate with the superior and middle thyroid veins, and empty into the left and right innominate veins. The middle thyroid veins arise from the venous plexus on the lateral surface of the gland, and empty into the lower end of the jugular vein. Similar to thyroid arteries, thyroid veins measure approximately 1 to 2 mm in diameter. Lower or inferior veins can measure up to 7 to 8 mm in diameter (see Figure 20-3, *D*).

SONOGRAPHIC APPEARANCE

The normal thyroid gland is uniformly echogenic, with medium- to high-level echoes similar to those of the liver and testes. It is more echogenic than the contiguous muscular structures and vasculature (see Figure 20-9). Branches of the inferior and superior thyroid arteries and veins appear as anechoic tubular structures with bright thin walls (Figure 20-7). Color Doppler sonography is helpful in identifying intrathyroidal and extrathyroidal arteries and veins (see Figure 20-3, *B* and *C*).

On transverse images, the CCA and IJV are seen as circular anechoic areas with hyperechoic walls, adjacent to the lateral border of the thyroid gland. The neck muscles (infrahyoid, sternocleidomastoid, and longus colli) are hypoechoic relative to the thyroid gland. The LCM is triangularly shaped. The esophagus is visualized slightly to the left of midline, adjacent to the trachea, and appears as a circular hypoechoic structure with an echogenic center representing mucosa. The vagus nerve is visualized as a hypoechoic dot lateral to the thyroid lobe, usually located between the carotid artery and jugular vein. The recurrent laryngeal nerve is a circular hypoechoic structure with an echogenic rim located between the esophagus, trachea, and posterior thyroid lobe (Figures 20-8 and 20-9). In the sagittal plane of imaging, the infrahyoid and sternocleidomastoid muscles are anterior to the thyroid, and the LCM is posterolateral (Figure 20-10).

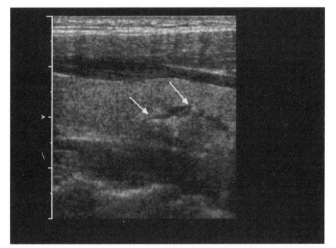
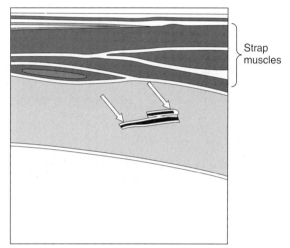

Figure 20-7 Sagittal view, axial section of thyroid gland; 1- to 2-mm tubular structures *(arrows)* represent intrathyroidal artery or vein.

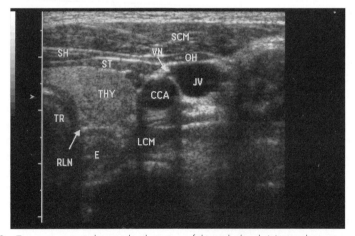

Figure 20-8 Transverse view, longitudinal section of thyroid gland. Note adjacent anatomic structures. *THY*, Thyroid; *CCA*, common carotid artery; *JV*, jugular vein; *E*, esophagus; *TR*, trachea; *LCM*, longus colli muscle; *RLN*, recurrent laryngeal nerve; *VN*, vagus nerve; *SH*, sternohyoid muscle; *ST*, sternothyroid muscle; *SCM*, sternocleidomastoid muscle; *OH*, omohyoid muscle.

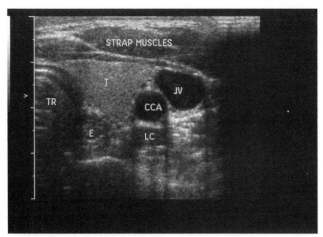

Figure 20-9 Longitudinal section of left lobe of thyroid gland. Note the anatomic relationship and shapes of the trachea *(TR)*, esophagus *(E)*, and longus colli muscle *(LC)*. *T,* Thyroid; *CCA,* common carotid artery; *JV,* jugular vein.

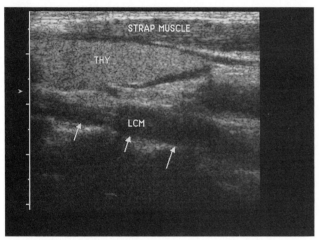

Figure 20-10 Axial sections of the strap muscle and longus colli muscle *(LCM) (arrows)*. Note their relationship to the thyroid gland *(THY)*.

SONOGRAPHIC APPLICATIONS

Determining composition of nonfunctioning "cold nodule" on scintigraphy

Determining the nature of a neck mass(es) (origin, number, composition, size)

Determining thyroid agenesis or dysgenesis in neonates

Detecting recurrent carcinoma after thyroidectomy

Screening patients with histories of head and neck irradiation

Monitoring the size of nodules under treatment (thyroid suppression therapy)

Delineating a thyroid nodule during pregnancy

Ultrasound-guided thyroid cyst aspiration(s)

NORMAL VARIANTS

An accessory lobe called the **pyramidal lobe** is present in approximately 10% to 40% of the population. It ex-

tends cephalad from the isthmus and ascends as far as the hyoid bone. A pyramidal lobe may extend from the right or left side of the isthmus; however, it arises more frequently on the left (see Figure 20-3, *A* and *E*). Other variations include absence of the isthmus, asymmetry (right lobe may be twice the size of the left lobe), or absence of lateral lobes. Complete agenesis or dysgenesis of the gland resulting in hypothyroidism is seldom noticed until a few weeks after birth, because the fetus is supplied, through the placenta, with sufficient maternal thyroid hormone to permit normal development.

REFERENCE CHARTS

■ ■ ■ ASSOCIATED PHYSICIANS

Surgeon: Specializes in surgery, a branch of medicine that treats diseases, deformities, and injuries by operative methods.

Endocrinologist: Specializes in medical diseases of the endocrine system. Principal endocrine glands include the thyroid, parathyroid, adrenal, pituitary, testes, and ovaries.

Radiologist: Specializes in the diagnostic interpretation of imaging modalities that assess thyroid and parathyroid abnormalities.

Interventional Radiologist: Specializes in invasive radiographic procedures for diagnosis and treatment.

Pathologist: Specializes in the interpretation of tissue biopsies and blood tests.

■ ■ ■ COMMON DIAGNOSTIC TESTS

Evaluation of the thyroid gland requires both physiologic and morphologic information in the treatment of thyroid disease. Various diagnostic tests available to achieve diagnostic efficacy include scintigraphy (radionuclide scanning), high-resolution sonography, computed tomography (CT), magnetic resonance imaging (MRI), and aspiration biopsy.

Scintigraphy: Scintigraphy is the diagnostic modality of choice for patients with palpable thyroid masses. It is the most common screening technique used in conjunction with ultrasound for the evaluation of thyroid function and morphology. A radioactive tracer or agent (^{123}I, ^{131}I, or ^{99m}Tc pertechnetate) is administered that targets the thyroid gland. It is monitored and photographed to assess thyroid function and differentiate between normal and abnormal thyroid tissue. This test is performed by a nuclear medicine technologist. Interpretation of the test is by the radiologist. The spatial resolution of this technique makes it difficult to delineate and characterize small nodules. Multiple nodules may be present within the gland when scintigraphy indicates only a solitary nodule. A major role of scintigraphy is to determine whether a lesion is "hot" (hyperfunctioning or more uptake than the normal thyroid gland) or "cold" (nonfunctioning or less uptake than the normal thyroid gland). On ^{123}I scintigraphy, hot nodules have a 1% to 4% risk of malignancies, whereas cold nodules have a 10% to 25% of malignancies. On ^{99m}Tc scintigraphy, hot nodules have 29% malignancies. [131] scintigraphy is often used to detect metastasis in patients with a thyroid cancer.

Ultrasound: Ultrasound uses high-frequency (7.5 to 15 MHz) sound waves to image and characterize thyroid parenchyma and adjacent anatomic structures. Resolution is between 0.7 and 1.0 mm. Linear transducers are preferred to sector transducers because of the wider field of view. In patients with large necks and/or an enlarged thyroid gland, a 5- to 8-MHz convex transducer provides a quick and accurate assessment of thyroid size and volume. Routine examination of the thyroid gland is performed with the patient supine. The neck is extended with a pad or pillow placed under the shoulders. The head is turned slightly away from the side being examined. This provides excellent anatomic access to image the thyroid gland, particularly in patients with short thick necks. Cross-sectional and sagittal images of the thyroid gland and relevant anatomy are obtained to differentiate normal from abnormal echo patterns. Ultrasound is the most definitive imaging technique used for determining whether a lesion is cystic or solid and whether it is intrathyroidal or extrathyroidal. It is also excellent for localizing nodules for aspiration and/or percutaneous biopsy. In selected cases, ultrasound biopsy can eliminate the need for surgery. Acoustic penetration is limited when evaluating the retrotrachea and substernal regions because acoustic walls or air-containing structures such as the trachea and lung preclude through sound transmission. This test is performed by a sonographer and sonologist. Interpretation of the test is by the sonologist.

Computed Axial Tomography (CT Scan): CT images the thyroid gland and adjacent anatomy in cross-section. A contrast material is usually administered to differentiate between pathology and normal anatomy. CT is less specific than sonography for establishing the cystic nature of nodules. However, it overcomes sound penetration limitations and provides anatomic definition in the substernal and retrotracheal regions. CT, like magnetic resonance imaging (MRI), is useful in assessing the overall extent of a mass. Less desirable features of CT imaging include streak artifacts from the shoulder girdle, use of intravenous iodinated contrast material, and exposure to ionizing radiation. This test is performed by a radiologic technologist. Interpretation of the test is by the radiologist.

Magnetic Resonance Imaging (MRI): MRI involves magnetism and radio waves. A surface coil is centered over the thyroid gland, providing high-quality images with a high signal-to-noise ratio. It provides multiplane imaging and may provide a contrast scale between normal and pathologic thyroid anatomy and adjacent anatomic structures. This technique permits excellent delineation of anatomic structures in the neck and thorax. For example, blood vessels are easily identified from adjacent lymph nodes. MRI is an excellent imaging modality for monitoring disease processes pretherapy and posttherapy. This test is performed by a radiologic technologist. Interpretation of the test is by the radiologist. CT and MRI are particularly useful when thyroid tissue extends into the mediastinum and cervical region.

Fine Needle Aspiration: Fine needle aspiration may provide the definitive diagnosis of thyroid nodules. With sonographic guidance, lesions a few millimeters in size can be biopsied. Such biopsies are easy to perform and well tolerated by the patient. With an experienced pathologist, a diagnostic sensitivity of 96% can be achieved. Complications are unusual, a small hematoma being the most common. This procedure is performed by a radiologist, an endocrinologist, or a surgeon. Interpretation of the test is done by a pathologist.

■ ■ ■ LABORATORY TESTS

Thyroid hormone production is modulated by a feedback control mechanism effected through the hypothalamus and the pituitary gland. Thyrotropin (TSH), secreted by the anterior pituitary, controls thyroid hormone production. Several laboratory tests are done to evaluate thyroid function. No one clinical test can be used alone to diagnose hypothyroidism or hyperthyroidism. Common tests include T_4, T_3, TSH (thyroid stimulating hormone), T_3 resin uptake, and RAI (radioactive iodine uptake). The following laboratory tests are performed by a licensed laboratory technologist. Interpretation of the tests is done by the pathologist.

Thyroxine: Thyroxine (T_4), with four iodine atoms, is the most abundant thyroid hormone produced. T_4 is commonly used for screening and follow-up of patients whose diagnosis is either hypothyroidism or hyperthyroidism. The test measures both free thyroxine and the portion carried by the thyroid-binding plasma protein. T_3 (triiodothyronine) contains three iodine atoms and represents a small portion of thyroid hormone, but it is more potent than T_4. Both T_3 and T_4 can also be measured indirectly by radioimmunoassay. This is a very sensitive method of determining the concentration of hormones in blood plasma. A venous blood sample is drawn and "tagged" with specific radioactive substances that specifically bind with either T_3 or T_4. The amount of radioactivity measured indirectly indicates the concentration of thyroid hormone indirectly. Increased levels of T_3 and T_4 are associated with hyperthyroidism, whereas decreased levels indicate hypothyroidism.

T_3 Resin Uptake: The T_3 resin uptake test measures the amount of T_4 indirectly by measuring the amount of T_3 that can be attached to the proteins that bind the thyroid hormones. The resin uptake test measures the amount of T_3 remaining and free to bind to the resin added to the blood sample. A measured amount of radioactive tagged T_3 and resin is added to a sample of the patient's blood. The resin is placed in a test tube to absorb any of the radioactive-tagged T_3 that cannot be taken up by the thyroid-binding globulin in the blood sample. Increased T_3 into the resin indicates hyperthyroidism; decreased T_3 into the resin indicates hypothyroidism.

Thyroid Stimulating Hormone: TSH (thyroid stimulating hormone) or thyrotropin, produced by the pituitary gland, controls the serum levels of the thyroid hormones. Measurement of TSH is useful in determining whether hypothyroidism is due to primary hypofunction of the thyroid gland (intrinsic thyroid disease) or to secondary hypofunction of the anterior pituitary gland, caused by insufficient stimulation by the pituitary. TSH also measures a patient's response to thyroid medication, particularly one with primary hypothyroidism, and pituitary hypothyroidism.

Radioactive Iodine Test: The radioactive iodine (RAI) uptake test evaluates thyroid function by measuring the amount of orally ingested ^{123}I or ^{131}I that accumulates in the thyroid gland after 6 and 24 hours. The largest portion of iodine is transported via the circulatory system to the thyroid gland. An external counting probe (gamma detector) measures the radioactivity in the thyroid as a percentage of the original dose, indicating the ability of the gland to trap and retain iodine. The normal range is about 10% to 15% at 6 hours and 15% to 30% at 24 hours. This test is performed by a nuclear medicine technologist. Interpretation of the test is done by the radiologist.

■ ■ ■   **LABORATORY VALUES**

Resin T$_3$ Uptake (RT$_3$U) (Specimen S): 25%-35%.
Thyroid Stimulating Hormone (Specimen S): 5-10 u U/ml.
Thyroxine (T$_4$) (Specimen S): 4.5-13$_{ug}$/dl.
Triiodothyronine: 75-195 ug/dl (pregnancy and oral contraceptives tend to increase values).

■ ■ ■   **NORMAL MEASUREMENTS**

Adult Thyroid Gland: 4-6 cm in length, 1.3-1.8 cm in anteroposterior diameter, 1.5-2 cm in width.
Isthmus: 0.2-0.6 cm in anteroposterior diameter
Newborn and Children: 2-3 cm in length, 0.2-1.2 cm in anteroposterior diameter, 1-1.5 cm in width.

■ ■ ■   **VASCULATURE**

Superior Supply: External carotid artery—superior thyroid artery—superior thyroid veins—internal jugular veins.
Inferior Supply: Thyrocervical artery—inferior thyroid artery—inferior thyroid veins—middle thyroid veins—right and left innominate veins.

■ ■ ■   **AFFECTING CHEMICALS**

Thyroid Stimulating Hormone (TSH): Stimulates the thyroid to make and release thyroid hormones.

PARATHYROID GLANDS

Parathyroid glands are small, encapsulated, oval bodies attached to the posterior surfaces of the lateral lobes of the thyroid gland. Most people have four symmetric parathyroid glands located adjacent to the thyroid gland (see Figures 20-1 and 20-3, *A*). Parathyroid glands secrete **parathyroid hormone** to maintain homeostasis of blood calcium levels.

PRENATAL DEVELOPMENT

The parathyroid glands develop from the third and fourth pharyngeal pouches, epithelial entodermal-lined cavities that give rise to a number of vital organs. Parathyroid-3 tissue descends and rests on the dorsal surface of the thyroid gland and forms the inferior parathyroid gland. It originates from the third pouch in conjunction with the thymic primordium in the fifth embryonic week. These primordia lose their connection with the pharyngeal wall and migrate together caudally to lie in a lower position in the neck. Parathyroid-4 loses its contact with the wall of the pharynx and attaches to the caudally migrating thyroid. It eventually rests on the dorsal surface of the upper thyroid gland and forms the superior parathyroid gland (Figure 20-11). The **thymus** descends to the thorax and lies behind the sternum and anterior to the pericardium and great vessels.

LOCATION

Parathyroid glands are typically located posterior to the thyroid gland and anterior to the LCM. Superior parathyroid glands are situated more posteriorly and

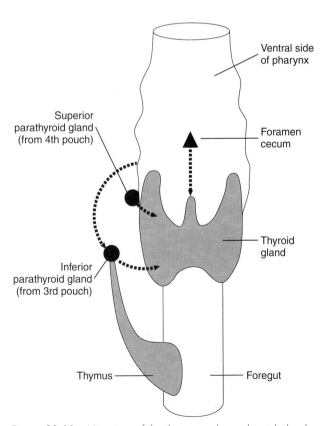

Superior parathyroid gland (from 4th pouch)

Inferior parathyroid gland (from 3rd pouch)

Ventral side of pharynx

Foramen cecum

Thyroid gland

Thymus

Foregut

Figure 20-11 *Migration of the thymus and parathyroid glands.*

medially than inferior parathyroid glands. They normally lie at the thyroid's mid to upper portion. Inferior parathyroid glands are situated more anteriorly than superior parathyroid glands. They are found on the posterior lateral surface of the thyroid gland, anterior and medial to the recurrent laryngeal nerve and inferior thyroid artery. Inferior parathyroid glands may also be imbedded within the thyroid tissue.

The majority of parathyroid masses appear in the area of an anatomic "triangle" formed by the thyroid gland, LCM, CCA, and IJV (see Figures 20-1 and 20-8). The MINVB is the only anatomic structure that lies in this region and measures 5 mm in diameter.

SIZE

Normal parathyroid glands measure approximately 5 to 7 mm in length, 3 to 4 mm in width, and 1 to 2 mm in thickness (5 × 3 × 1 mm). They weigh between 10 and 75 mg, with a mean average of 35 to 40 mg.

GROSS ANATOMY

Parathyroid glands are composed of masses of chief cells, with some wasserhelle (water-clear) and oxyphil cells arranged in a columnar fashion. The color of parathyroid glands varies from light yellow in older patients to a reddish or light brown in young patients, depending on the amount of fat within the gland.

The shape of parathyroid glands varies. They are generally oval, bean shaped, or spherical (83%), or sometimes elongated (11%), bilobulated (5%), or multilobulated (1%) (Figure 20-12).

The nerve supply is abundant; it arises from the thyroid branches of the cervical sympathetic ganglia.

PHYSIOLOGY

Parathyroid glands secrete **parathyroid hormone,** also called PTH or **parathormone.** As mentioned, their primary function is to help maintain homeostasis of blood calcium concentration by promoting calcium absorption into the blood, preventing hypocalcemia. When

serum calcium levels are low, the parathyroid hormone raises serum calcium by releasing calcium from the bone, increasing calcium absorption in the gut, and decreasing renal calcium by decreasing renal phosphate excretion.

BLOOD SUPPLY

The superior and inferior parathyroid glands are supplied by separate small branches of the superior and inferior thyroid arteries and by branches from the longitudinal anastomoses between these vessels (see Figure 20-3, A). Venous drainage is into the thyroid plexus of the veins. The lymphatic channels drain with those of the thyroid gland.

SONOGRAPHIC APPEARANCE

Normal parathyroid glands can be seen occasionally, especially in young patients, by using newer high-frequency transducers. A single gland is identified as a flat hypoechoic structure posterior to the thyroid gland and anterior to the LCM.

Since most normal adult parathyroid glands are not generally identified with ultrasound unless they are abnormal, this discussion will focus on the sonographic appearance of parathyroid adenomas, a common parathyroid gland abnormality appreciated sonographically. These adenomas generally appear as hypoechoic to anechoic, oval or bean-shaped, homogeneous structures without through transmission that measure slightly greater than 1 cm (Figure 20-13). Parathyroid adenomas are virtually never more echogenic than the thyroid gland. With enlargement, changes include lobulation, acoustic inhomogeneity (heterogeneous echo texture), cystic degeneration, and occasional calcifications (Figures 20-14 to 20-16).

Studies using color Doppler have studied vascularity to differentiate thyroid lesions from parathyroid adenomas. One study observed that thyroid lesions tend to have some vascularity when only 5 mm in size, and parathyroid adenomas are avascular until they reach almost 2 cm.

Current state-of-the-art color flow imaging of parathyroid adenomas demonstrates intraparenchymal hypervascularization in approximately 90% of cases (Figure 20-17). In 10% of cases, parathyroid adenomas are avascular, according to the technology currently available. Flow is increased relative to the thyroid gland, which is mainly arterial (Figure 20-18). Color and power Doppler have an overall accuracy of 94% in locating parathyroid adenomas. The presence of an extrathyroidal artery leading to an abnormal gland aids in the detection of an otherwise inconspicuous parathyroid adenoma (Figure 20-19).

It is of paramount importance to have a thorough understanding of the normal sonographic appearance

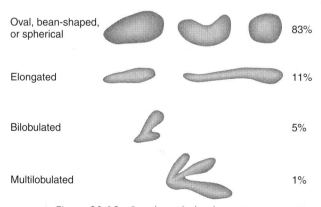

Oval, bean-shaped, or spherical	83%
Elongated	11%
Bilobulated	5%
Multilobulated	1%

Figure 20-12 Parathyroid gland variations.

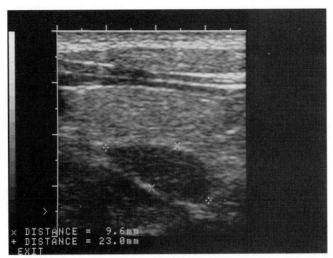
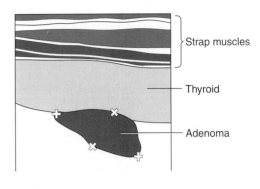

Figure 20-13 Longitudinal section of the thyroid gland demonstrating a typical parathyroid adenoma; hypoechoic, oval, and located posterior to the thyroid lobe. Calipers measuring the length and AP diameter. Note the position of calipers (+,x).

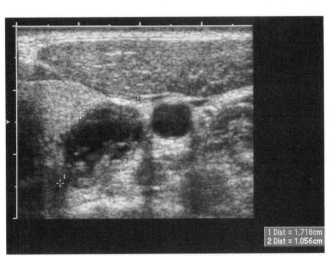
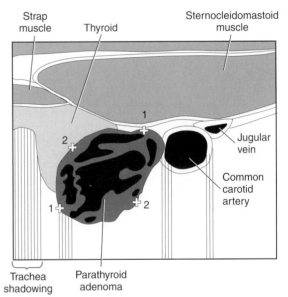

Figure 20-14 Transverse section through the mid left lobe of the thyroid demonstrating a heterogeneous parathyroid adenoma. Calipers measuring the width and AP diameter. Note the position of calipers (Dist 1 and Dist 2).

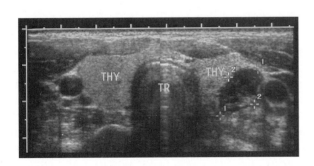
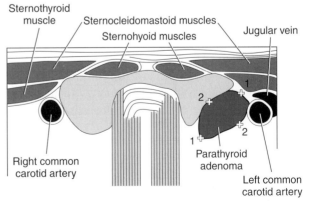

Figure 20-15 Transverse section through both thyroid lobes showing a left parathyroid adenoma. Calipers measuring the width and AP diameter. Note the position of the calipers (Dist 1 and Dist 2). Note the heterogeneity of the thyroid gland.

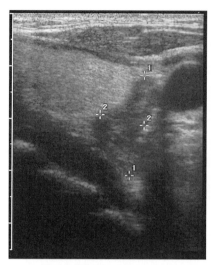
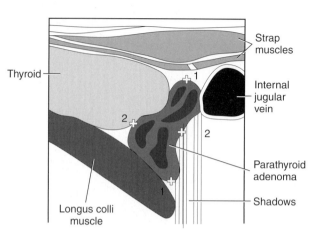

Figure 20-16 Longitudinal section of the lower lobe of the right thyroid gland showing a lobulated parathyroid adenoma, posteroinferior to the thyroid gland and anterior to the LCM. Note the position of the measurement calipers (Dist 1 and Dist 2) and that the longest axis of the adenoma is seen anteroposteriorly.

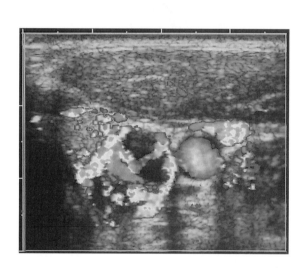
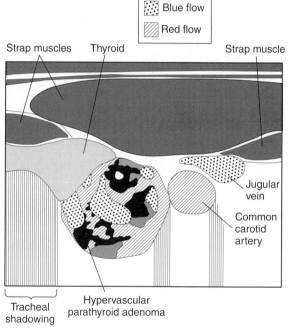

Figure 20-17 Color Doppler transverse image of a mid left parathyroid adenoma. Note the hypervascularization of the adenoma. Color-void areas represent cystic areas. Note the relationship of the adenoma to the thyroid gland, common carotid artery, and jugular vein. (See Color Plate 29.)

of relevant adjacent anatomic structures in the neck, to avoid pitfalls when imaging the parathyroid glands. Normal cervical structures can mimic parathyroid adenomas, producing false positive results.

In the sagittal imaging plane, the LCM runs the length of the thyroid gland and is hypoechoic compared with the thyroid (see Figure 20-10). In the transverse plane the LCM appears triangular in shape and is often mistaken for a parathyroid adenoma, particularly when

the gland is elongated (see Figure 20-9). An anechoic parathyroid adenoma located medial to a collapsed jugular vein could be mistaken for a normal IJV. The esophagus has also been mistaken for a large parathyroid adenoma (see Figure 20-9).

Other cervical structures that may simulate parathyroid adenomas include small **extrathyroidal veins and arteries** that lie adjacent to the posterior and lateral aspects of the thyroid, enlarged cervical lymph nodes, and

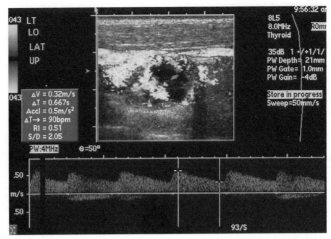

Figure 20-18 Color Doppler longitudinal section of a left parathyroid adenoma demonstrating hypervascular arterial flow.

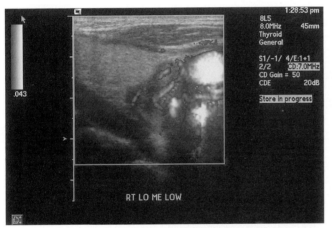

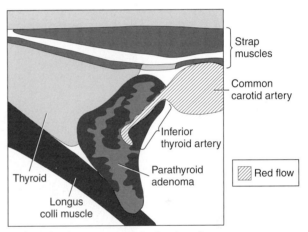

Figure 20-19 Color Doppler image of an inferior parathyroid adenoma. Note the feeder inferior thyroid artery supplying the adenoma. (See Color Plate 30.)

any coexisting thyroid nodules. Color Doppler imaging can differentiate vascular from nonvascular structures in the neck (Figure 20-20, *A* and *B*). Enlarged cervical lymph nodes appear oval and exhibit low-intensity echoes. They often have an echogenic band or hilum composed of fat, vessels, and fibrous tissue. These nodes usually lie laterally in the neck adjacent to the jugular vein, away from the thyroid gland (Figures 20-21 and 20-22). Occasionally, parathyroid adenomas can be found laterally in the carotid sheath, and percutaneous biopsy may be necessary to distinguish a parathyroid adenoma from an abnormal lymph node.

When a thyroid nodule protrudes from the posterior aspect of the thyroid, it can mimic a parathyroid adenoma. An imaging sign that is helpful in this situation is a thin echogenic line that separates the parathyroid adenoma from the gland itself. Thyroid nodules, which arise from within the gland, do not demonstrate this tissue plane of separation. Also, the sonographic appear-

ance of many thyroid nodules is heterogeneous or mixed, compared with parathyroid adenomas, which tend to be homogeneous and hypoechoic.

SONOGRAPHIC APPLICATIONS

The most common clinical indication for parathyroid imaging is hypercalcemia (serum calcium levels greater than 10.5 mg/dl).

Patients newly diagnosed with hyperparathyroidism. Both primary and secondary hyperparathyroidism result in hypercalcemia.

Ultrasound-guided parathyroid cyst aspiration(s).

Patients undergoing repeat surgical neck exploration.

NORMAL VARIANTS

Most people (about 80%) have four parathyroid glands located in a symmetric position contiguous with the thyroid gland (see Figures 20-1 and 20-3, *A*). Eighty to

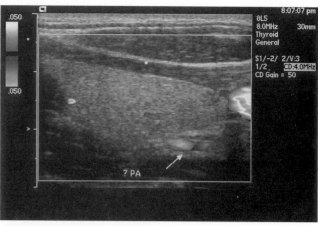

Figure 20-20 **A,** Longitudinal section showing a 0.6-cm flat hypoechoic structure simulating a small parathyroid adenoma, posterior to the lower pole of the thyroid gland. Note placement of calipers. **B,** Color Doppler image of A. Note the hypoechoic structure fills with color, indicating a vascular structure and not a parathyroid adenoma. (See Color Plate 31.)

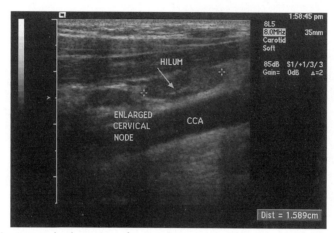

Figure 20-21 Longitudinal section of an enlarged hypoechoic cervical lymph node with echogenic hilum *(arrow)* adjacent to the common carotid artery. Note the position of calipers. (See Color Plate 32.)

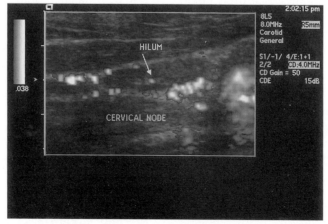

Figure 20-22 Color Doppler image of an enlarged cervical lymph node. Note the vascular flow within the hilum. (See Color Plate 33.)

eighty-five percent of parathyroid adenomas are found adjacent to the thyroid gland. As many as 13% to 15% of persons have more than five parathyroid glands, and 5% will have only three glands.

Ectopic Glands

Ectopic parathyroid glands account for approximately 15% of the total. They are frequently found within the thymus or perithymic tissues (10%). Other aberrant locations include the carotid bulb and sheath (1%), the retroesophageal space (1% to 3%), and intrathyroidal (1%) (Figure 20-23).

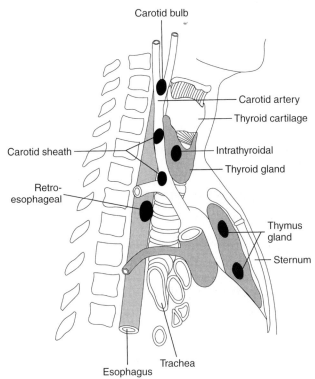

Figure 20-23 *Lateral section of mediastinum and neck illustrating aberrant locations of parathyroid glands. Dark circles indicate aberrant locations: thymus gland, carotid bulb, retroesophageal, intrathyroidal, carotid sheath.*

REFERENCE CHARTS

■ ■ ■ ASSOCIATED PHYSICIANS

Surgeon: Specializes in surgery, a branch of medicine that treats diseases, deformities, and injuries by operative methods.

Endocrinologist: Specializes in medical diseases of the endocrine system. Principal endocrine glands include the thyroid, parathyroid, adrenal, pituitary, testes, and ovaries.

Radiologist: Specializes in the diagnostic interpretation of imaging modalities that assess thyroid and parathyroid abnormalities.

Interventional Radiologist: Specializes in invasive radiographic procedures for diagnosis and treatment.

Pathologist: Specializes in the interpretation of tissue biopsies and blood tests.

■ ■ ■ COMMON DIAGNOSTIC TESTS

Several diagnostic tests are used to localize and evaluate parathyroid glands. Most commonly used imaging modalities include high-resolution sonography (7.5 to 15.0 MHz), scintigraphy using technetium-99m sestamibi, and magnetic resonance imaging (MRI). Current less commonly used modalities include computed tomography (CT), angiography, and selective venous sampling. Initial studies being evaluated for parathyroid localization include transesophageal ultrasound and positron emission tomography.

Each of these techniques alone has a sensitivity of between 60% and 80%, and a specificity of between 90% and 95% in revealing abnormal parathyroid glands. The combined use of ultrasound with either computed tomography, magnetic resonance, or radionuclide scanning raises the sensitivity to approximately 88%.

Ultrasound: Ultrasound is the imaging modality recommended for the initial evaluation of patients with primary hyperparathyroidism who have not had surgery, and after elevated calcium levels and parathormone levels have been identified. High-resolution sonography (7.5 to 15 MHz) is performed in both longitudinal and transverse planes beginning at the sternal notch and progressing to the angle of the mandible. Images are obtained medial to lateral, evaluating thyroid lobes, adjacent muscles, and vasculature in search of abnormal parathyroid glands. Routine examination for abnormal parathyroid glands is performed with the patient supine. The neck is extended, with a pad or pillow placed under the shoulders. The head is turned slightly away from the side being examined. This provides excellent anatomic access to the neck, particularly in patients with a short stocky body habitus. When locating inferior parathyroid adenomas, have the patient swallow. This briefly raises the gland upward and permits acoustic access to the most inferior aspect of the thyroid lobe. Patients with thick muscular necks may benefit from scanning with a 5-MHz transducer to increase acoustic penetration. Ultrasound is not a screening modality for parathyroid glands; there must be a specific indication for performing the examination such as hypercalcemia. This test is performed by a sonographer and sonologist. Interpretation of the test is done by the sonologist. When sonography fails to identify abnormal parathyroid glands preoperatively, the combined use of either scintigraphy or magnetic resonance imaging (MRI) is recommended to identify parathyroid adenomas in ectopic locations. The sensitivity of other imaging techniques such as MRI and CT is superior compared with ultrasound in locating parathyroid adenomas in the retroesophageal and substernal regions. Ultrasound is a sensitive technique in verifying whether or not tissue consistent with an abnormal parathyroid gland exists in a particular aberrant location such as the carotid bulb or sheath. Parathyroid aspiration biopsy under ultrasound guidance is helpful in postoperative localization of parathyroid adenomas, with a reported sensitivity of 91%.

Scintigraphy: With scintigraphy, 20 mCi of Tc-99m MIBI (technetium sestamibi) is administered intravenously and taken up by the patient's thyroid and parathyroid glands. Early (10-minute) and delayed (2-hour) images are compared. Technetium sestamibi "washes out" of the thyroid gland quickly, and focal uptake persists in abnormal parathyroid glands. The sensitivity of this technique ranges from 88% to 100%. This test is performed by a nuclear medicine technologist. Interpretation of the test is by the radiologist.

Computed Axial Tomography (CT Scan): CT imaging of parathyroid glands occurs in the following sequence: contrast material is injected that helps distinguish the vasculature from other structures such as lymph nodes. Axial scans are performed from the base of the skull to the sternal notch at 5-mm increments. Abnormal parathyroid glands will be enlarged. This test is performed by a radiologic technologist. Interpretation of the test is by the radiologist.

Magnetic Resonance Imaging (MRI): MRI uses an anterior surface coil with increased detail to image parathyroid glands. Axial and sagittal views are taken from the base of the skull to the sternal notch at slice thicknesses of 4 to 5 mm. Abnormal parathyroid glands tend to have a high-intensity signal in contrast to surrounding tissue. This test is performed by a radiologic technologist. Interpretation of the test is done by the radiologist. If the patient has had previous parathyroid surgeries that have failed to identify abnormal glands or has had recurrent hyperparathyroidism with negative noninvasive test results, digital angiography followed by selective venous sampling is helpful.

Selective Venous Sampling: Selective venous sampling tends to lateralize the site of abnormal parathyroid glands by providing access to the venous system (primarily the superior, inferior, and middle thyroid veins) so that parathyroid hormone assays can be obtained to determine abnormal calcium levels. Because parathyroid adenomas may arise anywhere in the cervical and mediastinal regions, sampling may be necessary from the internal jugular veins inferiorly to the level of the renal veins. This test is performed by an interventional radiologist. Interpretation of the test is by the radiologist and a pathologist.

Serum Calcium: An elevated serum calcium level, or hypercalcemia, is usually a clue to hyperparathyroidism. Hypercalcemia can be life-threatening when serum calcium levels reach 14.5 mg/dl or higher. Most cases of primary hyperparathyroidism are diagnosed by documenting a simultaneous increase in blood levels of both bone calcium and parathyroid hormone (PTH). Other general laboratory tests used in the differential diagnosis of the hypercalcemic patient include phosphorus, alkaline phosphatase, uric acid, chloride, serum protein, urinalysis, and 24-hour calcium. General laboratory tests are performed by a licensed laboratory technologist. Interpretation of the test is by a pathologist.

Urinary Calcium: Approximately 75% of patients with primary hyperparathyroidism have elevated urinary calcium

levels. A low serum phosphorus level is seen in about 50% of patients. An increased serum phosphorus level in the absence of renal failure or excessive intake of phosphorus suggests a nonparathyroid cause of hypercalcemia. Alkaline phosphatase levels are elevated in about 10% of patients with primary hyperparathyroidism. Serum chloride levels are increased in about 40% of patients. Serum protein and serum uric acid levels are also increased in many patients.

■ ■ ■ LABORATORY VALUES

Alkaline Phosphorus (Specimen S): 1.5-4.5 Bodansky units/dl; 0.8-2.9 BLB units.
Calcium (Specimen S): Adult 8.4-10.2 mg/dl; child 8.8-10.7 mg/dl.
Chloride (Cl): 98-106 mmol/L (specimen S); 110-250 mmol/L (CSF).
Phosphorus (Specimen S): 2.7-4.5 mg/dl.
Protein (Total): 6.5-8.3 g/dl (Specimen S); 0.5% of plasma (CSF).
Uric Acid (Specimen S): Male 3.5-7.2 mg/dl; female 2.6-6.0 mg/dl.

■ ■ ■ NORMAL MEASUREMENTS

Adult Parathyroid Gland: 5-7 mm in length, 3-4 mm in width, 1-2 mm in thickness.

■ ■ ■ VASCULATURE

Superior Supply: External carotid artery—superior thyroid artery—superior thyroid veins—internal jugular veins.
Inferior Supply: Thyrocervical artery—inferior thyroid artery—inferior thyroid veins—middle thyroid veins—right innominate veins.

■ ■ ■ AFFECTING CHEMICALS

Parathormone (PTH): A hormone that affects parathyroid function and homeostasis.

BIBLIOGRAPHY

Anderhub B: *Superficial parts: manual of abdominal sonography,* Baltimore, 1984, University Park, pp 188-204.

Anderson K: High-resolution water-path scanning of the parathyroid glands, *Med Ultrasound* 6:11-17, 1982.

Anthony CP. The endocrine system. In Anthony CP, editor: *Textbook of anatomy and physiology,* ed 10, St Louis, 1979, Mosby, pp 318-347.

Barton T: The thyroid gland: a review for sonographers, *Med Ultrasound* 4:127-134, 1980.

Butch J, Simeone JF, Mueller PR: Thyroid and parathyroid ultrasonography, *Radiol Clin North Am* 23:57-71, 1985.

Clark OH: Hyperparathyroidism. In Clark OH, editor: *Endocrine surgery of the thyroid and parathyroid glands,* St Louis, 1985, Mosby, pp 172-240.

Cole-Beuglet C: New high-resolution ultrasound evaluation of diseases of the thyroid gland, *JAMA* 249: 2941-2944, 1983.

Cole-Beuglet C: Ultrasonography of thyroid, parathyroid, and neck masses. In Sarti DA, editor: *Diagnostic ultrasound,* ed 2, Chicago, 1987, Yearbook, pp 608-655.

Corbett JV: *Laboratory tests and diagnostic procedures with nursing diagnoses,* ed 2, Los Altos, 1987, Appleton & Lange, pp 347-391.

Fugazzola C., Bergamo AI, Solbiati L: Parathyroid glands. In Solbiati L, Rizzatto G, editors: *Ultrasound of superficial structures,* 1995, Churchill Livingstone, pp 87-113.

Gary H: Parathyroid and thyroid glands. In Clemente CD, editor: *Gray's anatomy of the human body,* ed 30, Philadelphia, 1984, Lea & Febiger, pp 1596-1615.

Gavin AG: Thyroid physiology and testing of thyroid function. In Clark OH, editor: *Endocrine surgery of the thyroid and parathyroid glands,* St. Louis, 1985, Mosby, pp 1-34.

Gooding GAW: Sonography of the thyroid and parathyroid, *Radiol Clin North Am* 31(5):967-989, 1993.

Gooding GAW, Clark OH: Use of color Doppler imaging in the distinction between thyroid and parathyroid lesions, *Am J Surg* 164: 51-56, 1992.

Gooding GAW, Okerlund MD, Stark DD, Clark OH: Parathyroid imaging: comparison of double-tracer (TI-210, TC-99m) scintigraphy and high-resolution US, *Radiology* 161:57-64, 1986.

Gooding GAW, Clark OH, Stark DD, et al: Parathyroid aspiration biopsy under US guidance in the post-operative patient, *Radiology* 155:193-196, 1985.

Guyton AC: The thyroid metabolic hormones. In *Textbook of medical physiology,* ed 7, Philadelphia, 1986, WB Saunders, pp 897 -906.

Healy JE, Seybold WD: *The neck: a synopsis of clinical anatomy,* Philadelphia, 1969, WB Saunders, pp 10-39.

Hickey J, Goldberg FID: Neck and head: salivary, thyroid, and parathyroid glands. In *Ultrasound review of the abdomen, male pelvis, and small parts,* Lippincott, 1999, pp 151-168.

Higgins CB, Auffermann W: MR imaging of thyroid and parathyroid glands: a review of current status, *Am J Radiol* 151:1095-1106, 1988.

Hopkins RC, Reading CC: The parathyroid glands. In Rumack CM, Wilson SR, Charboneau JW, editors: *Diagnostic ultrasound,* ed 2, St Louis, 1988, Mosby, pp 731-750.

Lane MJ, Desser TS, Weigel RJ, Jeffrey RB, Jr: Use of color and power Doppler sonography to identify feeding arteries associated with parathyroid adenomas, *Am J Radiol* 171:819-823, 1998.

Langman J: Special embryology, head and neck. In *Medical embryology,* ed 4, Baltimore, 1981, Williams & Wilkins, pp 268-297.

Leisner B: Ultrasound evaluation of thyroid diseases, *Horm Res* 26: 33-41, 1987.

Netter FH: The thyroid and parathyroid glands. In *Ciba collection of medical illustrations: endocrine system and selected metabolic diseases,* vol 4, Edison, NJ, 1965, Ciba Pharmaceutical, pp 41-73.

Oates E: Improved parathyroid scintigraphy with TC-99m MIBI, a superior radiotracer, *Applied Radiol* March, 37-40, 1994.

Odwin CS, Dubinsky T, Fleischer AC: *Ultrasonography examination review and study guide,* Los Altos, 1987, Appleton & Lange, p 144.

Randel SB, Gooding AW, Clark OH, et al: Parathyroid variants: US evaluation, *Radiology* 165: 191-194,1987.

Sakaguchi T, Arakawa A, Takahashi M: Appropriate use of ultrasonography in the neck. *Semin Roentgenol* 35(1):54-62, 2000.

Schorzman L: High-resolution ultrasonography of superficial structures. In Hagen-Ansert SL, editor: *Textbook of diagnostic ultrasonography,* ed 3, St Louis, 1989, Mosby, pp 320-326.

Siegel ML: Neck. In Siegel ML, editor: *Pediatric sonography,* New York, 1991, Raven Press, pp 63-87.

Simeone JF, Mueller PR, Ferrucci JT, et al: High-resolution real-time sonography of the parathyroid, *Radiology* 141:745-751, 1981.

Solbiati L, Livaghi T, Ballaratti E, et al : Thyroid gland. In Solbiati L, Rizzatto G, editors: *Ultrasound of superficial structures,* 1995, Churchill Livingstone, pp 49-85.

Solbiati L, Charboneau JW, Meredith JE, Hay ID: The thyroid gland. In Rumack CM, Wilson SR, Charboneau JW, editors: *Diagnostic ultrasound,* ed 2, St Louis, 1998, Mosby, pp 703-729.

Solbiati L, Cioffi V, Ballarati E: Ultrasonography of the neck, *Radiol Clin North Am* 30(5):941-954, 1992.

Willinsky RA, Kassel PW, Cooper HB, et al: Computed tomography of lingual thyroid, *J Comput Assist Tomogr* 11(1):182-183, 1987.

Woodburne RT: The head and neck. In *Essentials of human anatomy,* ed 3, New York, 1965, Oxford University Press, pp 77-89.

CHAPTER 21

Breast Sonography

LISA STROHL

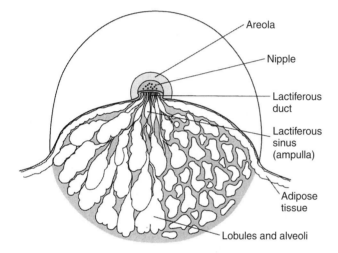

Areola

Nipple

Lactiferous duct

Lactiferous sinus (ampulla)

Adipose tissue

Lobules and alveoli

OBJECTIVES

Describe the function of the breast.
Define the location of anatomy related to the breast.
Describe the size relationships of normal breast anatomy.
Describe the sonographic appearance of normal breast anatomy.
Describe the associated physicians, diagnostic tests, and related laboratory values.
Define the key words.

KEY WORDS

Acini/acinus	Hypothalamus
Alveoli	Lactation
Anterior pituitary gland	Lactiferous ducts
Breast	Mammary layer
Breast parenchyma	Mammary pit
Connective tissues	Mammary ridges
Cooper's ligaments	Mammography
Estrogen	Montgomery's glands
Exocrine	Oxytocin

Parenchymal elements	Prolactin-inhibiting factor
Pectoralis major muscle	Retromammary layer
Progesterone	Stromal elements
Prolactin	Subcutaneous layer

The mammary glands are modified sweat glands. They are **exocrine** organs whose main function is the secretion of milk during pregnancy **(lactation)** (Figure 21-1).

PRENATAL DEVELOPMENT

The mammary glands develop along two strips of ectoderm, the **mammary ridges,** which run along each side of the developing embryo. These are visible by 6 weeks' gestational development (Figure 21-2).

By 8 weeks' gestation, a bud has developed in the ectoderm along the mammary ridges and extends into the underlying connective tissue. This bud will continue to develop, and by the fourth month of gestation it will begin to extend outward into secondary buds. These will further develop into the **lactiferous ducts** during puberty. Further development will occur during pregnancy due to hormonal stimulation (Figure 21-3).

In the early fetus, the nipple site on the mammary gland externally is recessed slightly. This is called the **mammary pit.** By birth, this will be slightly raised on the skin surface. Further development of breast tissue will not continue until puberty.

LOCATION

The **breast** is anterior to the pectoralis major, serratus, and external oblique muscles and the sixth rib. It is bounded medially by the sternum and is bordered laterally by the margin of the axilla. The superior border consists of the second and third ribs. The inferior border is the seventh costal cartilage. The breast is bordered laterally by the axilla (Figure 21-4).

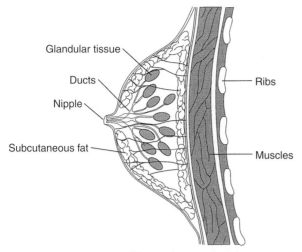

Figure 21-1   Cross-section of breast demonstrating basic anatomy.

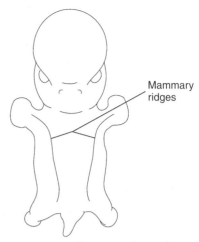

Figure 21-2   Mammary ridges seen during the prenatal development of the fetus.

A

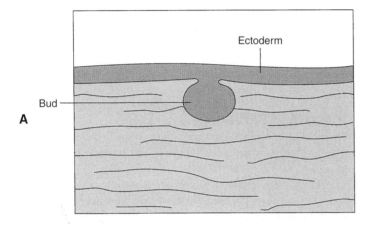

B

Figure 21-3   **A,** Connective tissue bud seen at approximately 10 weeks' gestational age. **B,** Outward extensions into lactiferous ducts seen at approximately 4 months' gestational age.

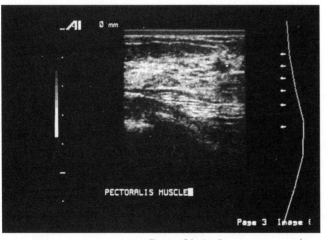

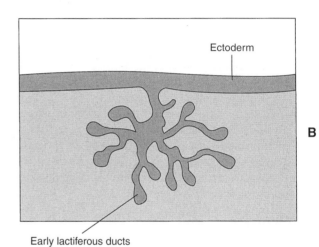

Figure 21-4   Breast anatomy showing posterior pectoralis muscle.

SIZE

The size of the normal breast varies depending on the age, functional state, and amount and arrangement of stromal and parenchymal elements of the individual.

There is an increase in development of breast tissue owing to stimulation by **estrogen** during puberty and, later, during the childbearing years and pregnancy. With the decrease in hormonal stimulation after menopause, the normal breast will atrophy to some degree.

GROSS ANATOMY

Anatomically, the breast is composed of parenchymal and stromal elements. The **parenchymal elements** include the lobes, lobules, ducts, and **acini.** The **stromal elements** include all of the **connective tissue** and fat.

The breast has three layers. The **subcutaneous layer** contains the skin and all of the subcutaneous fat; the **mammary layer** contains the glandular tissues, ducts, and connective tissues; and the **retromammary layer** contains the retromammary fat, muscle, and deep connective tissues.

The normal breast is composed of 15 to 20 lobes separated by adipose tissue. Each lobe has an external drainage pathway into the nipple. The lobes are further divided into lobules, each of which contains glandular tissue elements **(alveoli).**

Support of breast tissue is provided by the suspensory ligaments of Cooper **(Cooper's ligaments),** which run between each two lobules from the deep muscle fascia to the skin surface (Figure 21-5).

PHYSIOLOGY

Breast development is stimulated by estrogen, as stated earlier. This stimulation causes the development of stromal and parenchymal elements throughout the breast. The glandular tissues of the breast become active due to hormonal stimulation present during pregnancy. Increased levels of **progesterone** stimulate the development of the breast lobules and alveoli.

Both the production of milk and its absence are controlled by hormones produced within the **hypothalamus** and **anterior pituitary gland.** The hypothalamus produces **prolactin-inhibiting factor,** which prevents the release of prolactin until milk production becomes necessary following childbirth. At this time, the anterior pituitary gland will secrete **prolactin,** which stimulates development of the secretory system of the breast.

After the placenta has been expelled and estrogen levels have decreased, the prolactin levels will begin to increase to a level that allows the production of milk. The infant's suckling stimulates the secretion of **oxytocin** from the posterior pituitary gland. This causes contraction of the lactiferous ducts, and lactation begins.

The function of the alveoli is to secrete milk into the secondary tubules. All secondary tubules from each lobule converge to form a lactiferous duct. Each lactiferous duct has an ampulla or expanded region called **Montgomery's glands** near the nipple, where milk can be stored until released during suckling. Secretions from the areolar glands keep the nipple area pliant.

SONOGRAPHIC APPEARANCE

The sonographic appearance of the breast depends on several factors, primarily the age of the woman and the functional state of the breast.

Breast tissue is visualized as three distinct layers. The most anterior layer is the subcutaneous layer, which contains the skin, the most anterior connective tissue components, and fat lobules. The middle layer is the mammary layer, which contains the **breast parenchyma.** Fat is seen between the parenchymal elements. This layer varies according to maternal age and breast function.

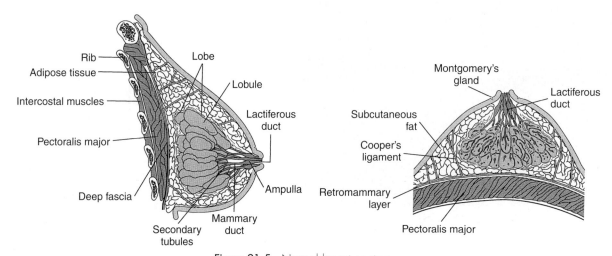

Figure 21-5 Normal breast anatomy.

The most posterior layer is the retromammary layer, which contains fat lobules and the deeper connective tissue components. This layer is bordered posteriorly by the **pectoralis major muscle** (Figure 21-6).

Although all three layers of breast tissue are affected by natural processes, the mammary layer demonstrates the greatest changes sonographically. The younger breast has a higher percentage of parenchyma compared with the percentage of fat within the breast. This higher percentage causes the younger breast to be more dense. Dense parenchyma is difficult to visualize with **mammography;** therefore younger patients presenting with possible masses are often first evaluated by sonography.

With age, the breast parenchyma becomes replaced by fatty tissues. This causes the anterior subcutaneous layer to become more prominent as the mammary layer atrophies and occupies a smaller percentage of overall breast size.

The fat components appear hypoechoic to surrounding parenchymal breast tissue. Breast ducts and ductules appear as anechoic tubular structures. The fibrous components, such as Cooper's ligaments, demonstrate increased echogenicity and are seen as bright, linear echoes. The glandular or parenchymal tissues tend to appear homogeneous in texture, with medium-level to low-level echogenicity. When scanning directly anterior to the nipple, posterior shadowing is visualized (Figure 21-7).

The overall sonographic appearance should be consistent throughout each breast and between the two breasts. When the sonographic appearance is heterogeneous throughout the breast, it allows for differentiation of pathology.

SONOGRAPHIC APPLICATIONS
Sonography can be used to evaluate several aspects of breast structure. The most common application is to de-

termine the composition of a breast mass. The presence of large collections of calcifications may also be detected sonographically, but, again, each collection or individual calcification must be fairly large, at least a few millimeters in diameter.

It is important to remember that ultrasound is not capable of detecting the very small (approximately 1 mm) calcifications that are visible with mammography and often represent the first signs of breast cancer.

Other applications include ruling out the presence of lymph node masses that often accompany breast cancer and evaluating breast implants (Figure 21-8).

In many cases, ultrasound-guided procedures such as breast cyst aspirations and breast biopsies are used as alternatives to surgery.

NORMAL VARIANTS
Several normal variants can be appreciated sonographically. A variant common in women of childbearing age is the fibrocystic breast. Various fibrotic components and cystic areas may be distributed throughout the entire breast.

Another variation is the fatty breast, in which the fatty components are increased, with decreased echogenicity throughout the breast. Deposition of fat increases with age and parity. Breasts often appear more fatty after menopause because the fat components become more prominent as the mammary ducts begin to atrophy. Fatty breasts may demonstrate areas of bright echogenicity due to the connective tissues surrounding the mammary ducts.

The fibrous breast has increased amounts of connective tissue and therefore increased echogenicity. Compression sonography is most helpful in assessing this breast because it eliminates some of the posterior shadowing resulting from the increase in dense connective tissues (Figure 21-9). *Text continued on p. 392*

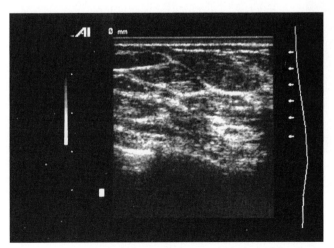 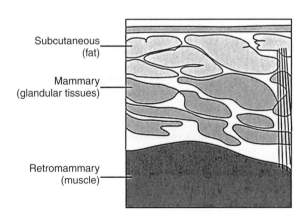

Figure 21-6 The anatomic layers of the breast. (Half-tone image courtesy Acoustic Imaging, Inc., Phoenix, AZ.)

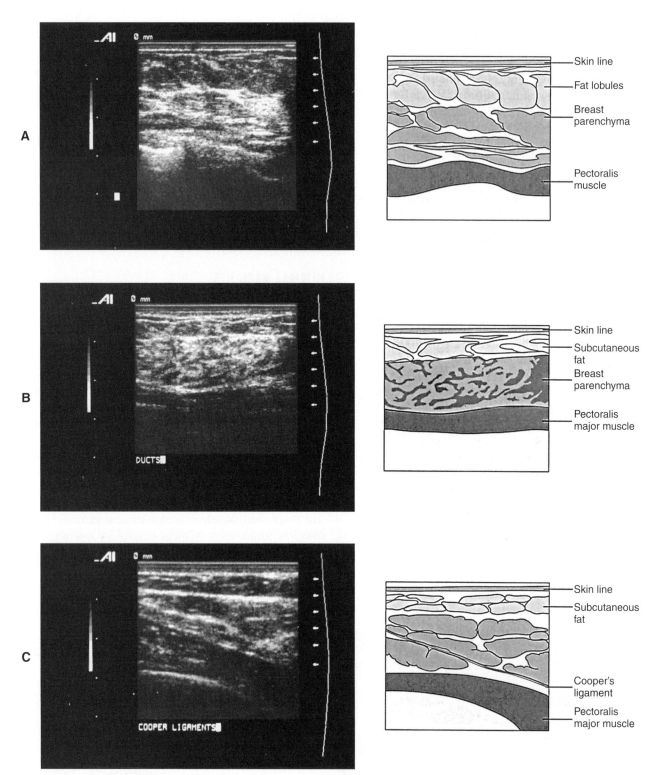

Figure 21-7 **A,** The fatty component of the breast. **B,** Ducts of the breast. **C,** The fibrous component of the breast (Cooper's ligament).

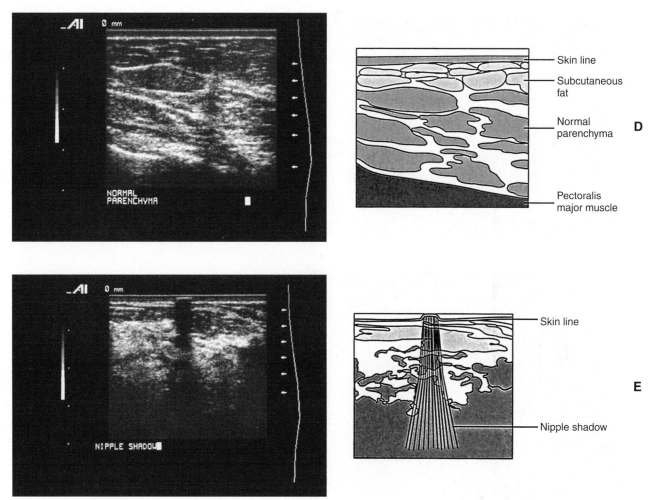

Figure 21-7, cont'd D, The glandular components of the breast. **E,** Posterior nipple shadow. (Half-tone images courtesy Acoustic Imaging, Inc., Phoenix, AZ.)

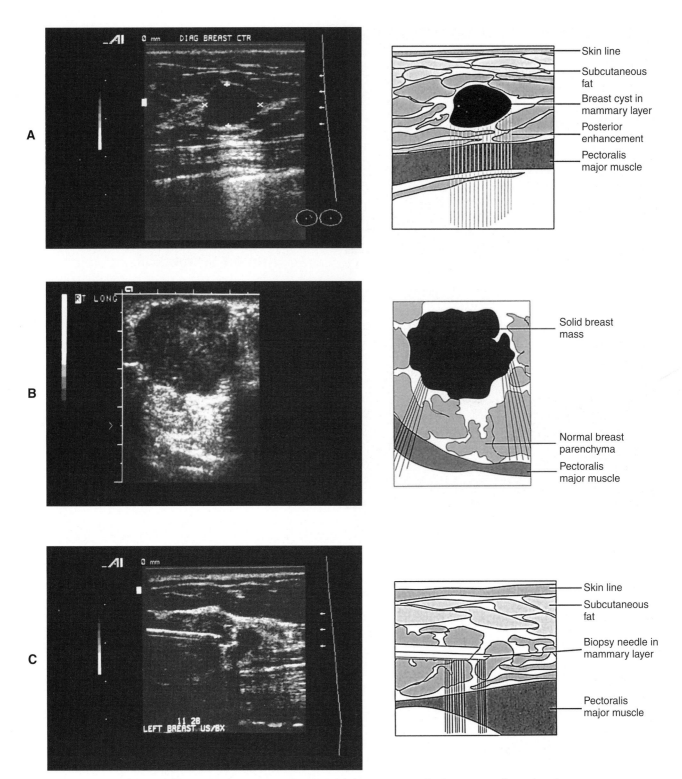

Figure 21-8 **A**, A breast cyst. **B**, A solid breast mass. **C**, Biopsy needle within breast parenchyma. (**A** and **C**, Half-tone images courtesy Acoustic Imaging, Inc., Phoenix, AZ. **B**, Half-tone image courtesy Acuson Corp., Mountain View, CA.)

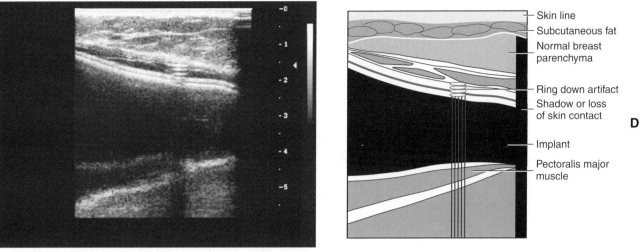

Figure 21-8, cont'd   D, Breast implant. (D, Image courtesy Johns Hopkins Hospital, Baltimore, MD.)

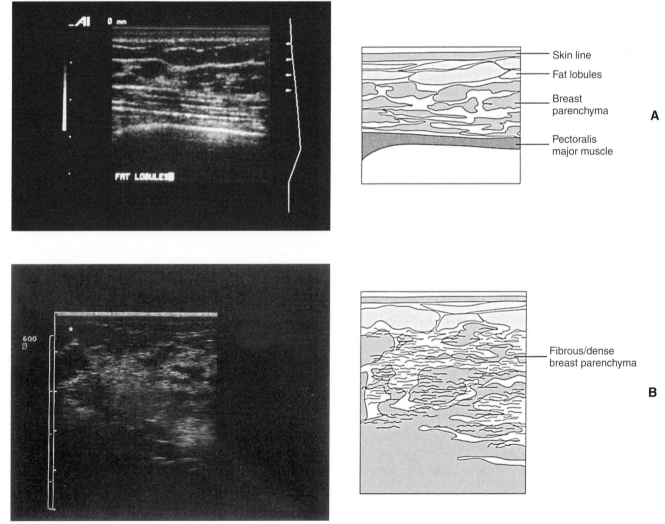

Figure 21-9   A, A fatty breast. B, A fibrous breast. (A, Half-tone image courtesy Acoustic Imaging, Inc., Phoenix, AZ. B, Half-tone image courtesy DePaul Medical Center, Norfolk, VA.)

HOW TO EXAMINE YOUR BREASTS

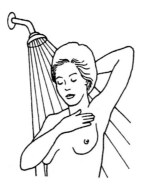

1 In the shower:

Examine your breasts during bath or shower; hands glide easier over wet skin. Fingers flat, move gently over every part of each breast. Use right hand to examine left breast, left hand for right breast. Check for any lump, hard knot or thickening.

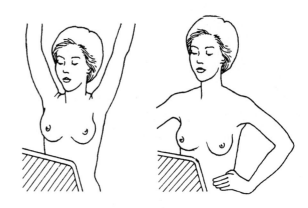

2 Before a mirror:

Inspect your breasts with arms at your sides. Next, raise your arms high overhead. Look for any changes in contour of each breast, a swelling, dimpling of skin or changes in the nipple.

Then, rest palms on hips and press down firmly to flex your chest muscles. Left and right breast will not exactly match – few women's breasts do.

Regular inspection shows what is normal for you and will give you confidence in your examination.

3 Lying down:

To examine your right breast, put a pillow or folded towel under your right shoulder. Place right hand behind your head – this distributes breast tissue more evenly on the chest. With left hand, fingers flat, press gently in small circular motions around an imaginary clock face. Begin at outermost top of your right breast for 12 o'clock, then move to 1 o'clock, and so on around the circle back to 12. A ridge of firm tissue in the lower curve of each breast is normal. Then move in an inch, toward the nipple, keep circling to examine every part of your breast, including nipple. This requires at least three more circles. Now slowly repeat procedure on your left breast with a pillow under your left shoulder and left hand behind head. Notice how your breast structure feels.

Finally, squeeze the nipple of each breast gently between thumb and index finger. Any discharge, clear or bloody, should be reported to your doctor immediately.

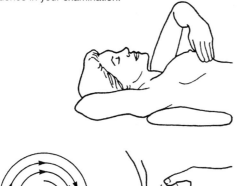

Figure 21-10   The correct procedure for self-examination of the breast. (Courtesy the American Cancer Society.)

REFERENCE CHARTS

■ ■ ■   ASSOCIATED PHYSICIANS

Gynecologist/Obstetrician: Specializes in the examination and treatment of women, including pregnancies. The physician often performs yearly breast examinations as part of a physical examination. Diagnostic tests based on the breast examination may be ordered. Often a referral to a surgeon will be made if follow-up is necessary.

Internist: Specializes in general health care. The physician may be involved in diagnostic testing or in referrals for further follow-up. The physician may be involved in surgical follow-up, if necessary.

Surgeon: Specializes in decision making and in surgical procedures, as well as follow-up made necessary by pathologic findings. This physician is generally responsible for performing surgical procedures such as biopsies, mastectomies, and lumpectomies.

Radiologist: Specializes in interpreting the diagnostic tests used to image the breast. The radiologist may perform procedures such as fine needle biopsies if questionable areas are seen on mammography.

Pathologist: Determines the presence of pathology through typing tissue obtained at biopsy or other surgical procedures, by means of microscopic cellular analysis.

■ ■ ■   COMMON DIAGNOSTIC TESTS

Self-Examination: This test should be performed regularly by all women more than 30 years of age, or by any woman whose family physician has determined that she is at risk for development of breast cancer. Changes of any sort should be reported and assessed by a physician as soon as possible (see Figure 21-10).

Mammography: This is a compression x-ray test used to visualize breast tissue. It easily demonstrates the small clusters of calcification that often indicate early breast cancer. It is recommended that women receive a baseline study at between 35 and 40 years of age, then according to their physician's guidelines. The test is performed by a radiologic technologist and interpreted by a radiologist.

Sonography: Sonography is a nonionizing imaging modality that uses sound waves to obtain diagnostic information. It is often done in conjunction with mammography. It is performed by a sonographer and interpreted by a radiologist.

Thermography: This test assesses breast tissue by indicating skin temperature, but is rarely used in the United States. It is based on the theory that the presence of cancerous tumors will cause the overlying skin to have a different temperature from normal areas. This test would be performed by a technologist and interpreted by a physician, most likely a radiologist.

■ ▪ ▪ LABORATORY VALUES

Carcinoembryonic Antigen (CEA): This antigen level is used following breast cancer. It is secreted by the liver, and may be elevated in cancer removal to rule out tumor recurrence. A decrease in the antigen level represents tumor removal. Antigen levels are then monitored to detect an increase in baseline levels, which would indicate tumor recurrence.

Alkaline Phosphatase: This enzyme may help rule out tumor metastasis in patients with identified breast cancer. It is secreted by the liver, and may be elevated in liver diseases as well as in bone, lung, and pancreatic carcinomas. Alkaline phosphatase is normally elevated during pregnancy and during the first year of life.

■ ▪ ▪ NORMAL MEASUREMENTS

Lactiferous Ducts: Nonpregnant women—2 mm; nursing women—8 mm.

■ ▪ ▪ VASCULATURE

Arterial blood is supplied through the internal thoracic or the internal mammary artery. The internal mammary artery originates off the subclavian artery and enters the breast through the second, third, and fourth intercostal spaces medially and through the lateral thoracic artery. That artery becomes the superficial mammary artery and supplies the more superficial breast structures.

Venous drainage from the breast occurs through a combination of superficial and deep venous systems. The veins course parallel to the arteries.

Lymph drainage from the breast originates in the connective tissues of the breast and follows three main pathways. The breast's lymphatic system originates in lymph capillaries within breast connective tissues.

Seventy-five percent of lymph drainage occurs through the axillary lymph nodes. These nodes are in close proximity to the axillary tail of the breast, which extends superolaterally to border the axilla. Twenty percent of lymph drainage occurs medially through the thoracic nodes, and 5% is subcutaneous through the intercostal nodes.

■ ▪ ▪ AFFECTING CHEMICALS

Prolactin: This hormone, secreted by the anterior pituitary gland, stimulates development of the breast's secretory system. Prolactin secretion is controlled by prolactin-inhibiting hormone, which is produced by the hypothalamus. After the decrease in estrogen that follows childbirth, prolactin levels increase and lactation becomes possible.

Estrogen: Estrogen, produced in the ovaries, stimulates the development of breast tissues and duct systems during puberty.

Oxytocin: This hormone, produced in the hypothalamus and stored in the posterior pituitary gland, causes duct contraction and allows for the flow of milk during nursing.

Progesterone: Progesterone is produced by the placenta. It stimulates development of the breast lobules and alveoli during pregnancy.

Insulin: Normal amounts of insulin, which is produced by the pancreas, are necessary for breast development during pregnancy.

Cortisol: This hormone, produced by the adrenal cortex, is necessary for breast development during pregnancy.

Thyroxine: Thyroxine is produced by the thyroid gland and is necessary for breast development during pregnancy.

Caffeine: A reduction in the level of caffeine may bring about a reduction in breast lumps, swelling, and soreness, especially in women with fibrocystic breast changes. Such a reduction will not affect risk factors for breast cancer.

Vitamin E: This vitamin affects the levels of fat and hormones in the blood and may help relieve pain and swelling of breast tissues.

Danazol: Danazol is a male hormone that may help to decrease pain and swelling of the breast. It suppresses activity of the anterior pituitary gland, and is used to treat women with endometriosis. The hormone may be associated with side effects.

BIBLIOGRAPHY

Moore KL, Persaud TVN: *The developing human: clinically oriented embryology,* ed 6, Philadelphia, 1998, WB Saunders.

Thibodeau GA, Patton KT: *Anatomy and physiology,* ed 4, St Louis, 1999, Mosby.

SECTION **VII**

Introduction to Specialty Sonography

CHAPTER 22

The Neonatal Brain

BETTY BATES TEMPKIN AND REVA ARNEZ CURRY

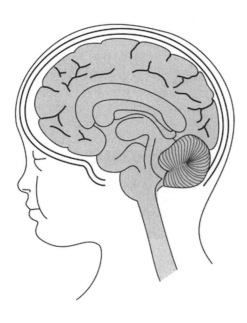

Cavum septum pellucidum
Cavum septum vergae
Centrum semiovale
Cerebellum
Cerebral peduncle
Cerebrospinal fluid (CSF)
Cerebrum
Choroid plexus
Choroidal fissure
Cingulate gyrus/sulcus
Circle of Willis
Cisterna magna
Corpus callosum
Falx cerebri
Foramen of Monro
Fourth ventricle
Frontal lobe
Germinal matrix
Globus pallidus
Glomus
Gyrus/gyri

Interhemispheric fissure
Interpeduncular cistern
Lateral ventricle
Massa intermedia
Medulla oblongata
Midbrain
Occipital lobe
Parietal lobe
Pons
Putamen
Quadrigeminal plate
   cistern
Sulcus/sulci
Sylvian fissure
Temporal lobe
Tentorium cerebelli
Thalamus/thalami
Third ventricle
Trigone
Vermis

OBJECTIVES

Describe the basic prenatal development of the human
   brain.
Identify the major structures in the neonatal brain.
Describe basic brain function.
Describe the sonographic appearance of the neonatal
   brain.
Describe normal structural variants seen sonographically.
Describe associated physicians, diagnostic tests, laboratory
   values, and normal measurements.
Identify the vasculature of the human brain.
Define the key words.

KEY WORDS

Anterior fontanelle
Basal ganglia
Brain stem

Calcarine fissure
Caudate nucleus
Caudothalamic groove

With the significant advances in the image quality and resolution of ultrasound seen in the 1980's, sonography has become the primary imaging study in evaluation of the neonatal brain. Currently, intracranial ultrasound imaging is performed exclusively using compact, high-resolution, real-time transducers. Its portability, low cost, and relative ease of performance make ultrasound particularly advantageous, especially when evaluating unstable premature infants.

Sonographic cross-sectional anatomy of the neonatal brain is best depicted with a series of both modified coronal and sagittal planes. In the past, axial scanning was also utilized, especially for obtaining accurate ventricular dimensions. However, now it is used primarily in Doppler imaging to investigate the **circle of Willis.** Because the **anterior fontanelle** is used as the primary

397

acoustic window, sonographic planes are different from those provided by computed tomography (CT) or magnetic resonance imaging (MRI). Therefore both coronal and sagittal ultrasound scans are angled from the fulcrum of the anterior fontanelle (Figures 22-1 and 22-2).

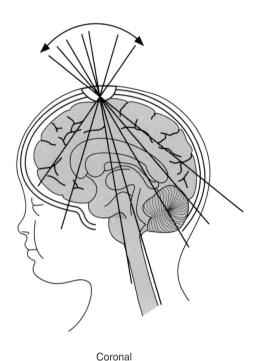

Coronal

Figure 22-1 Coronal survey from the fulcrum of the anterior fontanelle.

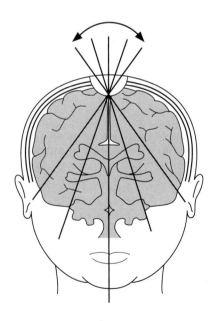

Sagittal

Figure 22-2 Sagittal survey from the fulcrum of the anterior fontanelle.

This chapter stresses especially the normal anatomy and sonographic appearance of the neonatal brain. Standard views and their anatomic landmarks have been described elsewhere and are not discussed here. However, a routine protocol that allows for comparable examinations should always be followed.

PRENATAL DEVELOPMENT

Brain development occurs in three specific stages, progressing from cytogenesis—the development of cells—to histogenesis—the formation of cells into tissues—to organogenesis—the formation of tissues into organs. Congenital malformations frequently result from an alteration of the normal events of organogenesis.

Organogenesis can be divided into several specific developmental events. The first major event, neural tube formation, has a peak occurrence at 3 to 4 weeks of gestation. The evolving neural plate folds in on itself and closes dorsally to form the embryonic neural tube, which gives rise to the early brain and spinal cord. By the end of this period, three primary brain vesicles are apparent: the forebrain (prosencephalon), the midbrain (mesencephalon), and the hindbrain (rhombencephalon) (Figure 22-3).

At 5 to 6 weeks of gestation, the most anterior brain vesicles, the prosencephalon, diverticulates (i.e., folds) to form the separate telencephalon (endbrain) and the diencephalon (in-between brain) (Figure 22-4). The telencephalon gives rise to the large cerebral hemispheres, the basal ganglia, and the lateral ventricles, and the diencephalon forms the thalamus and hypothalamus. The paired olfactory bulbs and optic tracts and unpaired pineal and pituitary glands also arise from the diverticulation of the forebrain (prosencephalon).

Another major event involves the proliferation of the developing brain's neurons (i.e., nerve cells). This occurs between the second and fourth months of gestation. All of the neurons are located in subependymal locations and thereby proliferate from both ventricular and subventricular areas. Unfortunately, very little is

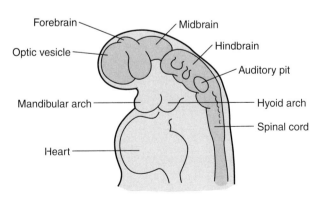

Figure 22-3 First stage in the early development of the brain at 3½ weeks.

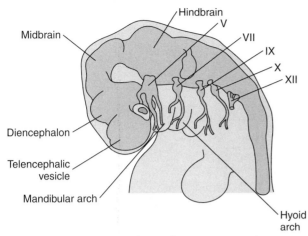

Figure 22-4 Developing brain at 5½ weeks.

known about the quantitative aspects of this event. Disorders of neuronal proliferation can result in either microencephaly or macroencephaly.

Neuronal migration occurs from primarily the third to fifth months of gestation. During this time, a remarkable series of occurrences takes place. Millions of neurons in their original ventricular and subventricular sites migrate to new locations within the central nervous system where they will reside permanently. Again, disorders in this major event result in severe neurologic disturbances.

From approximately the sixth month of gestation to several years after birth, major organizational events occur. These events settle the elaborate circuitry that distinguishes the human brain. One example of an organizational event is the proper alignment, orientation, and layering of the neurons of the cerebral cortex.

Finally, myelination, the laying down of a highly specialized myelin membrane, takes place. This event takes a very long time, continuing from the second trimester of pregnancy into adult life.

LOCATION

The location of the structures of the neonatal brain is discussed in the Sonographic Appearance section.

SIZE

Nonapplicable.

GROSS ANATOMY

The gross anatomy of the neonatal brain is identified and discussed in the Sonographic Appearance section.

PHYSIOLOGY

The human brain, the body's largest and most complex mass of nervous tissue, functions with remarkable abilities. It can be considered in terms of four major regions: cerebral hemispheres, diencephalon, brain stem, and cerebellum.

The brain's largest and most superior region, the paired cerebral hemispheres, exhibits elevated folds of tissue called **gyri,** and grooves called **sulci,** or fissures, which serve as important anatomic landmarks. The single deep **interhemispheric fissure,** for example, separates the hemispheres. Other fissures divide each hemisphere into four lobes. The cerebral cortical neurons (i.e., the outermost gray matter) are responsible for such functions as speech, memory, voluntary movement, logical reasoning, and emotional response. The **parietal lobe** contains the body's sensory receptors, which interpret the impulses that allow one to recognize such sensations as pain, cold, or a light touch (Figure 22-5). Importantly, because the sensory pathways are crossed pathways, the impulses from the body's right side are received by the left hemisphere's sensory cortex. This somatic sensory area is located posterior to the central fissure. Other cortical areas are responsible for interpreting impulses from the special sense organs. For example, the auditory area is adjacent to the sylvian fissure in the **temporal lobe,** and the olfactory area is deeper in the same lobe. The posterior part of the **occipital lobe** interprets visual impulses (see Figure 22-5).

The primary motor area is located anterior to the central fissure in the **frontal lobe.** This area controls the movements of the conscious skeletal muscles, such as those in the face, mouth, and hands. The motor pathways are crossed pathways as in the somatic sensory cortex.

The anterior part of the frontal lobes is believed to house the higher intellectual reasoning function. Complex memories are probably stored in both the temporal and frontal lobes. The speech function is located at the junction of the temporal, parietal, and occipital horns (see Figure 22-5).

The diencephalon (i.e., interbrain) rests superior to the brain stem and is enclosed by the cerebral hemispheres. Three distinct structures make up the diencephalon: the thalamus, hypothalamus, and epithalamus. The thalamus serves as a relay station for upward-moving sensory impulses. As a result, we can experience a crude recognition of both pleasant and unpleasant sensations. The hypothalamus, lying under the thalamus, plays a role in regulating body temperature, fluid balance, and metabolism. Additionally, it functions as the center for such drives as thirst, appetite, and sex.

The structures of the **brain stem,** the **midbrain, pons,** and **medulla oblongata** provide a pathway for ascending and descending fiber tracts. Additionally, they have small areas (i.e., nuclei) that are involved in such vital activities as swallowing and blood pressure. The pons, for example, contains nuclei involved in the control of breathing, and the medulla oblongata helps control heart rate, breathing, and vomiting, among others.

The **cerebellum** functions to provide balance and equilibrium to the body by adjusting the timing of

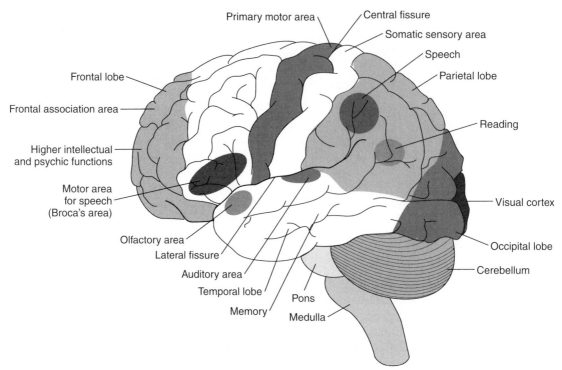

Figure 22-5 Lateral view of the brain. Some functional areas of the cerebral hemispheres.

skeletal muscle activity. As a result, body movements are coordinated and smooth.

SONOGRAPHIC APPEARANCE

When the neonatal brain is examined, the relative echogenicity of various intracranial structures, along with their locations, can be described. Appreciation of the normal anatomic structures becomes essential when ruling out intracranial pathology.

Sonographically, the bones comprising the cranial vault appear highly echogenic. The parenchyma of the large cerebral hemispheres reveals a mostly homogeneous texture of relatively low echogenicity. Interspersed throughout the cerebral cortex are thin echogenic lines representing various sulci and/or fissures that separate the cerebral folds (i.e., gyri).

When the neonatal brain is viewed in a modified coronal plane, the normal frontal horns and bodies of the **lateral ventricles** appear as thin, crescentlike, fluid-filled bilateral spaces. The hypoechoic **corpus callosum** forms their superior margin in the midline. The longitudinal echogenic line seen extending from the superior edge of the brain in the midline marks the **falx cerebri** within the interhemispheric fissure (Figure 22-6).

Anterior to the frontal horns, in the frontal cerebral cortex, a symmetric, echogenic area can be noted. Commonly referred to as the normal periventricular "blush" or "halo," this area corresponds to the frontal periventricular white matter area. The echogenic orbital cones can be seen inferiorly (Figure 22-7).

The frontal horns of the lateral ventricles are separated by the septum pellucidum, which forms their medial margins in the midline. The anechoic **cavum septum pellucidum** is a normal variant sometimes noted here in the neonate. The moderately hyperechoic head of the **caudate nucleus** forms the inferolateral margin of the anterior horns (Figure 22-8). It represents the more superior aspect of the gray matter of the **basal ganglia.** Immediately lateral and inferior to the caudate nucleus, the **putamen** and **globus pallidus** of the basal ganglia can be noted as areas of increased echogenicity relative to the surrounding parenchyma (Figure 22-9). The hypoechoic anterior corpus callosum forms the superior margin of the frontal horns. The superior margin of the corpus callosum is marked by the echogenic pericallosal sulcus. Superior to this is the hypoechoic **cingulate gyrus** and then the hyperechoic **cingulate sulcus** (see Figure 22-6).

The area of the **foramen of Monro** can be shown just posterior to the frontal horns. The bilateral foramina lie inferomedial to the bodies of the lateral ventricles and mark the communication between the lateral and third ventricles (Figure 22-10). The **third ventricle,** filled with **cerebrospinal fluid (CSF),** lies inferior to the foramina in the midline. It can be difficult to visualize in its transverse dimension when normal in size; however, it is clearly noted as an anechoic structure when dilated. The moderately hyperechoic body of the caudate nucleus marks the inferolateral margin of the bodies of the lateral ventricles. Also noted at this level are the lateral echogenic **sylvian fissures,** which divide the frontal and

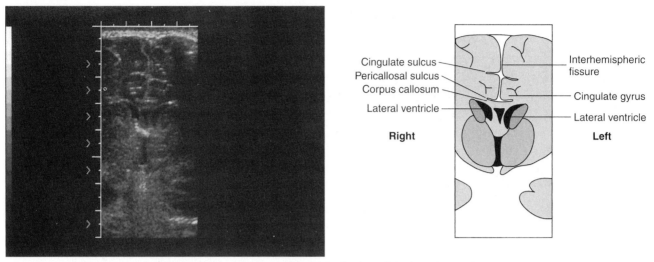

Figure 22-6 Coronal image of the bodies of the lateral ventricles.

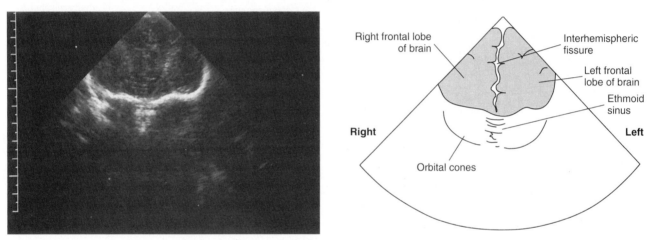

Figure 22-7 Coronal image of the frontal cerebral cortex.

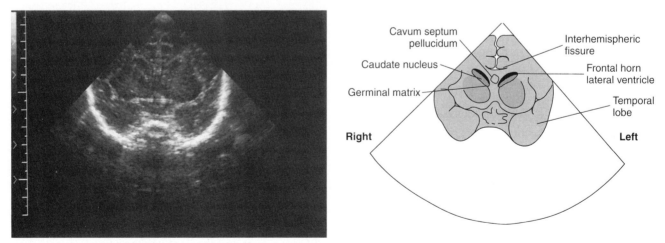

Figure 22-8 Coronal image of the frontal horns of the lateral ventricles showing the head of the caudate nucleus.

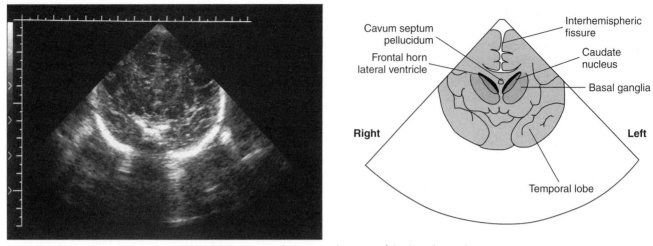

Figure 22-9   *Coronal image in the area of the basal ganglia.*

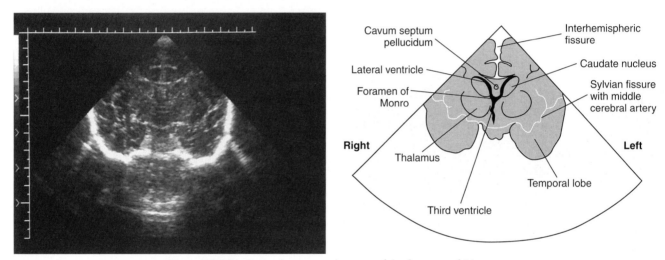

Figure 22-10   *Coronal image in the area of the foramen of Monro.*

temporal lobes of the cerebral cortex. The middle cerebral arteries lie here and are frequently seen pulsating on a real-time image. The echogenic **interpeduncular cistern** is also noted inferiorly. Near this cistern, the pulsations of the basilar artery are also frequently seen during the real-time examination (see Figure 22-9).

Another coronal view shows the homogeneous **thalami,** which can be seen lying inferior to the bodies of the lateral ventricles. The posterior aspect of the slitlike third ventricle lies between them. The anterior extent of the highly echogenic **choroid plexus** can be noted in the groove between the lateral ventricles. Choroid plexus also lies in the roof of the third and fourth ventricles. A pair of hypoechoic structures can be shown inferior to the thalami and just above the highly echogenic **tentorium cerebelli** and **choroidal fissures.** These represent the **cerebral peduncles.** The tent-shaped tentorium cerebelli separates the cerebellum from the more superior structures (Figure 22-11). This view also reveals the moder-

ately echogenic pons and medulla oblongata of the brain stem (seen inferiorly).

A coronal view through the **quadrigeminal plate cistern** reveals an echogenic, star-shaped structure inferior to the lateral ventricular bodies. The lateral extensions meet with the choroidal fissures, the brightly echogenic curving arcs, and the tentorium is noted inferiorly. Sometimes evident at this level is the **fourth ventricle,** a rectangular anechoic space in the midline (Figure 22-12). It lies just anterior to the vermis of the cerebellum in the posterior fossa. Sonographically, the **vermis,** the midline portion of the cerebellum, is quite echogenic, whereas the lateral cerebellar hemispheres are noticeably less echogenic. The anechoic **cisterna magna** is seen in the space between the inferior vermis and the occipital bone (see Figure 22-12).

Scanning more posteriorly reveals the **trigone** region of the lateral ventricles, where the bodies, occipital horns, and temporal horns converge. Most noticeable is the highly echogenic **glomus** of the choroid plexus within the trigones, which should generally demonstrate smooth margins (Figure 22-13). The lateral ventricles diverge laterally at this level and are divided by the posterior corpus callosum, which appears as an echogenic line between the ventricles. The area of increased periventricular echogenicity appears lateral to the trigones and should be less echogenic than the adjacent choroid plexus (see Figure 22-13).

Viewing the neonatal brain posterior and cephalad to the trigones reveals the symmetric, moderately echogenic "blush" of the posterior periventricular white matter (i.e., **centrum semiovale**). This area is visible on either side of the echogenic interhemispheric fissure. Also noted is the echogenic **calcarine fissure** coursing perpendicular from the interhemispheric fissure. A number of echogenic superficial cortical sulci extend from the lateral margins of the brain (Figure 22-14).

Viewing the neonatal brain in sagittal sections from the fulcrum of the anterior fontanelle also reveals several important anatomic landmarks. The hypoechoic, crescent-

shaped corpus callosum, for example, can be clearly recognized in the midline. It lies just superior to the anechoic cavum septum pellucidum and **cavum septum vergae,** when they are present. The echogenic pericallosal sulcus surrounds the corpus callosum and contains the pericallosal arteries. The thin, hyperechoic curved line superior to the pericallosal sulcus represents the cingulate sulcus, which separates the hypoechoic cingulate gyrus from the more superficial gyri. Pulsations from the anterior cerebral arteries are often seen just anterior to the corpus callosum during real-time scanning. Lying inferior to the cavum septum pellucidum and vergae (when present) is the normal slit—like third ventricle. The **massa intermedia,** a homogeneous, soft tissue structure, can be noted in a dilated third ventricle. The echogenic band lying posterior to the third ventricle represents the quadrigeminal plate cistern. Marking the inferior end of this cistern is the highly echogenic cerebellar vermis. Again, the anechoic cisterna magna arises just inferior to the vermis. Indenting the anterior vermis is the anechoic fourth ventricle, which ap-

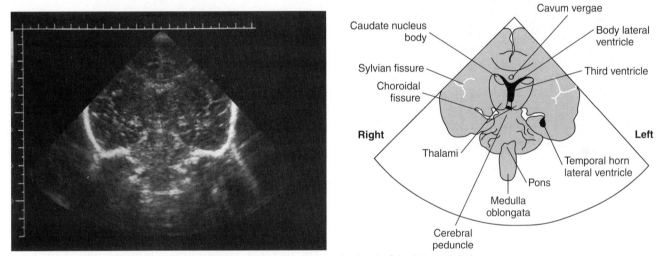

Figure 22-11 Coronal image at the level of the bilateral thalami.

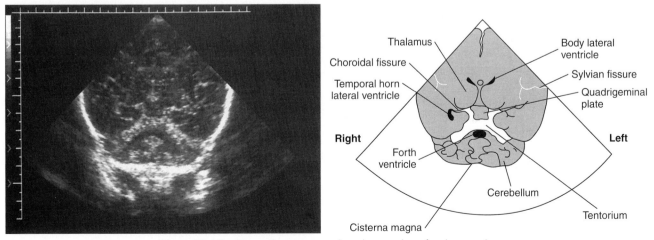

Figure 22-12 Coronal image revealing the anechoic fourth ventricle.

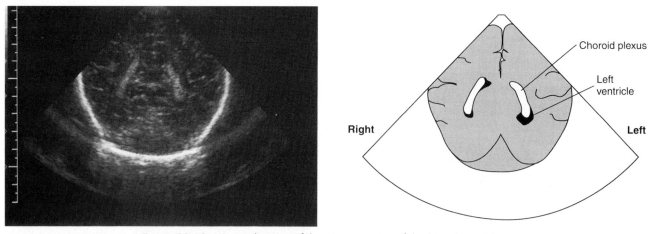

Figure 22-13   Coronal image of the trigone region of the lateral ventricles.

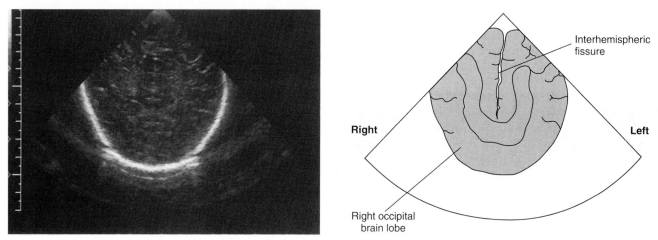

Figure 22-14   Coronal image posterior and cephalad to the trigones.

pears triangular in this plane. The moderately echogenic pons and medulla oblongata of the brain stem occupy the area anterior to the fourth ventricle (Figure 22-15).

Another important anatomic landmark, the **caudothalamic groove,** is clearly shown on a sagittal view. This groove is seen as a thin, brightly echogenic arc positioned between the head of the caudate nucleus and the thalamus (Figure 22-16). It marks the area of **germinal matrix,** which is found more anterosuperiorly. Being composed of a fine network of blood vessels and neural tissue, the germinal matrix is highly susceptible to hemorrhage in the premature infant. (Pressure and metabolic changes can lead to rupture of these small vessels.) Although the germinal matrix lies in the subependymal layer of the ventricular system in early fetal life, it regresses to the area over the head of the caudate nucleus by 6 months' gestation. It cannot be seen as a distinct structure at term by ultrasound. The caudate nucleus, lying more anteriorly, is normally slightly more echogenic than the thalamus.

A sagittal view can also simultaneously reveal all the horns of the lateral ventricles. The amount of CSF present in them varies greatly; however, the normal anechoic ventricles are often seen as slitlike structures. This area can also be characterized by the highly echogenic glomus of the choroid plexus present in the trigone region of the lateral ventricles (Figure 22-17). The normal choroid tapers as it courses anteriorly toward the foramen of Monro and should display a smooth contour. Surrounding the lateral ventricles are the frontal, parietal, temporal, and occipital lobes of the **cerebrum.** The echogenic periventricular "blush" should again be noted posterior to the occipital horns. This corresponds to an area of the posterior periventricular white matter.

A sagittal view to the far lateral left or right reveals the echogenic sylvian fissure and the temporal lobe of the cerebral cortex (Figure 22-18). Again, the middle cerebral arteries can commonly be seen pulsating in the sylvian fissures. Numerous echogenic linear and curvilinear sulci can be seen in the term infant at this level.

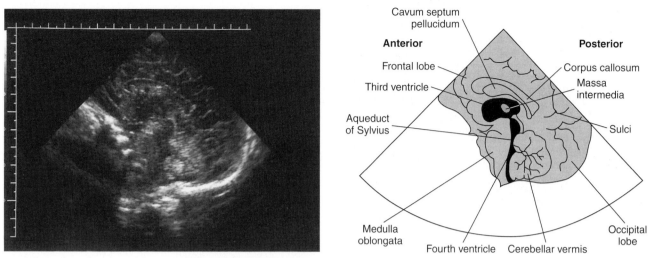

Figure 22-15 Sagittal image in the midline of the brain.

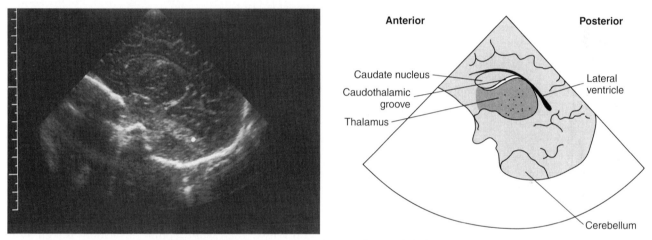

Figure 22-16 Sagittal image showing the caudothalamic groove.

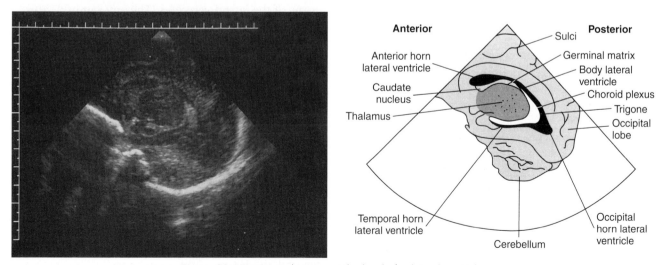

Figure 22-17 Sagittal image at the level of a lateral ventricle.

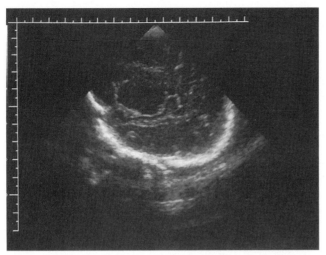

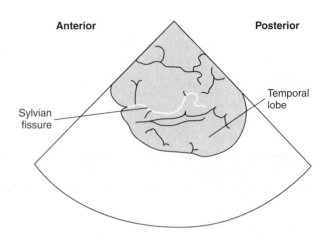

Figure 22-18 Sagittal image revealing a lateral sylvian fissure.

The echogenic "blush" from the periventricular area is again noted.

SONOGRAPHIC APPLICATIONS

Common considerations when performing sonography of the neonatal brain include Doppler evaluation of cerebral blood flow abnormalities and detection of:

1. Congenital anomalies
2. Intracranial hemorrhage
3. Intracranial masses
4. Venous malformations
5. Hydrocephalus (i.e., ventricular size)
6. Intracranial infections
7. Infarction and/or edema

NORMAL VARIANTS

Normal variants of the neonatal brain are typically associated with gestational immaturity.

Lateral Ventricles

Asymmetry in the size of the lateral ventricles is a common normal variant. Approximately 40% of premature infants and less than 20% of term infants reveal some asymmetry. The left lateral ventricle is generally larger than the right. The occipital horns are particularly susceptible (Figure 22-19). Interestingly, ventricular size varies with the age of the infant. As the infant matures, the lateral ventricular size decreases in relation to the size of the cerebral cortex.

Cavum Septum Pellucidum and Cavum Septum Vergae

Two common variants frequently noted in the normal infant are the cavum septum pellucidum and the cavum septum vergae. The cavum septum pellucidum is seen as an anechoic, fluid-filled space between the anterior horns of the lateral ventricles, whereas the cavum septum vergae lies most posterior, between the bodies (Figure 22-20). Al-

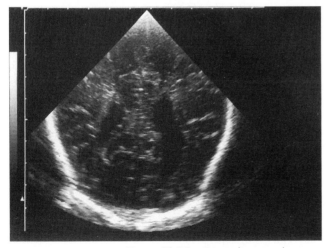

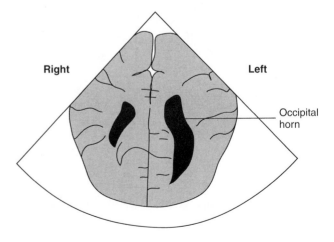

Figure 22-19 Coronal image showing asymmetry in the size of the occipital horns.

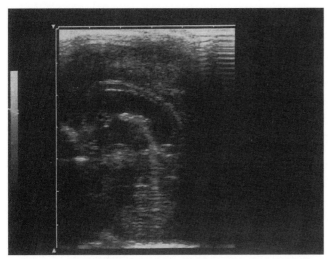

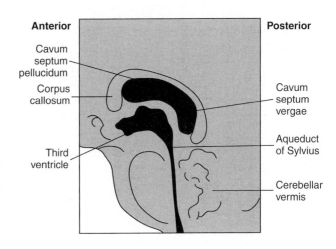

Figure 22-20 Sagittal image of a normal brain with the cavum septum pellucidum and cavum septum vergae.

though these structures communicate with each other, they do not connect with the ventricular system.

The cavum septum vergae closes from posterior to anterior beginning in the sixth month of gestation. So, while this structure can be seen in a premature infant, it is infrequently seen in the term infant. On the other hand, the cavum septum pellucidum begins to close near term. Therefore it can be noted alone until approximately 2 months of postnatal life.

REFERENCE CHARTS

■ ■ ■   ASSOCIATED PHYSICIANS

Radiologist: Specializes in the diagnostic interpretation of imaging modalities that assess central nervous system pathology.
Neurologist: Specializes in the diagnosis and treatment of disorders of the nervous system.
Neonatologist: Specializes in the diagnosis and treatment of disorders of the newborn infant.

■ ■ ■   COMMON DIAGNOSTIC TESTS

Computed Axial Tomography (CT Scan): Provides cross-sectional (i.e., axial) x-ray images of the brain to assess anatomy. A contrast medium is often administered to differentiate between pathology and normal anatomy. This test is performed by a radiologic technologist or radiologist. Interpretation of the test is by the radiologist.
Magnetic Resonance Imaging (MRI): Provides valuable information about the body's biochemistry when the patient is placed in a magnetic field. Provides axial, sagittal, and coronal images of the brain directly. This diagnostic imaging technique does not require exposure to ionizing radiation. The test is performed by a radiologic technologist or radiologist and interpreted by the radiologist.

Electroencephalography (EEG): Records changes in electric potential (i.e., activity) in various locations of the brain by means of electrodes placed on the scalp. This test is performed by a technologist and interpreted by a neurologist.

■ ■ ■   LABORATORY VALUES

Hematocrit: This laboratory test measures the percentage of blood that is composed of red blood cells, expressed as volume percent. A decreasing hematocrit can be an indication of a possible intracranial hemorrhage.

■ ■ ■   NORMAL MEASUREMENTS

VENTRICULAR SIZE
Ventricular Depth: In a coronal plane at the level of the foramen of Monro, the bodies of the lateral ventricles are measured from wall to wall (Figure 22-21). This measurement is the widest line perpendicular to the longest axis of the ventricles.
NORMAL MEASUREMENT: 4 mm or less.
Midline to Lateral Dimension: In the same coronal plane, this measurement is the horizontal distance from the midline (i.e., falx) to the most lateral aspect of the lateral ventricles (see Figure 22-21).
NORMAL MEASUREMENT: 12 mm or less.

■ ■ ■   VASCULATURE

The internal carotid and vertebral arteries supply blood to the brain (Figure 22-22).
A) Aorta—brachiocephalic (rt.)—common carotid artery—INTERNAL CAROTID ARTERY—anterior cerebral artery—anterior communicating artery—middle cerebral artery—posterior communicating artery.

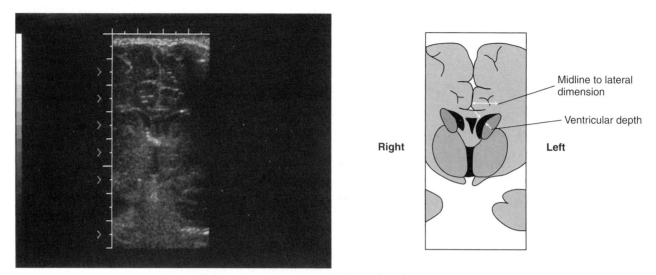

Figure 22-21 Coronal image at the level of the foramen of Monro.

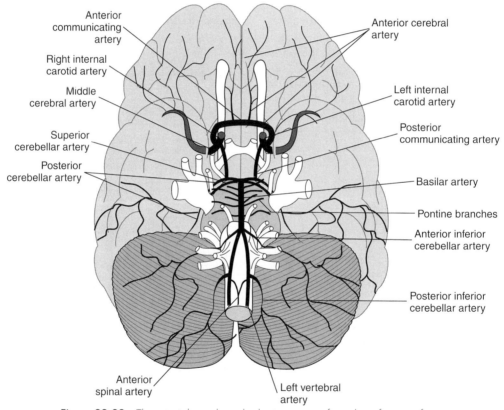

Figure 22-22 The arterial supply to the brain as seen from the inferior surface.

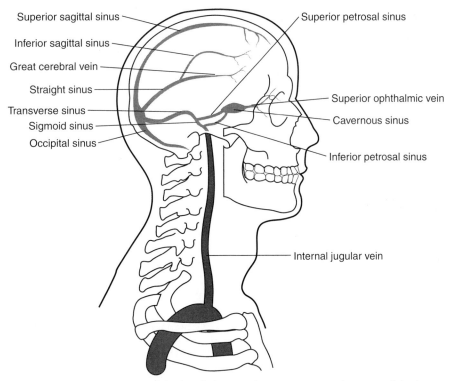

Superior sagittal sinus
Inferior sagittal sinus
Great cerebral vein
Straight sinus
Transverse sinus
Sigmoid sinus
Occipital sinus

Superior petrosal sinus
Superior ophthalmic vein
Cavernous sinus
Inferior petrosal sinus
Internal jugular vein

Figure 22-23 Lateral view of the head showing the major venous drainage of the brain.

B) Aorta—brachiocephalic (rt.)—rt. subclavian artery—VERTEBRAL ARTERY—anterior spinal artery—basilar artery—posterior inferior cerebellar artery—anterior inferior cerebellar artery—superior cerebellar artery—posterior cerebral artery.

Large veins, called sinuses, found in the brain's tough covering (i.e., the dura mater), drain the brain (Figure 22-23).

Superior sagittal sinus—inferior sagittal sinus—great cerebral vein of Galen—straight sinus—occipital sinus—transverse sinus—sigmoid sinus—superior ophthalmic vein—cavernous sinus—superior petrosal sinus—inferior petrosal sinus—internal jugular vein.

■ ■ ■ **AFFECTING CHEMICALS**

Nonapplicable.

BIBLIOGRAPHY

Dykstra-Downey K: Neonatal brain scanning protocol. In Tempkin BB: *Ultrasound scanning: principles and protocols,* Philadelphia, 1993, WB Saunders, pp 234-245.

Grant EG, editor: *Neurosonography of the pre-term neonate,* New York, 1986, Springer-Verlag.

Marieb EN: *Essentials of human anatomy and physiology,* ed 3, Redwood City, CA, 1991, Benjamin/Cummings.

Naidich TP, Quencer RM, editors: *Clinical neurosonography: ultrasound of the central nervous system,* New York, 1987, Springer-Verlag.

Rumack CM, Charboneau JW, Wilson SR, editors: *Diagnostic ultrasound,* ed 2, St. Louis, 1998, Mosby.

Sauerbrei EE, Digney M, Harrison PB, Cooperberg PL: Ultrasonic evaluation of neonatal intracranial hemorrhage and its complications, *Radiology* 139:677-685, 1981.

Siegel MI, editor: *Pediatric sonography,* New York, 1991, Raven Press.

Teele RL, Share JC: *Ultrasonography of infants and children,* Philadelphia, 1991, WB Saunders.

Tempkin BB: *Ultrasound scanning: principles and protocols,* ed 2, Philadelphia, 1998, WB Saunders.

Volpe JJ: *Neurology of the newborn,* ed 2, Philadelphia, 1987, WB Saunders.

CHAPTER 23

Pediatric Echocardiography

VIVIE MILLER

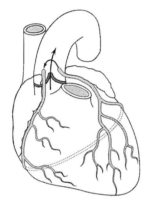

The pediatric heart.

OBJECTIVES

Describe the function of the heart.

Describe the size and position of the heart in the normal child.

Name the chambers, great veins, and great arteries of the heart.

Describe the flow of blood through the heart of a fully developed fetus including the fetal shunts and their purpose.

Describe the flow of blood through the heart of a normal neonate after closure of the fetal shunts.

Describe the sonographic appearance of the pediatric heart.

Describe the associated physicians.

Describe the associated diagnostic tests.

Define the key words.

KEY WORDS

Aorta (ascending, transverse, descending)	Atrioventricular node (AV node)
Aortic valve	Atrium (left, right)
Apex	Base
Bundle of His	Papillary muscles
Cardiac veins	Pericardium (parietal, visceral)
Chordae tendineae	Pulmonary artery (main, left, right)
Common carotid artery (left, right)	Pulmonary valve
Coronary arteries	Pulmonary veins
Coronary sinus	Purkinje fibers
Diastole	Semilunar valves
Ductus arteriosus	Sinoatrial node (SA node)
Ductus venosus	Sinuses of Valsalva
Endocardium	Subclavian artery (left, right)
Foramen ovale	Superior vena cava
Inferior vena cava	Systole
Innominate artery	Tricuspid valve
Interatrial septum	Ventricle (left, right)
Interventricular septum	
Mitral valve	
Myocardium	

The structures of the heart include four chambers, four main valves, two great veins, four smaller veins, two great arteries, septa, and muscle.

The heart is the muscular pump of the body's cardiovascular system, providing the force that propels blood through all the vessels. The heart and vessels are a distribution and collection system in general, providing transportation for the distribution of nutrients, gases, minerals, vitamins, hormones, and blood cells to the tissues and collection of waste products for excretion from the body.

1. The tissues of the body receive oxygen and nutrients.

2. The tissues of the body have a disposal service for the collection and excretion of waste products such as carbon dioxide and other toxic materials.

3. The tissues of the body can release secretory materials or hormones that can quickly exert an influence on body parts distant from the source.
4. Medications injected into the body are distributed quickly throughout all areas of the body.
5. The body's defense system, which includes antibodies and white blood cells, moves to areas of infection and inflammation.

PRENATAL DEVELOPMENT

In the 3-week-old embryo, the heart arises as two cords, called cardiogenic cords. These cords will canalize to form two heart tubes. The heart tubes will gradually move toward each other and fuse to form a single heart tube (Figure 23-1). The tube elongates and develops alternative dilatations and constrictions, which indicate the development to come. The bulbus cordis and ventricle

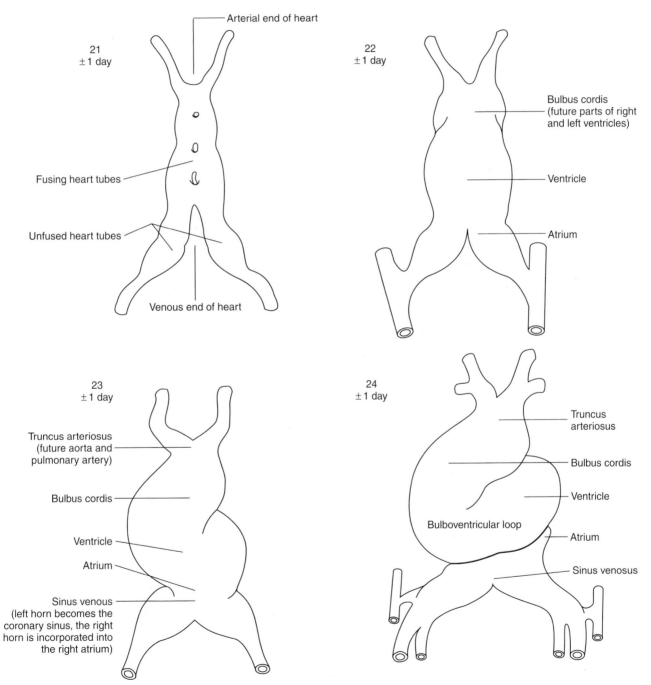

Figure 23-1   Ventral views of the developing heart at 20 to 25 days, showing fusion of the endocardial heart tube to form a single tube. Note bending to form the bulboventricular loop.

grow faster than other regions, causing the heart tube to bend upon itself and form a bulboventricular loop. Normal looping is toward the right. The result is that the atrium and the sinus venosus (which will later form right and left horns) come to lie posterior and superior to the bulbus cordis, truncus arteriosus, and ventricle.

Beginning in the fourth week of embryologic development and by the end of the seventh week, the heart is completely partitioned into two atria, two ventricles, two great arteries, and veins.

Partitioning of the atrioventricular canal begins during the fourth week of embryologic development (Figure 23-2). Swellings called endocardial cushions form on the dorsal and ventral walls of the atrioventricular canal. These cushions develop and grow toward each other, fusing during the fifth week. The heart is now divided into a right and left atrioventricular canal.

The partitioning of the common atrium is accomplished by the formation of two septa, the septum primum and the septum secundum (Figure 23-3). A thin, crescent-shaped membrane called the septum primum (the first septum) grows toward the fused endocardial cushions, beginning at the dorsocranial wall of the primitive atrium. As this curtainlike septum grows toward the endocardial cushions, a large opening, the foramen primum, forms. This opening eventually closes as the septum primum continues to grow toward and fuse with the endocardial cushions. However, before the foramen primum is closed, perforations, or fenestrations, appear in the dorsal part of the septum primum and form another, second, opening called the foramen secundum. At about this time, the septum primum joins or fuses with the left side of the endocardial cushions to completely close the foramen primum. By the end of

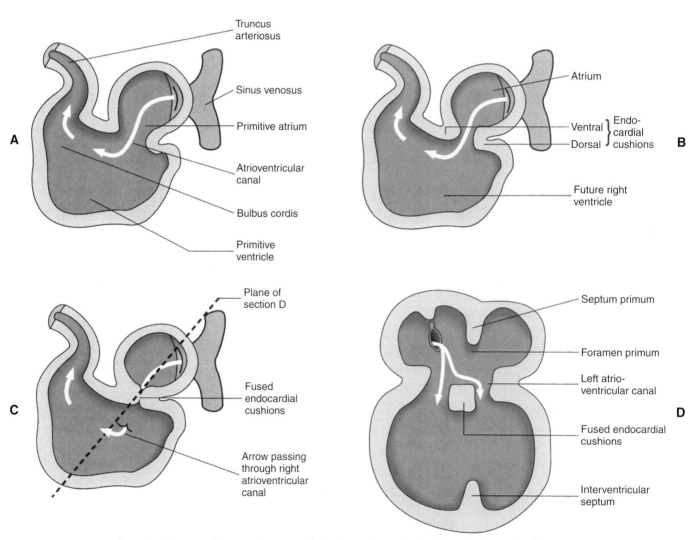

Figure 23-2 A to C, Sagittal sections of the heart during the fourth and fifth weeks, illustrating division of the atrioventricular canal. D, Coronal section of the heart at the plane shown in C. Note that the interatrial and interventricular septa have also begun to develop.

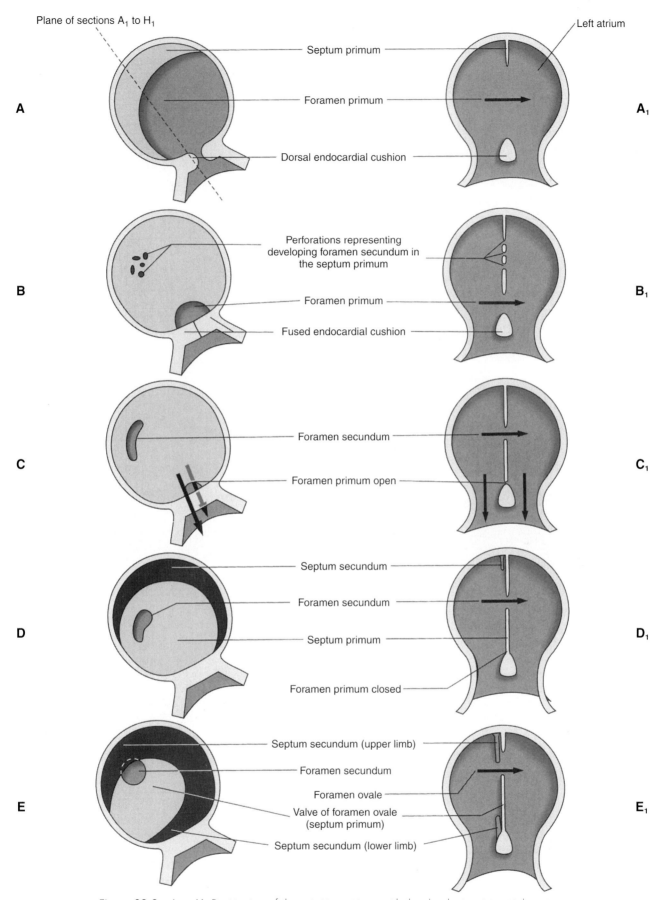

continued

Figure 23-3 **A** to **H,** Partitioning of the primitive atrium, with the developing interatrial septum viewed from the right side. **A₁** to **H₁,** Coronal sections of the developing interatrial septum at the plane shown in **A.** Note that as the septum secundum develops, it overlaps the opening in the septum primum (foramen secundum). The valvelike nature of the foramen ovale is illustrated in **G** and **H.** When pressure in the right atrium exceeds that in the left atrium (as in the fetus), blood passes from the right to the left side of the heart. When the pressures are equal or higher in the left atrium (as is normal after birth), the septum primum closes the foramen ovale.

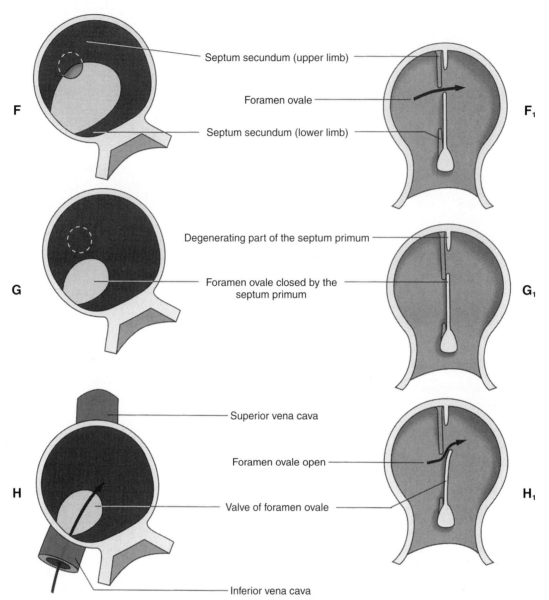

Figure 23-3, cont'd   **A** to **H,** Partitioning of the primitive atrium, with the developing interatrial septum viewed from the right side. **A₁** to **H₁,** Coronal sections of the developing interatrial septum at the plane shown in **A.** Note that as the septum secundum develops, it overlaps the opening in the septum primum (foramen secundum). The valvelike nature of the foramen ovale is illustrated in **G** and **H.** When pressure in the right atrium exceeds that in the left atrium (as in the fetus), blood passes from the right to the left side of the heart. When the pressures are equal or higher in the left atrium (as is normal after birth), the septum primum closes the foramen ovale.

the fifth week, another crescentic membrane grows from the ventrocranial wall of the atrium, immediately to the right of the septum primum. This is the septum secundum, or second septum. As it grows, it covers or overlaps the foramen secundum that formed in the septum primum to form an oval opening, the **foramen ovale.** The cranial part of the septum primum gradually disappears. The remaining part of the septum attaches to the endocardial cushions to form the flap of the foramen ovale. This is one of three fetal shunts.

Partitioning of the primitive ventricle begins with a muscular ridge in the floor of the single ventricle near the apex (Figure 23-4; see Figure 23-7). This foramen is subsequently closed with ridges extending from the right and left sides of the bulbus cordis, called bulbar ridges, and the endocardial cushions (Figure 23-5). The thin, small, membranous interventricular septum is derived from an extension of tissue from the right side of the fused endocardial cushions. This tissue merges with the aorticopulmonary septum (fused bulbar ridges) and the thick mus-

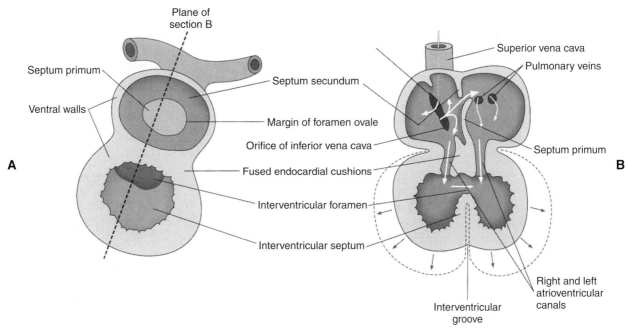

Figure 23-4 Partitioning of the primitive heart. **A,** Sagittal section in the fifth week, showing the cardiac septa and foramina. **B,** Coronal section at a slightly later stage, illustrating the direction of blood flow through the heart and expansion of the ventricles. Note the formation of the interventricular septum and the interventricular foramen in both diagrams.

cular interventricular septum. After closure of the interventricular septum, the **aorta** communicates with the left ventricle, and the pulmonary trunk communicates with the right ventricle. There is now no direct communication between the newly formed right and left ventricles.

The bulbus cordis and truncus arteriosus begin partitioning into the aorta and pulmonary artery during the fifth week. The growth of cells in the wall of the bulbus cordis results in bulbar ridges. Truncal ridges form in the truncus arteriosus and are continuous with the bulbar ridges (Figure 23-6). The spiral formation of these ridges results in a spiral aorticopulmonary septum. In Figure 23-6, *B* and *F,* this septum is shown oriented right/left at level 3. At level 2, it is oriented dorsoventrally or anterior/posterior. It twists again and at level 1 it is again oriented right/left. In Figure 23-6, *E* and *H,* the septum has divided the bulbus cordis and truncus arteriosus into the aorta and pulmonary trunk. Because of the spiraling of the aorticopulmonary septum, the pulmonary trunk twists around the aorta.

The bulbus cordis is absorbed into the ventricles (Figure 23-7). It becomes the conus arteriosus, or infundibulum, of the right ventricle. In the left ventricle it is called the aortic vestibule, which is the part just proximal to the aortic valve.

Another fetal shunt, the **ductus arteriosus,** is a connection between the dorsal aorta and the left pulmonary artery. Both the ductus arteriosus and the left pulmonary artery are derivatives of the left sixth aortic arch (see Figures 23-6, *A* and Figure 23-9).

The inferior vena cava is derived from four segments of the primitive veins of the embryonic trunk. It enters the inferior posterior part of the right atrium. The superior vena cava is derived from two primitive veins of the embryo, the right anterior cardinal vein and the right common cardinal vein. It enters the posterior superior part of the right atrium.

The four pulmonary veins are derived from the primitive pulmonary vein and its four main branches (Figure 23-8). As the primitive vein is incorporated into the left atrium, the four main branches remain, each one entering the left atrium separately.

Fetal Circulation

Circulation through the fully developed normal fetal heart is shown in Figure 23-9. Oxygenated blood from the mother, via the placenta, enters the umbilical vein and passes through the **ductus venosus** to the inferior vena cava and into the right atrium of the fetal heart. The ductus venosus, one of the three fetal shunts, enables oxygenated blood from the mother to pass almost directly into the fetal heart, bypassing the liver. After birth it will fibrose and become the ligamentum venosum.

Much of the blood from the inferior vena cava is directed across the foramen ovale, the second shunt, into the left atrium. From here the blood enters the left ventricle and then exits through the aorta.

Some blood from the inferior vena cava remains in the right atrium and mixes with blood from the superior vena cava and **coronary sinus** (the large cardiac vein draining

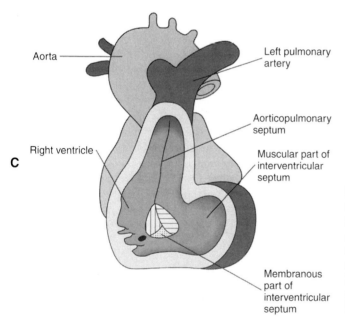

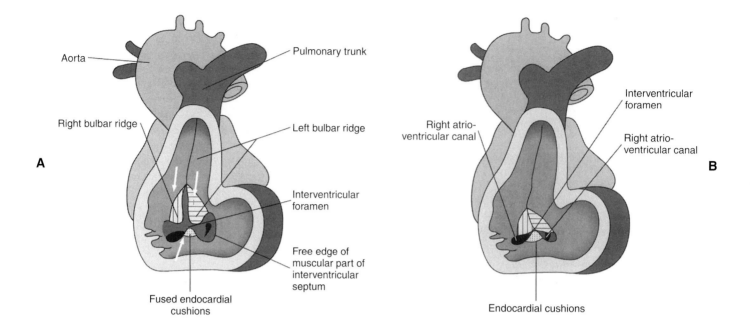

Figure 23-5 Closure of the interventricular foramen and formation of the membranous part of the interventricular septum. The walls of the truncus arteriosus, bulbus cordis, and right ventricle have been removed. **A,** At 5 weeks, showing the bulbar ridges and the fused endocardial cushions. **B,** At 6 weeks, showing that proliferation of subendocardial tissue diminishes the interventricular foramen. **C,** At 7 weeks, showing the fused bulbar ridges and the membranous part of the interventricular septum formed by extensions of tissue from the right side of the endocardial cushions.

Figure 23-6 Partitioning of the bulbus cordis and truncus arteriosus. **A,** Ventral aspect of the heart at 5 weeks. **B,** Transverse sections through the truncus arteriosus and bulbus cordis, illustrating the truncal and bulbar ridges. Note that the orientation is of looking down into the truncus arteriosus from above, keeping in mind the dorsal and ventral aspects of the truncal tube as the aorticopulmonary septum spirals within it. **C,** The ventral wall of the heart and truncus arteriosus have been removed to demonstrate these ridges. **D,** Spiral form of the aorticopulmonary septum. **E,** Ventral aspect of the heart after partitioning of the truncus arteriosus. **F,** Sections through the newly formed aorta *(Ao)* and pulmonary trunk *(PT),* showing the aorticopulmonary septum. **G,** At 6 weeks, the ventral wall of the heart and pulmonary trunk have been removed to show the aorticopulmonary septum. **H,** The great arteries twisting around one another as they exist in the normal neonatal heart.

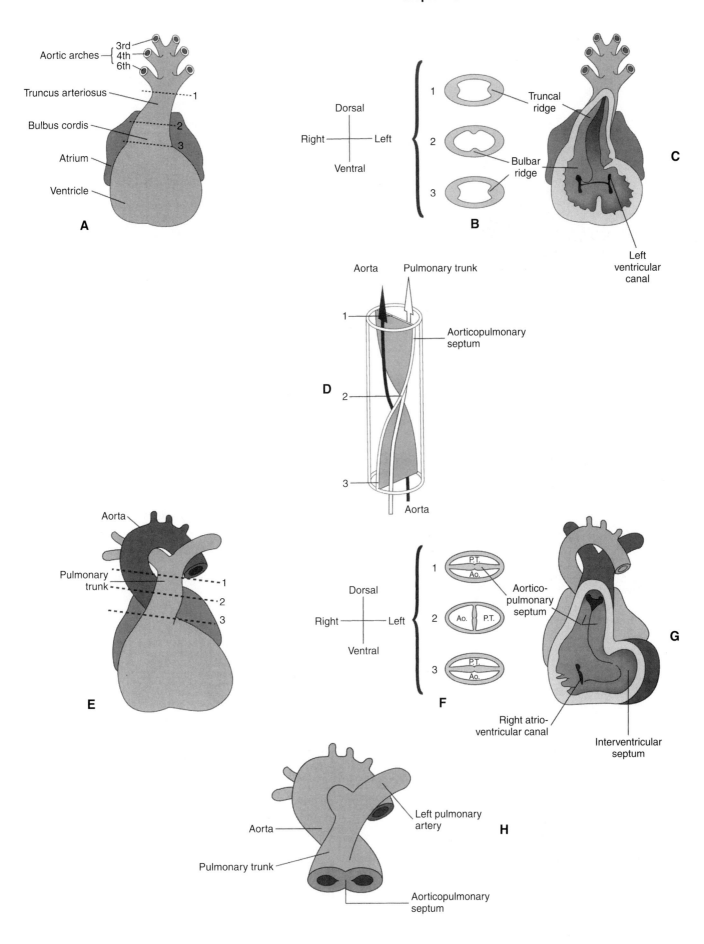

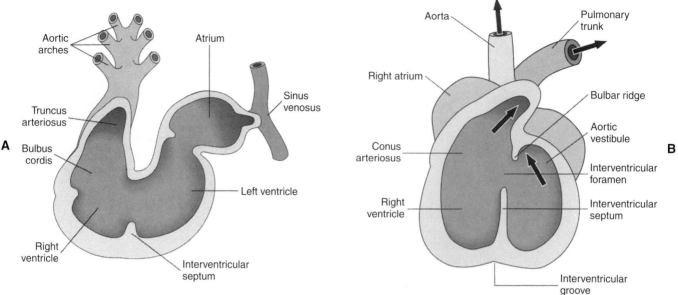

Figure 23-7 Incorporation of the bulbus cordis into the ventricles, and partitioning of the bulbus cordis and truncus arteriosus into the aorta and pulmonary trunk. **A,** Sagittal section at 5 weeks, showing the bulbus cordis as one of the five primitive chambers of the heart. **B,** Coronal section at 6 weeks, after the bulbus cordis has been incorporated into the ventricles to become the conus arteriosus (infundibulum) of the right ventricle and the aortic vestibule of the left ventricle.

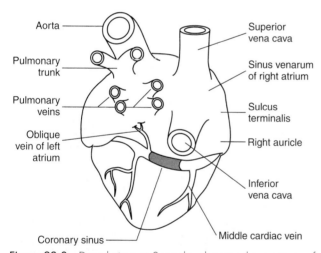

Figure 23-8 Dorsal view at 8 weeks, showing the positions of the superior and inferior venae cavae with respect to the right atrium. The pulmonary veins, each with separate openings into the left atrium, are also shown.

the heart muscle) and passes into the right ventricle. This blood then exits the pulmonary trunk, some going to the lungs for development, but most going through the ductus arteriosus, the third shunt, to the aorta.

LOCATION

The heart, as the name implies, is roughly heart shaped. It is positioned in the lower anterior chest, posterior to the sternum and anterior to the thoracic vertebrae and esophagus. It rests on the diaphragm in the middle mediastinum, bounded laterally by the right and left lungs. Two thirds of the heart lie to the left of midline and one third lies to the right. The **apex** of the heart is the bluntly pointed inferior or caudal end that is directed to the left and anteriorly. It is partially obscured by the left lung. The **base** is the broad end directed to the right posteriorly and cranially (Figure 23-10).

SIZE

The heart is approximately the size of a child's clenched fist. The pediatric internal dimensions of the structures vary with age and weight. Normal values for these structures are presented in Table 23-1.

GROSS ANATOMY

Structurally, the heart is as follows: divided into upper and lower chambers, and divided into right-sided and left-sided chambers (Figure 23-11).

The two upper chambers, the atria, are the filling chambers of the heart. There is a **right atrium** and a **left atrium,** of roughly equal size, thin walled, and separated by a partition called the **interatrial septum.** After birth, there is normally no direct communication between these two chambers.

The two lower chambers, the ventricles, are the pumping chambers of the heart. There is a **right ventricle** and a **left ventricle** separated by the **interventricular septum.**

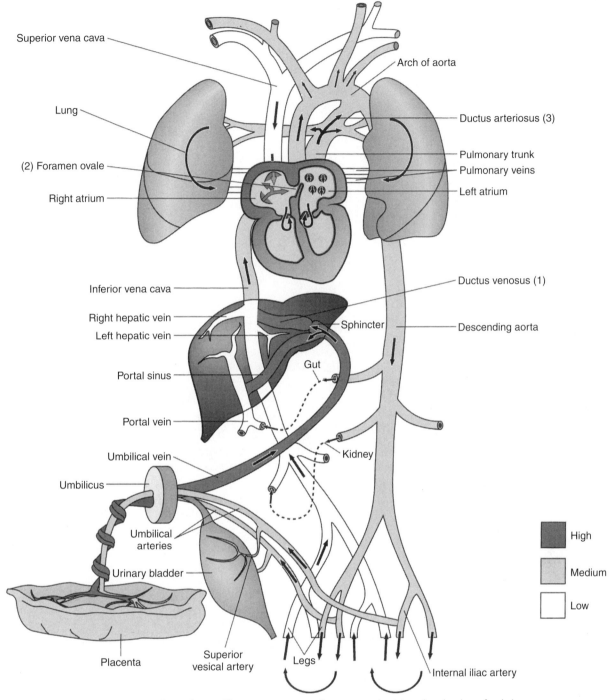

Superior vena cava

Lung

(2) Foramen ovale

Right atrium

Arch of aorta

Ductus arteriosus (3)

Pulmonary trunk
Pulmonary veins
Left atrium

Inferior vena cava

Right hepatic vein
Left hepatic vein

Portal sinus

Portal vein

Umbilical vein

Umbilicus

Umbilical arteries

Urinary bladder

Placenta

Superior vesical artery

Legs

Internal iliac artery

Ductus venosus (1)

Descending aorta

Sphincter

Gut

Kidney

High

Medium

Low

Figure 23-9 Fetal circulation. The organs are not drawn to scale. Note that the three fetal shunts permit most of the blood to bypass the liver and the lungs: *(1)* the ductus venosus, *(2)* the foramen ovale, and *(3)* the ductus arteriosus.

The atrium and the ventricles on each side are separate; however, they communicate through openings controlled by an atrioventricular (AV) valve. The ventricles, in turn, are connected to outflow tracts with semilunar (half-moon shaped) valves controlling the exit of blood from the heart.

The inner lining of the cavities of the heart is called the **endocardium.** The outer covering of the **myocardium,** or muscle of the heart, is called the epicardium. It is composed of two linings or membranes. The inner membrane, the **visceral pericardium,** adheres to the myocardium. The outer membrane is the **parietal pericardium.** The space

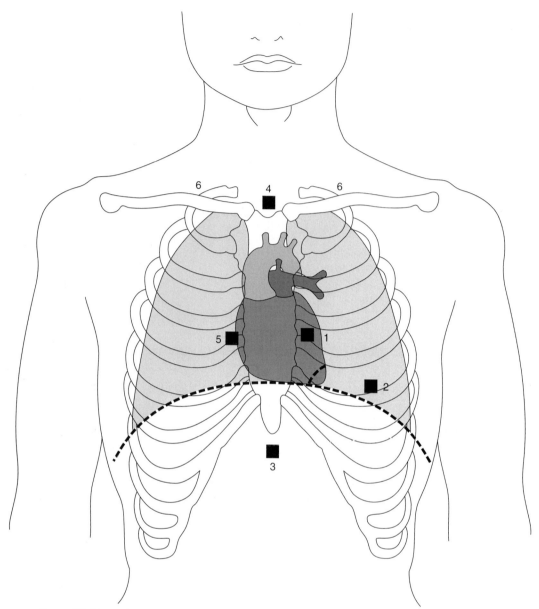

Figure 23-10 Relative position of the heart with respect to other organs within the chest cavity. Note blocks denoting transducer positions that provide "windows" for imaging the heart. *(1)* Parasternal long axis and parasternal short axis positions. *(2)* Apical four chamber, apical five chamber, and apical long axis. *(3)* Subcostal or subxiphoid position. *(4)* Suprasternal notch position. *(5)* Right parasternal position. *(6)* Although not indicated by blocks, the supraclavicular fossa (right and/or left) is also sometimes used in obtaining echocardiographic images.

between them is the pericardial cavity containing a thin, watery fluid that allows the heart to move easily as it beats.

The beating heart makes distinctive sounds. There are two major heart sounds. The first sound, S1, is caused by closure of the AV valves; the second, S2, is caused by the semilunar valves closing. There is a normal splitting of the second sound, the first being that of the aortic valve before the closure of the pulmonary valve component.

Structural differences of the chambers are very helpful in evaluating the pediatric heart. These differences help to determine situs (position), atrioventricular concordance, and ventriculoarterial concordance. The right atrium is normally connected to the two great veins, the **superior vena cava** and the **inferior vena cava.** The left atrium normally receives four pulmonary veins.

The right AV valve is called the **tricuspid valve,** and has three fan-shaped leaflets connected to three sets of

■ ■ ■ **Table 23-1** Normal Values for Children Arranged by Weight

	Weight (lbs)	Mean (cm)	Range (cm)	Number of Subjects
RVD	0-25	.9	0.3-1.5	26
	26-50	1.0	0.4-1.5	26
	51-75	1.1	0.7-1.8	20
	76-100	1.2	0.7-1.6	15
	101-125	1.3	0.8-1.7	11
	126-200	1.3	1.2-1.7	5
LVID	0-25	2.4	1.3-3.2	26
	26-50	3.4	2.4-3.8	26
	51-75	3.8	3.3-4.5	20
	76-100	4.1	3.5-4.7	15
	101-125	4.3	3.7-4.9	11
	126-200	4.9	4.4-5.2	5
LV and IV septal wall thickness	0-25	0.5	0.4-0.6	26
	26-50	0.6	0.5-0.7	26
	51-75	0.7	0.6-0.7	20
	76-100	0.7	0.7-0.8	15
	101-125	0.7	0.7-0.8	11
	126-200	0.8	0.7-0.8	5
LA dimension	0-25	1.7	0.7-2.3	26
	26-50	2.2	1.7-2.7	26
	51-75	2.3	1.9-2.8	20
	76-100	2.4	2.0-3.0	15
	101-125	2.7	2.1-3.0	11
	126-200	2.8	2.1-3.7	5
Aortic root	0-25	1.3	0.7-1.7	26
	26-50	1.7	1.3-2.2	26
	51-75	2.0	1.7-2.3	20
	76-100	2.2	1.9-2.7	15
	101-125	2.3	1.7-2.7	11
	126-200	2.4	2.2-2.8	5
Aortic valve opening	0-25	.9	0.5-1.2	26
	26-50	1.2	0.9-1.6	26
	51-75	1.4	1.2-1.7	20
	76-100	1.6	1.3-1.9	15
	101-125	1.7	1.4-2.0	11
	126-200	1.8	1.6-2.0	5

From Rudolph AM, et al: *Rudolph pediatrics*, ed. 19, East Norwalk, 1991, Appleton and Lange, p 1340.

chordae and two papillary muscles. The left ventricular myocardium is relatively thicker than its counterpart on the right because it is pumping against higher pressures. The left ventricle has an ellipsoid shape and smooth endocardial surface. All of these characteristics help differentiate the right heart from the left heart.

The **semilunar valves,** which are the **aortic valve** and **pulmonary valve,** have three leaflets or cusps so named because they are half-moon shaped. The aorta has a right coronary cusp, a left cusp, and a noncoronary cusp. Immediately distal to these cusps are recessed pockets, or outpouchings, of the aorta, called **sinuses of Valsalva.** These sinuses house the openings, or ostia, of the coronary arteries. There are three sinuses, each of which is associated with one cusp of the aortic valve. The right sinus is related to the coronary cusp where the ostium of the right coronary artery is located. The left sinus is behind the left cusp and houses the ostium of the left coronary artery. The noncoronary cusp is so named because no coronary artery is associated with its sinus.

The greatest volume of blood entering the right and left atria from their respective veins flows passively through the open AV valves into the ventricles. The pressure in the ventricles begins to rise. As the pressure rises, the AV valves begin to close. The atria contract, forcing the AV valves to reopen and the remainder of blood in the atria to be propelled into the ventricles. This is **diastole.**

The pressure in the ventricles is now greater than that in the atria. The AV valves close, the semilunar valves open, and the cycle continues. This is **systole.** The ventricular pressure is now less than the atrial pressure because blood is continuously filling the atria. The semilunar valves close, the AV valves open, and the cycle continues.

The right heart is concerned with the pulmonary circulation, moving blood to the lungs for oxygenation. The left heart is concerned with the systemic circulation, delivering oxygenated blood to the tissues (Figure 23-12; see Figure 23-11).

The flow of blood through the heart is as follows. Blood from the superior vena cava, inferior vena cava, and coronary sinus (draining the heart) empties into the right atrium. It then flows through the tricuspid valve into the right ventricle. From here the blood flows through the pulmonary valve into the main **pulmonary artery.** The main pulmonary artery branches into a right pulmonary artery to the right lung and a left pulmonary artery to the left lung. This is the pulmonary circulation.

Oxygenated blood returns to the left atrium via four **pulmonary veins.** From the left atrium it passes through the mitral valve into the left ventricle and through the aortic valve into the **ascending aorta.** Blood fills the head and neck vessels and travels along the **descending aorta** to the tissues. This is systemic flow.

chordae tendineae that are, in turn, connected to three **papillary muscles.** The tricuspid valve has a more inferior or apical insertion point than does its counterpart on the left side. The right ventricle is triangular. It has a more heavily trabeculated endocardial surface, a moderator band in the lower third of the chamber, and an infundibular muscle band, or conus, in the right ventricular outflow tract.

On the other side, the left AV valve is called the **mitral valve,** and has two fan-shaped or triangular leaflets inserted more superiorly on the septum toward the base of the heart. Normally the mitral valve has two sets of

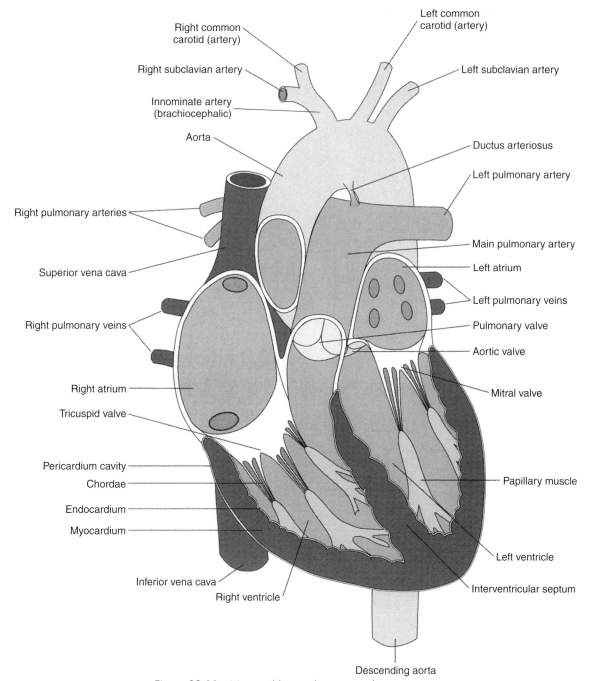

Figure 23-11   Neonatal heart, showing cardiac structure.

Cardiac Perfusion and Drainage

The **coronary arteries** perfuse the heart muscle and inner structures, and are so named because they form a corona, or crown, around the heart. There are two main coronary arteries: the right coronary artery arises from the right sinus of Valsalva, and the left coronary artery arises from the left sinus (Figure 23-13, *A*).

The right coronary artery courses in the atrioventricular groove separating the atria from the ventricles. It gives

off a muscular branch and a marginal branch, and continues around the heart posteriorly until it anastomoses with, or joins, the left circumflex coronary artery. At this anastomosis, the right coronary artery gives off a branch called the posterior descending coronary artery, which travels along the posterior interventricular septum.

The left main coronary artery divides almost immediately into the left circumflex and the left anterior descending coronary arteries. The left circumflex extends

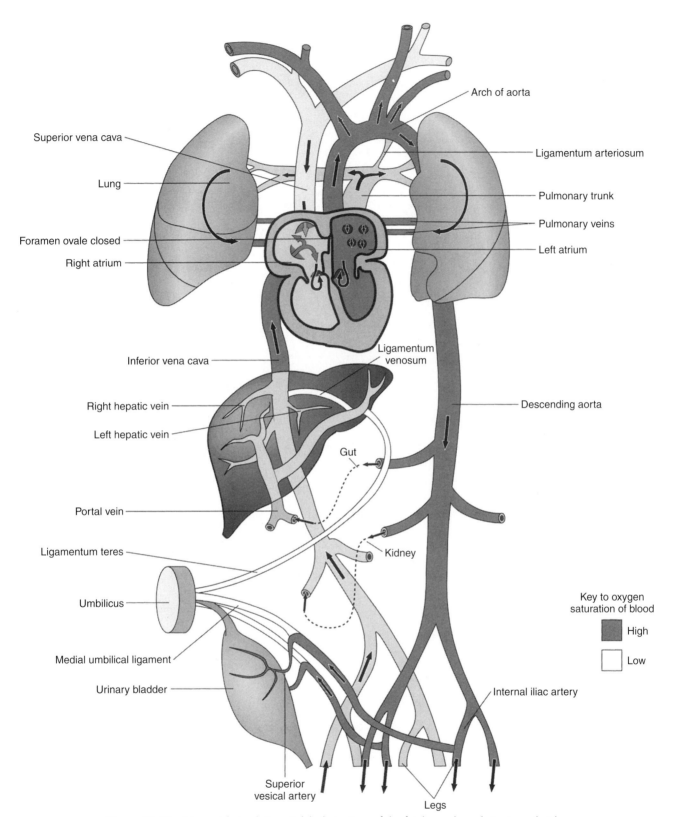

Figure 23-12 Neonatal circulation. Adult derivatives of the fetal vessels and structures that become nonfunctional at birth are also shown. Arrows indicate the course of the neonatal circulation. The organs are not drawn to scale. After birth, the three shunts that short circuited the blood during fetal life cease to function, and the pulmonary and systemic circulations become separated.

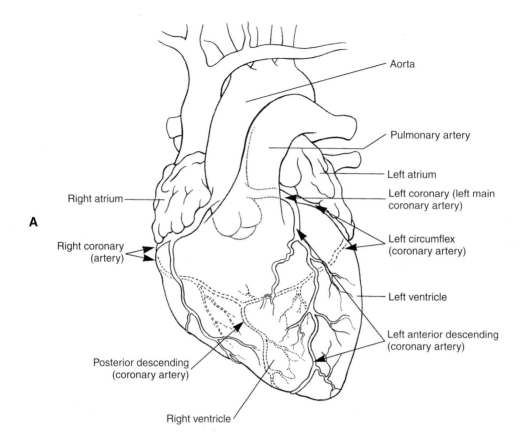

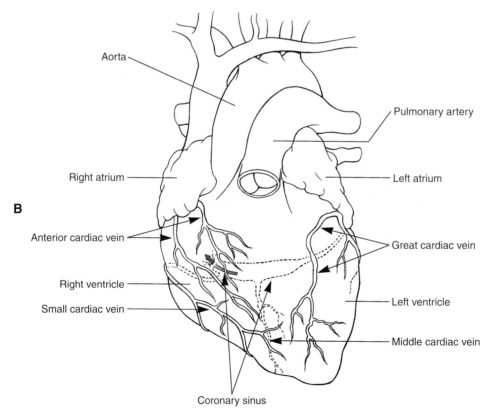

Figure 23-13 **A,** Coronary arteries and their positions on the heart. **B,** Cardiac veins. These are anterior, or ventral, views. The dashed lines indicate the position of the vessels as viewed from the posterior, or dorsal, surface of the heart.

around the heart posteriorly until it joins the right coronary artery, as mentioned. The left anterior descending coronary artery travels downward anteriorly along the interventricular septum, giving off muscular branches, or septal perforators. It curves posteriorly to meet the posterior descending coronary artery.

The veins that drain the heart do not form a corona, though they usually course with the arteries. They are simply called **cardiac veins** (Figure 23-13, *B*). Most of the veins drain into the coronary sinus, a large vein that serves as a reservoir. From here it empties into the right atrium through the thesbian valve. The veins that do not drain into the sinus drain directly into the right atrium.

Normal variations in coronary artery anatomy and perfusion must be taken into account when an evaluation of them is needed for diagnostic purposes.

Cardiac Conduction

The cardiac conduction system is the mechanism by which the heart is made to effectively pump blood through the vessels. The muscle fibers of the heart have the inherent ability to contract without a nerve stimulus. However, if each fiber contracted independently, the heart would not be very effective in getting blood to the tissues.

The cardiac conduction system is a specialized group of cardiac muscle, nodes, tracts, and fibers that can generate and conduct electrical impulses through heart muscle, causing a synchronous, coordinated contraction or heartbeat (Figure 23-14).

The **sinoatrial node,** or **SA node,** sets the pace of the heart. It is therefore called the pacemaker of the conduction system. The electrocardiogram (ECG or EKG) measures the electrical activity of the conduction system and indirectly myocardial activity. As the SA node fires, electrical impulses travel through internodal tracts to both atria, SA_1. On the ECG this is reflected by the P-wave signaling that atrial contraction is about to take place. Contraction occurs at once.

At the same time that impulses are passing through the atria, they also travel to the **atrioventricular node,** or **AV node,** located in the medial wall of the right atrium. There is a very brief delay in the activation and transmission of the AV node. This is reflected on the ECG as the end of the P-wave, labelled 2 on the tracing and AV_2 on the heart diagram. After this delay the AV node fires, sending impulses along the **bundle of His** located superficially on the interventricular septum. From here the impulses travel through the **Purkinje fibers** into the myocardium. The ventricles contract at once from above downward. The QRS deflection on the ECG reflects this transmission and is numbered 3 and 4 on the tracing. BH_3 and Pf_4 on the heart diagram reflect this electrical activity.

The T-wave indicates a recovery of electrical charge in the ventricles or return of the myocardium to a resting state. The next cycle begins with another P-wave.

Normal pacemaker (SA node) rates (beats/min) at various ages are as follows:

SA node rate	100-180	110-180	60-120	55-110	50-100
Age	0-1 mo	1 yr	5 yrs	10 yrs	Adult

Cardiac muscle, as mentioned earlier, has the inherent ability to contract without a nerve stimulus. However, stimulation by the autonomic nervous system (ANS) affects the rate of SA node firing and also the coronary arteries.

The sympathetic fibers of the ANS cause an increase in the heart rate. The parasympathetic division, specifically the vagus nerve, or tenth cranial nerve, causes the heart rate to slow down.

PHYSIOLOGY

The heart is the primary organ of the circulatory system, providing the force that propels blood through all the vessels of the body.

The basic function of the heart is to receive deoxygenated blood from the head and body for transportation to the lungs and distribution of oxygenated blood to all parts of the body.

SONOGRAPHIC APPEARANCE

In sonography of the heart, we use different ultrasonic techniques to get the most complete, accurate diagnostic information: 2-D, M-mode, color Doppler, pulsed wave (PW) Doppler, and continuous wave (CW) Doppler. (See Chapter 2 for an explanation of these techniques.) Of note, regarding the color flow imaging, the color sector is usually narrowed or "coned" as much as possible to see only the area of interest. This yields better resolution. Structures outside of the "coned" area may be seen poorly or not at all depending upon the equipment used and how the color wedge is presented.

All of these techniques have their advantages and disadvantages. However, in doing an echocardiogram, all are needed to perform a thorough examination that will give the clinician the information needed to properly diagnose the patient.

On the two-dimensional image, the heart muscle (myocardium) has a soft, homogeneous, even-textured echogenicity. The appearance ranges from medium to low intensity. The valves and chordae appear more echogenic than the myocardium. The valves will appear as thin, flexible lines that are freely mobile. The pericardium is the most echogenic structure, having a smooth, fluidlike, linear appearance.

Figure 23-15 shows the plane of sound through the heart in the parasternal long axis view. Figure 23-16 shows echocardiographic images in the parasternal long

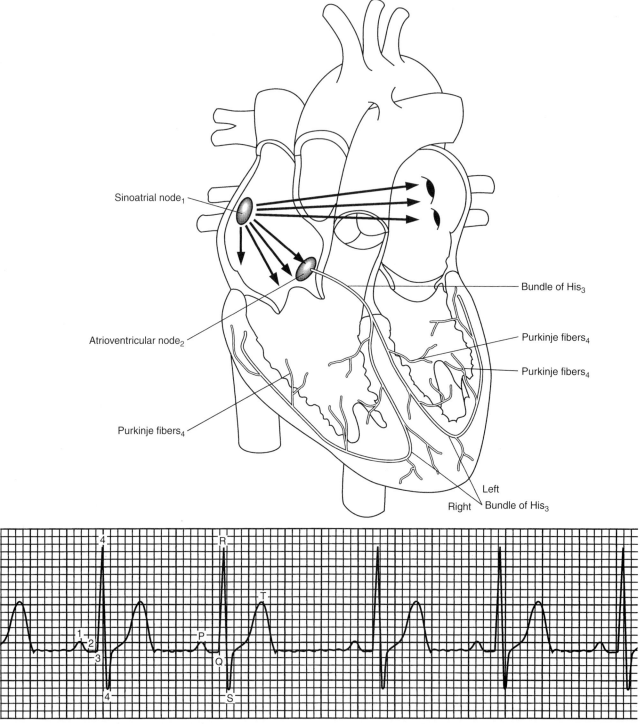

Figure 23-14 Cardiac conduction system and an electrocardiogram (ECG) tracing. The numbers on the ECG corresponding with the numbers indicated on the heart diagram relate the electrical activity of the heart to the waveform of the ECG.

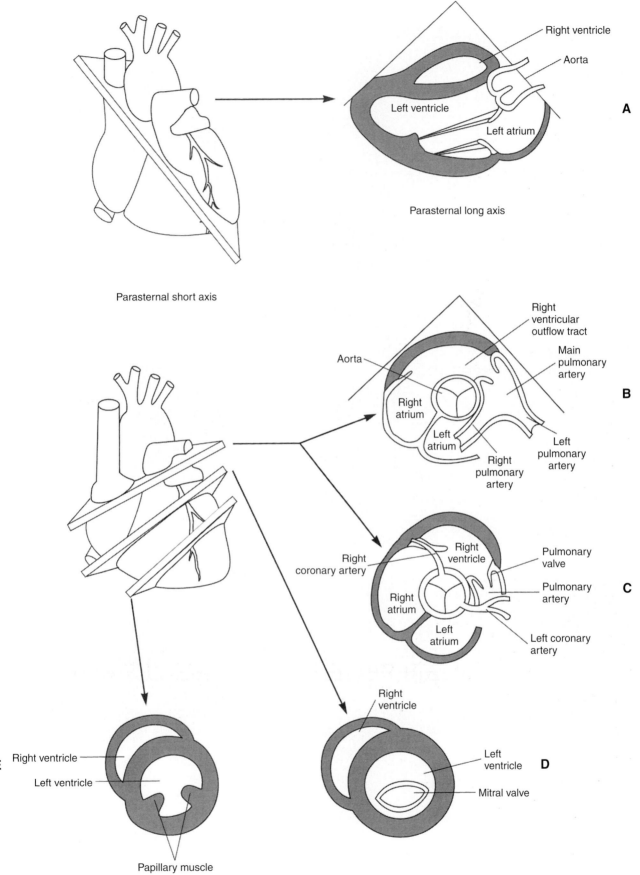

Figure 23-15 Parasternal long axis and short axis planes, or cuts, through the heart. **A,** Echocardiographic sketch of the parasternal long axis view. **B,** Parasternal short axis view at the level of the aortic valve. **C,** Short axis view showing the coronary arteries. **D,** Short axis view at the level of the mitral valve. **E,** Short axis view at the level of the papillary muscles.

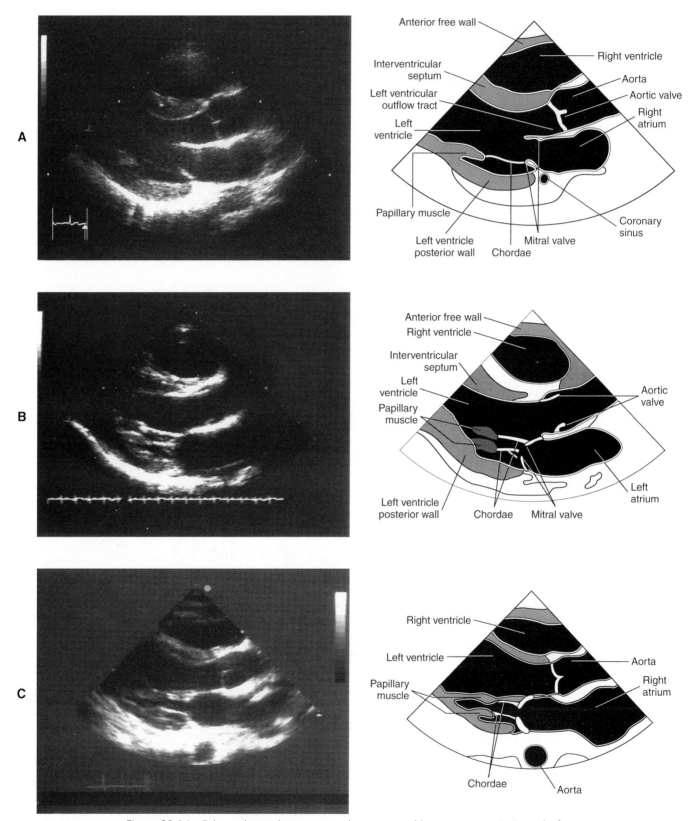

Figure 23-16 Echocardiographic images in the parasternal long axis view. **A,** Diastolic frame. **B,** Systolic frame. **C,** Late diastolic frame.

axis view and their schematic representations, respectively. Note the structures and their positions relative to one another. Also note that the left ventricular apex is not seen in this view.

Basic M-mode (for time-motion mode) includes measurements taken at the aortic valve level, the mitral valve level, and the chordal level in the left ventricle (Figure 23-17).

Figure 23-18 shows an M-mode tracing of the left ventricle. Note the chordae on the inner surface of the left ventricular posterior wall. Figure 23-19 is a tracing at the mitral valve level. The echogenic areas seen in the right ventricle after each QRS complex are artifacts caused by inspiration of air into the lungs. The tracing of the aortic valve is shown in Figure 23-20 taken from the short axis view.

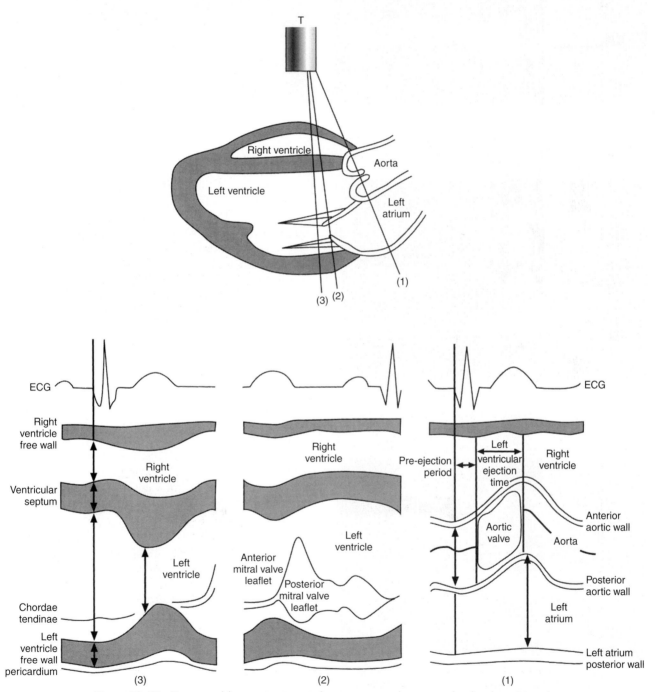

Figure 23-17 Parasternal long axis view, indicating cuts at the various levels where M-mode tracings will be recorded. The lower diagram is a schematic of an M-mode tracing at the various levels shown in the upper diagram. Currently, M-mode tracings are also being done in parasternal short axis views.

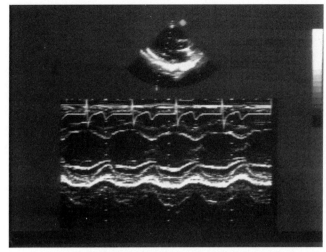

A

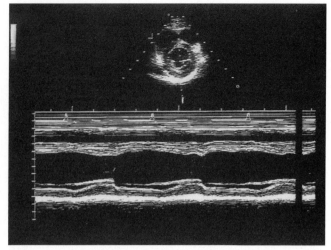

B

Figure 23-18   A, M-mode of the left ventricle in the parasternal long axis view. B, M-mode of the left ventricle in the parasternal short axis view.

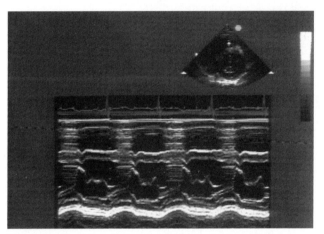

Figure 23-19   M-mode tracing of the mitral valve in the parasternal short axis view.

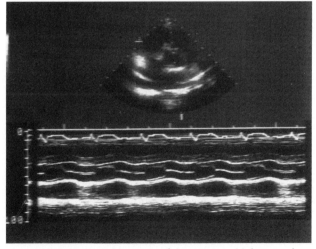

Figure 23-20   M-mode tracing of the aorta and left atrium from the parasternal short axis view.

The planes of the short axis views through the heart are shown in Figure 23-15.

Figure 23-21 shows the echocardiographic image in the parasternal short axis view at the aortic valve level. Note that the commissure, or closure line, between the noncoronary and left coronary cusp of the aortic valve is not well-visualized. This occurs because of the orientation of the plane of sound, which strikes the structure parallel rather than perpendicularly. Figure 23-21, C and D show color flow in this short axis view. Flow is seen in the right atrium passing through the tricuspid valve into the right ventricular outflow tract. It then moves through the pulmonary valve into the main pulmonary artery. From here, the blood flows into the right and left pulmonary artery branches toward their respective lung. Figure 23-21, E is a PW Doppler tracing of the pulmonary valve. The velocity is within normal limits.

The mitral valve level is seen in Figure 23-22. The left ventricle should appear as a concentric circle; the anterior and posterior mitral valve leaflets should appear within the circle toward the posterior aspect of the cavity. In real time, the leaflets should open symmetrically and appear unrestricted in their movement. The left ventricular outflow tract is seen anterior to the mitral valve. The left ventricular walls should contract and relax concentrically and smoothly. The right ventricle is often seen in this view. It should look like a half moon, adjacent to the interventricular septum. The moderator band may also be visualized.

The echocardiographic image and schematic of the papillary muscle level are shown in Figure 23-23. Again, the left ventricle should appear as a concentric circle. The anterolateral papillary muscle is seen at its usual position, 3 or 4 o'clock. The posteromedial papillary muscle is most often positioned at 8 o'clock. Note the

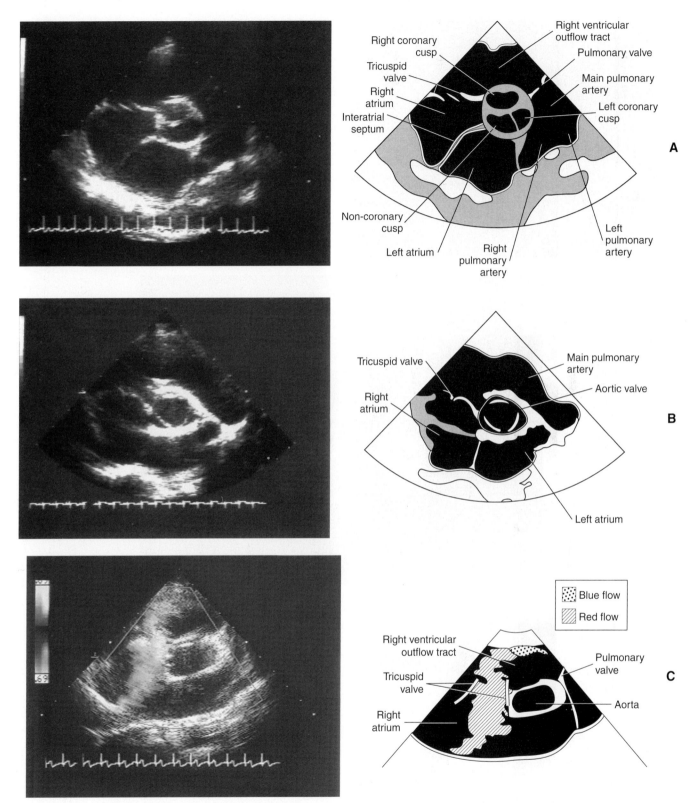

Figure 23-21 Echocardiographic images in the parasternal short axis view at the aortic valve level. **A,** With the valve closed. **B,** With the valve open. **C,** Parasternal short axis view showing color flow through the tricuspid valve. Note the blue color as the flow turns to move away from the transducer. (See Color Plate 34.)

continued

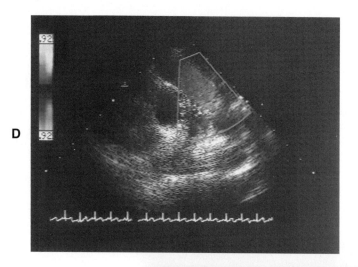

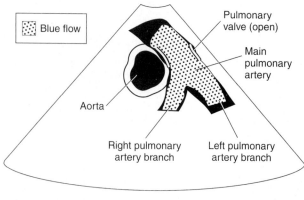

Blue flow

Pulmonary valve (open)

Main pulmonary artery

Aorta

Right pulmonary artery branch

Left pulmonary artery branch

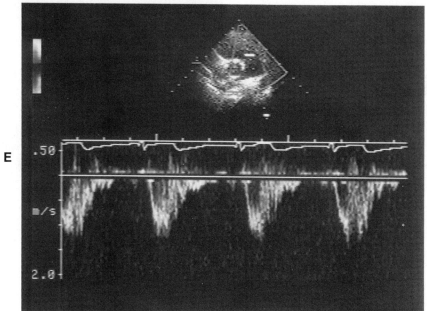

Figure 23-21, cont'd   **D,** As flow continues from **C,** it is going away from the transducer through the pulmonary valve and into the right and left pulmonary branches. (See Color Plate 35.) **E,** Pulsed wave Doppler at the pulmonary valve with normal velocity.

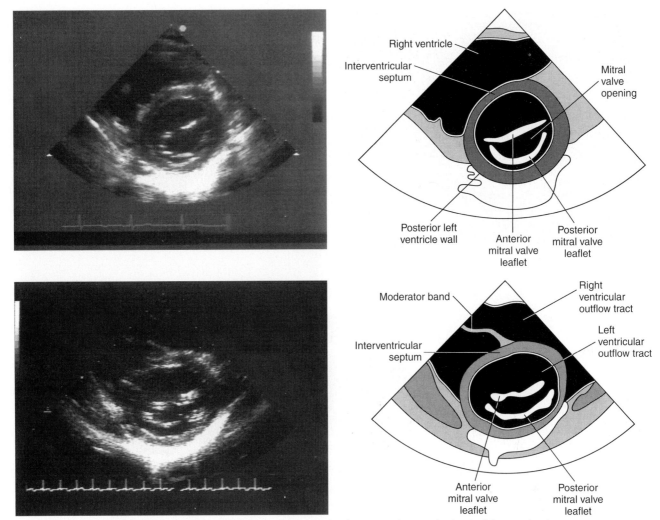

Figure 23-22 Echocardiographic images in the short axis plane at the level of the mitral valve.

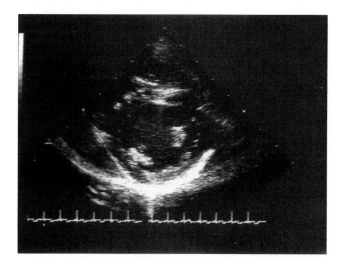

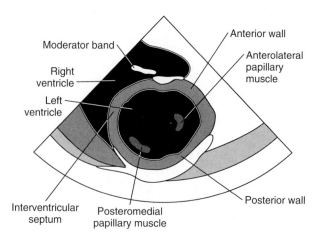

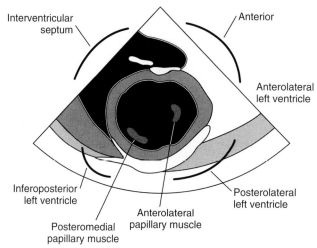

Figure 23-23   Echocardiographic image of the left ventricle at the papillary muscle level.

areas of the interventricular septum, the anterior and anterolateral walls, the posterior lateral wall, and the inferoposterior wall of the left ventricle.

The apical views include the apical four chamber, the apical five chamber, and the apical long axis (Figure 23-24). There is also an apical two-chamber view, not shown, visualizing the left atrium and ventricle only.

Echocardiographic images of the four-chamber view are shown in Figure 23-25. All four cardiac chambers are visualized as well as the tricuspid and mitral valves. There may be an artifactual dropout of echoes in the midportion of the interatrial septum. The interventricular septum is usually seen in its entirety. It is usually possible to visualize the four pulmonary veins entering the left atrium. However, confirmation can be realized only by Doppler examination. Figure 23-25, *A* shows a color flow image in this view. The flow is across the mitral valve. Figure 23-25, *B* is an image of the PW

Doppler tracing of the mitral valve in a different patient. In the apical long axis view, note the left atrium, mitral valve, left ventricle, left ventricular outflow tract, the aortic valve, and the ascending aorta (Figure 23-26).

Subcostal views provide a wealth of information (Figure 23-27).

The subcostal four-chamber view is used mainly to interrogate the interatrial septum. In this view the septum is perpendicular to the plane of sound, giving the best possible image of the structure (Figure 23-28). The entire heart and surrounding area can be seen very well in this view, making it excellent for determining situs and optimum for detecting pericardial effusions (Figure 23-29).

Figure 23-30 visualizes the suprasternal planes; see Figure 22-30, *A* for the long axis view of the aorta.

Figure 23-31 shows echocardiographic images and simplified diagrams, respectively, of the long axis of the

Text continued on p. 442

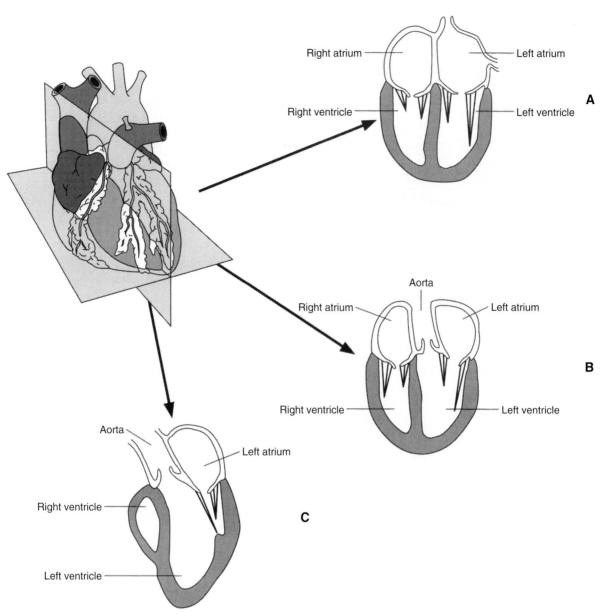

Figure 23-24   Scanning planes of the apical views of the heart. A, Four-chamber view. B, Five-chamber view. C, Apical long axis view.

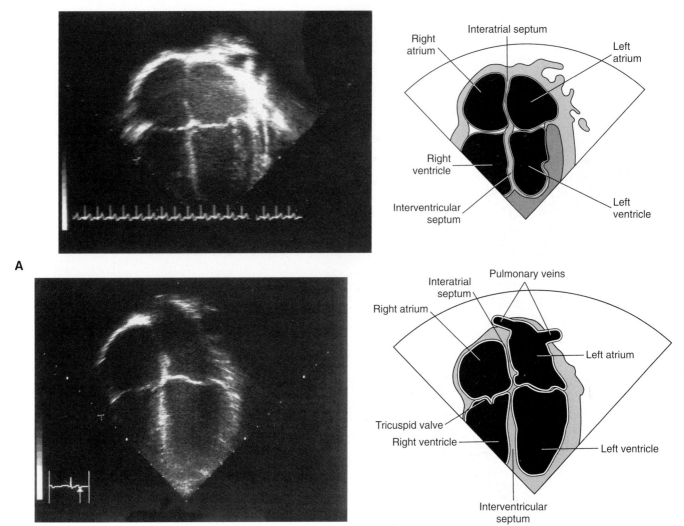

A

Figure 23-25　**A,** Echocardiographic images of the apical four-chamber view.

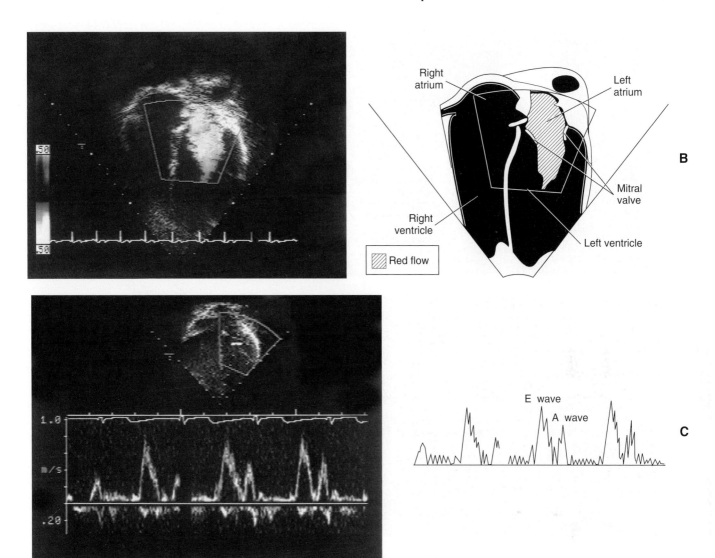

Figure 23-25, cont'd **B,** Color flow Doppler of the mitral valve. Echocardiographic image of inflow from the left atrium through the mitral valve into the left ventricle. The flow is red because it is moving toward the transducer positioned at the apex. Note the laminar flow (no turbulence). (See Color Plate 36.) **C,** Pulsed wave Doppler of the mitral valve. Pulsed wave Doppler of mitral inflow. Again, note the laminar flow indicated by lack of echoes between the waves.

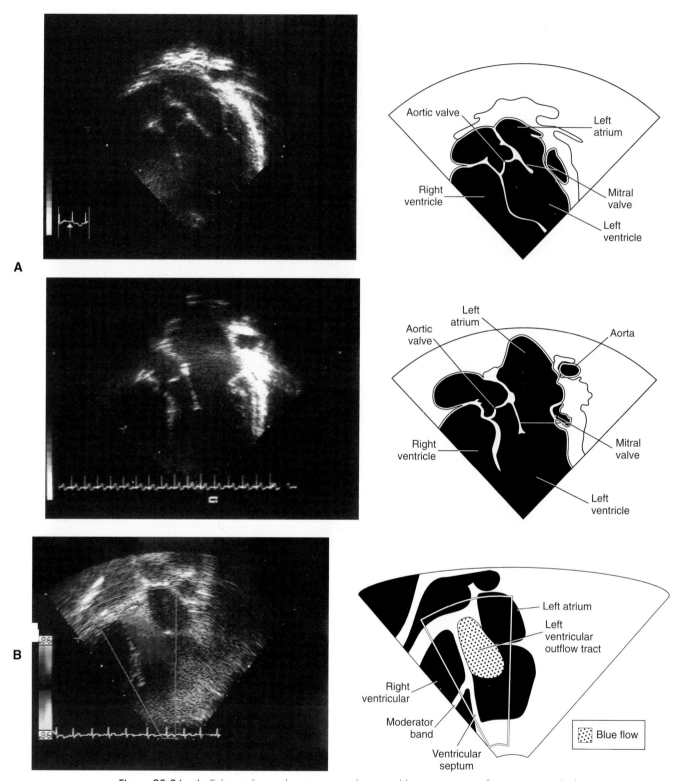

Figure 23-26 **A,** Echocardiographic images in the apical long axis view of two patients. Both are shown in the anatomically correct position. **B,** Apical long axis view showing color flow in the left ventricular outflow tract, through the aortic valve and a limited section of the ascending aorta. The transducer is at the apex of the heart, with the flow moving away from it. Therefore the blood flow is shown in blue. (See Color Plate 37.)

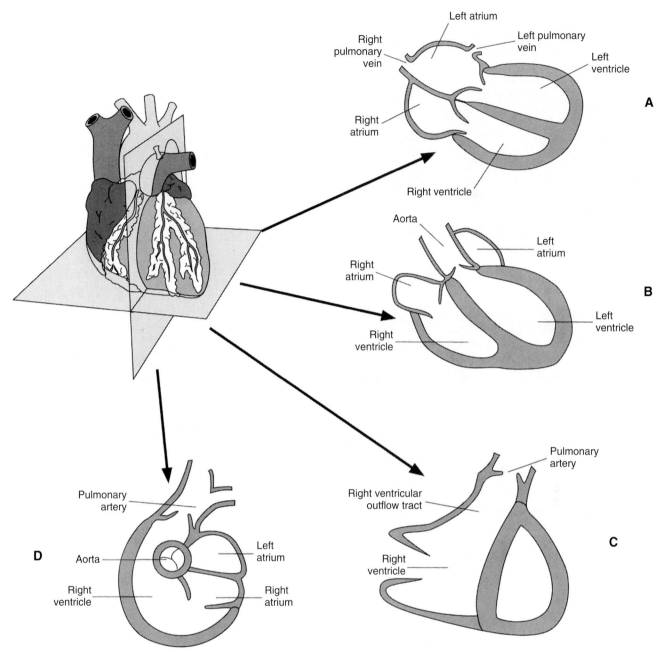

Figure 23-27 Four planes in the subcostal position are shown. **A,** Four chamber. **B,** Five chamber. **C,** Long axis of right ventricular outflow tract. **D,** Short axis at aortic valve level.

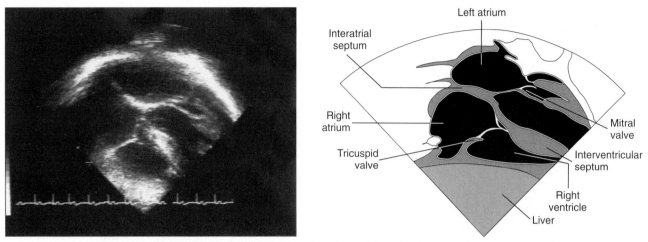

Figure 23-28 Echocardiographic image in the subcostal four-chamber view for interrogation of the interatrial septum.

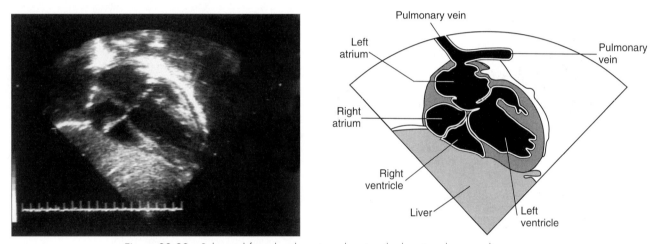

Figure 23-29 Subcostal four-chamber view showing the heart and surrounding area.

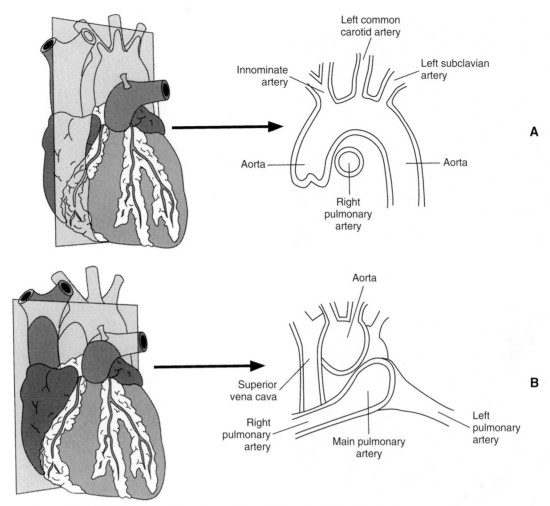

Figure 23-30 Schematic of the planes of sound through the heart in the suprasternal position. **A,** Long-axis view. **B,** Short-axis view.

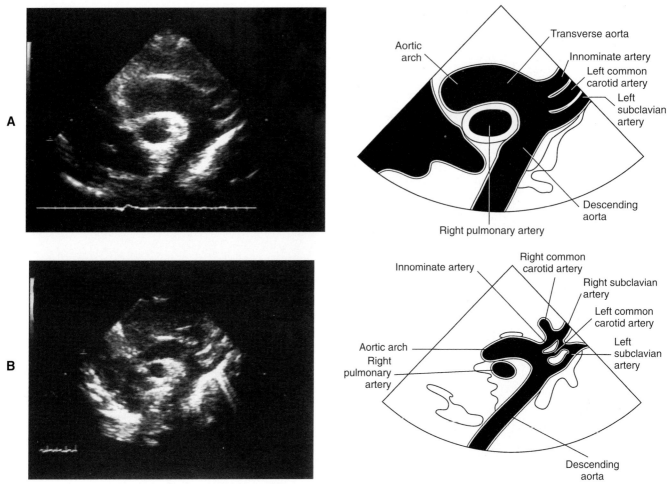

Figure 23-31 *A* and *B,* Echocardiographic images of the aortic arch in long axis. *B,* Note the bifurcation of the innominate artery into the right subclavian and right common carotid arteries.

aorta. The ascending aorta, transverse arch, and descending aorta are shown. The **innominate artery, left common carotid artery,** and **left subclavian artery** are visualized leaving the arch. The right pulmonary artery is cut in cross-section and is seen as a circular structure in the inner curvature of the arch.

The long axis of the right ventricular inflow tract is shown in Figure 23-32. It offers an excellent image of the right ventricular inflow tract. In some patients, all three papillary muscles and chordae may be seen. Note the eustachian valve in the right atrium marking the entrance of the inferior vena cava. See Figure 23-32, *C* for a color flow image across the tricuspid valve.

The long axis view of the right ventricular outflow tract is shown in Figure 23-33. It includes the right ventricular outflow tract, pulmonary valve, main pulmonary artery, and the right and left pulmonary artery branches.

Views of the coronary arteries from the parasternal, short axis view, aortic valve level are shown in Figure 23-34.

The long axis of the coronary sinus as it empties into the right atrium is seen in Figure 23-35.

Figure 23-36 shows sagittal cuts. Figure 23-36, *A* is at the level of the long axis view of the left ventricular outflow tract, aortic valve, and ascending aorta. Figure 23-36, *B* is of the right ventricular outflow tract and the pulmonary valve. Figure 23-36, *C* is a short axis view of the heart at the aortic valve level.

The long axis of the superior and inferior venae cavae entering the right atrium is shown in Figure 23-37.

SONOGRAPHIC APPLICATIONS

Sonography is an aid in diagnosing congenital structural and flow abnormalities in the heart such as ventricular septal defect, patent ductus arteriosus, tetralogy of Fallot, transposition of the great arteries, and others. It helps in ruling out intracardiac masses and tumors. Sonography is helpful in assessing and monitoring heart size and function in patients on continual medical therapy that may affect the heart, such as chemothera-

Text continued on p. 447

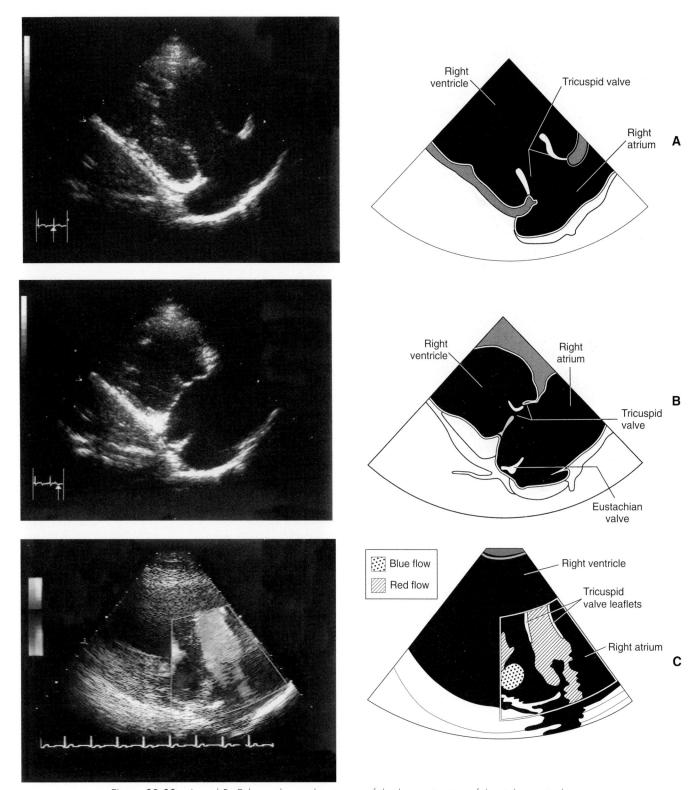

Figure 23-32 **A** and **B**, Echocardiographic image of the long-axis view of the right ventricular inflow tract. **A**, Diastolic image. **B**, Systolic frame. **C**, Color flow Doppler of the right ventricular inflow tract. The flow is toward the transducer from the right atrium through the tricuspid valve into the right ventricle. (See Color Plate 38.)

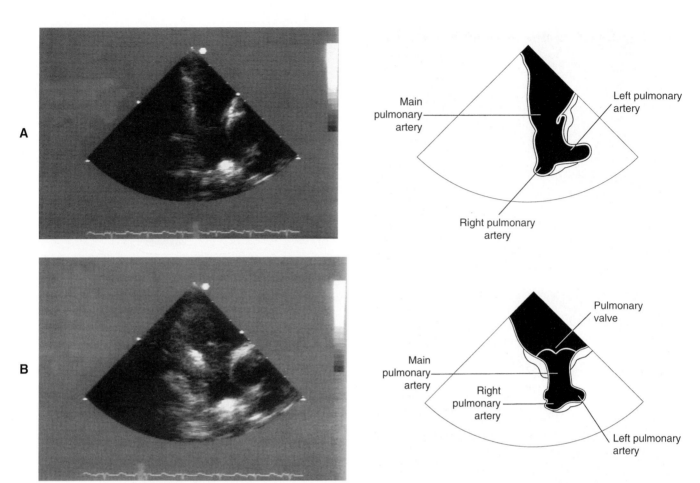

Figure 23-33 Echocardiographic image of the parasternal long axis of the right ventricular outflow tract. **A,** Systolic frame with the pulmonary valve open. **B,** Diastolic frame with the pulmonary valve closed.

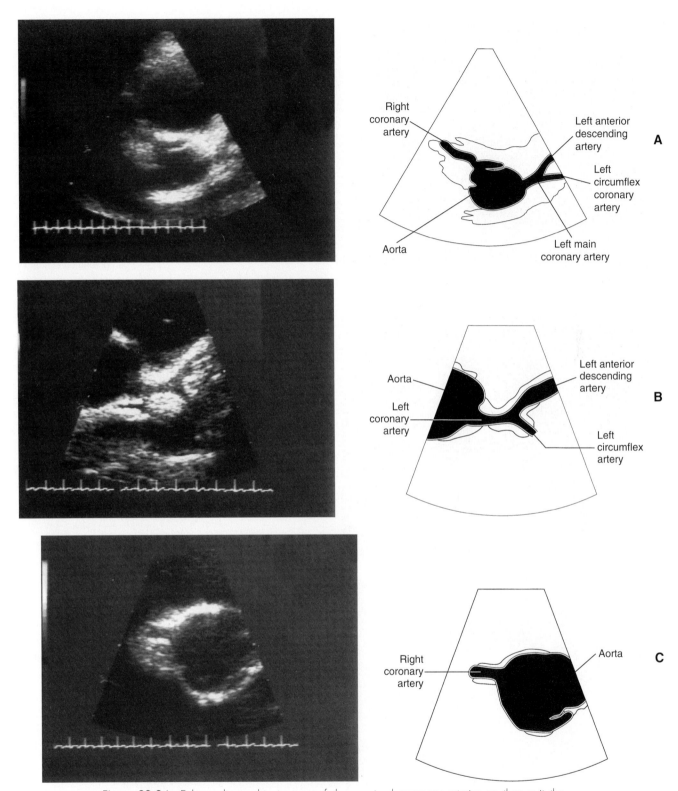

Figure 23-34 Echocardiographic images of the proximal coronary arteries as they exit the aorta. **A,** View of the RCA, LCA and bifurcation, LAD, and LCX. Part of the aortic valve leaflets is seen within the aorta. **B,** Image of the LCA and branches. **C,** RCA. *RCA,* Right coronary artery; *LCA,* left coronary artery; *LAD,* left anterior descending coronary artery; *LCX,* left circumflex coronary artery.

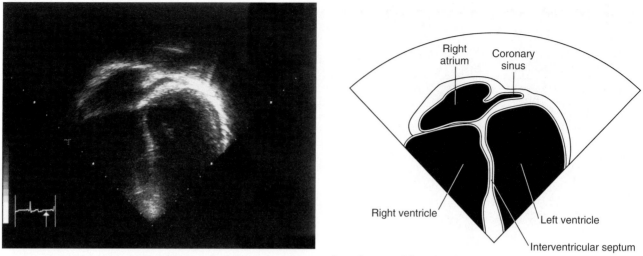

Figure 23-35 View of the coronary sinus from the apical four-chamber position.

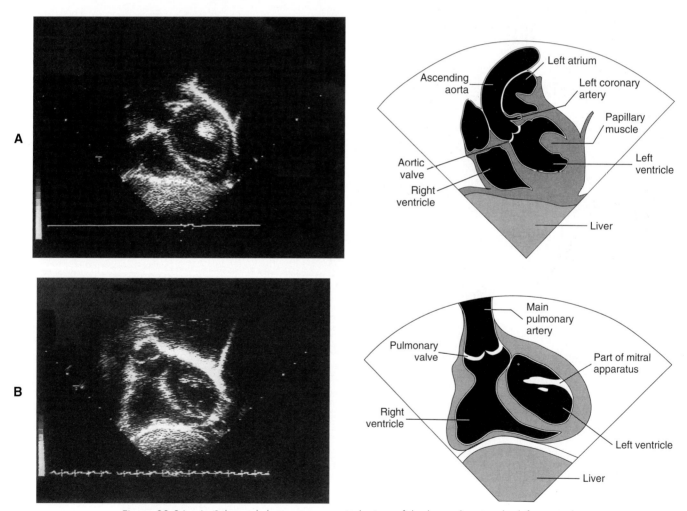

Figure 23-36 **A,** Subcostal short axis, or sagittal, view of the heart showing the left ventricular outflow tract, aortic valve, and ascending aorta. Note the left main coronary artery. **B,** Subcostal or subxiphoid short-axis view, demonstrating the right ventricular outflow tract, pulmonary valve, and main pulmonary artery.

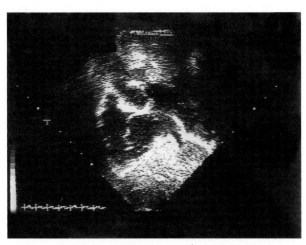

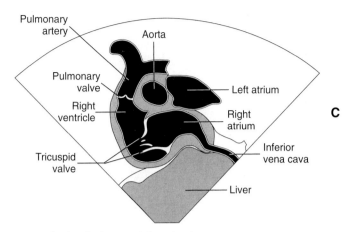

Figure 23-36, cont'd   C, Subxiphoid short axis, aortic valve level, showing left and right atrium, tricuspid valve, right ventricular outflow tract, and main pulmonary artery.

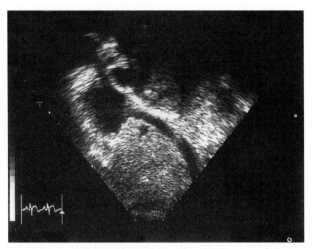

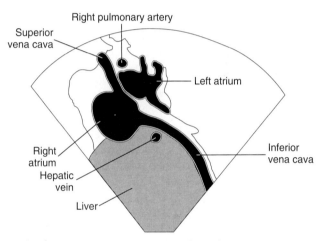

Figure 23-37   Subxiphoid view of the superior and inferior venae cavae entering the right atrium.

peutic drugs. Echocardiography is used to evaluate and monitor patients with conditions that directly or indirectly affect the heart, such as sickle cell anemia and Kawasaki disease. Sonography is used to evaluate the results of medical treatment and surgical repair of diseases of the heart.

NORMAL VARIANTS
Dextrocardia
Dextrocardia is a condition in which the heart is located in the mediastinum as a mirror image of its normal position, the ventricular apex being rightward.

Mesocardia
This is a condition where the apex is directed to the left as normal, but with the heart itself being more medially positioned within the chest.

REFERENCE CHARTS

■ ■ ■   **ASSOCIATED PHYSICIANS**

Radiologist: Specializes in the diagnostic interpretation of imaging modalities that aid in the diagnosis of heart disease.
Cardiologist: Specializes in the diagnosis and treatment of the diseases of the heart and related vessels.
Thoracic Surgeon: Specializes in the structural modification of the heart in the treatment of heart disease.

■ ■ ■   **COMMON DIAGNOSTIC TESTS**

Chest X-ray Study: This test, recorded on photographic film, provides a picture of the ribs, lungs, and heart. If the possibility of congestive heart failure is considered, this study aids in determining whether the heart is abnormally enlarged and there is fluid in the lungs. The test is performed by a radiologic technologist and interpreted by a radiologist.

Electrocardiogram (EKG or ECG): This test monitors or measures the electrical activity of the heart and indirectly the heart muscle. Electrodes are placed on various positions on the chest and on each wrist and ankle. The electrodes are connected to a machine that amplifies the electrical impulses of the heart and records them on graph paper. A stress ECG may be done to measure the electrical activity of the heart during exertion, such as exercise on a treadmill. This test is usually performed by an ECG technician or a cardiologist and interpreted by a cardiologist.

Cardiac Scan: This scan involves the injection of a radioactive substance while a special camera traces its movement, through the heart. "Hot spot" imaging shows areas of heart muscle damage due to an infarct by increased activity in the area. A thallium scan will indicate areas where heart muscle is not receiving oxygen. A blood pool scan will reveal how efficiently blood is moving through the heart. This test is performed by a nuclear medicine technologist and interpreted by a radiologist or cardiologist.

Electrophysiologic Study (EPS): A catheter with electrodes attached to the end is placed through the femoral vein and guided to the heart. One electrode is placed near the sources of electrical activity, the SA node, and the bundle of His. Another electrode may be guided through the subclavian vein into the right ventricle. This study maps the electrical activity of the heart and is used to help diagnose patients with various arrhythmias. It is more accurate than an ECG because the electrodes are closer to the source of the electrical activity. This test is performed by an EPS technician and cardiologist. It is a sterile procedure.

Cardiac Catheterization: Catheterization is a sterile procedure in which one or more catheters are introduced into a vein or artery and guided to the heart. The catheter can be used to assess intracardiac pressures, retrieve samples of blood for testing (oxygen content), and inject contrast agent to render the heart visible on film. This test is used to evaluate chambers, valves, and coronary arteries. Cardiac catheterization is performed by cardiologists assisted by radiologic/cardiac technicians. The examination is interpreted by the cardiologist.

Transesophageal Echocardiography (TEE): In this procedure, a very small probe (transducer/endoscope combination) is placed in the mouth and advanced into the esophagus down to the stomach. Images of the heart in multiple planes are taken from the stomach and the esophagus. From these positions within the body, the view of the heart is unobstructed by bone, small rib spaces, increased body mass, and air in the lungs. Heart structures are well visualized, especially posterior structures that are not well seen from a transthoracic approach. The study is performed by a cardiologist with the help of a sonographer who operates the ultrasound equipment. The cardiologist interprets the study.

Stress Echocardiography: This is a procedure in which the echocardiogram is performed while the patient is stressed (the heart rate is caused to be increased by some method). There are three basic types or methods of increasing the heart rate: treadmill, bicycle, and pharmacologic. There are many indications for doing a stress echocardiogram. A major indication is visualization of wall motion abnormalities in coronary artery disease. The study is performed by a cardiologist or designate, a treadmill technologist, and a sonographer. A cardiologist interprets the study.

■ ■ ■   **LABORATORY VALUES**

The laboratory values for the heart are shown in Figure 23-38. Note that the oxygen content in the pulmonary circuit is lower than in the systemic circuit. Normal oxygen content on the right side is usually between 65% and 80%. Oxygen content on the left side ranges between 95% and 100%.

The pressures on the left side are normally higher than those on the right side, with right-sided systolic pressures being about one fourth to one fifth of those on the left.

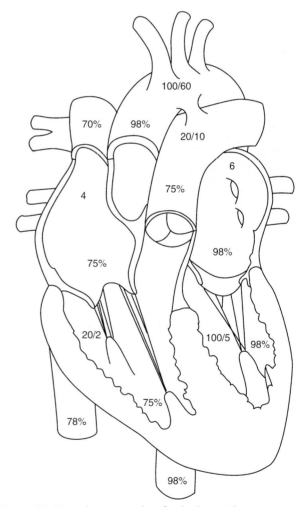

Figure 23-38 Laboratory values for the heart. The percentages show the relative oxygen saturations of the blood in the various vessels and cavities of the heart. The numbers with the slash between them show the normal systolic and diastolic pressures, respectively. The pressure values in the atria are diastolic since they have no systolic pressure.

■ ▨ ▨ NORMAL MEASUREMENTS

Normal measurements are presented in Table 23-1 on p. 421.

■ ▨ ▨ VASCULATURE

Aorta—right and left coronary arteries—Right and left coronary artery branches—Heart muscle and structures—Capillaries—Cardiac veins—Right atrium or coronary sinus—to Right atrium.

■ ▨ ▨ AFFECTING CHEMICALS

Epinephrine: A hormone secreted by the adrenal medulla that causes an increase in the heart rate and an increase in the blood pressure.

Thyroid Hormone: A hormone secreted by the thyroid gland that regulates overall body metabolism and causes an increase in the heart rate.

BIBLIOGRAPHY

Elson M: *It's your body,* New York, 1975, McGraw-Hill, p 479.

Feigenbaum H: *Echocardiography,* ed 4, Philadelphia, 1986, Lea & Febiger.

Fink BW: *Congenital heart disease: a deductive approach to its diagnosis,* ed 2, Chicago, 1985, Year Book.

Mallett M: *Handbook of anatomy and physiology for students of medical radiation technology,* ed 3, Mankato, 1981, Bumell, pp 129-137.

Monaghan MJ: *Practical echocardiography and Doppler,* Chichester, England, 1990, Wiley.

Moore KL: *The developing human,* ed 4, Philadelphia, 1988, WB Saunders, pp 286-333.

Rudolph AM, et al: *Rudolph's pediatrics,* ed 19, East Norwalk, 1991, Appleton and Lange, p 1340.

Snider A, Serwer GA: *Echocardiography in pediatric heart disease,* Chicago, 1990, Year Book.

Williams G, et al: *Echocardiographic diagnosis of cardiac malformations,* Boston, 1986, Little, Brown.

CHAPTER 24

Adult Echocardiography

J. CHARLES POPE III

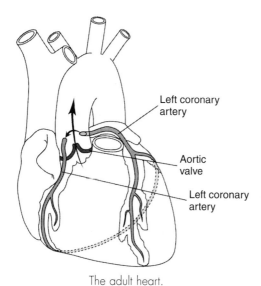

The adult heart.

Describe the location of the heart in the chest.
Describe the sonographic appearance of the heart.
Describe the imaging planes of the heart.
Identify cardiac anatomy in the various imaging planes.
Describe cardiac hemodynamics and physiology.
Describe the phases of the cardiac cycle, and relate them to intracardiac events.
Learn the normal values for heart chamber sizes, wall thickness, and Doppler flow velocities.
Identify normal Doppler flow patterns.
Discuss the indications for transesophageal echocardiography (TEE).
Identify the most common reasons for obtaining a TEE.
Select patients who most likely will require TEE for diagnosis of their condition.
Discuss the intraoperative use of TEE.
Describe the standard TEE echocardiographic images.
Define the key words.

KEY WORDS ■■■■■■

Aortic valve	Moderator band
Apex	Myocardium
Apical	Papillary muscles
Appendage	Parasternal
Atrioventricular (AV) node	Pericardium
Atrioventricular valves	Pulsed wave (PW)
Atrium (left and right)	Pulmonary arteries (right,
Base	left, and main) and veins
Bundle of His	Pulmonic valve
Chordae tendineae	Purkinje fibers
Continuous wave (CW)	Semilunar valves
Coronary arteries	Sinoatrial (SA) node
Coronary sinus	Subcostal (subxiphoid)
Diastole	Superior vena cava
Doppler	Suprasternal
Electrocardiogram	Systole
(ECG, EKG)	Transesophageal echocar-
Endocardium	diography (TEE)
Epicardium	Transthoracic echocardio-
Eustachian valve	graphy (TTE)
Inferior vena cava	Tricuspid valve
Interventricular septum (IVS)	Two-dimensional
Mitral (bicuspid) valve	echocardiogram
M-mode	Ventricle (left and right)

The heart is the center of the cardiovascular system. It is a muscular organ, about the size of your fist, that beats over 100,000 times every day. The heart's main function is to pump unoxygenated blood to the lungs and oxygenated blood to the vessels and tissues of the body.

The echocardiogram is a noninvasive diagnostic test used to evaluate the structural and hemodynamic relationships within the heart. It is an important tool used to assess overall cardiac function.

PRENATAL DEVELOPMENT

See Chapter 23.

LOCATION

The heart lies within the thoracic cavity, obscured by bone and lung. Located posterior to the sternum, the heart is situated between the right and the left lung within a space called the middle mediastinum (Figure 24-1). The heart lies at a 45-degree angle, between the third and fifth intercostal spaces.

The heart sits within a sac called the **pericardium.** This sac contains a small amount (10 to 20 ml) of serous fluid that lubricates the heart as it beats.

The lower border of the heart forms a blunt point called the **apex.** The apex is formed by the tip of the left ventricle. It is directed to the left of the midline and sits more inferiorly and anteriorly than the **base** of the heart, where the great vessels arise.

The superior border of the heart is formed by the atria. The inferior portion is almost entirely right ventricle and only a small portion of the left ventricle.

The anterior surface of the heart is composed almost entirely of right ventricle, though a small portion of the right atrium and left ventricle can be seen. The left heart covers the posterior surface.

The right atrium makes up the right border of the heart, and the left ventricle, along with a small portion of the left atrium, covers the left border.

SIZE

The size of the heart depends on a person's age, weight, and sex. The American Society of Echocardiography has set standards by which the heart should be measured.

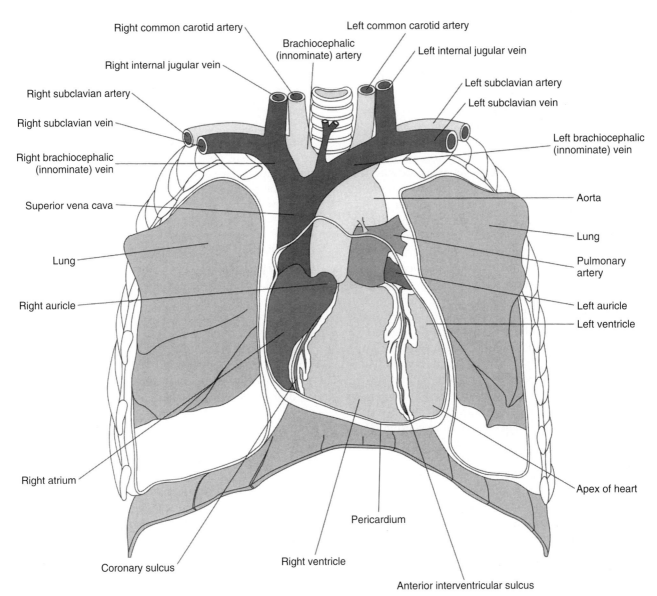

Figure 24-1 The external structures and location of the heart in the thoracic cavity.

These measurements will be discussed further in the section on M-mode echocardiography.

GROSS ANATOMY

The heart is a muscular four-chambered pump located in the center of the chest. Internally it is divided into two collecting chambers (atria) and two pumping chambers (ventricles). A system of connecting arteries and veins allows the heart to move blood from systemic to pulmonary circulation and back (Figure 24-2).

The walls of the heart consist of three layers: (1) the **epicardium,** the smooth, thin outer layer; (2) the **myocardium,** the thick layer of contractile muscle; and (3) the **endocardium,** the thin layer of endothelial tissue lining the internal surface.

The two upper cavities of the heart are the **right** and **left atria.** From the superior portion of each atrium is a small triangular extension called an **appendage.** The appendages are also called auricles (because they resemble ears). Within the appendages and extending out to the anterior surfaces of the atria are the pectinate muscles. The remaining endocardial surfaces of the atrial walls are smooth.

The atria are separated medially by the interatrial septum. Along this septum is a thinner oval region known as the fossa ovalis. This corresponds to the foramen ovale in the fetal heart.

The right atrium receives deoxygenated blood from all parts of the body including itself. The blood returning from the peripheral tissues enters the heart via the inferior and superior venae cavae. The coronary sinus also enters the right atrium and drains the vessels that had supplied the heart. The left atrium, on the other hand, receives blood from the lungs via four pulmonary veins.

The two inferior chambers are the **right** and **left ventricles.** The ventricles are thicker walled than the atria, with the left ventricle being almost three times thicker than the right. This is because the pressure is greater in the left heart than in the right. The right ventricle is also more trabeculated than the left and contains four prominent muscular bands; (1) parietal band, (2) crista supraventricularis, (3) septal band, and (4) **moderator band** (often seen with ultrasound). Medially, the ventricles are separated by the **interventricular septum (IVS).**

On the external surface of the heart, the ventricles are separated by the anterior and posterior interventricular sulci. The ventricles are then separated from the atria by the coronary sulcus. The sulci are grooves that contain the coronary vessels, all of which are embedded in fat. The fat serves to protect the vessels.

Located within the heart are four one-way valves. Their function is to maintain a uniform direction of blood flow. These valves are divided into two groups; atrioventricular and semilunar. The **atrioventricular valves** are located between the atria and the ventricles,

and are anchored at one end to the annulosus fibrosus. **Chordae tendineae** attach the tips of the leaflets to **papillary muscles** located in the ventricles. Normally this arrangement keeps blood flowing in one direction only.

The **semilunar valves** are located at the junction where the ventricles meet the great vessels. They are called semilunar because each of the three leaflets is shaped like a half moon. The pocket shape of the leaflets, as well as the pressure exerted during diastole, closes the semilunar valves and prevents blood from moving backward.

The right-sided atrioventricular valve is called the **tricuspid valve** because it has three leaflets: anterior, posterior, and septal. The left-sided atrioventricular valve is called the **mitral** (or **bicuspid**) **valve** because of its similar appearance to a bishop's miter. It has two leaflets: anterior and posterior.

The two semilunar valves are the **aortic valve** and the **pulmonic valve.** The aortic valve is located at the junction of the left ventricle and the aorta. Its three cusps are the right coronary cusp, the left coronary cusp, and the noncoronary cusp. The pulmonic valve is located at the junction of the right ventricle and the pulmonary artery. It has three cusps: anterior, right, and left. Just distal to the aortic valve in the proximal aortic root are outpouchings known as the sinuses of Valsalva.

Just as there are three cusps to the valve, there are three sinuses. This is where the **coronary arteries** originate. The right and left coronary arteries arise from the right and left sinuses of Valsalva. The noncoronary sinus has no artery associated with it.

PHYSIOLOGY

Circulatory System

As blood circulates throughout the body, it carries valuable nutrients and the oxygen required for survival of the tissues. Circulation of the blood is controlled by the heart.

Right heart circulation begins in the right atrium, which collects deoxygenated blood from the entire body (Figure 24-3). Blood returning from the upper portion of the body enters the right atrium via the **superior vena cava.** Deoxygenated blood from the lower body enters the right atrium by way of the **inferior vena cava.** The heart also drains deoxygenated blood from itself through the **coronary sinus.** This blood also enters the right atrium.

Once the right atrium is full, the oxygen-depleted blood flows through the tricuspid valve and into the right ventricle. The right ventricle then pumps the blood past the pulmonic valve and into the **main pulmonary artery.** The main pulmonary artery shortly thereafter bifurcates into the **right** and **left pulmonary arteries.** These in turn enter each of the lungs, where the blood is reoxygenated in the pulmonary circuit.

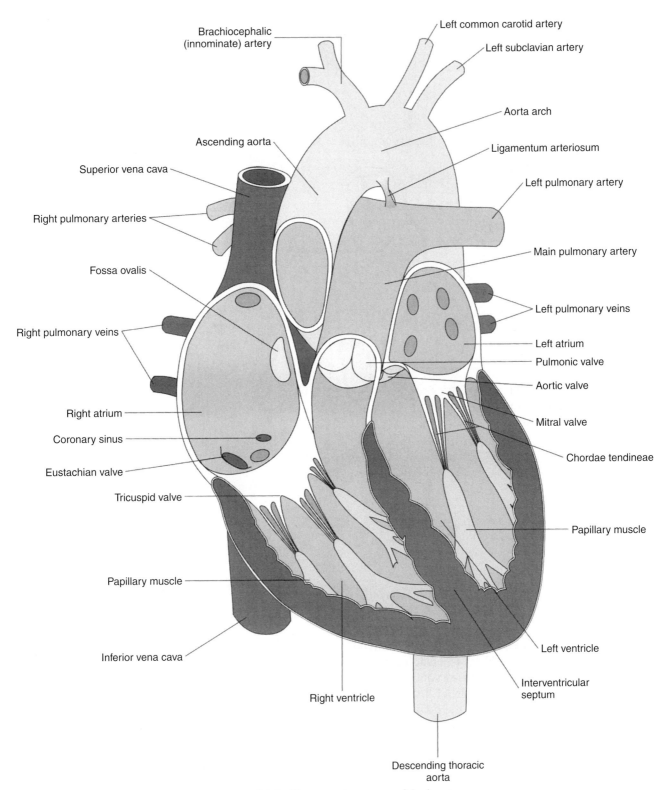

Figure 24-2 The internal structures of the heart.

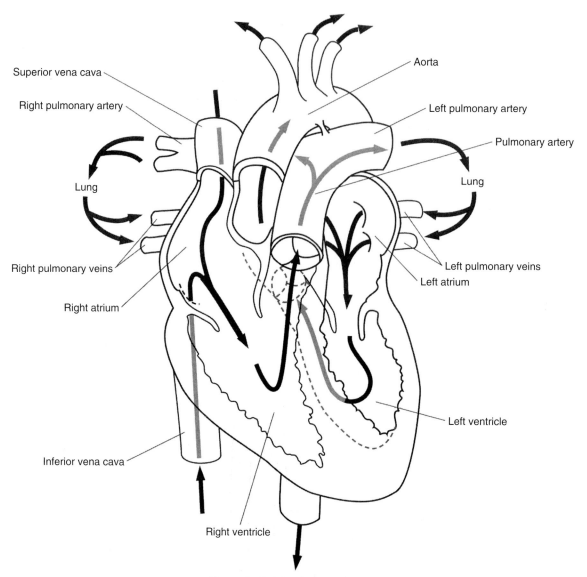

Figure 24-3 Cardiac circulation.

Once the blood has passed through the pulmonary capillary circuit and has been reoxygenated, it needs to be collected and distributed to the heart and the rest of the body. This is the function of the left heart. Freshly oxygenated blood is returned from the lungs to the left atrium through the four **pulmonary veins.** The blood then passes from the left atrium, through the mitral valve, and into the left ventricle. The left ventricle then pumps the blood past the aortic valve and into the aorta. From here, the oxygenated blood is distributed to the heart and the rest of the body through the arterial system. This is the start of systemic circulation.

Cardiac muscle tissue needs a constant supply of fresh blood to remain viable. It accomplishes this through the coronary arterial system. There are two major coronary arteries: the right and the left main coronary arteries. The origin of the coronaries is the aortic root just posterior to the valve in the region of the right and left sinuses of Valsalva.

The left coronary artery differs from the right in that shortly after its origin, the left main artery bifurcates, forming the left anterior descending artery, which usually supplies the anterior left ventricular wall, apex, and a portion of the interventricular septum with oxygenated blood. The other branch is the left circumflex coronary artery, which mainly supplies the left atrium and the lateral and posterior walls of the left ventricle.

The right coronary artery also branches into the posterior descending artery, which supplies portions of the right and left ventricles with oxygenated blood, and the marginal artery, which supplies the right atrium and some of the right ventricle.

The heart also has a venous system that courses over its surface and drains into the coronary sinus. The specific pattern of the arteries and veins may vary among individuals.

Conduction System

The heart has an intricate electrical system composed of highly specialized cardiac muscle tissue. The conduction system is designed to provide continuous electrical stimulation to the heart, ensuring that the various segments of the cardiac cycle progress in the normal, sequential manner.

The conduction system is composed of four major sections; the **sinoatrial (SA) node,** the **atrioventricular (AV) node,** the **bundle of His** (pronounced hiss), and the **Purkinje fibers** (Figure 24-4). Each section has a

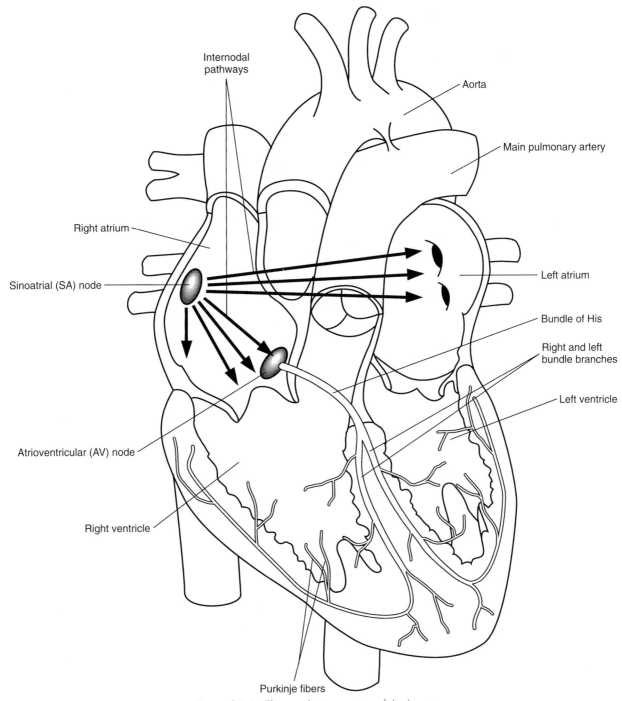

Internodal pathways

Aorta

Main pulmonary artery

Right atrium

Sinoatrial (SA) node

Left atrium

Bundle of His

Right and left bundle branches

Left ventricle

Atrioventricular (AV) node

Right ventricle

Purkinje fibers

Figure 24-4 The conduction system of the heart.

specific task to perform in regulating the cardiac cycle. In addition to its specific tasks, each portion of the conduction system has its own intrinsic rate of discharge. This allows the different sections of the conduction system to regulate the cardiac cycle in the event of a primary pacemaker failure. The dominant pacemaker of the heart is going to be the one discharging at the highest rate.

Normally the SA node is the pacemaker. It therefore sets the basic pace for the heart rate with a discharge rate of between 60 and 100 beats per minute. Located in the upper portion of the right atrium, near the entrance of the superior vena cava, the SA node receives input from both the sympathetic and parasympathetic nervous systems. Electrical impulses from the SA node spread over both atria by way of internodal pathways, causing them to contract at the same time (atrial systole). This impulse is responsible for the P wave of the electrocardiogram and, in turn, causes the AV node to depolarize.

The AV node is the second section of the conduction system. It is located near the inferior portion on the right side of the interatrial septum. Its primary task is to delay transmission of the SA nodal impulse long enough to give the ventricles time to repolarize and fill completely. The AV node is responsible for the P-R interval of the electrocardiogram, with an intrinsic discharge rate of 55 beats per minute. In the event of SA node failure, the AV node is the backup pacemaker for the heart.

The impulse is then delivered to the final segments of the conduction system, the bundle of His and the Purkinje fibers. The bundle of His divides into the right and left bundle branches, which run down the interventricular septum. The Purkinje fibers innervate the ventricular myocardium. Together they are responsible for distributing the electrical impulse to the ventricular muscle fibers, thereby causing mechanical contraction. This transmission is responsible for the QRS complex noted on the electrocardiogram. The bundle of His and the Purkinje fibers (with discharge rates of 40 to 30, respectively), are next in line in the event of pacemaker failure, with the ventricular myocardium (discharge rate of 20 beats per minute) acting as a final backup in the event of total pacemaker failure.

The Electrocardiogram

The **electrocardiogram (ECG, EKG)** is composed of a number of different waveforms that represent the electrical impulses of the cardiac cycle. These impulses can be detected on the surface of the body; when electrodes are placed on the skin, the change in the electrical field can be measured. Three distinct waves are recognized and labeled, with letters P, Q, R, S, and T (Figure 24-5).

The P wave and the P-R interval represent the final portion of the cardiac cycle, known as diastole. The P wave appears as a small upward bump. This reflects

atrial depolarization caused by the SA node, as the electrical impulse travels through atrial muscle tissue. The atria contract, resulting in atrial systole. The P-R interval reflects the delay in transmission caused by the AV node.

The next downward deflection represents the beginning of the QRS complex, which continues in an upward direction and ends in a downward motion. This reflects the electrical stimulation of the ventricular myocardium, caused by the distribution of the electrical impulse through the bundle of His and the Purkinje fibers. The QRS complex represents the beginning of the portion of the cardiac cycle known as systole.

The T wave of the ECG represents the ventricular repolarization (relaxation) phase of the cardiac cycle, and marks the start of the diastolic portion of the cardiac cycle. The S-T segment is a refractory period and begins at the end of ventricular systole to the time of repolarization.

By study of the variations in the sizes of the deflections and the time intervals of the ECG, abnormal cardiac rhythms and conduction patterns can be diagnosed.

Systole/Diastole

The cardiac cycle is categorized into two separate and distinct segments: systole and diastole. Both segments contribute significantly to maintaining the cardiac output. A thorough understanding of the systolic and diastolic phases of the cardiac cycle as well as the hemodynamics (the movement of blood) associated with them will allow the sonographer to think through the echocardiographic examination.

Diastole is the left ventricular relaxation and filling phase of the cardiac cycle. Diastole occurs from the end of the T wave until the beginning of the next QRS complex. During this portion of the cardiac cycle the atria are filling with blood. The AV valves are closed and the ventricular pressures are at or near 0 mm Hg. As pressure in the atria rises to a point above the ventricular pressures, the AV valves open to eject the volume of blood into the ventricles. This is known as the rapid filling phase of the cardiac cycle. At that point, ventricular myocardium is relaxed. As pressures rise in the ventricle and fall in the atria, the AV valves begin to drift shut. Just prior to ventricular systole, the atria contract (corresponding to the P wave on the ECG) to eject their final volumes of blood into the ventricles. This increases the amount of stretch on ventricular muscle fibers, thereby increasing the force of muscle contraction. During this period of time, the semilunar valves are closed and pressure in the ventricles increases just as the volume of blood increases, prior to systole.

Systole is the ventricular ejection phase of the cardiac cycle and occurs from the onset of the QRS complex to the end of the T wave. The ventricular muscle fibers contract. The increase in pressure causes the AV valves to close, preventing backflow of blood and causing the

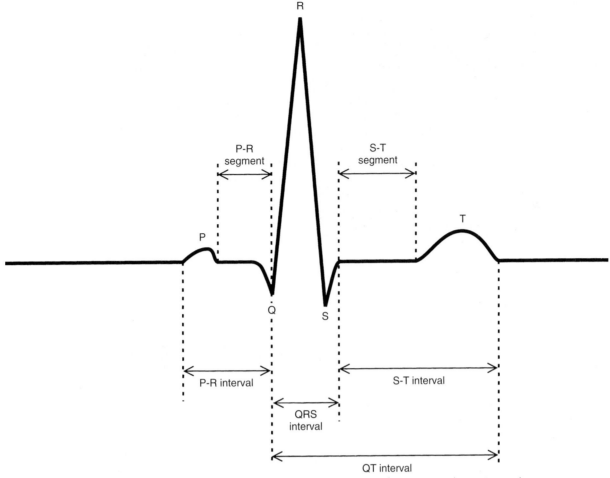

Figure 24-5 Single beat on a normal electrocardiogram (ECG) demonstrating the QRS complex.

semilunar valves to open. The blood is ejected from the ventricles and enters the aorta and pulmonary artery. As the blood is ejected, the pressure in the ventricles starts to decrease and, in turn, pressure in the atria starts to increase. This sets the stage for the next cardiac cycle.

SONOGRAPHIC APPEARANCE
Two-Dimensional Echocardiography
Sonographically, the pericardium is the most echogenic structure of the heart and is often seen as bright or white in color. Blood or any other fluids appear anechoic or black. The myocardium and papillary muscles are homogeneous and appear sonographically to be composed of medium-gray shades. The thin, mobile leaflets, or valve cusps, have a slightly increased echogenicity when compared with heart muscle, depending on the angle of the ultrasound beam. The views presented here reflect the standards set by the American Society of Echocardiography for **two-dimensional echocardiograms.**

A **parasternal** long axis view transects the heart from the base to the apex (Figure 24-6). Most anteriorly, the right ventricle will be visualized. This is separated from the left ventricle by the interventricular septum (IVS).

The IVS is continuous with the anterior portion of the aortic root. Only two of the aortic valve leaflets are visualized from this view. The more anterior leaflet is the right coronary cusp, and the more posterior leaflet is the noncoronary cusp. Posterior to the aortic root is the left atrium. The posterior portion of the aortic root is continuous with the anterior mitral valve leaflet. The posterior mitral valve leaflet attaches to the valve annulus, near the atrioventricular groove. Attached to the posterior wall of the left ventricle, the posteromedial papillary muscle may be visualized. The chordae tendineae can be seen to extend from this muscle to the tips of the mitral valve leaflets. The area from the tips of the mitral valve leaflets to the aortic valve is considered the left ventricular outflow tract (LVOT). At the level of the atrioventricular groove a small, echofree area may be noticed. This represents the coronary sinus. Posterior to the heart another anechoic area is seen. This represents a cross-section of the descending thoracic aorta.

During diastole, the mitral valve is in the open position, allowing the left ventricle to fill with blood, and the aortic valve is closed (Figure 24-7, *A*). As the ventricle fills with blood, the distance between the septal and

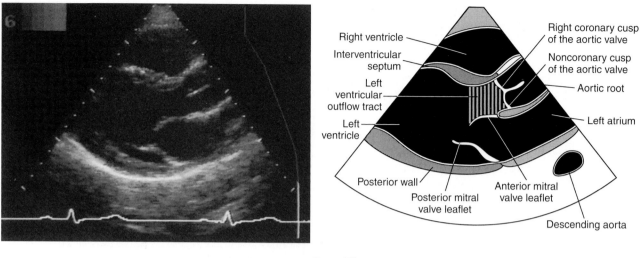

Right ventricle
Interventricular septum
Left ventricular outflow tract
Left ventricle
Posterior wall
Posterior mitral valve leaflet
Anterior mitral valve leaflet
Right coronary cusp of the aortic valve
Noncoronary cusp of the aortic valve
Aortic root
Left atrium
Descending aorta

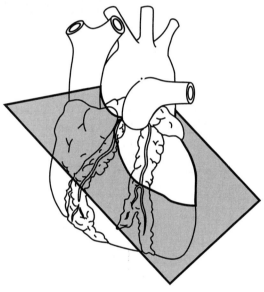

PLANE OF SECTION

Figure 24-6 Parasternal long axis view.

posterior walls increases. During systole, the left ventricle contracts and the walls squeeze closer together. The mitral valve is now closed and the aortic valve is open, allowing blood to leave the left ventricle and enter the aortic root (Figure 24-7, *B*). The patient is connected to an ECG monitor that runs simultaneously along the image. This helps to assist in timing the cardiac cycle.

In a parasternal short axis view at the level of the aortic valve, the great arteries of the heart are visible (Figure 24-8). Centrally located in this view is the aortic valve. This should appear as a circle with a Y in the middle, representing the aortic valve cusps in the diastolic phase of the cardiac cycle, when the leaflets are normally closed. At this point in the cardiac cycle one can easily visualize the right, the left, and the noncoronary cusps. During systole, the valve leaflets open to form a triangle (Figure 24-9). The origin of the coronary arteries may be

seen at this level near the right and left coronary cusps. Posterior to the aorta, the left atrium can be seen. In some instances, the left atrial appendage may be seen jutting off to the right of the screen. The right atrium can be seen on the left side of the screen separated from the left atrium by the interatrial septum (IAS). Moving anteriorly along the left side of the screen, the next structure noted is the tricuspid valve, which separates the right atrium from the right ventricle. The right ventricle is most anterior and can be seen wrapping around the aorta. The right ventricle is separated from the pulmonary artery, which is seen on the right side of the screen, by the pulmonic valve.

The mitral valve can be visualized from a parasternal short axis view. The heart appears as a circle, with the anterior and posterior valve leaflets seen in the center of the image (Figure 24-10). As the leaflets open and close

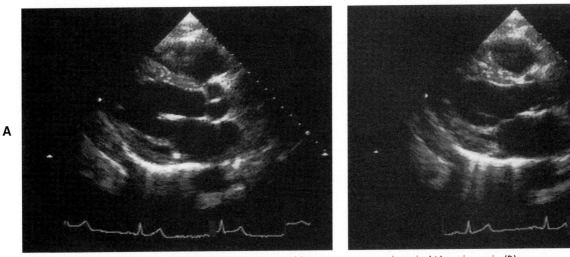

Figure 24-7 Parasternal long axis view in diastole **(A)** and systole **(B)**.

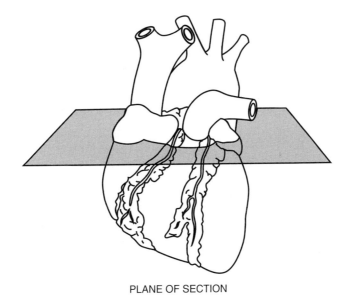

Right ventricular outflow tract

Right coronary cusp of the aortic valve

Pulmonic valve

Pulmonary artery

Tricuspid valve

Left coronary cusp of the aortic valve

Noncoronary cusp of the aortic valve

Left atrium

Right atrium

Interatrial septum

Descending aorta

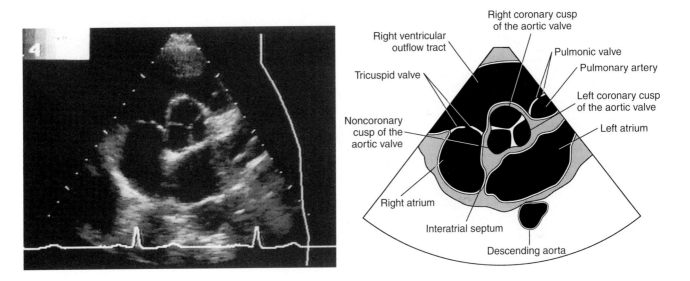

PLANE OF SECTION

Figure 24-8 Parasternal short axis view at the level of the aortic valve during diastole.

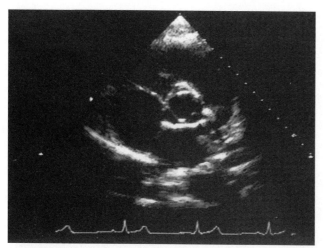

Figure 24-9   Parasternal short axis at the level of the aortic valve during systole.

during the cardiac cycle, they look somewhat like a fish's mouth. Anterior to the left heart is the right ventricle. These structures are separated by the IVS.

At the level of the papillary muscles, the left ventricle again appears as a circular structure, and the papillary muscles protrude from the inner surface of the ventricular wall. Two papillary muscles are visible (Figure 24-11). The posteromedial muscle is seen on the left of the screen and the anterolateral is seen on the right of the screen. The anechoic area within the left ventricle then takes on the shape of a mushroom. The right ventricle is again anterior to the left ventricle and is separated by the IVS.

Figure 24-12 is an **apical** four-chamber view displaying all four chambers of the heart. The ventricles are displayed at the top of the screen and the atria are displayed at the bottom of the two-dimensional sector

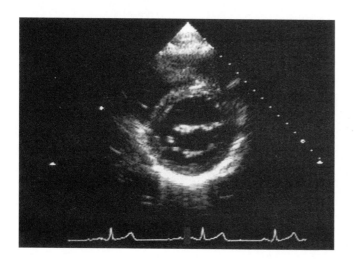

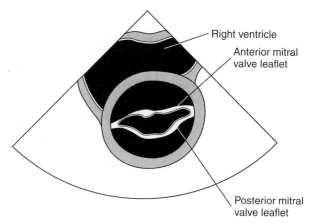

Right ventricle

Anterior mitral valve leaflet

Posterior mitral valve leaflet

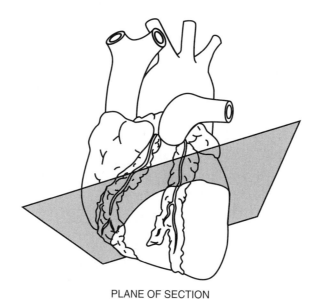

PLANE OF SECTION

Figure 24-10   Parasternal short axis view at the level of the mitral valve.

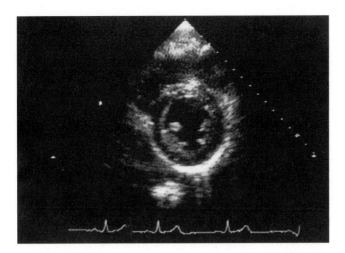

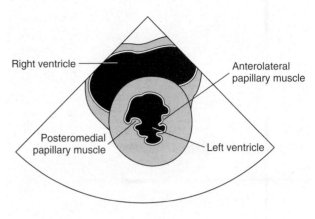

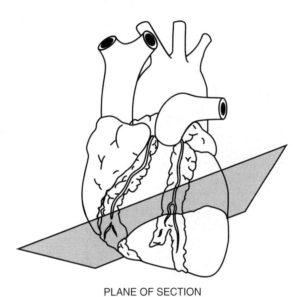

PLANE OF SECTION

Figure 24-11 Parasternal short axis view at the level of the papillary muscles.

image. The left ventricle and left atria are displayed on the right side of the screen. The right ventricle and right atria are displayed on the left side of the screen. Wall motion can be evaluated from the apical view by further subdividing the left ventricle into basal (proximal), mid, and apical (distal) walls (Figure 24-13).

The interventricular septum separates the left from the right ventricle. Deep in the right ventricle, near the apex, the moderator band can be seen to cross from the right ventricular free wall to the interventricular septum. The interatrial septum separates the left from the right atria. The pulmonary veins can be seen entering the inferior portion of the left atrium. Both the anterior and posterior mitral valves can be seen in the left heart, while only two of the tricuspid leaflets can be seen in the right heart. The septal leaflet of the tricuspid valve is situated slightly closer to the apex of the heart (normally no more than 1 cm) than the anterior leaflet of the mitral valve.

The aortic root can be imaged along with the other four chambers. This is referred to as an apical five-chamber view (Figure 24-14).

An image of the ascending and descending aorta and the aortic arch, as well as the vessels that arise from it, can be visualized from a **suprasternal** orientation (Figure 24-15). The vessels in descending order are (1) brachiocephalic (or innominate) artery, (2) left common carotid artery, and (3) left subclavian artery.

Posterior to the arch, a cross-sectional view of the right pulmonary artery can be seen. In some instances, the left atrium can be seen posterior to this.

M-Mode Echocardiography

Two-dimensional imaging is a very powerful diagnostic tool and has superseded the qualitative role of M-mode in the echocardiographic examination. Yet M-mode is still an important supplement to the cardiac examination. It

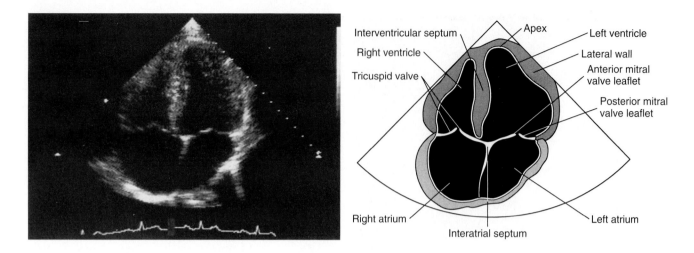

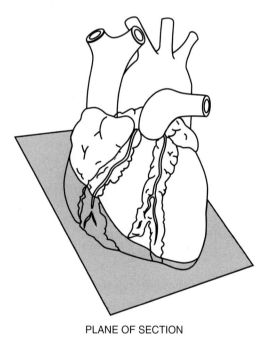

PLANE OF SECTION

Figure 24-12 Apical four-chamber view.

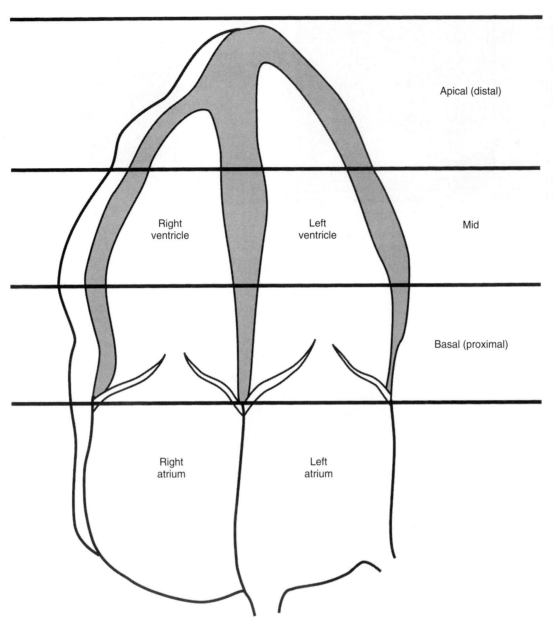

Figure 24-13 The subdivisions of the left ventricular walls from an apical four-chamber view.

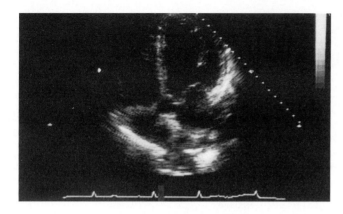

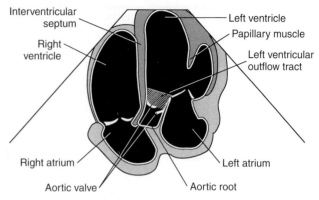

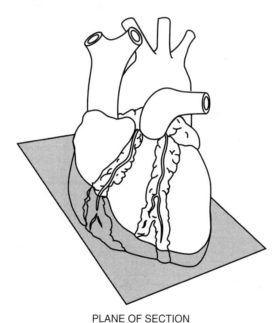

PLANE OF SECTION

Figure 24-14 Apical five-chamber view.

provides a quantitative system through which measurements of cardiac structures can be obtained. Where a structure should be measured and what is considered normal are based on the recommendations of the American Society of Echocardiography. This makes the practice of assessing an M-mode examination consistent.

M-mode is also a tool for evaluating subtle changes or rapid movements of the heart that the eye may not see during the real-time examination. Simply put, the *M* in M-mode stands for motion. Imagine drawing a line through the heart. Everything along that line is portrayed on a graph, creating a one-dimensional reproduction of the cardiac structures.

An M-mode is a measure of distance over time. Distance is presented on the X axis and is calibrated by a series of dots that are 1 cm apart. Time is displayed across the Y axis. Here a series of dots 0.5 second apart are used for calibration (Figure 24-16).

The M-mode is most commonly scrolled on paper from a strip chart and appears as a black tracing on a white background.

The anatomy seen at the level of the aortic valve includes the right ventricle anteriorly, the anterior wall of the aortic root, the posterior wall of the aortic root, and the left atrium. The aortic valve is seen with the aortic root. Only two cusps are seen from this view: the right coronary cusp, anteriorly, and the noncoronary cusp, posteriorly (Figure 24-17). These cusps can be seen to form a sort of box during systole as blood is ejected from the left ventricle. The closed valve appears as a straight line during diastole.

The mitral valve is a biphasic valve caused by the rapid filling phase of the LV and the atrial "kick" in the latter part of the cardiac cycle (Figure 24-18). The valve is open during diastole and closed during systole. Its biphasic quality causes the motion of the anterior

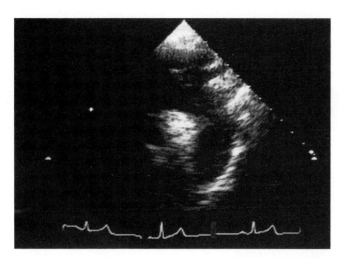

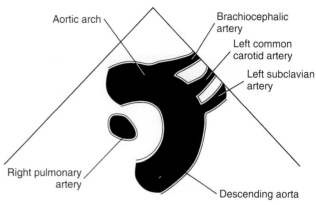

Aortic arch

Brachiocephalic artery

Left common carotid artery

Left subclavian artery

Right pulmonary artery

Descending aorta

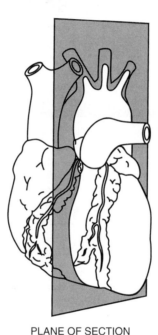

PLANE OF SECTION

Figure 24-15   Aortic arch from the suprasternal notch.

leaflet to appear in the shape of an M. The posterior leaflet mirrors the anterior and appears as a W.

The anterior leaflet of the mitral valve is labeled alphabetcially to correspond with the various phases of diastole (Figure 24-19). To begin with, the D point represents the opening of the valve during disastole and the E point represents the maximum excursion of the leaflet. This occurs during the passive filling phase. The anterior leaflet then begins to close. The point where it stops moving posteriorly is the F point. The next peak anterior motion of the mitral valve is the A wave. This corresponds to atrial contraction and the P wave on the ECG. Valve closure is appropriately represented by the C point. In some situations, such as diastolic dysfunction

of the left ventricle, an additional bump may occur between the A and C points. This abnormal closure of the valve creates what is known as a B notch.

M-mode sampling from the left ventricle is seen in Figure 24-20. Starting anteriorly, the anatomy seen is the right ventricle, the IVS, the left ventricle, and the posterior wall of the left ventricle.

Other areas of the heart can be evaluated by M-mode. Generally, the only other structures seen are the valve leaflets from the tricuspid and pulmonary valves. Normally, only one tricuspid valve leaflet is seen with M-mode (Figure 24-21.). The pulmonic valve is most difficult to visualize, but can be especially helpful in patients with pulmonary stenosis or hypertension (Fig-

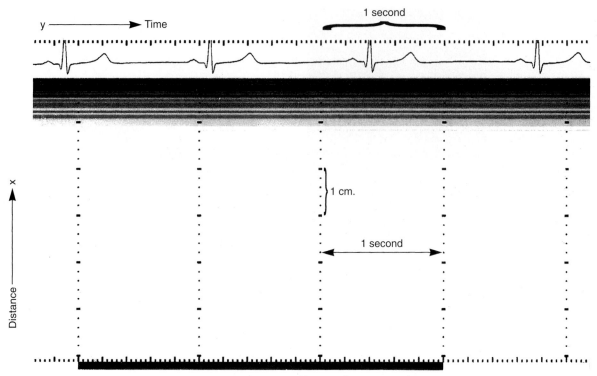

Figure 24-16 Proper calibration for an M-mode.

ure 24-22). The pulmonic valve is also labeled using letters A through F.

Doppler Echocardiography

Spectral Doppler and color flow mapping are two forms of **Doppler** used to derive hemodynamic information about the heart. Spectral Doppler is divided into two forms: **pulsed wave (PW)** and **continuous wave (CW).** Each has its advantages and disadvantages but should be used in conjunction to realize their full potential.

Normal Doppler Waveforms. Normal flow within the heart has a characteristic appearance. When interrogating each valve, it is important to recognize these normal patterns so that any type of disturbance can be fully evaluated. Abnormal flow within the heart indicates increased velocities, regurgitation, and turbulence.

It is also important to note the direction of flow. Blood moving toward the transducer will be represented above the baseline on the Doppler strip, and flow moving away from the transducer will fall below the baseline. When evaluating a profile, it is important to look at the pattern, velocity, direction of flow, and timing, in accordance with the cardiac cycle.

Doppler is best evaluated when flow is parallel to the transducer. This is not necessarily where the best two-dimensional image is obtained.

Mitral Valve. Normal mitral flow is biphasic, taking the shape of an M. Like the M-mode tracing, the E wave is higher than the A wave. In the apical four-chamber view, flow moves toward the transducer from the left atrium to the left ventricle. Mitral flow therefore is above the baseline and occurs during diastole (Figure 24-23).

Aortic Valve. Normal aortic flow is systolic and is shaped like a bullet. When sampled from the apical five-chamber view, blood moves away from the transducer, from the left ventricle to the aortic root. Here the profile would appear below the baseline (Figure 24-24).

Aortic Arch. Either the ascending or the descending aorta may be evaluated from the suprasternal notch. Depending on how the transducer is angled, flow will appear above the baseline within the ascending aorta and below the baseline within the descending aorta. Flow will be systolic and bullet shaped (Figure 24-25).

Tricuspid Valve. Normal triscuspid flow is also shaped like an M. It occurs during diastole and appears above the baseline. The velocity range is lower than that for the mitral valve. This is due to lower pressures found in the right heart (Figure 24-26).

Pulmonic Valve. The systolic flow of the pulmonic valve appears below the baseline and has a bullet shape (Figure 24-27).

In addition to a duplex Doppler evaluation, which provides an image of the heart along with the Doppler waveform, a dedicated CW Doppler probe may be used (Figure 24-28). This specialized probe provides only the spectral waveform, without the two-dimensional image.

Text continued on p. 473

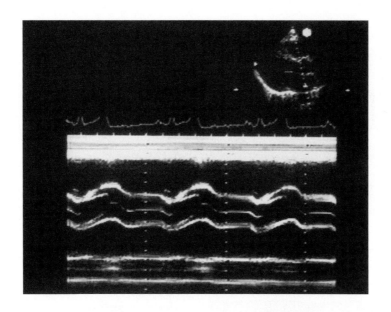

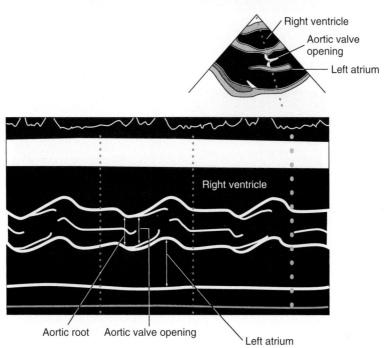

Figure 24-17 M-mode at the level of the aortic valve.

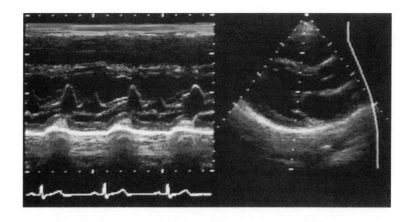

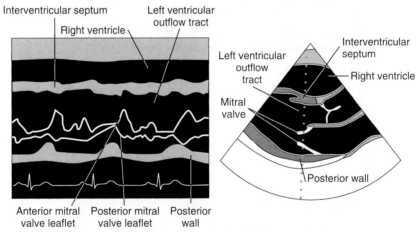

Interventricular septum

Right ventricle

Left ventricular outflow tract

Left ventricular outflow tract

Interventricular septum

Right ventricle

Mitral valve

Posterior wall

Anterior mitral valve leaflet

Posterior mitral valve leaflet

Posterior wall

Figure 24-18 M-mode at the level of the mitral valve.

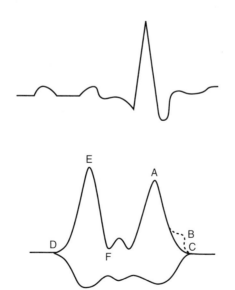

E

A

D

F

B

C

Figure 24-19 Proper labeling of the mitral valve.

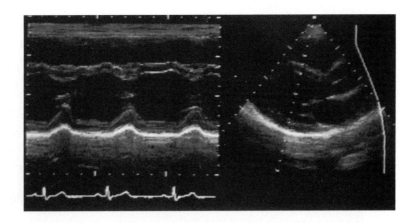

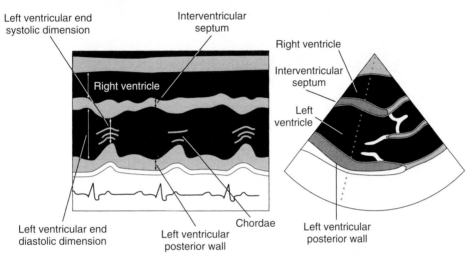

Figure 24-20 M-mode at the level of the left ventricle.

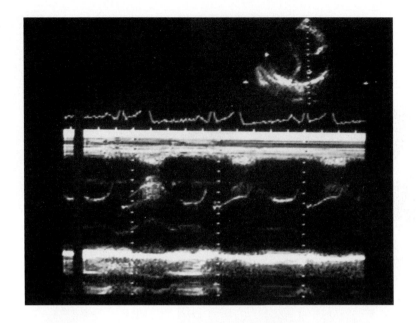

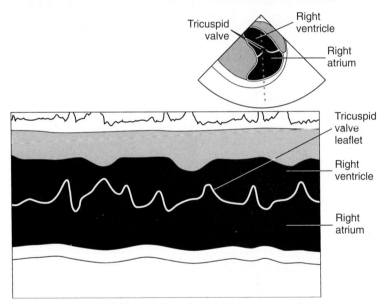

Figure 24-21 M-mode through the tricuspid valve.

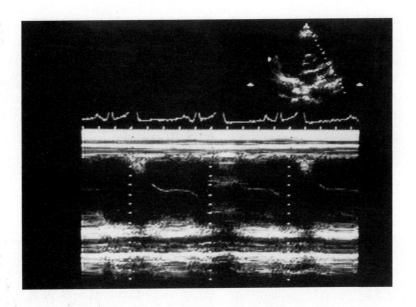

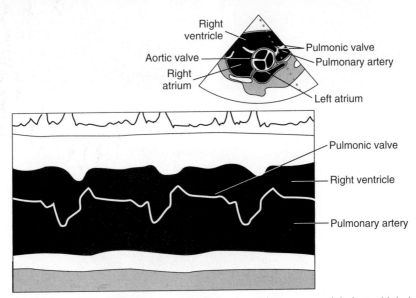

Figure 24-22   M-mode through the pulmonic valve with its proper alphabetical labels.

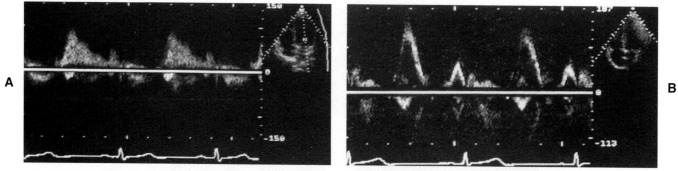

Figure 24-23 Doppler flow profiles of the mitral valve in both continuous wave (**A**) and pulsed wave (**B**).

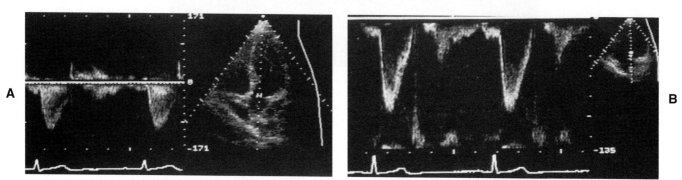

Figure 24-24 Doppler flow profiles of the aortic valve in both continuous wave (**A**) and pulsed wave (**B**).

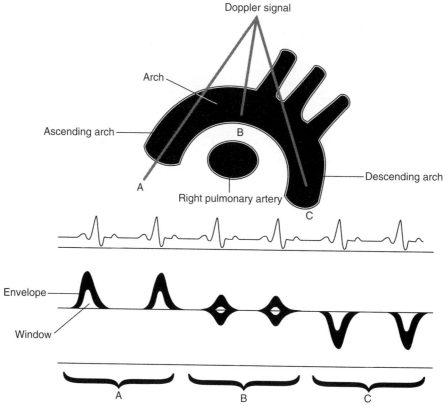

Figure 24-25 Doppler flow in the aortic arch. As flow moves toward the transducer in the ascending aorta, it appears above the baseline; as flow moves away in the descending aorta, it falls below the baseline.

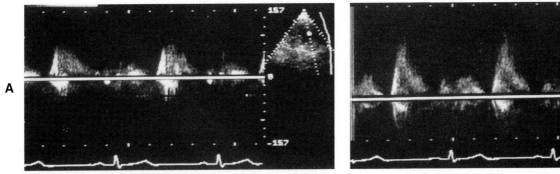

Figure 24-26 Doppler flow profiles of the tricuspid valve in both continuous wave **(A)** and pulsed wave **(B)**.

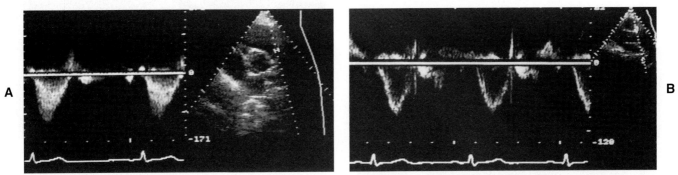

Figure 24-27 Doppler flow profiles of the pulmonic valve in both continuous wave **(A)** and pulsed wave **(B)**.

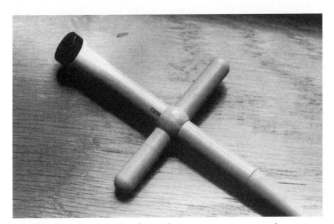

Figure 24-28 Dedicated continuous wave probe.

Transesophageal Echocardiography (TEE)

Although **transthoracic echocardiography (TTE)** remains the cornerstone of echocardiographic imaging and diagnosis, **transesophageal echocardiography (TEE)** is increasing in use because it provides information not obtainable by the transthoracic approach.

In most labs, the most common indication for TEE is evaluation for cardiac source of embolus. Other common indications include evaluation of prosthetic valves and native valvular disease, infective endocarditis, aortic

pathology including aortic dissection, intracardiac masses, and congenital heart disease. Other indications include patients with lung disease; critically ill patients, especially those on a ventilator; and patients with sternal infections or thoracic deformities.

Technically inadequate surface examinations may be the result of a poor acoustic window from the patient's body habitus or other skeletal abnormalities, or chronic obstructive pulmonary disease with hyperinflated lungs. Patients on ventilators or status post–open heart surgery with sternal bandanges or open sternum are also candidates for TEE. Critically ill patients and patients on ventilators who often have very limited acoustical windows are good candidates for TEE.

Applying the probe requires the patient to be lying in the left lateral decubitus position or in an upright position. The probe is advanced to the oropharynx and the patient is asked to swallow several times. The neck is flexed. The probe is advanced 30 to 35 cm from the incisors into position.

Midesophageal views are short or horizontal views from a longitudinal scan obtained at approximately 30 to 35 cm. At roughly 35 to 40 cm, the four chambers of the heart can be identified (Figure 24-29). Transgastric long-axis and short-axis views at the 40 to 45 cm range are where the descending thoracic aorta is evaluated with about a 180-degree counter-clockwise rotation. The left ventricle and chamber size can be assessed as well (Figure 24-30). On basilar views at approximately the same range, the aorta, right and left atria, and interatrial septum can be demonstrated (Figure 24-31). Contrast enhancements may be performed using agitated saline with rapid intravenous injection to rule out any shunting abnormalities.

TEE is often used in the intraoperative setting. It can be used to evaluate valve replacement or repair. TEE can detect air or fat emboli—complications that may occur from operative procedures. Although not recommended as a routine procedure, TEE can be also be used to monitor high-risk coronary artery disease to identify wall motion abnormalities that may indicate abnormal left ventricular function.

SONOGRAPHIC APPLICATIONS

Echocardiography is commonly used in the evaluation of the following: cardiac anatomy, cardiac size, acquired heart disease (stenosis, valve replacement), congenital heart disease, coronary heart disease, pericardial diseases, cardiac tumors/thrombi, diseases of the aorta, cardiomyopathies, and hemodynamic information.

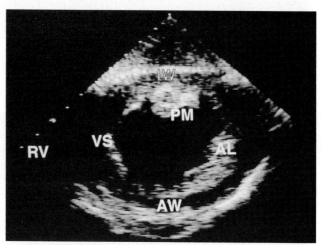

Figure 24-30 TEE transgastric view. Trangastric view demonstrating the walls of the left ventricle and chamber size. Note the ventricular septum separating left and right ventricles.

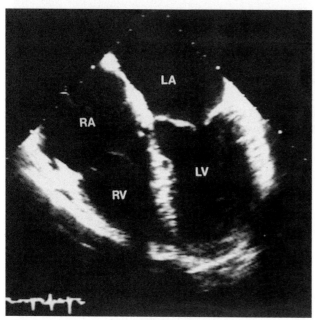

Figure 24-29 TEE midesophageal view. Four chambers of the heart are demonstrated. The left and right atria and ventricles are seen. Note the mitral valve is more visible than the tricuspid valve.

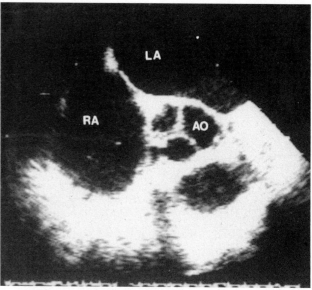

Figure 24-31 TEE basilar view. Basilar view of the aorta, left and right atria, and the interatrial septum.

NORMAL VARIANTS
Eustachian Valve
The **eustachian valve** can be seen in the right atrium near the entrance of the inferior vena cava. In the fetus, it was a functional valve covering the entrance to the IVC. Only a remnant of the valve is now seen. It is best visualized in the right ventricular inflow view.

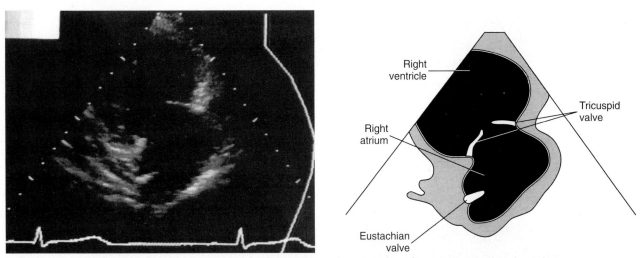

Figure 24-32 Eustachian valve as seen in the right ventricular inflow view. Found in the right atrium, it is a normal variant.

Moderator Band
The moderator band is a normal tissue structure that extends from the anterior free wall of the right ventricle to the IVS. It provides a quick path for the conduction system to reach the ventricular wall. The moderator band is best visualized in the apical four-chamber view.

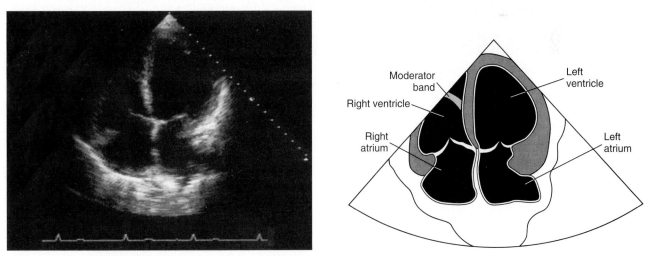

Figure 24-33 Moderator band as seen in the apical four-chamber view. It is a normal structure found in the right ventricle.

Chiari Network
The Chiari network appears as a fine mobile fiber within the right atrium that originates near the entrance of the inferior vena cava and often extends to the crista terminalis. This can be seen in any of the views in which the right atrium is pictured.

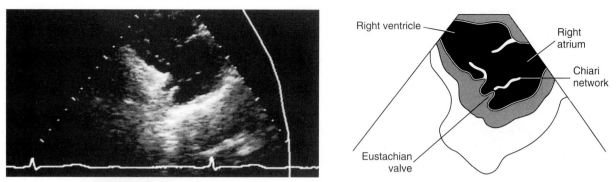

Figure 24-34 Chiari network as seen in the right ventricular inflow view. It is a normal variant found in the right atrium.

Ectopic Chordae

Ectopic chordae are thin fibrous strands that extend from one ventricular wall to another. They can be found in either ventricle and are best visualized in the apical views.

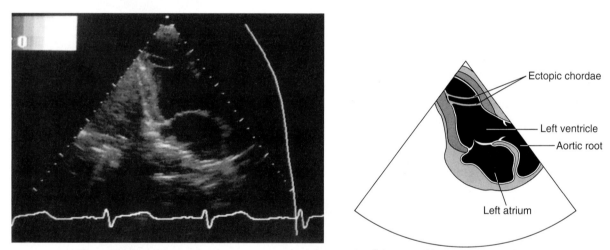

Figure 24-35 Ectopic chordae as seen in the left ventricle of the apical long axis view. These are normal variants and can be found in either ventricle.

Interatrial Septal Aneurysm

An interatrial septal aneurysm appears as a bulge in the atrial septum that moves to and fro with respiration. This is best seen in either the apical four-chamber view or the **subcostal** four-chamber view.

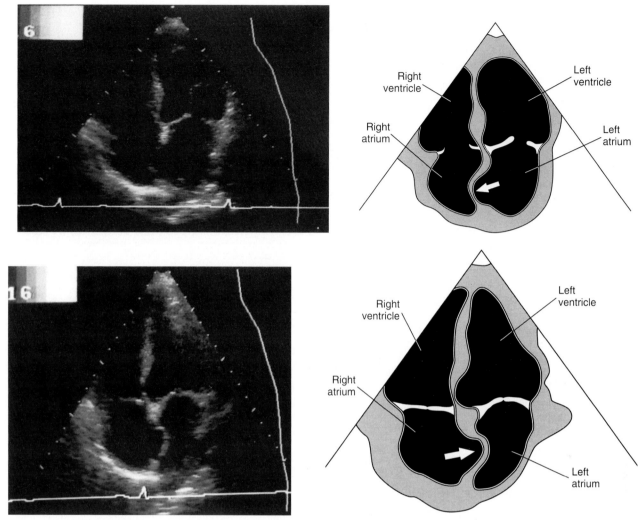

Figure 24-36 Interatrial septal aneurysm as seen in the apical four-chamber view. This is considered a normal variant and moves to and fro with respiration.

REFERENCE CHARTS

■ ■ ■ ASSOCIATED PHYSICIANS

Cardiologist: Specializes in the medical treatment of patients with heart disease.

Radiologist: Specializes in the diagnostic interpretation of imaging modalities; therefore some radiologists may also read echocardiograms.

■ ■ ■ COMMON DIAGNOSTIC TESTS

Transesophageal Echocardiography (TEE): Provides information regarding the heart and associated vessels not obtainable by the transthoracic approach. The personnel involved in TEE usually include a cardiologist, cardiac sonographer, nurse, and possibly cardiovascular physician's assistant. The laboratory should be equipped with suction equipment, oxygen, crash cart, and blood pressure monitoring. Imaging equipment includes the ultrasound unit and a transesophageal probe, usually with multiplane capabilities.

The probe is basically a gastroscope with an imaging PISA electric crystal at the tip. The frequency is typically between 5 and 6.5 MHz. The TEE scope consists of a control head with deflection controls. The device usually has a large inner wheel and a smaller outer wheel for antegrade and retrograde flexion and for lateral and medial angulations. The flexible shaft is similar to that seen in gastroscopy.

Patient preparation includes a thorough history and cardiac examination. The patient should be asked about any gastrointestinal symptoms. Preoperative orders include approximately 4 hours of fasting prior to the procedure. Just before the examination, intravenous access is established and a topical anesthesia is applied to the oropharynx to diminish the gag reflex. Sedation is also administered. Outpatients should have a responsible person drive them to and from the hospital.

Risks of TEE are extremely low, although a few deaths have been reported when rare cardiac arrhythmias have occurred. Additional possible complications are uncommon, but may include hypotension, laryngospasm and arterial hypoxia (rare), drug reactions, and endocarditis.

History and Physical Examination: The cardiologist questions the patient to gather a good history and performs a full physical examination. This can help determine the diagnosis.

Auscultation: Listening to the sounds of the heart with the aid of a stethoscope.

Chest X-ray Study: This provides information on the size and structure of the heart. At times the cardiac silhouette is diagnostic for specific abnormalities. The test is performed by a technician but is interpreted by either the radiologist or the cardiologist.

Electrocardiogram (ECG): Provides information on the electrical behavior of the heart during the cardiac cycle. A technician performs the test, which is then interpreted by a cardiologist.

Exercise Stress Test: The patient may be exercised on a bicycle or treadmill when coronary artery disease is suspected. During the stress test an ECG is done. This provides information on functional changes in the heart and determines the degree of stimulus that will provoke an adverse reaction. Thallium can also be used. It is a radionuclide that traces the path of the blood as it flows through arteries and perfuses the myocardial cells. A stress test is not performed when valvular disease is suspected. The technician performs the test in the presence of a cardiologist, who then interprets the results.

Computed Axial Tomography (CT) and Magnetic Resonance Imaging (MRI): These are two other imaging studies that can be used in the evaluation of heart disease. They are most useful in evaluating cardiac masses, tumors, or effusions. They are often performed by a technician but may be done in the presence of a physician. These tests are interpreted by a radiologist.

Cardiac Catheterization: An invasive technique in which the tip of a long catheter is introduced into either an artery or a vein through an arm or leg. The catheter is then threaded into the heart. This is an important clinical test used to evaluate coronary artery disease, ventricular and valvular function, pressures within the chambers and across the valves, and the oxygen content of the blood (important in cases of septal defects). The test is performed and interpreted by a cardiologist.

■ ■ ■ LABORATORY VALUES

Creatine Phosphokinase (CPK): An enzyme found in all muscle tissue. The MB fraction of CPK helps in assessing the presence of myocardial infarction. Elevation of CK-MB indicates that an infarct is present. The CK-MB should peak within 24 hours.

Lactic Dehydrogenase (LDH): LDH is also found throughout the body and a certain percentage is used to assess myocardial infarction. LDH usually peaks within 24 to 48 hours and when elevated indicates the presence of an infarct.

■ ■ ■ NORMAL M-MODE MEASUREMENTS

Aortic root dimension: 1.9-4.0 cm
Aortic cusp separation: 1.5-2.6 cm
Left atrial dimension: 1.9-4.0 cm
Mitral valve excursion: 1.6-3.0 cm
Mitral valve EF slope: 70-150 mm/sec
Left ventricular end diastolic dimension: 3.5-5.7 cm
Left ventricular ejection fraction: >55%
Left ventricular fractional shortening: >25%
Interventricular septal thickness: 0.6-1.2 cm
Posterior left ventricular wall thickness: 0.6-1.2 cm
Right ventricular dimension: 0.7-2.7 cm

■ ■ ■ NORMAL DOPPLER VELOCITIES IN ADULTS

Mitral valve: 0.6-1.3 m/sec
Aortic valve: 1.0-1.7 m/sec
Tricuspid valve: 0.3-0.7 m/sec
Pulmonic valve: 0.6-0.9 m/sec
Left ventricular: 0.7-1.1 m/sec

■ ■ ■ AFFECTING CHEMICALS

Epinephrine: Produced by the adrenal medulla, it increases the excitability of the SA node, thereby increasing the heart rate and the strength of the contractions.

Potassium: Can interfere with nerve impulse generation; therefore it decreases heart rate and the strength of the contractions.

Sodium: Also may decrease heart rate and contraction strength since it tends to interfere with calcium participation in muscular contraction.

Calcium: As with sodium, a high amount of calcium can increase the heart rate and the strength of its contractions.

BIBLIOGRAPHY

Allen MN: How to perform a transesophageal exam. In *Diagnostic medical sonography: a guide to clinical practice of echocardiography*, ed 2, Philadelphia, 1999, Lippincott, pp 207-223.

Feigenbaum H: *Echocardiography*, ed 5, Philadelphia, 1994, Lea & Febiger.

Feigenbaum H: Echocardiography. In Braunwald E, editor: *Heart disease: a textbook of cardiovascular medicine*, ed 2, Philadelphia, 1984, WB Saunders, pp 88-105.

Felner JM: Echocardiography and Doppler techniques. In Hurst JW, et al, editors: *The heart*, ed 6, vol 2, New York, 1986, McGraw-Hill, pp 1926-1973.

Hatle L: Doppler ultrasound in cardiology. In Hatle L, Angelsen B, editors: *Physical principles and applications*, ed 2, Philadelphia, 1985, Lea & Febiger.

Henry WL, et al: Report of the American Society of Echocardiography Committee on nomenclature and standards in two-dimensional echocardiography, *Circulation* 62:212-217, 1980.

Netter FH, Yonkman FF, editors: *The Ciba collection of medical illustrations: the heart*, vol 5, Summit, NJ, 1978, Ciba Pharmaceutical, Division of CIBA-GEIGY, pp 2-14; 48-50.

Otto CM: *Textbook of clinical echocardiography*, ed 2, Philadelphia, 2000, WB Saunders, pp. 59-79.

Paluides DS, Hauser AN, Stewad JR, et al: Contribution of transesophageal echocardiography to patient diagnosis and treatment: a perspective analysis, *Am Heart J* 120:910-914, 1990.

Phillips J: Transesophageal ecocardiography: the cardiac sonographer's role, *J Am Soc Echocardiogr* 3:73-74, 1989.

Sahn DJ, DeMaria A, Kisslo J, Weyman A: The Committee on M-mode standardization of the American Society of Echocardiography. Recommendations regarding quantitation in M-mode echocardiographic measurements, *Circulation* 58:1072-1082, 1978.

Schuster AH, Nanda NC: Doppler exam of the heart, great vessels and coronary arteries. In Nanda NC, editor: *Doppler echocardiography*, Tokyo, 1985, Igaku-Shoin, pp 93-129.

St John Sutton M, Plappert T, Oldershaw P: Normal Doppler echocardiographic examination. In St John Sutton M, Olderstrom P, editors: *Textbook of adult and pediatric echocardiography and Doppler*, Boston, 1989, Blackwell Scientific, pp. 47-75.

Weyman AE: Cross sectional echocardiography, Philadelphia, 1982, Lea & Febiger, pp 98-136.

CHAPTER 25

Vascular Technology

MARSHA M. NEUMYER

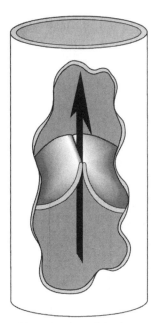

Venous valves of the leg.

OBJECTIVES

Define the role of indirect and direct noninvasive techniques used for the evaluation of vascular disease.

Describe the anatomy of the extracranial carotid and vertebral arteries, and the peripheral arterial and venous systems.

Describe the function of the cerebrovascular, peripheral arterial, and venous systems.

Describe the sonographic appearance of the carotid and vertebral vessels, and the lower extremity peripheral arterial and venous vasculature.

Define the hemodynamic patterns and Doppler spectral waveforms found in the normal vasculature.

Define the key words.

KEY WORDS ■

Accuracy	Negative predictive value
Area reduction	(NPV)
Boundary layer separation	Positive predictive value
Diameter reduction	(PPV)
Direct/indirect noninvasive	Prevalence
vascular diagnostic tests	Sensitivity
Doppler color flow imaging	Specificity
Doppler time-velocity	Spectral bandwidth/
waveform	spectral broadening
Duplex technology	Systolic window
False negative (FN)	Transmural pressure
False positive (FP)	Triphasic Doppler spectral
High-resistance vascular	waveform
bed	True negative (TN)
Linear reflectivity	True positive (TP)
Low-resistance vascular	
bed	

Noninvasive diagnostic vascular technology has evolved rapidly over the past two decades from the use of the simple hand-held continuous wave Doppler velocimeter to the sophisticated and complex technology found in duplex and triplex ultrasound systems. Vascular laboratory evaluations complement the clinical impression by providing information about the location and severity of cerebrovascular, peripheral arterial, and venous disease.

Noninvasive vascular diagnostic tests are divided into two types: **indirect** and **direct.** The indirect physiologic test procedures indicate the presence of significant occlusive disease by demonstrating pressure or volume changes downstream from the area of disease. They are an integral part of vascular laboratory evaluations. The direct procedures, in contrast, evaluate the flow patterns in vessels at the location of disease. This is most often accomplished with the use of B-mode ultrasound imaging of the vessel with Doppler velocity spectral analysis of blood flow patterns. These technologies may be complemented by **Doppler color flow imaging,** which encodes the Doppler-shifted frequencies within the gray scale image of the surrounding tissues.

This presentation focuses on the direct ultrasound examination of the cerebrovascular, peripheral arterial, and venous vascular systems.

EXTRACRANIAL CEREBROVASCULAR SYSTEM
Common Carotid Arteries, Internal Carotid Arteries, External Carotid Arteries, and Vertebral Arteries

The extracranial cerebrovascular system comprises the common carotid arteries, the internal carotid arteries (ICAs), the external carotid arteries (ECAs), and the vertebral arteries. The system is symmetric on each side of the neck (Figure 25-1).

The carotid arteries supply blood flow principally to the anterior cerebral hemispheres, the eye, and muscles of the face, forehead, and scalp. The vertebral arteries carry blood to the posterior cerebrum, meeting to form the basilar artery at the level of the foramen magnum. Intracranially, the carotid arterial system anastomoses with the vertebral-basilar system to form the circle of Willis, an arterial ring around the base of the brain (Figure 25-2). Each extracranial carotid system has a common carotid artery that bifurcates, most often at the level of the superior thyroid cartilage, into an ICA and ECA.

On the right side of the body, the common carotid artery arises from the innominate, or brachiocephalic, artery, which also branches into the subclavian artery.

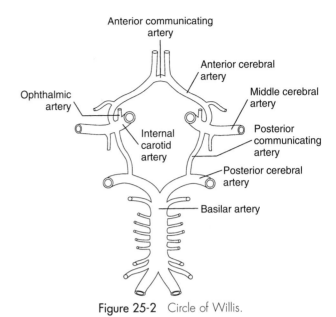

Figure 25-2 Circle of Willis.

On the left, the subclavian and common carotid arteries arise separately from the aortic arch. Variations may include absence of the innominate artery with the right subclavian and common carotid originating from the arch, or the presence of a left innominate artery; or the aorta may arch to the right with the normal arterial arrangements reversed.

The common carotid arteries pass cephalad into the anterolateral aspect of the neck slightly behind the thyroid gland. The level of the carotid bifurcation and the arrangement of the ICA and ECA may vary. In most patients, the ICA is posterior and lateral to the ECA. The ICA normally has no branches in the neck, but intracranially gives rise to the ophthalmic artery, which supplies blood flow to the eye, and to the middle and anterior cerebral arteries. The ECA has branches that supply blood flow to the neck, face, and scalp. These branches sonographically help to distinguish the ECA from the ICA. Anatomic variations may include the absence of the common carotid artery, with the ICA and ECA arising directly from the aortic arch, or the absence of a carotid bifurcation.

The vertebral arteries arise as the first branch of the subclavian arteries and pass cranially through the foramina of the transverse processes of the upper six cervical vertebrae. The vertebrals pass superiorly to the atlas, winding around the lateral mass of the atlas, and enter the vertebral canal anterior to the spinal cord. The two vertebral arteries enter the skull through the foramen magnum and join to form the basilar artery, which supplies structures in the posterior fossa.

Size of the Extracranial Cerebrovascular Vessels. The normal common carotid artery is approximately 5 to 6

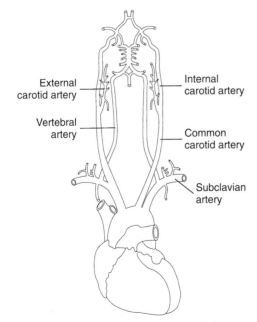

Figure 25-1 The extracranial cerebrovascular system.

mm in diameter. This vessel may decrease in transverse diameter due to atherosclerotic occlusive disease, which prevents antegrade blood flow.

The extracranial portion of the ICA measures approximately 4 to 5 mm in width. The vessel decreases in diameter as it enters the brain.

The ECA is usually of smaller diameter than the ICA, measuring approximately 3 to 4 mm.

The vertebral arteries are approximately 2 to 3 mm wide at their origin, decreasing in diameter as they course cephalad.

Sonographic Appearance of the Extracranial Carotid and Vertebral Arteries. Using an anterior oblique or posterior oblique longitudinal scan plane, the skin, platysma, and fascia will lie between the probe and the carotid artery.

The lateral lobe of the thyroid gland is identified posterior to the common carotid artery. The jugular vein lies lateral to the common carotid artery and displays characteristic movement varying with respiration and cardiac activity (Figure 25-3). Transverse pulsatility of the carotid artery will be noted to be in phase with the cardiac cycle.

At the level of the carotid bifurcation, the dilatation (carotid sinus) of the carotid bulb can be identified and the division into the ICA and ECA noted (Figure 25-4). The relationship between these two vessels is variable and may depend on whether an antero-oblique or a postero-oblique scan plane has been used. The vessels can be further identified by their signature Doppler waveform.

The sonographic evaluation of the normal arterial wall will document the **linear reflectivity** associated with the echogenic properties of the collagen fibers that are found in the intima and media of arteries (Figure 25-5). Examination of the walls of the jugular vein will fail to reveal this reflectivity.

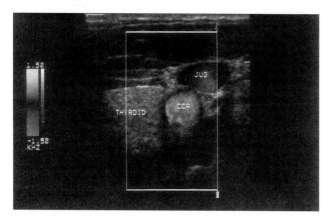

Figure 25-3 Transverse section, Doppler color flow image of the common carotid artery, jugular vein, and thyroid gland. (See Color Plate 39.)

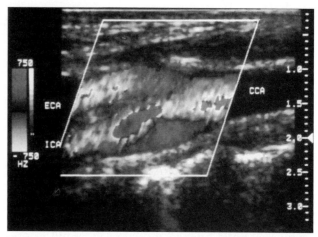

Figure 25-4 Long axis section, Doppler color flow image of the carotid bifurcation demonstrates the common, external, and internal carotid arteries. Note the zone of retrograde flow in the carotid bulb caused by boundary layer separation. (See Color Plate 40.)

The vertebral arteries may be visualized using an anteroposterior approach in the midcervical segment of the neck as they course through the fossae of the transverse vertebral processes. The origin of the vertebral vessels can be documented using a transverse approach to the subclavian artery at the level of the common carotid origin (Figure 25-6).

Hemodynamic Patterns of the Extracranial Carotid and Vertebral Arteries. The common carotid artery supplies approximately 80% of its flow to the ICA and about 20% to the ECA.

As the ICA supplies the **low-resistance vascular bed** of the brain and eye, the flow will be cephalad throughout the cardiac cycle. In contrast, the ECA supplies the **high-resistance vascular bed** of the face, forehead, and scalp. The flow pattern for this vessel is characterized by forward flow in systole, and a low or reverse diastolic flow component.

A pressure-flow gradient develops as a result of dilatation of the carotid bulb, resulting in separation of the flow stream into central forward flow entering the ICA and reversed flow near the posterolateral wall (Figure 25-7). This is known as **boundary layer separation** and characterizes the normal blood flow patterns in the carotid bulb.

The vertebral arteries supply blood flow, by way of the basilar artery, to the posterior cerebral hemispheres. Therefore their flow patterns will be similar to those seen in the ICA with constant forward diastolic flow.

The red blood cells move through the arteries in layers or laminae. The laminae slide over each other, impeded by friction from within the fluid or from movement against the arterial wall. Velocity profiles, in general, will

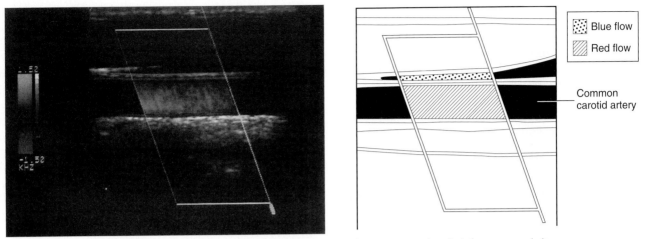

Figure 25-5 Long axis section of the common carotid artery. Arterial wall definition reveals linear reflectivity resulting from the echogenicity of collagen found in the intima and media. (See Color Plate 41.)

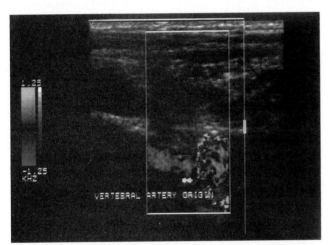

Figure 25-6 Doppler color flow image of the vertebral artery origin. The subclavian artery is seen in the transverse plane just distal to the origin of the right common carotid artery. (See Color Plate 42.)

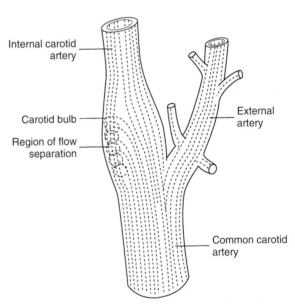

Figure 25-7 Carotid bifurcation demonstrating boundary layer separation in the carotid bulb.

be influenced by tapering or curvature of the vessel, entrance and exit effects on inertia of blood as the vessel widens and dilates, and the presence of turbulence caused by anatomic abnormality or disease.

The velocity spectral information must be collected at an angle of insonation of 60 degrees with respect to the blood flow vector in order to accurately evaluate the hemodynamic patterns. Remember the Doppler equation:

$$F = \frac{2VF_0 \cos \Theta}{c}$$

Where F = Doppler shifted frequency, V = velocity of red cell movement, F_0 = carrier Doppler frequency, $\cos \Theta$ = angle of insonation with respect to the blood flow vector, and c = constant for speed of sound in soft tissue (1,540 m/sec).

Doppler Velocity Spectral Waveforms. The common carotid artery has a Doppler velocity spectral waveform that mimics both the internal carotid and external carotid waveforms. The blood flow pattern is characterized by a sharp systolic upstroke, a rapid systolic deceleration, and constant forward diastolic flow. There is a "window," an area absent of Doppler shifts, under the systolic component. During systole, the red blood cells will move at a uniform velocity with an undisturbed flow profile in a normal common carotid artery. This flow pattern is characterized by a very narrow Doppler velocity spectrum (Figure 25-8).

During the deceleration phase of systole, the velocity will decrease, and the viscous drag on the cells nearest the wall will result in the movement of the cells over a slightly broader range of velocities. This is manifested by a thickening of the velocity spectral envelope. This **spectral broadening** becomes more evident during diastole.

If frequency information is desired, the carrier Doppler frequency and angle of insonation (60 degrees) must be known. The normal velocity in the carotid artery is approximately 100 cm/sec, but a wide range of normal velocities from 30 to 110 cm per second has been documented (Table 25-1).

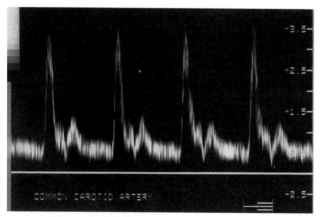

Figure 25-8 Doppler time-velocity waveform from a normal common carotid artery.

■ ■ ■ Table 25-1 Diagnostic Doppler Velocity Criteria for Determining Degree of Carotid Artery Diameter Reduction

Diameter Stenosis (Category)	Peak Systolic Velocity (cm/sec)	End Diastolic Velocity (cm/sec)
0% (Normal)	<110	<40
1-39% (Mild)	<110	<40
40-59% (Moderate)	<130	<40
60-79% (Severe)	>130	>40
80-99% (Critical)	>250	>100
100% (Occlusion)	N/A	N/A

N/A, not applicable.

The ICA is characteristically a high-flow, low-resistance vessel. The Doppler velocity waveform from this artery demonstrates a quasi-steady flow with blunt systolic peak and constant forward diastolic flow (Figure 25-9). A **systolic window** is present in the absence of disease or vessel tortuosity.

In contrast, the ECA is a low-flow, high-resistance vessel. The Doppler velocity waveform exhibits multiphasicity with sharp systolic upstroke, rapid deceleration, and low diastolic flow (Figure 25-10). In the presence of ICA occlusion, the ECA may mimic the internal carotid waveform due to collateral compensatory flow to the brain offered by the ECA.

The **Doppler time-velocity waveform** from the carotid bulb will vary with position of the Doppler sample volume (Figure 25-11). If the sample volume is placed in the region of the flow divide, the waveform will demonstrate forward diastolic flow. As the sample volume is stepped across the lumen of the carotid bulb to the posterior wall, the waveform will exhibit reverse flow in the region of the separation of the boundary layers.

The spectral display from the normal vertebral arteries should resemble that recorded from the ICA with constant forward flow demonstrated during diastole. The vertebrals are high-flow, low-resistance vessels.

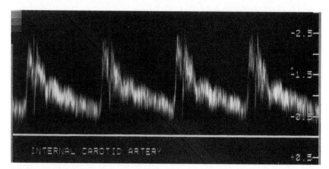

Figure 25-9 Doppler time-velocity waveform from a normal internal carotid artery demonstrating constant forward diastolic flow.

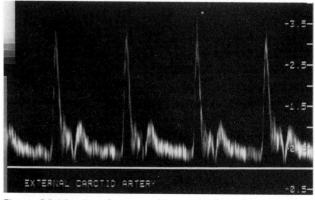

Figure 25-10 Doppler time-velocity waveform from a normal external carotid artery. Note the low diastolic flow component.

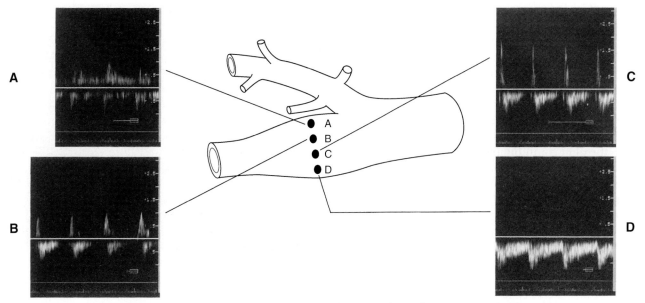

Figure 25-11 Montage of carotid bulb and Doppler spectral waveforms. **A,** Recorded from the region of the flow divide with primarily forward flow. **B,** Recorded from the boundary layer showing separation of the flow stream into forward and reverse flows. **C,** The beginning of the reverse flow phase. **D,** Reverse flow occurring along the posterolateral wall of the bulb.

THE LOWER EXTREMITY ARTERIAL SYSTEM
Common Iliac, External Iliac, Common Femoral, Deep Femoral, Popliteal, and Tibial Arteries

The lower extremity peripheral arterial vessels can be divided into three systems: aortoiliac (inflow), femoropopliteal (outflow), and tibioperoneal (run-off) (Figure 25-12).

The aortoiliac system begins at the aortic bifurcation and ends at the level of the inguinal ligament. It comprises the distal abdominal aorta and the common iliac, external iliac, and internal iliac (hypogastric) arteries. Blood flow through this system supplies the buttocks, pelvis, and thighs. The aortoiliac system is the second most common site for lower extremity arterial occlusive disease.

The femoropopliteal system begins at the level of the inguinal ligament and ends at the trifurcation of the popliteal artery in the popliteal fossa behind the knee. This system comprises the common femoral, deep femoral (profunda femoris), superficial femoral, and popliteal arteries. The thighs and calves receive blood flow through these major vessels. This system is the most common site for atherosclerotic occlusive disease of the lower extremities.

The tibioperoneal system begins at the termination of the popliteal artery in the popliteal fossa and ends at the ankle where these vessels anastomose with the plantar and metatarsal vessels of the foot. These arteries make up the supply system for blood flow to the calves and feet.

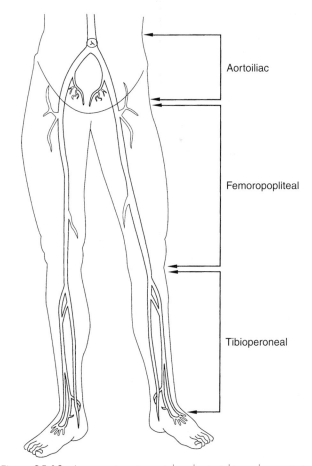

Figure 25-12 Lower extremity peripheral arterial tree demonstrating the aortoiliac, femoropopliteal, and tibioperoneal systems.

Sonographic Appearance of the Lower Extremity Peripheral Arterial Vessels. The bifurcation of the abdominal aorta takes place on the left side of the body of the fourth lumbar vertebra. The common iliac arteries pass posterolaterally from the termination of the aorta to the margin of the pelvis and divide opposite the last lumbar vertebra and the sacrum into the external and internal iliac arteries (Figure 25-13).

The peritoneum, small intestine, and ureter lie anterior to the right common iliac artery. The common iliac veins and the psoas magnus muscle lie posteriorly with the inferior vena cava, sharing a lateral relationship.

The left common iliac artery lies posterior to the ureter and peritoneum. It is anterior to the left common iliac vein. The psoas magnus muscle borders the left common iliac artery laterally. The location of the aortic bifurcation is subject to variation as is the point of division of the common iliac arteries. On occasion, the common iliac artery may be absent, with the external and internal iliac arteries arising directly from the aorta.

The external iliac artery is larger than the internal iliac artery. This vessel passes obliquely posterolateral to the inner border of the psoas muscle from the bifurcation of the common iliac to Poupart's ligament, where it enters the thigh and becomes the common femoral artery. The common and external iliac arteries are frequently difficult to image due to overlying bowel gas.

The common femoral artery commences posterolateral to Poupart's ligament between the anterior superior spine of the ilium and the symphysis pubis and courses down the medial aspect of the thigh through Scarpa's triangle as the superficial femoral artery, where it is contained in Hunter's canal. This vessel terminates in the lower third of the thigh at the opening of the adductor magnus, where it becomes the popliteal artery (Figure 25-14). It is bordered on its medial side by the superficial femoral vein and lat-

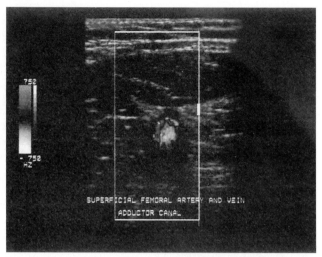

Figure 25-14 Transverse section, Doppler color flow image of the superficial femoral artery and vein in Hunter's canal. (See Color Plate 44.)

erally by the adductor muscle. On rare occasions the superficial femoral artery may divide into two trunks below the origin of the profunda femoris, reuniting in the adductor canal to form the popliteal artery.

The popliteal artery commences at the termination of the superficial femoral artery in Hunter's canal and passes obliquely behind the knee joint to the lower border of the femur, where it divides into the anterior and posterior tibial arteries. It is bordered medially by the inner head of the gastrocnemius and posteriorly by the popliteal vein. Occasionally the popliteal artery divides prematurely into its branch vessels (Figure 25-15).

The anterior tibial artery commences at the bifurcation of the popliteal artery and passes through the interosseous membrane to the deep part of the front of the leg lying close to the inner side of the neck of the fibula. At the lower third of the limb, it lies on the tibia and on the anterior ligament of the ankle joint, where it moves superiorly to become the dorsalis pedis artery. The anterior tibial artery is accompanied by the anterior tibial veins that lie on each side of the artery.

The posterior tibial artery extends obliquely downward along the lateral (tibial) side of the leg, lying posterior to the deep transverse fascia. It is accompanied by the two posterior tibial veins (Figure 25-16).

The peroneal artery lies along the posteromedial side of the fibula. It arises from the posterior tibial trunk about an inch below the border of the popliteus muscle, passing obliquely outward to the fibula (see Figure 25-16). The peroneal veins lie on either side of the artery.

In the absence of disease, the lumen of the peripheral arteries will be anechoic, with linear reflectivity apparent along both the posterior and anterior walls of the vessels. Transverse pulsation of the arteries is notable and may become quite pronounced in tortuous segments of the lower extremity arterial tree.

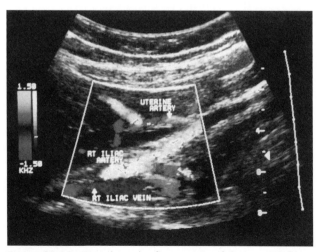

Figure 25-13 Doppler color flow image of the aortic bifurcation. (See Color Plate 43.) (Courtesy Advanced Technology Laboratories.)

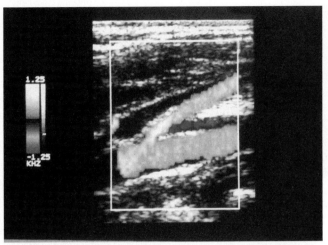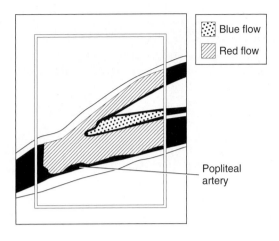

Figure 25-15 Long axis color flow image of the popliteal artery. (See Color Plate 45.)

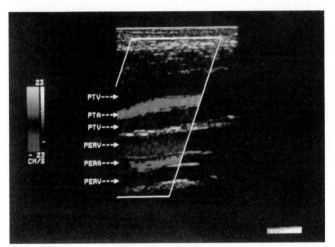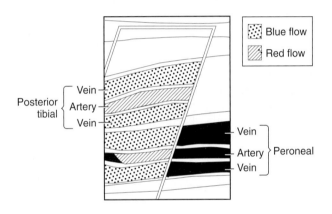

Figure 25-16 Long axis section, Doppler color flow image of the posterior tibial and peroneal arteries surrounded by their companion tibial veins of the same name. (See Color Plate 46.) (Courtesy Advanced Technology Laboratories.)

Size of the Lower Extremity Arteries

External iliac artery	0.79 cm
Common femoral artery	0.82 cm
Superficial femoral artery (proximal)	0.60 cm
Superficial femoral artery (distal)	0.54 cm
Popliteal artery	0.52 cm

Hemodynamic Patterns in the Lower Extremity Peripheral Arterial System. The pulsatile pressure wave that results from the pumping action of the heart is transmitted from the aortic root to the feet. During systole and left ventricular contraction, the walls of the aortic root will expand, creating a high-pressure wave. This wave is transmitted down the aorta and into the lower extremity arterial system. As the high-pressure wave travels peripherally, the lower extremity arterial walls will also expand and contract in a pulsatile manner.

The resistance to blood flow in the small-diameter tibial vessels is greater than that in the wide-diameter aorta, resulting in a pressure gradient between the aorta and the distal tibial arteries. In the absence of arterial occlusive disease, systolic pressure is greater in the tibial arteries than in the abdominal aorta.

As the primary high-pressure wave from the aortic root meets the high resistance of the tibial arterial tree, a secondary reflected pressure wave is created. The blood flow pattern to this high-resistance vascular bed is therefore triphasic. There is forward flow in systole, then early reverse diastolic flow, and a forward diastolic component in vessels with normal arterial wall compliance.

Doppler Velocity Spectral Waveforms. A **triphasic Doppler spectral waveform** is normally found in arteries from the level of the abdominal aorta to the tibial arteries at the ankle (Figure 25-17). In healthy, young

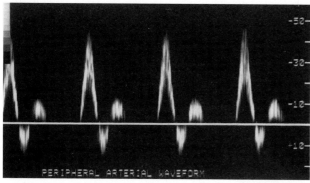

Figure 25-17 Doppler time-velocity waveform recorded from a lower extremity peripheral artery. Note the triphasic pattern of flow.

adults with marked elasticity of the vessel wall, an additional reverse flow component may be recorded. Vessel wall compliance may decrease with advancing age, and the peak systolic forward velocity and peak diastolic forward velocity may diminish slightly, resulting in a biphasic waveform. Velocity waveforms recorded from peripheral arteries of women will generally demonstrate lower peak diastolic velocities than those from men of the same age.

The **spectral bandwidth** will be narrow throughout the systolic and early reversed diastolic flow cycles. Spectral broadening may occur at bifurcations because of boundary layer separation and the presence of disturbed flow.

In the absence of proximal disease, the reverse flow component will be present, and a systolic window will be noted.

The peak systolic velocity decreases in the normal lower extremity arterial tree from the central to the peripheral vessels (Figure 25-18). In the normal abdominal aorta, the velocity averages 90 cm/sec and decreases between the external iliac artery and the proximal superficial femoral artery, and again between the superficial femoral and popliteal arteries to average 60 cm/sec in the popliteal artery.

THE LOWER EXTREMITY VENOUS SYSTEM

The veins of the lower extremity are divided into the deep, superficial, and perforating veins. The deep veins accompany the arteries and share the same names.

The Deep Venous System

The paired anterior tibial veins arise in the dorsal venous arch and accompany the anterior tibial artery up the calf (Figure 25-19, A). The anterior tibial veins pass posteriorly from the anterior compartment of the leg to penetrate the interosseous membrane and course between the tibia and fibula to meet the popliteal vein.

The posterior tibial veins arise from the plantar venous arch of the foot. They accompany the posterior tib-

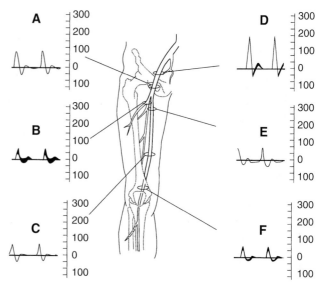

Figure 25-18 Normal velocity spectral waveforms. **A,** Waveforms from the common femoral artery. **B,** Waveforms from the profunda femoris artery. **C,** Waveforms from the distal superficial femoral artery. **D,** Waveforms from the external iliac artery. **E,** Waveforms from the proximal superficial femoral artery. **F,** Waveforms from the popliteal artery. Note the decreases in peak systolic velocity between the external iliac artery and proximal superficial femoral artery and between the proximal superficial femoral artery and the popliteal vessel.

ial artery through the leg and join the peroneal veins. The posterior tibial veins unite with the anterior tibial veins at the distal border of the popliteus muscle to form the popliteal vein.

The peroneal veins arise medial to the lateral malleolus. These veins follow the medial surface of the fibula in the lower half of the calf and then course medially to form the posterior tibial trunk in the upper third of the calf.

The posterior tibial and anterior tibial trunks at the level of the knee form the popliteal vein. From this location, the popliteal vein extends cephalad to the medial aspect of the femur, lying 1 to 2 cm from the posterior surface of the distal femur, and then passes through the adductor hiatus to become the superficial femoral vein. The popliteal vein accompanies the popliteal artery lying within a fascial sheath. The popliteal vein will course posterior and superficial to the popliteal artery. At the distal popliteal fossa, the vein lies slightly medial to the artery but crosses the artery to lie lateral to it as it ascends into the proximal part of the fossa. This vessel normally contains two valves.

The superficial femoral vein is the continuation of the popliteal vein. It accompanies the superficial femoral artery as it courses up the medial aspect of the thigh to the level of the inguinal ligament to form the common femoral vein. The superficial femoral vein normally contains two to five valves along its course.

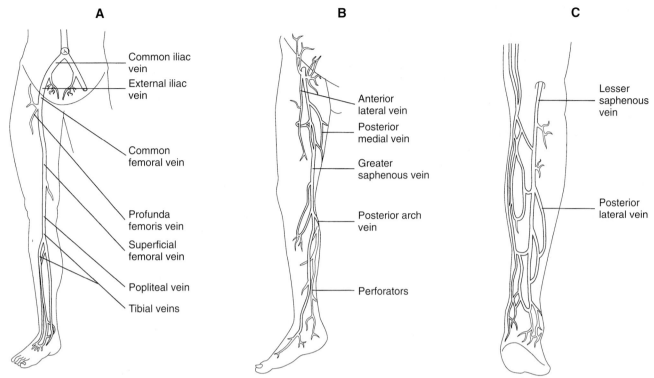

A, Common iliac vein, External iliac vein, Common femoral vein, Profunda femoris vein, Superficial femoral vein, Popliteal vein, Tibial veins

B, Anterior lateral vein, Posterior medial vein, Greater saphenous vein, Posterior arch vein, Perforators

C, Lesser saphenous vein, Posterior lateral vein

Figure 25-19   A, Lower extremity deep venous system. B and C, Greater and lesser saphenous veins.

Anatomic variations are common in the deep venous system. The most common anomalies seen include duplication of the popliteal and/or superficial femoral veins, duplication of the distal segment of the superficial femoral vein subsequently uniting to form a single vein in the mid to proximal thigh, and the presence of three or more popliteal or superficial femoral veins.

The Superficial Venous System
The major superficial veins are the greater saphenous and the lesser saphenous veins (Figure 25-19, *B* and *C*). These veins lie in subcutaneous tissue and are superficial to the deep fascia.

The greater saphenous vein arises from the medial aspect of the dorsal venous arch, continuing in the foot, and ascends in the ankle anteromedial to the medial malleolus.

It then moves posteriorly to cross behind the medial condyle of the femur at the level of the knee. It courses up the medial aspect of the thigh to drain into the common femoral vein about 3.5 cm below the inguinal ligament. There are usually four valves in the greater saphenous vein in the lower leg and up to six valves in the thigh.

The lesser saphenous vein begins at the lateral end of the dorsal venous arch and ascends in the ankle posterior to the lateral malleolus. This vein extends up the back of the calf to the distal popliteal fossa where it per-

forates the deep fascia, passing between the heads of the gastrocnemius muscle, and drains into the popliteal vein. The greater and lesser saphenous veins may communicate through the femoropopliteal vein.

The Perforating Veins
The deep and superficial venous systems are connected by the perforating, or communicating, veins.

The posterior group of perforators connects the lesser saphenous vein with the greater saphenous vein. The medial perforating veins connect the greater saphenous vein with the posterior tibial veins, and the lateral perforators join the greater saphenous vein with the anterior tibial and peroneal veins. There are up to six perforating veins in the medial thigh connecting the greater saphenous vein with the superficial femoral vein.

Size of the Deep and Superficial Veins
Average diameters of the deep veins are:

Tibial veins	approximately 5 mm
Popliteal vein	0.9 to 1.5 cm
Superficial femoral vein	0.9 to 1.0 cm
Common femoral vein	1.2 to 1.9 cm

Average diameters of the superficial veins are:

Greater saphenous vein	2 to 3 mm (calf)
	4 to 6 mm (thigh)
Lesser saphenous vein	4 to 7 mm

Sonographic Appearance of the Deep and Superficial Venous Systems

Every deep vein is accompanied by an artery that courses in close proximity to it.

The common femoral vein lies midway between the pubis and the iliac spine at the level of the inguinal crease. It should be found medial to the common femoral artery and slightly deeper than this vessel. The lumen of the normal common femoral vein is anechoic, and the walls of the vein will coapt entirely with gentle transducer pressure applied to the anterior vein wall from the transverse image plane.

The greater saphenous vein arises medially from the common femoral vein and courses superficially to the fascia of the thigh and calf to the dorsum of the foot.

The common femoral vein bifurcates into the superficial femoral vein and the deep femoral vein (profunda femoris) about 2 to 4 cm distal to the takeoff of the greater saphenous vein. The profunda femoris vein courses laterally and deep to the superficial femoral vein. It will lie in the same scan plane as the profunda femoris artery.

The superficial femoral vein will accompany the artery of the same name, lying deep to this vessel and medial to the profunda femoris. Both the superficial femoral vein and artery enter the adductor canal, crossing beneath the adductor fascia in the lower third of the thigh. The superficial femoral vein is duplicated, over at least a short length, in 15% to 20% of patients.

The superficial femoral vein becomes the popliteal vein at the level of the adductor canal. The vein will remain posterior to the popliteal artery; however, the vein is most easily interrogated from the popliteal fossa. From this image plane, the popliteal vein will appear superficial to its companion artery. The popliteal vein will be duplicated in approximately 35% of patients.

The lesser saphenous vein normally arises from the popliteal vein proximally at about midknee level. The vessel courses posterolaterally down the leg, terminating anterior to the lateral malleolus. The paired gastrocnemius veins also arise from the popliteal vein, originating from the distal segment of the vein, and run parallel to the popliteal artery.

The popliteal vein can be imaged to the proximal calf, where it bifurcates into the anterior tibial trunk and the tibioperoneal trunk, which lies deep to the gastrocnemius and soleus muscles. At this point, the veins duplicate. For each tibial artery there are at least two tibial veins.

The anterior tibial veins can be imaged from the anterior aspect of the leg as they emerge after crossing the interosseous membrane. They remain on top of the membrane as they course down the leg to cross the region of the ankle.

The posterior tibial veins can be imaged from the medial aspect of the calf at about midcalf to the level of the medial malleolus. They will lie superficially.

The peroneal veins can also be imaged from midcalf level, lying deeper than the posterior tibial veins and adjacent to the fibula.

Hemodynamic Patterns of the Lower Extremity Deep Venous System

The movement of blood in the lower extremity veins is influenced by respiratory variation, which causes changes in intraabdominal pressure, the calf muscle pump, and the presence of competent venous valves.

As one inhales, the diaphragm descends and the blood flow return from the lower extremities is impeded due to an increase in intraabdominal pressure. With expiration, the diaphragm rises, intraabdominal pressure decreases, and venous return is possible.

As much as 20% of the body's total blood volume may be pooled in the leg veins within 15 minutes of standing still. When a person is at rest, the energy for transport of venous blood from the legs to the heart is supplied by contraction of the left ventricle. This cardiac contraction alone is insufficient to move blood from the leg and is complemented by the calf muscle pump, which is activated with exercise. The calf muscle pump helps to control the hydrostatic pressure in the leg veins by continuously pumping blood out of these veins. The venous pressure in the feet of an exercising adult will therefore usually be less than 25 mm Hg.

The cephalad movement of blood in the lower extremities is a complex function of the calf muscles and the venous valves. With each step taken during walking, there are periods of relaxation and contraction of the calf muscles. When the calf muscles are relaxed, the blood flows into the lower pressure deep venous system from the high-pressure superficial venous system. As the muscle contracts, the blood moves from the deep calf veins into the deep thigh veins. Valves in the deep veins prevent the flow of blood toward the feet, and the valves in the perforating veins prevent blood from flowing from the deep to the superficial system.

One of the most remarkable characteristics of veins is the capacity to undergo tremendous volume changes with little change in **transmural pressure** (Figure 25-20, A). The venous wall is about one-tenth as thick as the arterial wall, with little elastin present in the media of the vein. The percentage of smooth muscle found in the media wall will vary depending on the location of the vein, with about 60% muscle being found in the veins of the foot—the veins subjected to the greatest hydrostatic pressure. The walls of the normal vein can be coapted with gentle transducer pressure during transverse imaging of the vein (Figure 25-20, B and C).

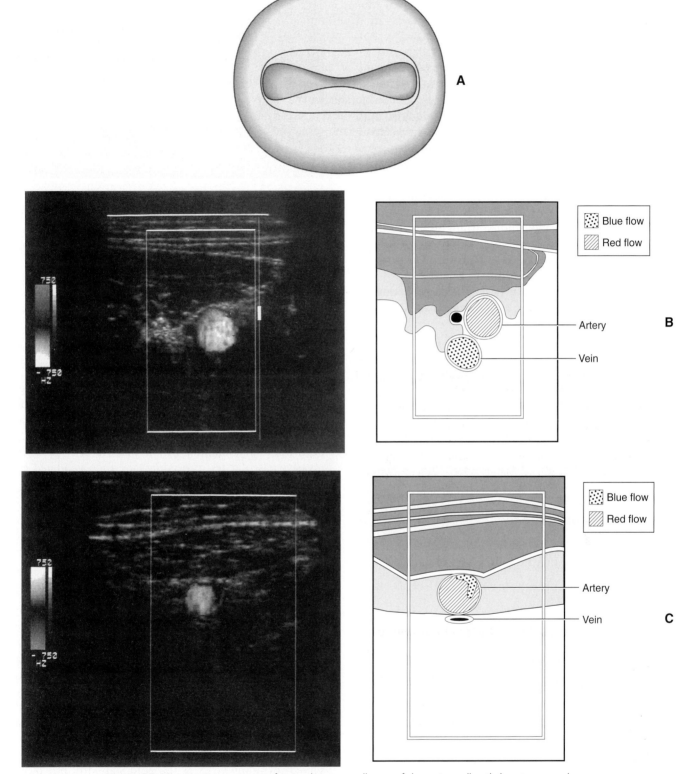

Figure 25-20 **A,** Cross-section of vein showing collapse of the vein wall with low transmural pressure. **B,** Transverse section, Doppler color flow image of the superficial femoral artery and vein. (See Color Plate 47.) **C,** Transverse section, Doppler color flow image of the superficial femoral artery and vein demonstrating coaptation of the venous walls that occurs with gentle transducer pressure. (See Color Plate 48.)

Doppler Spectral Analysis

Blood flow in the lower extremity veins is spontaneous and phasic with respiration, ceasing with inspiration and augmenting with expiration (Figure 25-21). Pulsatility of flow may be caused by increased central venous pressure due to fluid overload or tricuspid insufficiency or may be related to the proximity of the veins to the heart.

Flow can be augmented by compressing the limb proximally and impeded by distal compression (Figure 25-22). A Valsalva maneuver often will enlarge a vein, dramatically aiding in identification and localization of the vessel.

Because they lie deep in the pelvis and are usually noncompressible, veins proximal to the inguinal ligament cannot be reliably studied using **duplex technology** alone. The addition of color flow imaging to confirm luminal filling has complemented the examination procedure.

Valvular competence may be confirmed by noting the absence of retrograde venous flow with distal compression of the limb (Figure 25-23).

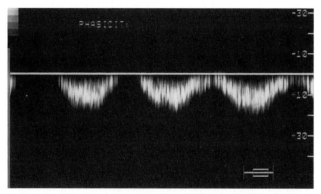

Figure 25-21 Doppler spectral waveform recorded from the normal common femoral vein. Note phasicity of flow, which varies with the respiratory cycle.

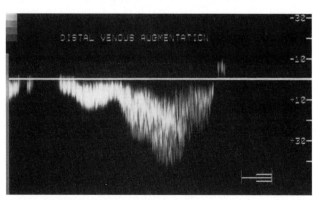

Figure 25-22 Doppler spectral waveform demonstrating augmentation of venous flow with manual compression of the limb proximal to the transducer position.

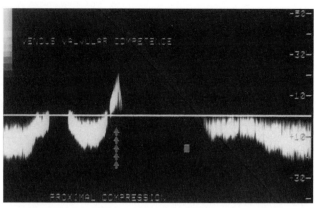

Figure 25-23 Doppler spectral waveform demonstrating the absence of retrograde venous flow when the limb is manually compressed distal to the transducer position. The valve is competent, preventing reflux of blood with distal compression.

In general, the following flow characteristics should be examined in each limb and the symmetry of flow patterns compared with the opposite limb with regard to spontaneity, phasicity, augmentation, competence, and absence of pulsatility.

QUALITY ASSURANCE IN VASCULAR TECHNOLOGY

Vascular ultrasonography allows us not only to recognize the presence of disease but also to determine the severity of the hemodynamic compromise. Categorization of disease severity is based upon criteria that have been internally validated by each laboratory. The noninvasive vascular test procedures are then validated by comparison with a "gold standard." In the case of cerebrovascular and extremity arterial test procedures, this has historically involved comparison with arteriography. Most recently, magnetic resonance imaging has been used as the standard for correlation of carotid and arterial noninvasive test results.

Measurements Used for Test Validation

Historically, laboratories have used measurement of the diameter of the residual lumen of the artery at the site of disease compared with the diameter of the more distal normal segment of the artery. These data are then compared with velocities associated with each of the chosen categories of disease. The majority of vascular laboratories have established criteria based on diameter reduction, and others have chosen area reduction as their standard for diagnostic criteria. In the case of venous duplex examinations, venography served for many years as the gold standard, but most recently, clinical outcome has been used as the means of choice for correlating the results of venous duplex examinations.

Diameter reduction was originally measured using the "best estimate" of the original arterial lumen diameter as the reference (Figure 25-24). This measurement was compared with the diameter of the residual lumen.

$$\text{\% Luminal diameter reduction} = (1 - \text{residual/original}) \times 100 = (1\text{-}4 \text{ mm/8 mm}) \times 100 = 50\% \text{ stenosis}$$

The technique for determining diameter reduction has changed in recent years as a result of the Asymptomatic Carotid Artery Stenosis (ACAS) and North American Symptomatic Carotid Endarterectomy Trial (NASCET) studies. Currently, the diameter of the normal distal arterial lumen is used as the reference for comparison with the diameter of the residual arterial lumen at the site of disease.

$$\text{\% Luminal diameter reduction} = (1 - \text{residual/distal}) \times 100 = (1\text{-}4 \text{ mm/4 mm}) \times 100 = 0\% \text{ stenosis}$$

If you look closely at this method of measurement, you can see how it would be possible to have disease with a resultant measurement of 0% stenosis or even a negative stenosis! **Area reduction** can be calculated from a single plane view or from two single plane views. When calculated from a single plane, the percent cross-sectional area reduction is:

$$(1\text{-}residual^2/original^2) \times 100$$

$$(1\text{-}4 \text{ mm}^2/8 \text{ mm}^2) \times 100$$

$$(1 - 16/64) \times 100$$

$$= 75\%$$

If the percent cross-sectional area reduction is calculated from two single plane views, the equation then becomes:

$$(1\text{-}residual_1 \times residual_2/original_1 \times original_2) \times 100$$

$$(1\text{-}2 \text{ mm} \times 4 \text{ mm/8 mm} \times 8 \text{ mm}) \times 100$$

$$(1\text{-}8/64) \times 100$$

$$= 88\%$$

Some laboratories attempt to use both diameter reduction and cross-sectional area reduction in hopes of achieving increased test sensitivity and optimization of the predictive values of noninvasive test procedures. It is important to recognize that a comparison of these methods of measurement requires an assumption that the lesion is uniform and circumferential, a feature rarely found with atherosclerotic disease. Careful study of the relationship between diameter and area reduction as shown in Table 25-2 will reveal how misunderstanding of the data and the nature of disease might lead to errors in diagnosis.

Statistical Correlation

Although the process of statistical correlation may seem quite complex, the steps are really straightforward. The first step in the validation process is to categorize the results of a noninvasive test as either positive or negative based on validated criteria. As an example, if you were evaluating the ability of cerebrovascular duplex scanning to detect ICA stenosis in the range 40% to 59% diameter reduction, a positive study would include only stenosis in that range, and a negative examination would include stenoses in all other categories and also normal arteries and those with total occlusions.

The next step is to compare (correlate) the individual test results with the "gold standard," using your chosen criteria for a positive or negative test result. Using the example described above, a positive carotid arteriogram would include only 40% to 59% diameter reducing stenoses, and negative test results would include all normals, all stenoses other than those in our chosen range, and all occlusions. The data are typically analyzed by using a 2 × 2 table as illustrated in Figure 25-24. The table compares the positive and negative noninvasive test results with the gold standard.

Understanding the Assigned Values

True positive (TP) tests are those in which the noninvasive test is positive for the disease category in question, and the gold standard is also positive for the same severity of disease. In other words, if we use our example, the noninvasive test and the gold standard are in agreement that 40% to 59% stenosis is present.

True negative (TN) tests are those in which the noninvasive test is negative for our chosen category of dis-

Gold standard results

		+	−
Noninvasive test results	+	TP	FP
	−	FN	TN

Figure 25-24 Positive and negative noninvasive test results compared with the gold standard.

■ ▨ ▨ **Table 25-2** Comparison of the Relationship Between Diameter Reduction and Area Reduction

Diameter Reduction	Area Reduction
10%	19%
20%	36%
30%	51%
40%	64%
50%	75%
60%	84%
70%	91%
80%	96%
90%	99%

ease, and the gold standard is also negative. Using our example, the duplex scan and the gold standard both agree that the ICA does not have 40% to 59% stenosis.

False positive (FP) tests are those in which the noninvasive test is positive for the chosen category, but the gold standard is not in agreement. In other words, the duplex scan demonstrates 40% to 59% stenosis, but the gold standard indicates that the narrowing is only in the category 20% to 39% diameter reducing.

False negative (FN) tests are those in which the noninvasive test is negative for the chosen category of disease, but the gold standard is positive for that degree of disease severity. Using our example, the duplex scan demonstrates 20% to 39% stenosis of the ICA, and the gold standard demonstrates 40% to 59% stenosis.

If we assume that the gold standard is always correct, then it is understood that TP and TN occur when the noninvasive test and the gold standard are in agreement, and FP and FN occur when the noninvasive test and the gold standard are in disagreement.

Understanding the Columns and Rows

If we assign numerical values to our example, we can then determine the ability of our carotid duplex examination to detect stenosis in the category 40% to 59% diameter reduction. If we have 64 patients who underwent carotid arteriography, we have a total of 128 ICAs to correlate with our gold standard. Of those 128 ICAs, duplex scanning said 16 had stenosis in the category 40% to 59%, but the arteriogram said 20 ICAs had that degree of stenosis (TP = 16). Therefore there must have been 0 FP. However, that leaves four that were FN (remember, the arteriogram said there were 20 arteries with the chosen category of disease severity and the

gold standard is assumed to be correct). The arteriogram and the ultrasound examination agreed that there were 108 ICAs that did not have disease in the category 40% to 59% diameter reduction (TN). If we fill these values into the 2 × 2 table, we can complete our analysis as shown in Figure 25-25.

Understanding the Calculations

Sensitivity is the ability of a noninvasive test procedure to detect disease by the gold standard when disease is present. Therefore the calculation indicates how "sensitive" a noninvasive test is in detecting the presence of disease.

$$\text{Sensitivity} = \frac{TP}{TP + FN} \times 100$$

In our example above, Sensitivity = (16/16 + 4) × 100 = 80%.

Specificity is the ability of a noninvasive test procedure to exclude disease by the gold standard when no disease is present. Therefore the calculation indicates how "specific" a noninvasive test is in determining when a patient is normal, or negative, for disease.

$$\text{Specificity} = \frac{TN}{TN + FP} \times 100$$

In our example, the Specificity = (108/108 + 0) × 100 = 100%.

Positive predictive value (PPV) allows us to determine the likelihood that when the noninvasive test is positive, the gold standard will also be positive. In other words, the calculated PPV indicates the predictive capability of a positive test to identify patients with disease.

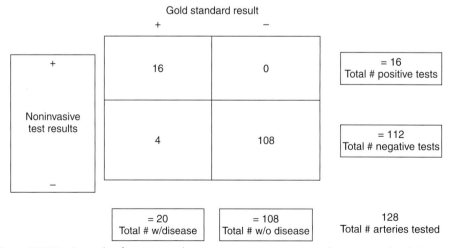

Figure 25-25 Example of positive and negative noninvasive test results compared with the gold standard.

You should note that this calculation takes into consideration only the "positive" tests.

$$PPV = \frac{TP}{TP + FP} \times 100$$

In our example, the PPV = (16/16 + 0) × 100 = 100%.
Negative predictive value (NPV) allows us to determine the likelihood that when the noninvasive test is negative, the gold standard will also be negative. In other words, the calculated NPV indicates the predictive ability of a negative test to identify patients without disease. You should note that calculation of the NPV takes into consideration only the "negative" tests.

$$NPV = \frac{TN}{TN + FN} \times 100$$

Using our example, the NPV = (108/108 + 4) × 100 = 96%.
Accuracy indicates the percentage, i.e., overall agreement, of all of the noninvasive studies that were correctly identified when compared with the gold standard. You should note that the numerator in this calculation comprises the "true positives" and "true negatives" (the number of tests that were in total agreement with the gold standard), and the denominator is the total number of noninvasive studies submitted for correlation with gold standard.

$$Accuracy = \frac{TP + TN}{TP + TN + FP + FN} \times 100$$

In our example, the accuracy of the noninvasive test for identification of carotid artery stenosis in the range of 40% to 59% would be represented as:

Accuracy = (16 + 108/16 + 108 + 0 + 4) × 100 = 97%.

Prevalence is the incidence of disease in the total population of patients that were studied noninvasively. The calculation indicates when disease is truly present in the population. Therefore the numerator of the equation is comprised of the "true positives" (the number of times the noninvasive test agreed with the gold standard that disease was really present) and the "false negatives" (the number of times the gold standard identified disease in the chosen category of severity but the noninvasive test failed to identify it).

$$Prevalence = \frac{TP + FN}{TP + TN + FP + FN} \times 100$$

In our example, Prevalence = (16 + 4/16 + 108 + 0 + 4) × 100 = 16%.

SUMMARY
Noninvasive vascular diagnostic methods have shown tremendous advancement over the past two decades with the development of sophisticated instrumentation and technology. Thus a large armamentarium of direct and indirect test procedures is available for identification and evaluation of cerebrovascular, peripheral arterial, and venous disease. The laboratory staff must not only be skilled in performance of each test, but also must recognize the capabilities and limitations of these test procedures and understand the pathophysiology of vascular disease. The goal of the vascular diagnostic laboratory is to provide accurate, cost-effective, noninvasive diagnostic procedures that will answer the following questions: Is vascular disease present? Where is it located? How severe is the vascular disorder? What is the prognosis? And, are therapeutic results being obtained?

REFERENCE CHARTS

■ ■ ■ ASSOCIATED PHYSICIANS

Vascular Surgeon: Specializes in the surgical and endovascular treatment of cerebrovascular, peripheral arterial, and venous disorders.
Neurologist: Specializes in the treatment of cerebrovascular disorders.
Vascular/Interventional Radiologist: Specializes in identification, diagnosis, localization, and endovascular treatment of cerebrovascular, peripheral arterial, and venous disorders. Treatment includes endovascular balloon dilation and stent placement.

■ ■ ■ COMMON DIAGNOSTIC TESTS

Vascular Angiography: A contrast medium is injected into an artery or vein and x-ray films are taken at specific intervals to observe blood flow patterns in vessels. Performed by interventional radiologists assisted by radiologic technologists; interpreted by the radiologists.

■ ■ ■ LABORATORY VALUES
Nonapplicable

■ ■ ■ NORMAL M-MODE MEASUREMENTS
Nonapplicable

■ ■ ■ VASCULATURE
Nonapplicable

■ ■ ■ AFFECTING CHEMICALS
Nonapplicable

BIBLIOGRAPHY

Bernstein EF, editor: *Vascular diagnosis,* ed 4, St Louis, 1993, Mosby.

Kremkau FW: *Doppler ultrasound: principles and instrumentation,* Philadelphia, 2000, WB Saunders.

Neumyer MM, Thiele BL: Evaluation of lower extremity occlusive disease with Doppler ultrasound. In Taylor KJW, Burns PN, Wells PNT, editors: *Clinical applications of Doppler ultrasound,* New York, 1988, Raven, pp 317-337.

Pick TP, Howden R, editors: *Gray's anatomy,* New York, 1977, Bounty Books.

Strandness DE Jr: *Duplex scanning in vascular disorders,* New York, 1990, Raven.

Sumner DS: Evaluation of noninvasive testing procedures: data analysis and interpretation. In Bernstein EF, editor: *Vascular diagnosis,* ed 4, St Louis, 1993, Mosby, pp 35-63.

Zweibel WJ, editor: *Introduction to vascular ultrasonography,* ed 3, Orlando, 2000, Grune & Stratton.

CHAPTER 26

Introduction to Ultrasound of Human Disease

KATHRYN A. GILL AND BETTY BATES TEMPKIN

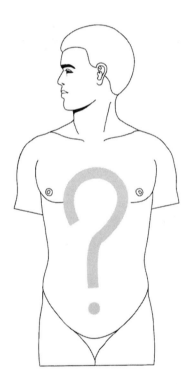

KEY WORDS

Acoustic shadows	Hypoechoic
Anechoic	Infiltrative
Ascites	Intrahepatic
Complex	Intraorgan pathology
Congenital	Isogenic
Cyst(ic)	Isosonic
Diffuse	Localized
Echogenic	Mass
Enhancement	Necrotic
Extrahepatic	Neoplasm
Extraorgan pathology	Parenchyma
Focal	Septations
Heterogeneous	Solid
Homogeneous	Through transmission
Hyperechoic	

Ultrasound is based on the concept that every soft tissue organ visualized by ultrasound has an individual normal textural appearance, shape, size, contour, and specific position within the body. This appearance is highly consistent among persons, with only small variations seen. The textural patterns help the sonographer to detect changes in organ tissue or **parenchyma** and the pathologic conditions that those changes might represent. All pathology visualized by ultrasound in some way disrupts the normal textural pattern of the organ involved and may alter its shape, size, contour, and position.

The primary responsibility of the sonographer is to evaluate areas of interest and identify the textural patterns visualized as part of the examination documentation process. This function includes differentiating abnormal echo textures from normal echo textures. This approach affords the interpreting physician with a description of the abnormality, which will help determine the diagnosis and ultimately the best treatment for the patient.

The purpose of this chapter is to aid the sonographer in accurately describing the sonographic appearance of abnormal findings to the interpreting physician. This specific need arises with the understanding that legally, a sonographer's responsibility is limited to documenting and describing the appearance of disease. By virtue of education, training, and legal parameters, physicians exclusively render diagnoses.

It is not necessary to be familiar with diseases to describe them sonographically. However, a sonographer benefits from having an understanding of diseases and their sonographic presentations. Many diseases affect more than one organ or system. Being aware of this can result in a more complete and effective ultrasound study. Although that is not within the focus of this chapter or book, the reader may want to explore other ultrasound textbooks regarding specific pathologic processes.

PRENATAL DEVELOPMENT

Some pathologic states arise because of a fault in prenatal development and are present at birth **(congenital).** The development of pathologic states, prenatal or otherwise, is not discussed because this is not the focus of this chapter.

LOCATION

Pathology can arise anywhere throughout the body. The sonographer's goal is to describe the accurate location of abnormal findings. Location is based on the origin of the pathology. In some cases, this may be difficult to determine depending on the extent of the pathologic process. In these instances, adjacent recognizable structures and descriptive divisions of the body (discussed in Chapter 4) are used in defining the primary pathologic site. The following image is a good example of how challenging it can be to determine the origin of a mass. It is difficult to determine from this single view whether the mass is part of the liver, right kidney, or right adrenal gland. A sonographer could describe the findings in this view as

"Right upper quadrant, primarily cystic, complex mass. 7 cm long axis measurement, 4.3 cm anteroposterior measurement. Right kidney and right adrenal gland not visualized."

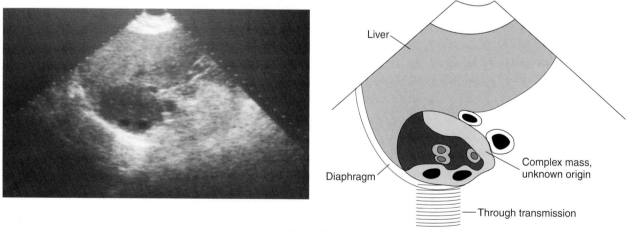

Figure 26-1

When determining the origin of pathology it may be helpful to classify disease as intraorgan or extraorgan. **Intraorgan** features to look for are (1) disruption of the normal internal architecture, (2) external bulging of organ capsules, and (3) displacement or shift of adjacent structures. The image below shows an intraorgan mass. The findings can be characterized as

"Primarily solid, 10 × 10 cm complex, **intrahepatic** mass. Central portion has irregular borders and appears hypoechoic and homogeneous except where it is interrupted anteroposteriorly by an anechoic fluid collection with irregular walls. Periphery appears hyperechoic with slightly irregular borders. There is a slight bulge of the liver capsule posterosuperiorly. The inferior vena cava is visualized."

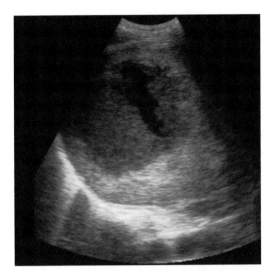
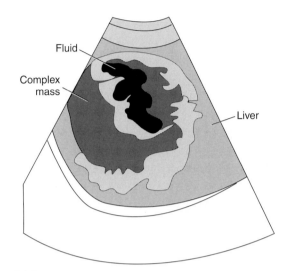

Figure 26-2

The features of **extraorgan** pathology that sonographers should look for include (1) displacement of other organs and structures, (2) obstruction of other organs or structures from view, (3) internal invagination of organ capsules, and (4) discontinuity of organ capsules. It may be impossible to determine the origin of a mass from any single view; however, for the sake of description, review of the next image demonstrates some conclusive determinations. This image showing an extraorgan mass could be described to the interpreting physician as

"Right upper quadrant, solid, homogeneous, hypoechoic mass. Borders appear uniform. Long axis measures 6.2 cm, anteroposterior measurement 5 cm. Mass appears **extrahepatic.** Evidence of discontinuity of liver capsule is visualized. Right adrenal gland is not visualized. Right kidney is seen inferiorly and separate from the mass."

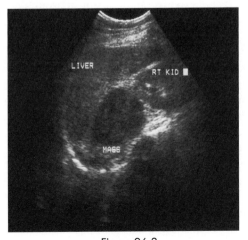

Figure 26-3

SIZE

Pathology may be further classified as localized or diffuse. The size of localized abnormalities such as neoplasms and cysts is variable and must be measured. Careful placement of measurement calipers provides accurate dimensions. In some cases, localized tumors such as uterine leiomyomas may affect the overall size of an organ (Figure 26-4). Diffuse or infiltrative disease may also affect overall organ size. With some cases of cirrhosis of the liver, for example, the right lobe shrinks and there is focal enlargement of the caudate lobe. Another example, end stage renal disease, causes the kidney to become smaller. Whether a change in size is easily recognizable or not, the organ in question must be measured and documented for the interpreting physician.

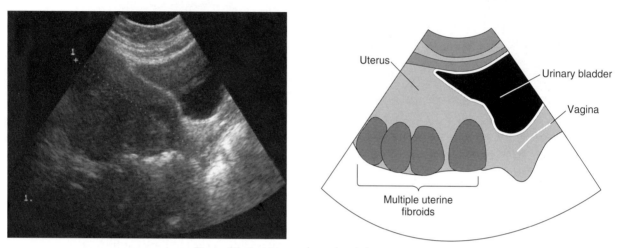

Figure 26-4 Uterus enlarged with leiomyomas.

GROSS ANATOMY

A discussion of pathologic gross anatomy is not within the focus of this chapter.

PHYSIOLOGY

Pathology arises from different pathways. Some are blood borne, as with hepatitis and other diffuse diseases. Some are hereditary, such as hereditary pancreatitis. Others arise as **neoplasms** (new, abnormal growth of existing tissues; either benign or malignant) and cysts, which are thought to originate internally from organs and the structures that compose them. Additionally, congenital abnormalities like Wilms' tumor of the kidney are believed to be the result of anomalous development. Still, other pathologic states arise having no identified etiology.

SONOGRAPHIC APPEARANCE

All soft tissue organs exhibit a normal textural appearance, which varies little among persons. Most organs display a uniform, or homogeneous, texture composed of low- to medium-level shades of gray. In Figure 26-5, notice the normal sonographic appearance, shape, and position of the liver and kidney. The organ parenchyma is homogeneous and the contours are smooth. Pathology disrupts the normal sonographic appearance of organs.

When the normal, homogeneous texture of an organ is interrupted by disease, the parenchyma assumes an irregular, or **heterogeneous,** pattern. In other words, the parenchyma no longer appears uniform and smooth. Key findings can be used to help detect parenchymal changes. The changes may be **diffuse** (**infiltrative** throughout the organ or **focal,** in a specific area[s]) or localized (single or multiple). An infiltrative change in the normal appearance of organ parenchyma suggests dif-

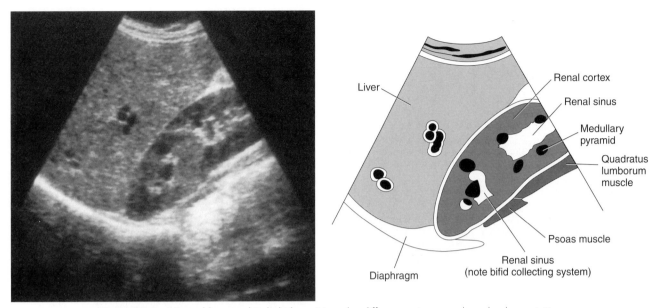

Figure 26-5 Normal liver and right kidney. Note the differences in parenchymal echogenicities between the outer renal cortex, the inner medulla, and the liver.

fuse disease. These diseases may present as subtle change to very obvious change, depending on the severity and progression of the disease. A **localized** change in the normal appearance of organ parenchyma represents a mass or multiple masses, which are restricted to a circumscribed area. A mass may be described as cystic, solid, or complex according to its composition.

Some disease processes are accompanied by the formation of calculi, which further interrupt the normal appearance of an organ. Typically, calculi or "stones" are distinguished by the fact that they reflect and absorb sound waves, creating an **echogenic** or bright anterior surface and dark to anechoic posterior shadow. These **acoustic shadows** generally have sharp, well-defined edges. The image below is a good example. This view shows calculi inside the gallbladder. A sonographer could describe the findings for the interpreting physician as

"Multiple echogenic foci visualized within the gallbladder. Anechoic distal shadowing is present."

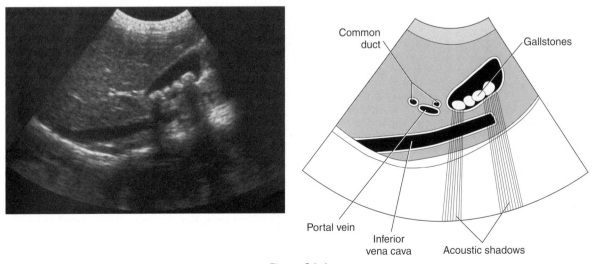

Figure 26-6

As another example, the findings in this next image could be characterized as "Intraluminal gallbladder density with well-defined posterior shadow."

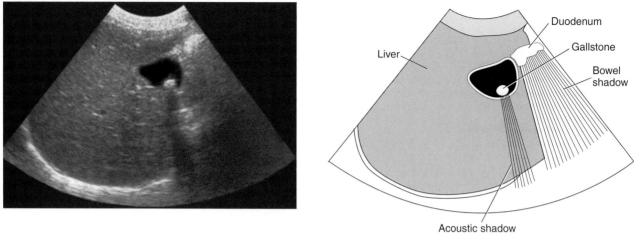

Figure 26-7

Not all distal shadows visualized with ultrasound are representative of pathology. Refracted shadows can occur at edge margins, especially on round structures. The fetal skull is a good example (Figure 26-8; see Chapter 1 to review the properties of ultrasound refraction). Refractive shadowing, however, is not limited to nonpathologic structures. True cysts, for instance, are generally round and may also exhibit refractive shadowing (Figure 26-9).

Describing Diffuse Disease

Generally, diffuse abnormalities, although varied in type, share similar characteristics in their sonographic presentation. The characteristics sonographers should look for are changes in organ echo texture, size, shape, and position, and any associated complications with adjacent structures. Each diffuse disease has its own distinctive criteria that may include all or only some of these characteristics. As noted earlier, it is not necessary to be familiar with these criteria to describe them sonographically.

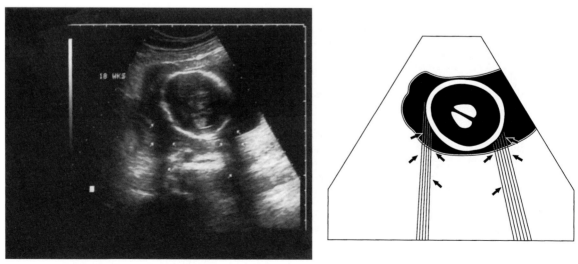

Figure 26-8 Fetal skull with refractive shadowing *(arrows)*. (Half-tone image courtesy the Group for Women, Norfolk, VA.)

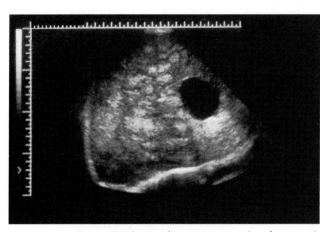
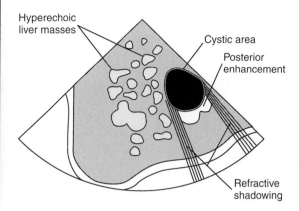

Figure 26-9 Intrahepatic cyst with refractive shadowing. (Half-tone image courtesy Acuson Corp, Mountain View, California.)

As previously discussed, changes in organ parenchyma appear as differences in texture and/or echogenicity compared with the normal sonographic appearance, so they should be described that way. With diffuse disease, organ texture may be described as heterogeneous (random pattern), rough, patchy, or coarse as opposed to smooth. With advanced diffuse disease, the appearance of the parenchyma may also be interrupted with **necrotic** (a visible breakdown or "death" of tissue) or blood-filled spaces that must also be noted. As discussed in Chapter 4, comparative terms used to describe echogenicity include **hyperechoic** (increased echogenicity), **hypoechoic** (decreased echogenicity), **isogenic** or **isosonic** (same relative echogenicity), and **anechoic** (echo free). In some cases, a change in parenchyma may be described as simply as

"The liver appears enlarged and hyperechoic compared with the pancreas."

In other cases, where disease is more progressive, a description of parenchymal change could be characterized as

"The liver appears coarse, with scattered increases in echogenicity and multiple fluid-filled, anechoic spaces."

Changes in the size, shape, and position of an organ affected by diffuse disease may be subtle and unrecognizable or immediately obvious. Either way, measurements of the organ including necrotic or fluid-filled components must be documented, with any change in shape or position described. For instance,

"Liver shape appears altered, with coarse, scattered increases in echogenicity and multiple fluid-filled, anechoic spaces, 1 to 5 mm in diameter."

A description of a renal study might include

"The kidneys are enlarged with smooth cortical margins. The right kidney is lower in position than normal and measures 16 cm long, 5.2 cm thick, and 6.5 cm wide. The left kidney is 14.4 cm long, 5 cm thick, and 6 cm wide."

When diffuse disease causes either generalized enlargement or focal areas of enlargement of an organ, the sonographer must determine the extent of enlargement and describe whether any adjacent structures exhibit associated complications. Infiltrative or focal enlargement of an organ may cause all or part of the organ to extend far beyond its normal boundaries and ultimately have an effect on the structures adjacent to it. This process can displace organs and other structures from their normal positions or block them from view. For example, diffuse infiltrative disease of the liver may cause compression of normal vasculature that is usually readily identified when evaluating the liver. In the image below, the findings can be described as

"Enlarged, hyperechoic right lobe. Few internal vascular structures noted. Right kidney appears compressed and displaced inferomedially."

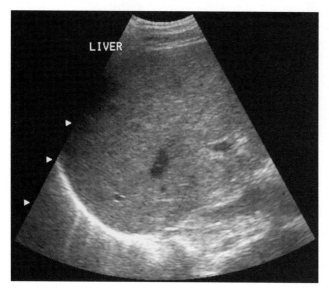 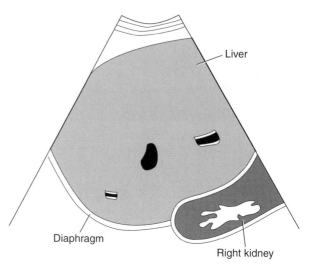

Figure 26-10

If the caudate lobe of the liver is also enlarged, it can exert pressure on the inferior vena cava, leading to vena caval hypertension, which may contribute to renal failure in some patients. Another example is diffuse infiltrative disease of the spleen that displaces the left kidney. A description could be

"Spleen appears enlarged, homogeneous, and hypoechoic to the liver. Splenic volume index is 50. Left kidney is displaced inferomedially with the upper pole flattened by the lumpy splenic contour."

An example of focal enlargement that affects adjacent structures is chronic pancreatitis with focal enlargement of the head, which can cause biliary duct obstruction (jaundice). Pressure from the enlarged head can obstruct, constrict, stenose, and dilate the common bile duct. Some of these cases present with duodenal obstruction as well. These findings, among others associated with chronic pancreatitis, could be described as

"Pancreas appears heterogeneous and hyperechoic. Small, shadowing calcifications throughout, and irregular outline are noted. Head appears focally enlarged: 6 cm anteroposterior. Common bile duct appears dilated: 12 mm. The duodenum is not visualized."

Clearly, a detailed observation can be reported to the interpreting physician without stating that the findings are consistent with pancreatitis.

Describing Localized Disease

A localized parenchymal change is described as a **mass,** defined according to composition. Regardless of composition, most masses are distinguishable because they are restricted to a circumscribed area. The characteristics sonographers should look for are number, composition, size, origin, and any associated complications with adjacent structures or systems. Each localized disease has its own criteria for diagnosis that may include all or only some of these characteristics. Again, it is not necessary to be familiar with these criteria to describe them sonographically.

Depending on the extent or type of localized disease, single or multiple masses may be visualized.

Each type of mass possesses distinctive sonographic characteristics that define its composition. The composition of a mass determines what it is: fluid filled, a **cystic** mass; tissue, a **solid** mass; fluid and tissue, a **complex** mass. The key to determining composition is technical, using time-gain compensation (TGC) (see Chapter 2). Never be fooled by the initial appearance of the composition of a mass. For instance, the mass may appear cystic but actually be a solid, hypoechoic mass. Sonographers can make this differentiation by adjusting the TGC from high to low while visualizing the mass. In fact, most scanning protocols recommend documenting high- and low-gain images, in at least two scanning planes, as part of the study for the interpreting physician.

The size of localized abnormalities is variable. All abnormal findings should be measured in at least two scanning planes to obtain a volume measurement. Measurement calipers must be placed at the greatest dimensions of a mass. The longest axis of the mass should be noted. As previously discussed, some localized tumors may affect the overall size of an organ (see Figure 26-4). In these cases, if the individual tumors can be differentiated from each other and organ parenchyma, they should be measured individually.

Masses are generally distinctive in appearance and unless very small, readily identified. In some cases, the organ that a mass arises from is obvious; in others, as noted earlier, it can be difficult to determine the origin. The close proximity of body structures, location, and size of a mass can make it hard to differentiate the primary site. Large masses usually present the greatest challenge, especially if their size obstructs the organ of origin and complicates adjacent structures. In the following image, the liver appears to be compromised by an extrahepatic, right lower quadrant mass. The right kidney is separate from the mass and the adrenal gland is not visualized. Although a conclusive determination cannot be made from this single view, it is highly probable that the mass is adrenal in origin and is obstructing the view of the small adrenal gland.

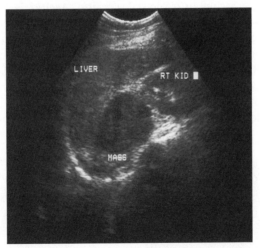

Figure 26-11

Describing Cystic Masses

To be considered a true cyst, the mass in question must meet three sonographic criteria. The first criterion is that it contain no internal echoes. This means the mass appears anechoic. It is possible to observe "cystic noise" within a true cyst; that is, low-level echoes may be located near the anterior wall. Echoes never occur in the posterior portion of a true cyst. The second criterion is that the walls of the cyst must be well-defined, thin, and smooth. The final criterion is that there be posterior through transmission, or **enhancement. Through transmission** refers to the appearance of the sound waves that pass unobstructed through and beyond fluid. This through transmission exhibits enhanced or bright echoes, which are hyperechoic to adjacent structures. For example, the following image could be described as

"2 cm anechoic mass superior pole, right kidney. 1 cm anechoic mass anterior edge, midportion of kidney. Both masses have smooth, well-defined walls and exhibit through transmission."

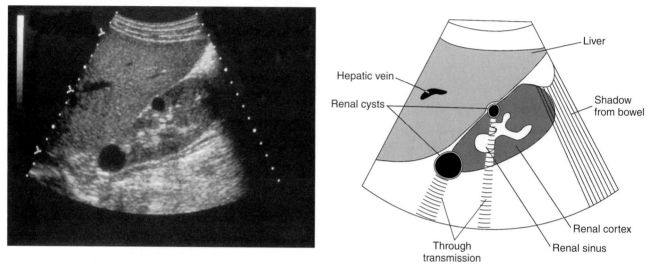

Figure 26-12 (Half-tone image courtesy Acuson Corp, Mountain View, California.)

If one of the three criteria is not met, the mass is not a true cyst. A mass that meets one or more of these criteria, but not all three, is said to be cystic in nature, although not a true cyst. An example of a cystic area that does not meet the requirements for a true cyst would be ascites or a pleural effusion. **Ascites** is an accumulation of serous fluid anywhere in the abdominopelvic cavity. A pleural effusion is a collection of fluid inside the lung. Both fluid collections are anechoic areas that may demonstrate posterior enhancement, but neither has well-defined, thin, smooth walls (Figure 26-13). There are two situations in which the enhancement criterion may be difficult to meet: (1) a cyst located deep in the body beyond the focal zone of the transducer, meaning there are not enough sound waves being generated to pass through the fluid to create the enhancement effect; (2) a cyst located immedi-

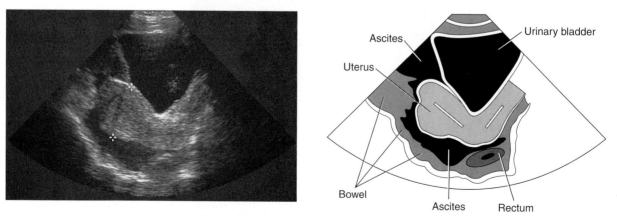

Figure 26-13 Ascites in the pelvic cavity.

ately anterior to a bony structure, which absorbs the sound waves and prohibits posterior enhancement.

A cystic structure that contains thin membranous inclusions is said to be septated. An example of how a multilocular renal cyst might be described sonographically is

"A solid, renal mass with multiple, 1- to 3-cm, fluid-filled structures separated by highly echogenic **septations.**"

Describing Solid Masses

Although there are numerous varieties of solid masses or neoplasms, they are all composed of one thing, tissue. A solid mass is visualized sonographically as echogenic shades of gray that represent its internal composition. The level of echogenicity and appearance of tissue texture depend on what type of localized disease is present, the degree of its echodensity, and its effect on internal architecture. In some respects, solid tissue masses are characterized sonographically in the same manner as soft tissue organs: hyperechoic or hypoechoic, isosonic, homogeneous, or heterogeneous. The image below shows multiple liver masses that appear brighter than surrounding parenchyma and single cyst. The ultrasound findings could be characterized as

"Right lobe of the liver appears heterogeneous. 1- to 3-cm multiple, solid, intrahepatic masses are hyperechoic, and coarse. 3 × 3 cm anechoic fluid collection located in the medial portion of the right lobe. Walls are well-defined and smooth. Posterior enhancement is visualized."

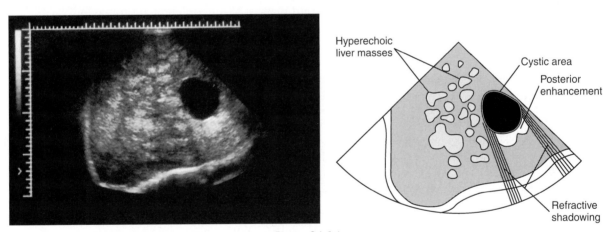

Figure 26-14

The next image shows a mass that appears darker than the parenchyma surrounding it. An example of how to characterize the findings is

"A solid, homogeneous, hypoechoic breast mass. 10 cm long axis measurement. 6 cm anteroposterior measurement."

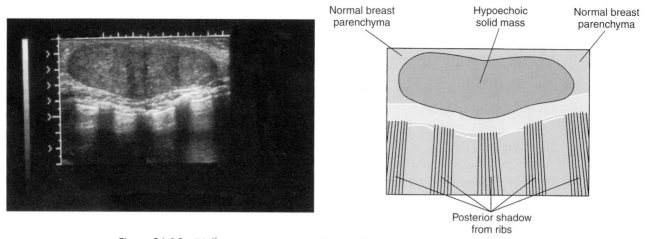

Figure 26-15 (Half-tone image courtesy Acuson Corp, Mountain View, California.)

A mass having the same echogenicity as the surrounding tissue is seen in the following image, which could be described as

"Left upper quadrant, single, solid, homogeneous mass, isosonic to the spleen. Mass lies inferior to the spleen and does not appear to be splenic in origin. 14 cm long axis measurement, 8 cm lateromedial measurement. Left kidney and left adrenal gland were not visualized."

Note that in some cases of isosonic solid masses, border differentiation may be the only clue to their presence.

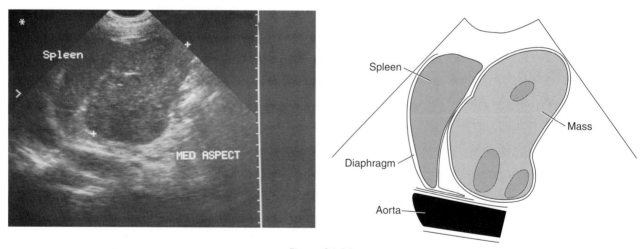

Figure 26-16

Describing Complex Masses

A mass that contains fluid and solid components is said to be complex. Complex masses may be primarily cystic or primarily solid. The combination of both appearances within the same structure gives rise to the term *complex*. The appearance of the walls varies from well-defined and smooth to poorly defined and irregular.

The internal composition of a mass may vary with time. This is especially true of vascular masses, which may appear anechoic when the blood is fresh, but become complex and even solid as the blood forms clots. Another example is a solid mass, which degenerates over time. This occurrence may be seen with uterine fibroids. These benign tumors may remain very stable for years and then, as a result of various hormonal changes, begin to change internally. This type of degenerating process usually means that a solid mass has begun to liquefy and thereby assume a more complex appearance. For example, the transverse image below could be characterized as

"A primarily cystic, complex, uterine mass. Posterior enhancement is noted. Borders appear smooth and thin. Measures 10 cm wide and 7 cm anteroposterior. Solid component appears heterogeneous with irregular borders and a posterior extension running along the posterior border of the mass. Measures 5 cm wide and 5.5 cm anteroposterior. Posterior extension measures 6 cm wide and 2 cm anteroposterior."

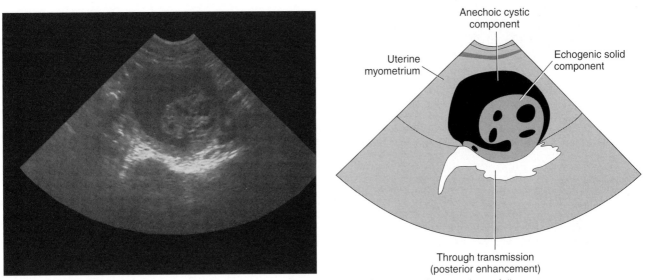

Figure 26-17 (Half-tone image courtesy Sentara Norfolk General Hospital, Norfolk, VA.)

The following image shows a complex breast mass that can be described as

"Single, primarily solid, complex breast mass. Appears hypoechoic, and heterogeneous, with slightly thick, irregular borders. 6 cm long axis measurement, 4 cm anteroposterior measurement. 1.5- to 2-cm multiple anechoic structures noted throughout."

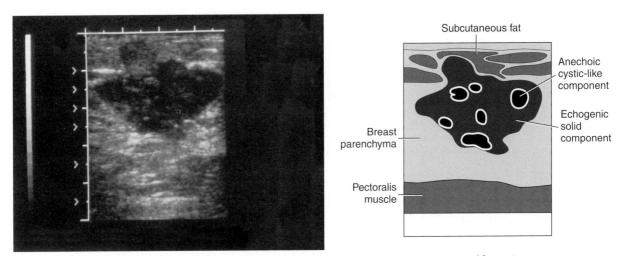

Figure 26-18 (Half-tone image courtesy Acuson Corp, Mountain View, California.)

Another example of a complex breast mass in a different patient is seen below. These findings could be related to the interpreting physician as

"Single, primarily solid, heterogeneous, complex breast mass. Border is relatively smooth and slightly thick. Long axis measurement 2.2 cm. Anteroposterior measurement 1.9 cm. Contains a centrally located 1.3 × 1.3 cm anechoic area with smooth, thin walls."

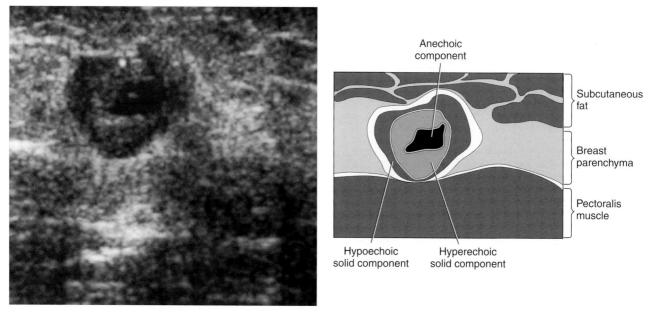

Figure 26-19

The complex intrahepatic mass seen in this next image could be described for the interpreting physician as

"A primarily solid, heterogeneous, 10 × 10 cm complex, intrahepatic mass. Central portion is hypoechoic, interrupted anteroposteriorly by an anechoic fluid collection with irregular walls. Periphery of mass appears thick, slightly irregular, uniform, and bright. There is a slight bulge of the liver capsule posterosuperiorly. The inferior vena cava is not visualized"

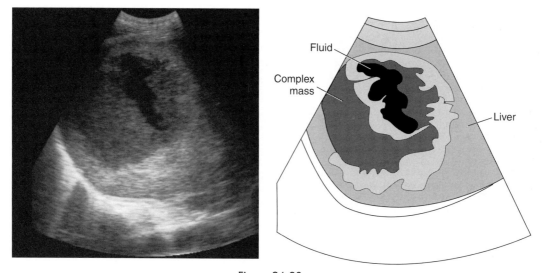

Figure 26-20

Notice the identification and description of the walls and border. It is very important to convey the appearance of mass borders to the interpreting physician. This means describing the borders as smooth or irregular in contour and thin or thick, and whether they appear uniform throughout the circumference of the mass. The following is a sagittal image and longitudinal section of the urinary bladder with a mass that could be characterized as

"Single, solid, heterogeneous, hyperechoic, bladder mass. 7.5 cm long axis measurement, 5 cm anteroposterior measurement. Superior, inferior, and anterior borders are markedly irregular. Anterior border rises to meet the anterior bladder wall. Posterior border is slightly irregular and adjacent to the posterior bladder wall. Borders appear thick posteriorly and inferiorly; slightly thinner anteriorly and superiorly. Anechoic fluid (urine) is noted superior and inferior to the mass."

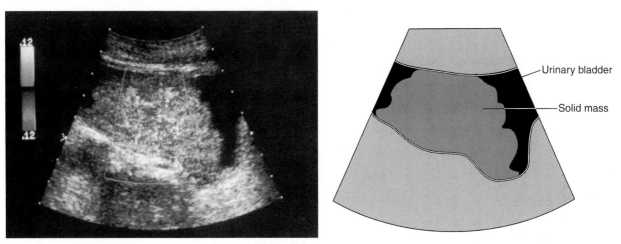

Figure 26-21   See also Color Plate 49. (Half-tone image courtesy Acuson Corp, Mountain View, California.)

The right upper quadrant mass seen in this next image could be related to the interpreting physician as

"A primarily solid, complex, intrahepatic mass. Long axis, anteroposterior measurement 9.5 cm. Superoinferior measurement 7 cm. Appears heterogeneous and coarse. Primarily hyperechoic compared with the liver, with an irregular, hypoechoic portion located posteroinferiorly. Measures 5 cm long axis, 4 cm anteroposterior. Additional small, scattered anechoic areas noted throughout the mass. Mass borders are markedly irregular and thin except for a portion of the superior and inferior borders, which appear slightly thicker."

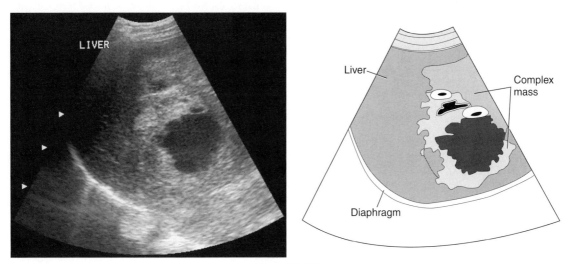

Figure 26-22

SONOGRAPHIC APPLICATIONS

This chapter demonstrates that in addition to image documentation, sonographers can precisely describe sonographic findings without compromising their legal position. The goal of this chapter is to provide the sonographer with the knowledge base necessary to relate abnormal sonographic findings to the interpreting physician in an accurate and professional manner.

NORMAL VARIANTS

The many aspects of pathologic variants are not within the focus of this chapter.

REFERENCE CHARTS

■ ■ ■ ASSOCIATED PHYSICIANS

Radiologist: Specializes in the diagnostic interpretation of imaging modalities that are used to determine the presence of pathologic processes. The physician may utilize invasive maneuvers to determine the exact nature of the demonstrated pathology, such as biopsies.

Pathologist: Specializes in determining the nature of pathologic tissues. This is usually done through biopsies and cellular examination.

Obstetrician/Gynecologist: Specializes in treating female patients, whether pregnant or not. The physician often performs and/or interprets the ultrasound examinations and may perform whatever follow-up is necessary.

Cardiologist: Specializes in the interpretation of cardiac testing methods, including the echocardiogram (ultrasound of the heart).

■ ■ ■ COMMON DIAGNOSTIC TESTS

Computed Axial Tomography (CT Scan): This test utilizes x-rays to demonstrate a cross-sectional image of the body. A contrast medium is often injected to help differentiate pathology from normal anatomic variants. The test is performed by a radiologic technologist and interpreted by a radiologist.

Magnetic Resonance Imaging (MRI): This imaging modality utilizes changes in magnetic fields to assess anatomy. The test may also require the injection of a contrast medium. A MRI is performed most often by a specially trained radiologic technologist and is interpreted by a radiologist.

■ ■ ■ LABORATORY VALUES

The laboratory findings vary from case to case and organ to organ. Some have been mentioned in previous chapters and further review is not presented in this chapter.

■ ■ ■ NORMAL MEASUREMENTS

All pathology should be imaged and measured in two planes, including the longest axis of a mass.

■ ■ ■ VASCULATURE

It is extremely important to determine the location of pathology relative to adjacent vasculature. Normal vasculature can be very helpful in describing the correct location of pathology for the interpreting physician. Adjacent vasculature must be assessed to determine if pathologic involvement or changes are present due to the pathologic state.

■ ■ ■ AFFECTING CHEMICALS

The chemicals affecting the potential for pathologic development, as well as those that can affect existing pathologies, vary from organ to organ and are not discussed further in this chapter. Refer to previous chapters for relevant information.

BIBLIOGRAPHY

Bega G: Three- and four-dimensional ultrasound imaging in the first trimester, section IV. In *The leading edge in diagnostic ultrasound program textbook,* Philadelphia, 2003, Jefferson Ultrasound Research and Education Institute, pp 19-24.

Bega G: Three- and four-dimensional ultrasound imaging in the second and third trimester, section IV. In *The leading edge in diagnostic ultrasound program textbook,* Philadelphia, 2003, Jefferson Ultrasound Research and Education Institute, pp 53-58.

Blass HG, Eik-Ness SH, et al: In vivo three-dimensional ultrasound reconstruction of embryos and early fetuses, *Lancet* 352(9135): 1182-1186, 1998.

Advances in Ultrasound

CHAPTER 27

Three-Dimensional Ultrasound

MICHAEL J. KAMMERMEIER AND REVA ARNEZ CURRY

OBJECTIVES

Define three-dimensional ultrasound.

Explain the sonographer's role in the three-dimensional examination.

Describe current methods and techniques on how to perform three-dimensional ultrasound.

Explain the importance of the following components of three-dimensional ultrasound: volume data sets, volume acquisition, multiplanar display, and three-dimensional rendering.

Identify examples of normal anatomy on three-dimensional images.

Describe the clinical applications of three-dimensional ultrasound.

Define four-dimensional ultrasound.

Describe the clinical applications of four-dimensional ultrasound.

KEY WORDS

Acquisition	Real-time three-dimensional (3D)
Automatic acquisition	
Four-dimensional (4D) ultrasound	Three-dimensional (3D) rendering
Manual acquisition	Three-dimensional (3D) ultrasound surface mode
Maximum mode	
Minimum mode	Volume data set
Multiplanar	

Ultrasound is a very progressive and ever-evolving imaging modality. **Three-dimensional (3D) ultrasound** is one of the latest innovations in this dynamic field. Most sonographers have seen incredible images of the fetal face on 3D. This is just one small aspect of 3D ultrasound. While 3D is beneficial in obstetrical scanning, it is also valuable in the evaluation of gynecologic, ab-

dominal, prostate, neonatal, small parts, musculoskeletal, and invasive ultrasound procedures. New applications for 3D ultrasound are still being identified.

3D ultrasound was first introduced in the late 1980's. It has only been recently, with the advent of faster processors and advances in ultrasound and transducer technology, that 3D ultrasound has become more widely accepted.

METHODS

The technologies behind 3D ultrasound are diverse. There are many companies developing 3D ultrasound and they are all different in technological research. Most new ultrasound scanners can be purchased with a 3D option. This simply means that the 3D software is integrated into the system. Other companies have designed off-line computers that connect to existing ultrasound systems and can process ultrasound data into 3D. More precise 3D systems use electromagnetic positioning sensors, which attach to the ultrasound transducer and offer more accurate data **acquisition.** Still others have dedicated 3D ultrasound transducers that are more bulky, but provide the easiest, most accurate, and reproducible 3D images at this time.

This presents a challenge to the sonographer, because some methods are more difficult than others, and the results between methods are different. This chapter will describe the common methods and try to simplify the explanation of the 3D examination procedure.

When performing 3D ultrasound, the patient's anatomy is acquired as a **volume data set.** This volume data set must be displayed on a flat screen. This is typically achieved in the **multiplanar** format. From this display, the sonographer defines the area of interest within the volume to be reconstructed in a process called **three-dimensional (3D) rendering.** Therefore 3D ultrasound can be divided into three basic steps: (1) volume acquisition, (2) multiplanar display, and (3) 3D rendering.

Volume Acquisition

When performing 3D ultrasound, the sonographer must first acquire a volume of the anatomy, the volume data set. This acquisition is the most important step. Without an accurate volume data set, the 3D reconstruction and rendering will not be accurate, and therefore not useful. There are two primary methods of acquiring volumes, **manual acquisition** and **automatic acquisition.**

The manual method is the most common and requires the sonographer to physically move the transducer across the region of interest. This movement is best performed in either a steady sliding motion or a pivoting motion. The two-dimensional (2D) slices are stored in a cineloop and compressed into a 3D volume data set. Because the method requires manual movement of the transducer, it is very operator dependent. The transducer must be moved a specific distance in a certain amount of time to acquire a quality volume data set. To compensate for the potential error in manually moving the transducer, some manufacturers have developed positioning sensors that can be attached to the transducer. Once calibrated, the computer can more accurately estimate the movement of the transducer, resulting in a more accurate data set acquisition. These sensors are sometimes subject to interference from other equipment in the room and may not be the best solution for every department.

The automatic volume method essentially removes the element of human error during the acquisition. This requires dedicated 3D transducers in which the elements within the transducer move while the sonographer holds the probe stationary. These transducers are often larger and more bulky than conventional transducers, but they provide a more accurate and reproducible volume data set.

Multiplanar Display

Once the volume data set has been acquired, the block of information must be displayed on a flat screen. This is typically achieved through multiplanar display. In order to display the information, three orthogonal planes are displayed, the longitudinal, transverse, and coronal planes. These planes can then be rotated and manipulated to create the optimal scan plane. This is accomplished by rotating each plane on the x-, y-, or z-axis. The multiplanar display, in conjunction with the 3D rendered image, provides the most clinical benefit. On some of the more advanced systems (sensor based and automatic acquisition), the operator can measure distances and even volumes in the multiplanar display.

3D Rendering

There are several different types of rendering algorithms that the operator can use to view different anatomy. We are probably most familiar with the fetal face demon-

strated with **surface mode,** which is used to generate a surface perspective of the anatomy (Figure 27-1). This is the most common, but there are other clinical uses. When viewing the volume data set, instead of telling the computer to look at the surface anatomy, we can tell the computer to display only the brightest intensity echoes within the volumes. This is called the **maximum mode.** This is used for assessment of fetal skeletal anatomy, as seen in Figure 27-2, as well as hyperechoic pathology, such as hemangiomas.

In contrast to the maximum mode, the **minimum mode** emphasizes the lowest intensity echoes within the volume. This is used for visualizing fluid-filled structures, such as vasculature, cystic areas, and other fluid-filled areas, such as fetal bladder, stomach, and amniotic fluid. Figure 27-3 demonstrates liver vasculature using minimum mode.

There are other algorithms available that can be useful for a specific evaluation. These rendered images can then be rotated to show the area of interest from any perspective.

SONOGRAPHIC APPLICATIONS

There are many applications available for 3D ultrasound. They include:

- Obstetrics
- Gynecology
- Abdominal
- Small parts

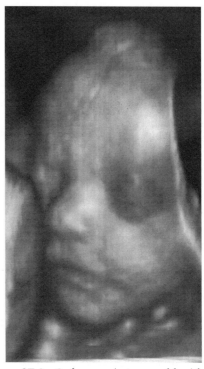

Figure 27-1   Surface mode image of fetal face.

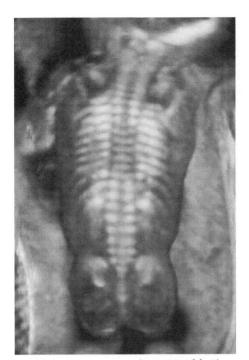

Figure 27-2 Maximum mode image of fetal spine.

Obstetrics

3D reconstruction can be used with a vaginal transducer for first trimester imaging. Fetal anatomy and length can be demonstrated (Figure 27-4). Evaluation of the nuchal fold can occur using 3D imaging even though the fetus is not in the optimal position. The data set can be rotated to create the best plane for imaging the fold.

Second and third trimester imaging is performed with abdominal transducers. Figure 27-5 shows second trimester fetuses, and Figure 27-6 demonstrates a fetus in the third trimester.

Gynecology

Using the endovaginal transducer, the nongravid uterus can be evaluated with 3D. In traditional endovaginal scanning, the operator is limited in the images that can be acquired. Using 3D ultrasound, imaging planes that best show the uterus, ovaries, and fallopian tubes can be utilized to get the most optimal image. 3D imaging can also be used during saline hysterosalpingography (Figure 27-7).

Abdominal

Volumetric abdominal imaging can be accomplished with 3D, allowing for a complete evaluation of organ systems. Organs such as the kidneys are more clearly delineated with 3D ultrasound than standard sonography, as seen in Figure 27-8. Another application of 3D imaging is that serial examinations of tumors are more accurate with pretreatment and posttreatment volumetric measuring.

Using the endorectal transducer, the prostate and seminal vesicles can be evaluated with 3D (Figure 27-9). A single acquisition can yield more information than a lengthy examination, because all of the views, coronal, transverse, and longitudinal, can now be manipulated.

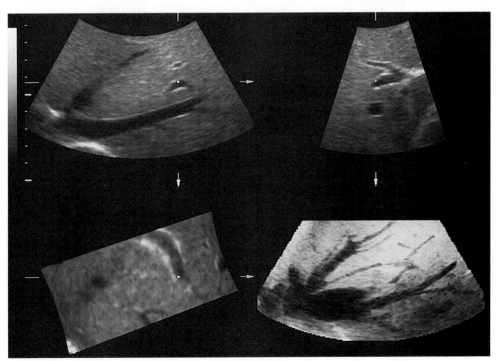

Figure 27-3 Minimum mode images of liver vasculature in an adult.

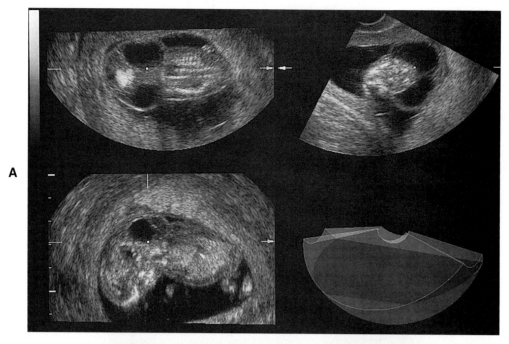

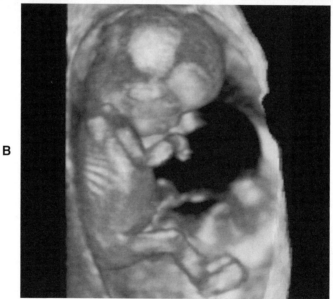

Figure 27-4 **A,** First trimester fetus with a cystic hygroma. **B,** Normal first trimester fetus in sitting position. Note the entire length of the fetus is demonstrated. The fetal face, upper extremities, lower extremities, rib cage, and umbilical cord are clearly shown.

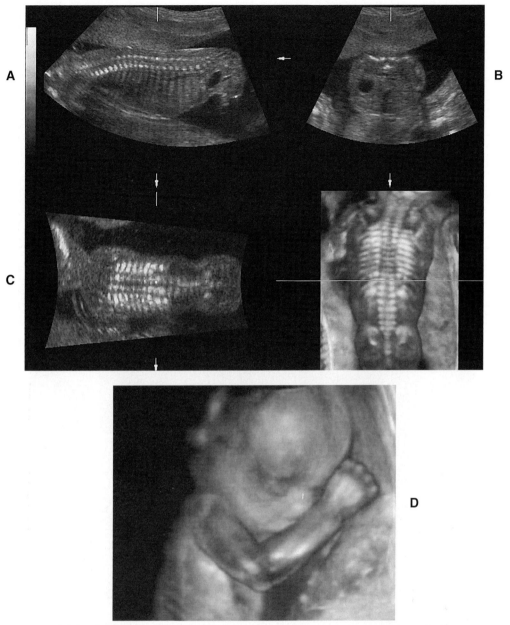

Figure 27-5 Thorax **(A)**, abdomen **(B)**, and pelvis **(C)** in a second trimester fetus. **D**, Face, upper extremity, and thorax in another second trimester fetus.

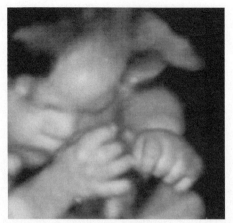

Figure 27-6 Face and hands in a third trimester fetus

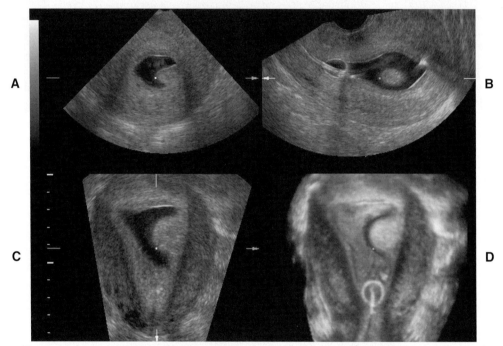

Figure 27-7 Endovaginal examination of the uterus during a saline hysterosalpingogram. **A** and **B,** Note the anechoic saline clearly delineating an endometrial polyp. **C,** Three distinctly different echogenicities: the circular, very hyperechoic catheter at the cervix, the hyperechoic endometrium, and the hypoechoic myometrium, are clearly demonstrated in this coronal view. **D,** Post saline absorption. Some residual saline is still visualized in the endometrium.

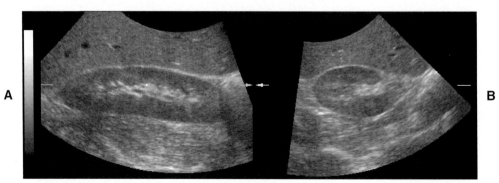

Figure 27-8 Longitudinal **(A)** and transverse **(B)** views of an adult kidney. Note the anterior liver.

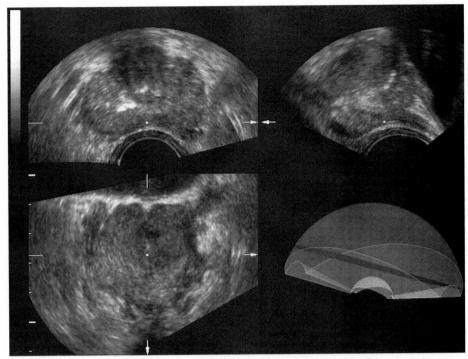

Figure 27-9 Endorectal examination of the prostate.

Small Parts

Using high-frequency linear transducers in a 3D evaluation enhances visualization of small parts such as the thyroid, breast, and testicles. The appearance and degree of echogenicity of breast masses can be better studied as demonstrated in Figure 27-10. Musculoskeletal structures can also be visualized.

In addition to 3D B-mode imaging, 3D acquisition can occur with color and power Doppler, allowing for complete visualization of the surrounding vasculature.

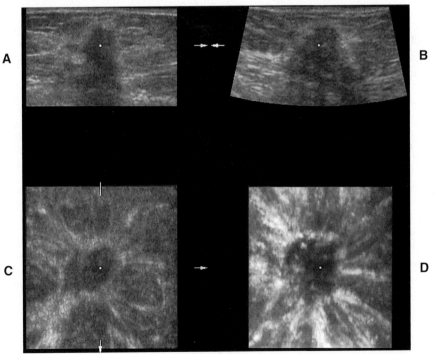

Figure 27-10 A and B, Breast with mass identified by tiny, echogenic dot applied during image processing. C and D, Magnified views of the same mass showing irregular borders and varying echogenicity.

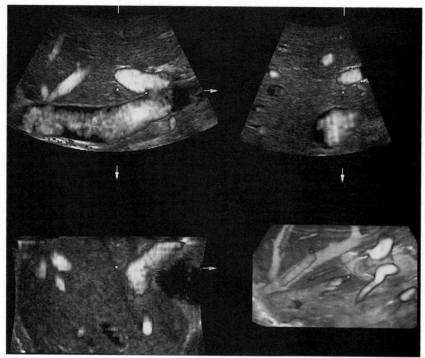

Figure 27-11 Multiple sections of the liver demonstrating vasculature using power Doppler. Note the hepatic veins and inferior vena cava in the upper left image.

This can be achieved with any structure, but is especially impressive in liver evaluation as shown in Figure 27-11.

SUMMARY

Clearly, 3D imaging is beneficial in everyday practice. It enables manipulation to occur for the most optimal imaging and for more accurate measurements. Recent advances include **real-time 3D,** sometimes called **four-dimensional (4D) ultrasound** (the fourth dimension is time). This is only available with the automatic acquisition technique and is accomplished with the operator holding the transducer still while the elements within the probe continuously acquire, process, and display the 3D real-time image. With this method, we can now observe fetal movement in 3D. Another advantage is more accurate needle guidance using real time multiplanar displays: the needle insertion can be followed live in all three dimensions. Other advances include 4D fetal and adult cardiac applications.

At this time, 3D imaging does not replace a thorough 2D examination, but when used in conjunction with 2D, it can provide enhanced visualization and ultimately more information. Sonographers can have greater confidence in the studies they produce and sonologists in their diagnoses. In addition to the benefit of more detailed studies, the scanning time in some applications such as rectal and endovaginal exams can be greatly reduced and at the same time improve the quality of the study. 3D scanning is an exciting new area in ultrasound technology and will only improve as more applications are investigated and introduced.

BIBLIOGRAPHY

Fenster A, Downey DD: Three-Dimensional Imaging Website, Imaging Research Laboratories, The J.P. Robarts Research Institute, Ontario, Canada. http://www.irus.rri.on.ca/~afenster/Papers

Gajonova VY, Zubarev AV: 3-D virtual US-angiography in evaluation of renal arteries. In *The leading edge in diagnostic ultrasound,* Philadelphia, PA, 2001, Jefferson Ultrasound Research and Education Institute.

Lev-Toaff AS: 2-D and 3-D sonohysterography. In *The leading edge in diagnostic ultrasound,* Philadelphia, 2001, Jefferson Ultrasound Research and Education Institute.

Nelson TR, Downey DD, Pretorius DH, Fenster A: *Three-dimensional ultrasound,* Philadelphia, 1999, Lippincott Williams & Wilkins.

Rawool NM: 3-D and other new horizons in musculoskeletal ultrasound. In *The leading edge in diagnostic ultrasound,* Philadelphia, 2001, Jefferson Ultrasound Research and Education Institute.

CHAPTER 28

Interventional and Intraoperative Ultrasound

BETTY BATES TEMPKIN

ULTRASOUND-GUIDED INTERVENTION

Ultrasound is routinely used for needle-guided biopsies, aspirations, and drainage procedures. The site of interest is easily located with ultrasound, and the needle can be imaged and tracked (Figure 28-1).

Ultrasound-guided biopsies facilitate needle placement for tissue sampling. The biopsy site is scanned to determine the best point of entry with the shortest distance and least angle. To monitor the procedure, the transducer may not have to be in the sterile field. If it does, sterile couplant gel and a sterile sheath to cover the transducer are used. Alternatively, some physicians prefer that the transducer and cord be wiped down with alcohol instead of using the sheath. Air bubbles can oc-

cur between the tip of the transducer and the sheath that affect image quality.

Most chest tumors, abdominal organ masses, retroperitoneal lymph node masses, and gastrointestinal tumors can be percutaneously biopsied. Other percutaneous biopsies include chorionic villi sampling, musculoskeletal lesions, thyroid masses, and breast lesions (Figures 28-2 and 28-3).

Ultrasound-guided aspirations assist needle placement for fluid sampling or total evacuation of fluid. The technique is very similar to the percutaneous biopsy procedure. The site is scanned and the most direct entry determined. If monitored in the sterile field, sterile gel is

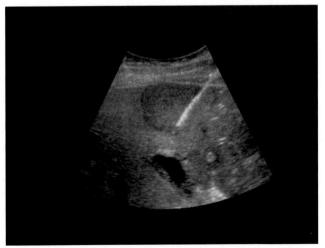
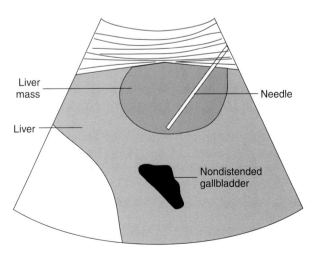

Figure 28-1   Ultrasound-guided biopsy of a liver mass. (Half-tone image courtesy Philips Medical Systems, Bothell, WA.)

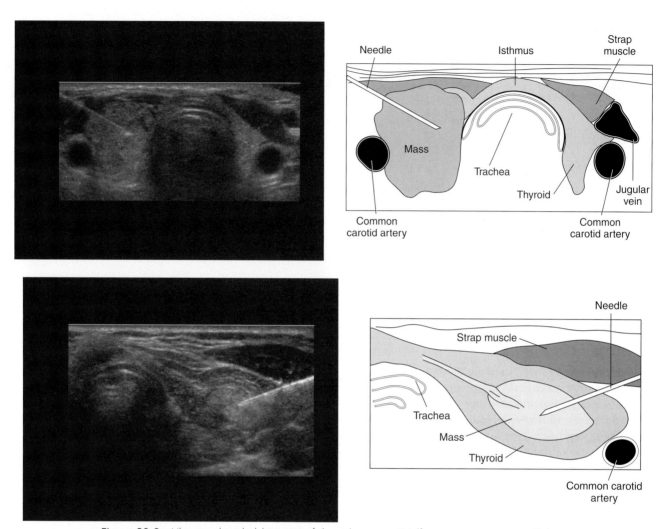

Figure 28-2 Ultrasound-guided biopsies of thyroid masses. (Half-tone images courtesy Philips Medical Systems, Bothell, WA.)

used as well as a sterile sheath or alcohol "bath" for the transducer and cord. Any change in shape or size of a fluid-filled structure can be visualized while the needle tip is inserted and fluid is sampled or evacuated. Aspiration procedures may apply to hepatic cysts, pancreatic pseudocysts, renal cysts, percutaneous cholangiograms, and amniocentesis.

Ultrasound-guided percutaneous drainage procedures aid needle and catheter placement for procedures that include abscess drainage, biliary drainage, and nephrostomy tube placement. A radiologist in a special procedures room with fluoroscopy performs the majority of these drainage techniques. Basically, ultrasound determines the entry site and monitors the placement of the needle and catheter. As with biopsies and aspirations, sterile procedure is utilized.

Interventional sonography has become a safe and accurate clinical tool as well as an attractive alternative to surgery in some cases.

INTRAOPERATIVE ULTRASOUND

Intraoperative ultrasound can provide crucial information to surgeons that may influence their choice of surgical technique. Ultrasound is a timely way to precisely localize and characterize structures. Because the transducer is in direct contact with the organ or vessel being examined, high-resolution images can be obtained that are not limited by overlying soft tissues, bone, or air. Other advantages include its noninvasiveness without radiation or the administration of contrast. Scans are instantaneous, repeatable, multidimensional, and magnified at will.

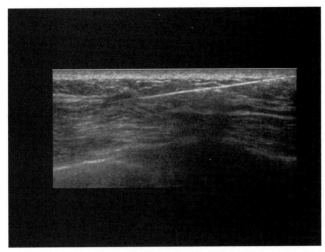 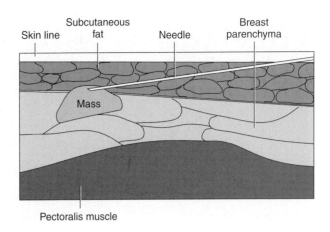

Figure 28-3 Ultrasound-guided breast mass biopsy. (Half-tone image courtesy Philips Medical Systems, Bothell, WA.)

Intraoperative ultrasound is best performed using routine mobile sonography equipment with dedicated transducers. Linear array probes have a small field of view with the best near-field definition, whereas sector probes give a larger field of view for small contact areas. Transducer choice depends on the structure(s) being imaged. Unlike conventional intraoperative sonography, laparoscopic sonography is performed using a flexible tip laparoscopic 5 to 7.5 MHz transducer.

To maintain the sterile operative field, sterile cover sheaths or gas sterilization are sterilizing options. Sheaths should fit snugly over the transducer head to reduce artifacts and tears. Acoustic gel is used as a couplant between the transducer and probe cover; however, it is not used as a scanning couplant. In most cases, natural surface moisture is sufficient to couple the transducer to the target organ. If more moisture is required, warm sterile saline may be used to improve surface contact. Because of potential contamination if the probe cover tears, some authorities recommend presoaking transducers in alcohol for 30 minutes. Alternatively, ethylene oxide gas can be used to sterilize the transducer, but because this approach requires 24 hours, it limits the use of the probe to once a day. Furthermore, some equipment manufacturers do not recommend this method as it may ultimately damage the delicate outer coating of the transducer head.

Intraoperative ultrasound can be utilized for a variety of surgical applications. Neurosurgical uses of intraoperative ultrasound involve the brain and spinal cord, whereas intra-abdominal applications of intraoperative ultrasound have focused primarily on the liver, pancreas, and biliary tree (Figures 28-4 and 28-5). Nonetheless, this technique is increasingly being used to evaluate breast and renal tumors and vascular and gynecologic

diseases (Figures 28-6 and 28-7). Some intraoperative applications are to guide relatively simple procedures, such as biopsies, aspirations, and drainages; other applications are sophisticated, such as tumor ablation. Laparoscopic ultrasound is used to identify and stage tumors, to detect retained biliary calculi in patients undergoing laparoscopic cholecystectomy, and to assist thoracoscopic procedures. Endoluminal ultrasound is being utilized to evaluate vessels and grafts during vascular surgical procedures.

Intraoperative ultrasound is used to facilitate surgery. The technique can provide significant additional information to the surgeon at the time of the operation and may contribute to operative decision-making and surgical planning.

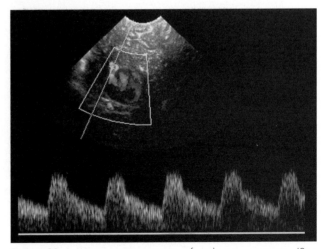

Figure 28-4 Intraoperative image of a brain aneurysm. (See Color Plate 50.) (Courtesy Philips Medical Systems, Bothell, WA.)

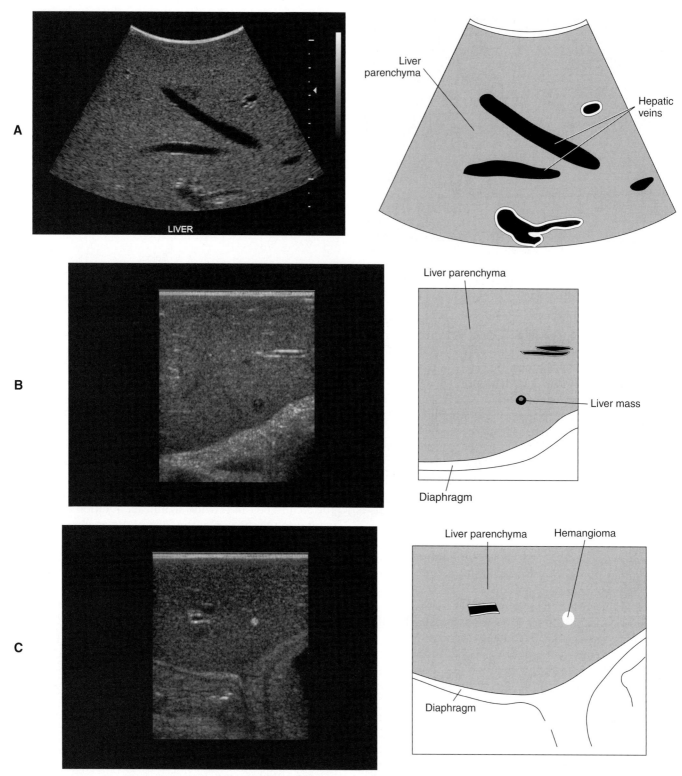

Figure 28-5 Intra-abdominal intraoperative ultrasound images. **A,** Transverse section of the liver. **B,** Intraoperative image of a small liver mass. **C,** Intraoperative image of a small liver hemangioma.

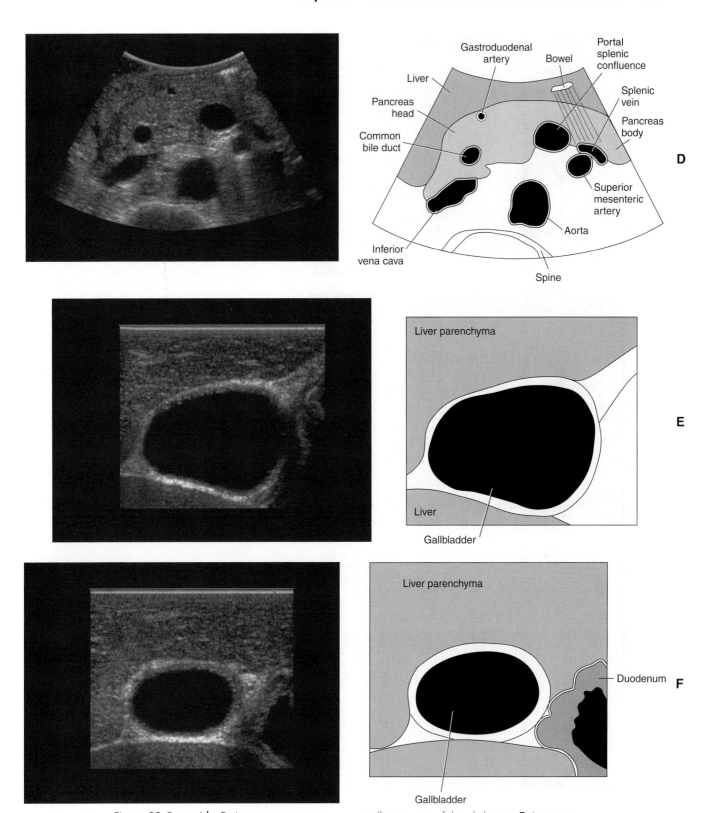

Figure 28-5, cont'd D, Intraoperative, transverse, midline section of the abdomen. E, Intraoperative view of the gallbladder. F, Intraoperative view of the gallbladder.

continued

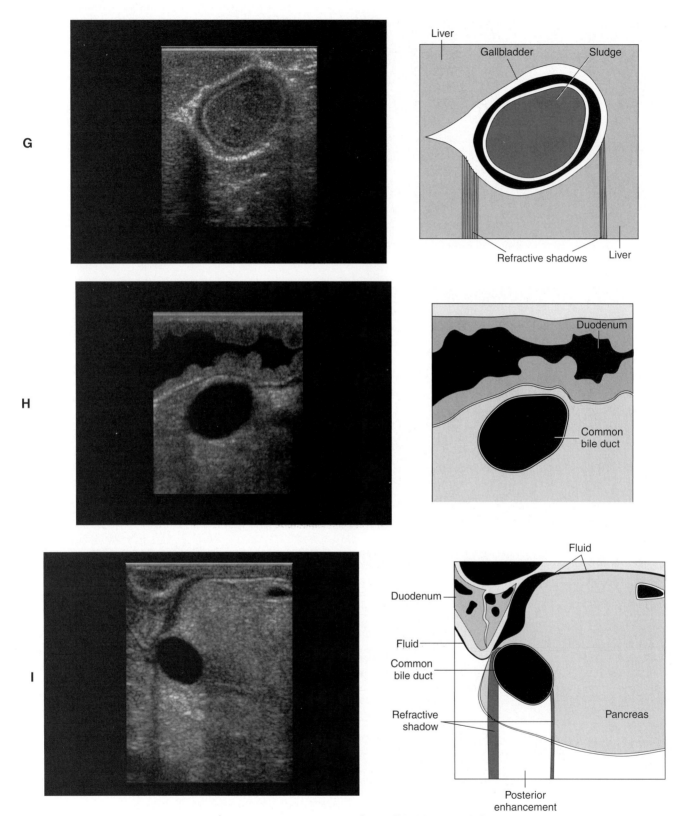

Figure 28-5, cont'd G, Intraoperative image of a gallbladder with sludge. H, Intraoperative view of the common bile duct and duodenum. I, Intraoperative image of the common bile duct.

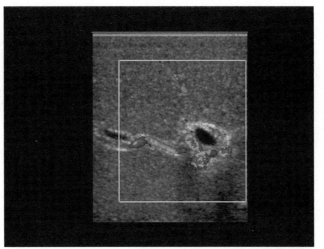

Figure 28-5, cont'd   J, Intraoperative, color Doppler image of the hepatic artery. (See Color Plate 51.) (Courtesy Philips Medical Systems, Bothell, Washington.)

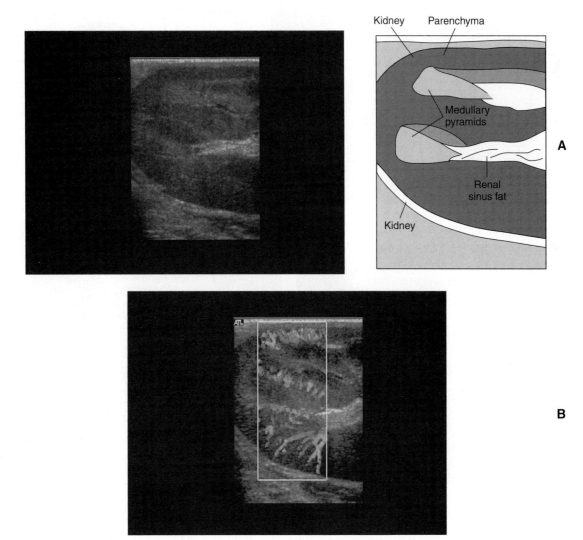

Figure 28-6   A, Intraoperative transverse section of the kidney. **B,** Color Doppler of the same section. (See Color Plate 52.) (Half-tone images courtesy Philips Medical Systems, Bothell, WA.)

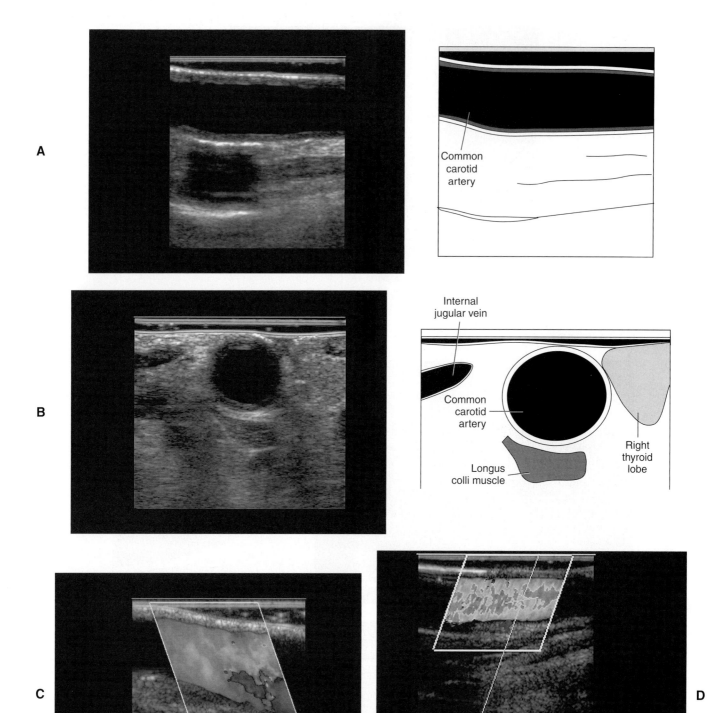

Figure 28-7 Vascular intraoperative ultrasound images. **A,** Longitudinal view of the internal carotid artery. **B,** Intraoperative transverse view of the internal common carotid artery. **C,** Intraoperative color Doppler image of the internal carotid artery. (See Color Plate 53.) **D,** Intraoperative color Doppler image of the internal carotid artery. (See Color Plate 54.)

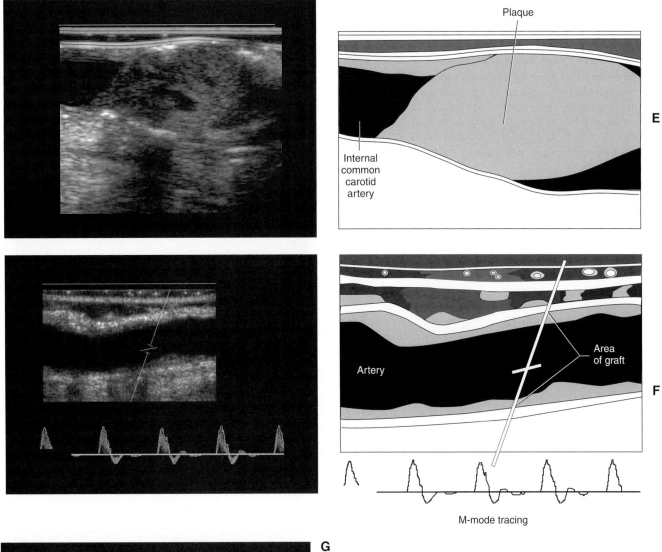

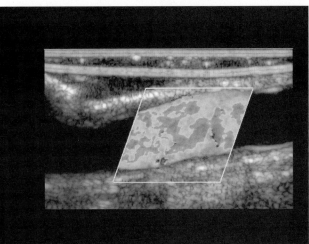

Figure 28-7, cont'd **E,** Intraoperative image of the internal carotid artery with plaque. **F,** Intraoperative image of an arterial graft with Doppler tracing. **G,** Intraoperative color Doppler image of an arterial graft. (See Color Plate 55.) (Half-tone image courtesy Philips Medical Systems, Bothell, WA.)

BIBLIOGRAPHY

Kruskal JB, Kane RA: Intraoperative sonography of the biliary system, AJR 177:395, 397, 2001.

Mittelstaedt CA: Intraoperative abdominal real-time ultrasound. In Abdominal ultrasound, New York, 1987, Churchill Livingstone, p 693.

Silas AM, Kruskal JB, Kane RA: Intraoperative ultrasound, Radiol Clin North Am 39(3):429-431, 2001.

Appendices

APPENDIX I

Ultrasound Documents Related to Patient Examination

LISA STROHL, KATHRYN A. GILL, AND BETTY BATES TEMPKIN

The ultrasound request form, patient chart, and final report are essential documents for ultrasound examinations. The following explanation should assist the entry-level sonographer in utilizing these materials.

ULTRASOUND REQUEST FORM AND PATIENT CHART

The sonographer usually reviews the ultrasound request form and patient chart before the ultrasound examination is performed. A request should include patient identification data, clinical symptoms, and the type of examination requested.

A sample request form is shown in Figure I-1. This form has four main sections. (Each institution uses a different type of request, dependent upon the information it requires.) The top right corner of this request is used to record patient identification. Adjacent to this section is the information needed to report preliminary results. To the far left is a check box for "stat" or portable procedures. Immediately beneath this area is a check box for patients who require isolation precautions.

The next section contains the referring physician's or clinic's name, address, and essential clinical data that explain the reason that the examination has been requested.

The following section contains space for additional patient history, a bar code for computerized entry into the department's data system, and space for the referring physician's signature and beeper number.

The last section of the form contains check-off boxes for the type of examination ordered. The lower left corner of the form contains space for sonographer identification and where the procedure was performed.

This request form stresses information needed in this particular tertiary care center. Notice the emphasis on providing assistance to referring physicians through preliminary reporting and listing the types of procedures that can be ordered.

Another document that sonographers review before an inpatient examination is the patient's chart. Refer to the accompanying list, in Appendix IV, of the different information that may be included in a chart. The most important items for sonographers are any type of assessment notes (the results of the physical examination, a listing of patient's symptoms, and the like) and laboratory test results. Most charts will contain labeled sections for easier reference.

Outpatient charts are kept in the referring physician's office; therefore it is essential that the ultrasound request contain the patient's clinical symptoms and the reason the ultrasound study was ordered. In addition to this, many ultrasound departments require sonographers to take a brief medical history of the patient before conducting the examination. In lieu of a detailed history provided on the request form, this may be the only means of obtaining pertinent information for outpatient examinations.

INTERPRETIVE REPORT (THE FINAL REPORT)

When the ultrasound examination is completed, the sonologist (usually a radiologist; always a physician) dictates a report, interpreting the ultrasound findings. The rendered diagnosis on the report can include a definitive diagnosis or a list of differential diagnoses (multiple pathologic conditions that may be indicated by the ultrasound findings) (Figure I-2). The final report is sent to the referring physician; a copy goes in the inpatient's chart, and a copy is kept in the patient's ultrasound file.

THE SONOGRAPHER'S TECHNICAL OBSERVATIONS

As part of the ultrasound study, it is the responsibility of the sonographer to collect pertinent clinical information along with documenting the appropriate images in order to provide the sonologist with the information

ULTRASOUND REQUEST

THOMAS JEFFERSON UNIVERSITY HOSPITAL

DEPARTMENT OF RADIOLOGY

DIVISION OF DIAGNOSTIC ULTRASOUND

MEDICAL RECORD #

NAME

☐ STAT

☐ PORTABLE

CALL PRELIMINARY REPORT TO:
DOCTOR
LOCATION
PHONE NO

ADDRESS

AGE

BIRTH DATE

PHONE NO.

ISOLATION PRECAUTION ☐ YES

REFERRING PHYSICIAN/CLINIC (NAME & ADDRESS)

PHONE NO.

ESSENTIAL CLINICAL FACTS • (MUST BE COMPLETED BEFORE EXAM IS PERFORMED)

REASON FOR EXAMINATION

RELEVANT MEDICAL HISTORY

A 3 4 1 4 7 6

PHYSICIAN'S SIGNATURE & BEEPER #   DATE

ABDOMEN	PELVIS	GYNECOLOGY
☐ **ABDOMEN COMPLETE**	☐ **RENAL TRANSPLANT**	☐ **PELVIS COMPLETE**
☐ LIVER	☐ URINARY BLADDER	☐ UTERUS
☐ GALLBLADDER	☐ PROSTATE	☐ OVARIES
☐ SPLEEN	☐ RECTUM	☐ FOLLICLE SIZE
☐ ASCITES	☐ SCROTUM	☐ IUD LOCALIZATION
☐ PALPABLE MASS	☐ DOPPLER	☐ DOPPLER
☐ DOPPLER	**HEAD AND NECK**	**OBSTETRICAL**
RETROPERITONEUM	☐ BRAIN	☐ **FETAL COMPLETE**
☐ **RETROPERITONEUM COMPLETE**	☐ URINARY BLADDER	☐ FETAL COMPLETE (INTERNAL GROWTH)
☐ PANCREAS	☐ URINARY BLADDER	☐ OBSTETRIC DOPPLER
☐ KIDNEYS	**HEART**	☐ AMNIOCENTESIS
☐ ADRENALS	☐ **COMPLETE ECHOCARDIOGRAM**	☐ SPECIAL (SPECIFY)
☐ AORTA/IVC	☐ M-MODE & 2D ECHOCARDIOGRAM	**SUPERFICIAL**
☐ LYMPH NODES	☐ DOPPLER ECHOCARDIOGRAM	☐ BREAST
☐ DOPPLER	**VASCULAR**	☐ PALPABLE
CHEST	☐ CEREBROVASCULAR COMPLETE	☐ JOINT/TENDON/MUSCLE
☐ MEDIASTINUM	☐ PERIPHERAL VASC. (ARTERIAL)	**INTERVENTIONAL**
☐ PLEURAL EFFUSION	☐ PERIPHERAL VASC. (VENOUS)	☐ BIOPSY (SPECIFY AREA BELOW)
☐ THORACENTESIS	☐ IMAGING ☐ IPG	☐ ASPIRATION (SPECIFY AREA BELOW)
	NOT LISTED	☐ ABSCESS DRAINAGE
	☐ (SPECIFY)	☐ INTRAOPERATIVE GUIDANCE
		AREA:

EXAM.	
TECH.	
ROOM	
DATE	

Figure I-1   Department request form.

FETAL AGE

DIAGNOSIS:

Findings compatible with complete spontaneous abortion, ectopic pregnancy, or very early intrauterine pregnancy.

COMMENT:

Real-time ultrasound of the pelvis was performed using transabdominal and endovaginal technique. No previous studies are available for review. The patient has a positive urine pregnancy test by history.

The uterus measures 10.2 x 4.2 x 5.0 cm. No intrauterine gestational sac is identified on transabdominal or endovaginal scan.

The left ovary is enlarged, measuring 4.2 x 2.9 x 3.6 cm. A cystic structure measuring less than 1 cm is seen in the left ovary.

The right ovary measures 2.6 x 1.1 x 2.8 cm. There are no right adnexal masses.

There is no free fluid in the cul de sac.

In light of the history of positive urine pregnancy test, the differential diagnosis for the above findings includes complete spontaneous abortion, ectopic pregnancy, or, less likely, very early intrauterine pregnancy. Correlation with serial beta-HCGs is advised.

Survey views of both kidneys reveal no hydronephrosis.

Figure I-2 Sonologist's final report on a fetal age study.

necessary to arrive at a diagnosis. Some institutions require sonographers to fill out a data sheet and also include a technical observation after the examination is completed. This information should include patient history, clinical symptoms, any laboratory test results, and any reports from other imaging tests or procedures. Technical observations should describe the sonographic appearance of the ultrasound findings, which include location, shape, size, and echogenicity.

Written documentation of any type, if retained, becomes part of the medical records. For this reason, the sonographer's technical observations should be documented in a way as not to be legally compromising. A sonographer could never "offer" a diagnosis simply because they have not had the curriculum to support that determination. However, a sonographer, based on knowledge and experience, can draw a conclusion from the ultrasound findings. A sonographer's conclusion regarding an ultrasound examination should never be part of the technical observations. The sonographer should comply with the heading "technical observations" by simply describing what is seen in sonographic terms. As discussed in Chapter 26, accurately describing the sonographic appearance of abnormalities is not dependent upon an understanding of diseases and their sonographic presentations.

In some cases, there is a fine line between describing something and drawing a conclusion. For example, one can describe the carotid artery as being stenosed. This is an *observation*. The cause of the stenosis may be a clot. This is a *conclusion*. A sonographer could describe the findings from a study to rule out an ectopic pregnancy as "Gestational sac with viable embryo visualized in the left adnexa." The sonographer might conclude but should never document that the findings are a viable ectopic pregnancy seen in the left adnexa. As another example, a sonographer can describe the liver as "enlarged." This is an observation. The sonographer cannot say that "The liver is enlarged due to primary hepatic carcinoma." The latter statement describes a conclusion regarding the cause of the enlargement.

Writing technical observations requires restraint and the careful selection of appropriate terminology. Keep in mind that technical observations are a summary of a sonographer's findings that may act as a reference for the interpreting physician; however, it is the documented images provided by the sonographer that the physician utilizes to render a diagnosis. If a sonographer fails to describe an abnormality in the technical observations, but demonstrates the abnormality on the images, he or she has performed within the legal guidelines of the scope of practice for diagnostic medical sonographers. The final interpretation of the ultrasound examination will always be the responsibility of the sonologist. By virtue of education, training, and legal parameters, physicians exclusively render diagnoses.

Additional examples of how to describe pathologies are listed below. Please refer to Chapter 26 for image reference. A clinical history has been added to the images to enhance the technical observations.

Example I: Figure 26-4
Clinical history: Heavy, prolonged periods, lumbar pain.
Sonographer technical observation: Uterus appears heterogeneous, enlarged, and markedly irregular in contour. Endometrial echo is not visualized.
Sonologist's diagnosis: Uterine fibroids.

Example II: Figure 26-6
Clinical history: RUQ (right upper quadrant) pain, N (nausea) and V (vomiting)
Sonographer's technical observation: Multiple echogenic foci within the gallbladder that shadow and move. (+) Murphy's sign during examination.
Sonologist's diagnosis: Cholecystitis with cholelithiasis (gallstones)

Example III: Figure 26-13
Clinical history: (+) pregnancy test, bleeding, and pelvic pain.

Sonographer technical observation: No evidence of an IUP (intrauterine pregnancy). Free fluid visualized superior and posterior to the uterus.

Sonologist's diagnosis: Ruptured ectopic pregnancy. Guidelines for writing technical observations have been developed by the Society of Diagnostic Medical Sonographers (SDMS) and the American Institute of Ultrasound in Medicine (AIUM). To obtain further information about technical observations, please contact either professional organization.

Ultrasound Instrumentation

LISA STROHL

This section describes the ultrasound system controls and explains how to operate them. Ultrasound systems are software-based systems and need to be configured correctly before some controls will appear on the touch panel or others will function as expected. Configuration is performed at installation by an ultrasound customer support representative.

Although hospitals around the world employ different types of ultrasound equipment, the basic "knobology" is the same. Here are a few of the common control buttons and their functions that may be used by an experienced professional performing the ultrasound examination.

KEYBOARD CONTROLS

Keyboard controls (alphanumeric) allow user to enter patient's name, ID number, and provide full screen annotation; they may also include specific function keys, for example:

1. **Annotation on/off,** which allows annotation to be entered from the keyboard onto the screen.
2. **Erase screen** will erase all user-entered annotations from the screen where the cursor is located.
3. **Backspace** will erase the last user-entered character to the left of the cursor.

Some systems employ a **HELP** menu to access and provide a quick reference manual to the system usage.

PRIMARY CONTROLS

Trackball. The basic functions of the trackball are to guide the cursor on the screen and position the measurement cursors during the freeze mode. In systems with cineloop, this control allows two-dimensional image review to be scrolled in real time. Depending upon the system, the trackball may serve various other functions.

Time Gain Compensation (TGC). TGC is used to equalize the differences in received echo amplitudes due to reflector depth. This is accomplished because the TGC provides a gradual increase in amplification with depth by compensating for attenuation of the signal strength over depth. This control adjusts the shape of the TGC curve. The TGC curve is displayed vertically to the right of the ultrasound image on the screen.

2-D/M Overall Gain. This controls the overall amplification or gain applied to the signals produced by the echoes returning from the body.

Focal Zone Position. This control positions the focal zone to the desired scan depth.

Focal Zone Depth. The depth range of the display is controlled by this function. Adjusting this will either increase or decrease the number of focal zones; however, the maximum allowed depth is dependent upon the scanhead selected.

Freeze Frame Key. Once the desired ultrasound image has been obtained, it may be stored in the system's memory by activating the freeze key. After the image is stored, measurements and calculations may be performed. Freezing automatically enables cineloop image review or Doppler review when applicable. Depress button when finished to restore frozen image to real time.

Print Key. Activates the resident multi-image camera to record the frozen image. The system will remain in freeze until the image is recorded. If the system was scanning before the print, it will resume scanning after the image is captured. If it was frozen before the print was taken, it will remain frozen.

Calc Key. Activates the appropriate calculations package.

Transducer Button (XCTR). This allows the operator to select different transducers and scan heads.

Image Direction. Depressing this button electronically reverses the scan direction of the displayed image.

Body Pattern. Used to display the body pattern to indicate patient positioning during the scan session.

New Patient Key. Will clear current patient ID, graphics, and comments so that new information may be entered.

Color Doppler/Power Doppler/Power Angio. These buttons allow the operator to activate the color or Power Doppler mode of the system.

Cine Loop. The memory of the ultrasound unit stores the recently scanned image frames before the freeze frame key is depressed. This allows for the images to be reviewed by the operator.

Measurement Keys
1. **Distance**—place cursor for distance measurements.
2. **Trace/Ellipse**—outline for curve or circumference measurements.
3. **Measure**—to complete above measurements and display results.
4. **Off**—to erase cursors, outlines, and measurement results.

Monitor Controls. Allows user to adjust the amount of detail in the ultrasound image.

Brightness. Adjusts the light output of the entire image.

Contrast. Adjusts the difference in light output between the light and dark parts of the image. CAUTION: Maintaining a very high display contrast level can damage your screen. Avoid using high-contrast settings for an extended period of time.

Needle/Biopsy Guide. This button activates a line display, which corresponds to the path of the needle used during invasive ultrasound procedures.

BASIC OPERATIONS
1. Enter patient name and ID. (Some machines may require depressing "new patient" soft key.)
2. After entering the information, press RETURN key to store patient information.
3. Place transducer on the patient with a generous amount of coupling gel.
4. Adjust TGC until desired image is obtained.
5. Adjust focal zones to cover the area of interest in the image.
6. Adjust image size by utilizing depth control.

Proper use of the above controls must be coupled with appropriate transducer selection. Below is a list of the basic types of transducers available with most modern machinery:
1. Flat linear array
2. Curved linear array
3. Electronic phases array
4. Annular array
5. Small footprint transducers

OTHER SPECIAL TRANSDUCERS PRODUCED TO HELP VIEW SPECIFIC AREAS OR FOR SPECIAL PROCEDURES:
1. Endocavital (Transvaginal and Transrectal)
2. Small Parts (5, 7, 10, 12 MHz)
3. Intraoperative
4. Endoluminal
5. Laparoscopic

Once the images have been stored, the next task is in the recording. Currently, there are a variety of ways in which images can be documented. Polaroid film makes it possible to record hard copies in black and white and even color. X-ray film can provide transparent or opaque hard copy images. Also, x-ray film can be used with a multi-image camera to record multiple images on a single sheet of film or photographic paper. Fiberoptic recorders using light-sensitive paper to produce black and white hard copy frozen images may also be used. Videotape recorders and video disk recorders are also being utilized to store information using a magnetic medium. The videotape recorder can store live or frozen images, and the newer video disk recorders are designed to store frozen images on mini diskettes. Many hospitals now use Picture Archival and Communications Systems (PACS). PACS captures images, which are stored on a hard drive and then sent to a computer work station to be reviewed and interpreted by a radiologist or sonologist. PACS is not limited to sending images to computers within a department or even a hospital; it has the capability of transmitting images to computers virtually anywhere.

Image Processing and Storage

LISA STROHL

Technology has rapidly moved image processing into the twenty-first century. Many hospitals and practices employ a range of film processing techniques, from the very basic to the most technologically advanced image processing and storage techniques. In this section we will cover the very basic film processing techniques as well as touch on some modern image processing and storage techniques.

Regardless of how competent a sonographer is, adequate visibility of necessary structures will not occur unless the film is properly developed. When employing basic film processing techniques, the individual developing the film must initially familiarize himself or herself with the darkroom layout upon entering the darkroom. First locate the processor and make sure it is on.

If it is not, there is usually a button about 5 inches under and to the left of the feeding tray that will turn the machine on. Next, locate the film bin but DO NOT OPEN. Doing so will expose the film inside and make it unusable. Before turning the lights out, orient the cassette so that changing the film will occur as rapidly and efficiently as possible. Turn on the safety light (usually red), and then turn off the overhead lights.

Lay the cassette on the counter. Begin to unload the cassette by pulling out the protective sheet on top of the cassette. This will slide right out if the tab is pulled. Turn down the safety strip located on the bottom of the cassette and slide the film out (Figure III-1, A). You will notice that the film has two different textured sides, a shiny side and

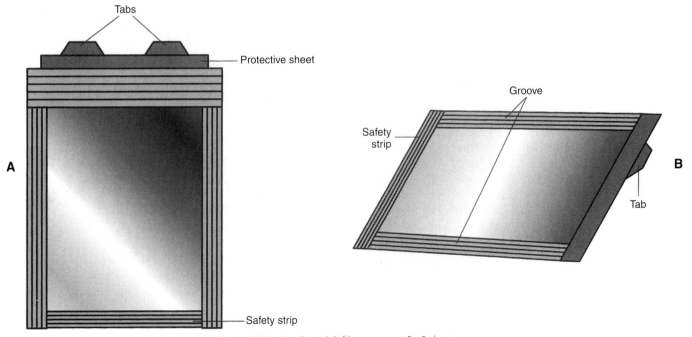

Figure III-1   A, 8 × 10 film cassette. B, Side view.

a dull side (the emulsion side). Place the film on the feeding tray of the processor with the shiny side down and push forward until the film is taken in by the processor's rollers. To avoid jamming the processor, a low-level bell will sound, indicating that the processor is now ready to accept another film. To reload the cassette, reach into the film bin for a single sheet of film. Place the shiny side down and slip it into the cassette, making sure the film is wedged between the two grooves along the length of the cassette. Flip up the safety strip and replace the protective sheet with the white border facing outward to show that the cassette contains unexposed film (Figure III-1, *B*). If both sides of the cassette are exposed, repeat this process. Before turning the lights back on, make sure the film bin is closed and that your film in the processor is secured from light exposure. (The low-level bell will ring.) Once this is checked, turn the lights on. Your film will drop into the receiving bin when it is fully developed.

The type of system described above is known as automatic processing and was developed in the 1950's. It increased efficiency and improved image quality, compared with the old way of developing film by hand. As film is fed into the film tray, the transport system begins to process the film. Excluding the entering rollers at the feed tray, most of the rollers in the transport system are positioned on a rack assembly. These racks are easily removable and provide for convenient, efficient maintenance of the processor. Completing this process is the dryer system, which thoroughly extracts all residual moisture from the processed film and drops it into the receiving bin either inside or outside the darkroom. This entire process takes 90 seconds.

Another type of processing system employed at some hospitals is commonly known as daylight processing. There is no manual loading or unloading of film necessary, and therefore the concept of a darkroom is eliminated. Instead, the system is divided into a modular dispenser and a modular unloader with automatic identification.

The dispenser is divided into two basic parts. The upper half is for unexposed film storage and dispensing, and the lower half accepts and lifts the empty cassette for loading one sheet of film. When an empty cassette is placed in the cradle of the dispenser and pressed against a pair of interlock switches, the cassette is automatically lifted to the load position. It is recommended that the cassette be inserted with the white side out; however, this switch will not close if the cassette is upside down. The arrow on the display panel appears as an indication that a film is being dispensed. The cassette is then lowered and ready for use. In addition to these features, a base for dispenser support and cassette storage is provided (Figure III-2).

To use the modular unloader, first observe on the display panel that the green power light is on. Insert the pa-

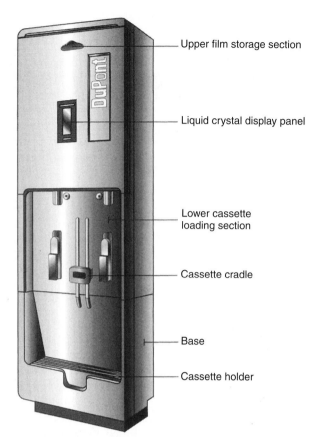

Figure III-2 Modular dispenser.

tient identification card into the slot provided with the image side down. Next, insert a cassette with the green-colored side toward the operator. A spring-loaded movable guide block adjusts automatically to match the width of the cassette. Press down on the cassette and observe the display panel to see an image of the film leaving the cassette. This will not occur if the cassette is upside down. When the above process is complete, remove the cassette and wait for your image to be processed (Figure III-3).

With either automatic processing or daylight processing systems, the sequence of events when processing a film is as follows:

1. **Wetting:** This step swells the emulsion to permit subsequent chemical penetration.
2. **Development:** This is the production of the manifest image from the latent image. The temperature during this stage is most critical and should remain constant at around 93° F.
3. **Stop bath:** During this time, the developmental process is finished and excess chemicals are removed from the film's emulsion.
4. **Fixing:** The fixer removes the remaining silver halide from the emulsion and hardens the gelatin covering the film.
5. **Washing:** This is the final removal of any excess chemicals before the ultimate step occurs.

Labels on Figure III-2:
- Upper film storage section
- Liquid crystal display panel
- Lower cassette loading section
- Cassette cradle
- Base
- Cassette holder

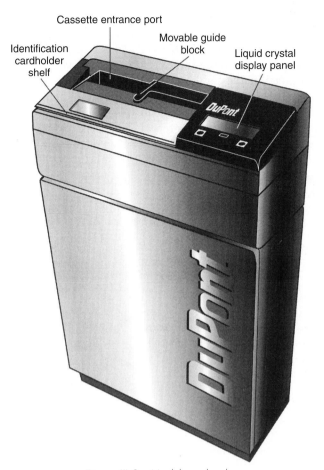

Identification
cardholder
shelf

Cassette entrance port

Movable guide
block

Liquid crystal
display panel

Figure III-3 Modular unloader.

6. **Drying:** It is during this step that excess water is removed and the film is prepared for viewing.

Film development is a chemical reaction, and it is governed by three physical properties: time, temperature, and concentration of the developer. Manufacturers of film and developing chemicals have carefully selected the conditions for these parameters to work optimally. Deviation from these recommendations will result in loss of image quality, possibly due to chemical or developmental fog.

As with any electromechanical device, maintenance is crucial. If the equipment is not properly maintained, it will malfunction when least expected, causing serious delays in providing optimal images by decreasing film quality.

Many larger hospitals employ a laser printing system that may link several imaging modalities on a network to a central laser printer. This is usually done with a keypad attached to the ultrasound machine, which is then networked to a centrally located laser printer.

A wave of the future is the filmless department that can be instituted by using a computer technology system called PACS, short for Picture Archiving and Communication System. This new computer technology allows for improved film resolution, increased sensitivity of Doppler, and faster frame rates. The ultrasound images are acquired digitally, and viewed and stored on a computer (Figure III-4). This system can be dedicated to the ultrasound department or utilized throughout the entire radiology department, hospital, or outside hospitals and other computers located virtually anywhere that are equipped with PACS capabilities.

PACS's ability to interface with other computer systems within the hospital allows the sonographer to communicate with the Hospital Information System (HIS) to capture the demographic information of the patient and the patient's medical record. It also may have the ability to interface with the Radiology Information System (RIS). Communicating with RIS via PACS provides the sonographer with images and reports from other imaging examinations that the patient may have had previously. Some of the main advantages of PACS are that it allows for quick and reliable retrieval of

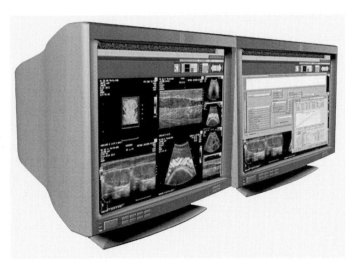

Figure III-4 Computer monitor employing PACS. (Courtesy McKesson Corp.)

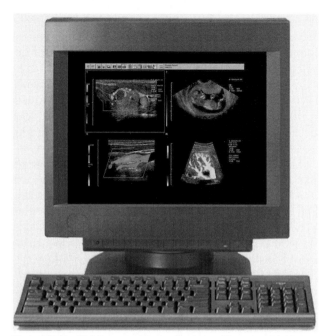

Figure III-5 PACS computer workstation. (Courtesy McKesson Corp.)

images, and that it allows ability to send images to remote locations for interpretation (teleradiology).

A PACS system works basically by capturing the ultrasound image, storing it locally on a hard drive, and then sending it to the computer work station. The images may then be interpreted at the work station by a radiologist or sonologist (Figure III-5). The images are then digitally stored, with or without a report, long term on magneto-optical (MO) disks or other digital storage media.

BIBLIOGRAPHY

Acuson XP: Acoustic Imaging AI 5200, ATL Ultramark 9, and General Electric Operator's Instrumentation Manuals.

Bushong SC: *Radiologic science for technologists,* ed 7, St Louis, 2001, Mosby, pp 225-240.

De Jong MR: *PACS: use in an ultrasound laboratory,* Johns Hopkins Hospital, September 1997.

EI Dupont De Nemours Co Inc: *Dupont Modular Daylight System Operations Manual: modular dispenser and modular unloader: auto ID,* Wilmington, 1987.

Pickney N: *A review of the concepts of ultrasound physics and instrumentation,* West Point, PA, 1991, Sonicor Inc.

Promotional material supplied by A.L.I. Technologies, Inc.

APPENDIX IV

Patient Chart Information: Medical/Surgical Assembly Order

LISA STROHL

The following lists the type of information found in inpatient charts. Items of particular importance to sonographers are in boldface type.

ROUTINE INPATIENT CHART

Diagnosis worksheet
Admission form
Consent for routine examination and treatment
Patient authorizations
Consent for operations, procedures, etc.
Consent for anesthesia
Release form
Living will
Preadmission forms
Physician's orders for admission
Discharge summary
Discharge summary sheet
Emergency room record
Patient care plan
Acute dialysis unit patient care plan
Patient problem list
Nursing transfer summary
History, physical progress notes
Social work evaluation and social work notes go in date order within progress notes
Respiratory care department, patient care record
Patient teaching record
Discharge planning record
Discharge planning assessment
Home IV therapy performance checklist
Instructions to patient
Discharge summary note
Consultations

Cardiac catheterization reports
    Preoperative nursing record
    Cardiac catheterization nursing
    Preliminary catheterization report
    Catheterization report
Operative reports: Perioperative nursing record
Preoperative anesthesia summary
Operative notes
Pathology
OR sponge/instrument count
Postanesthesia record
Recovery room record
Cardiopulmonary perfusion record
Endoscopy report
Fibroscopic bronchoscopy
Data mount
Clinical laboratory summary sheets
MRICU blood gas laboratory report
Radiology reports
Ultrasound reports
EKG rhythm strips
EEG
Nuclear medicine
Pulmonary function test
Request for blood components and testing
Antibody ID report
Blood component-ID tag
Miscellaneous
Energy expenditure—Nutrition department
Cardiopulmonary resuscitation record
Transfer order sheet
Adult total nutrient admixture physician's treatment sheet
Acute dialysis unit treatment sheet
Physician's treatment sheets
    Precatheterization orders
    Postanesthesia physician's treatment sheets
Physician's order sheet for antimicrobial agents

Lists of documents that comprise patient charts courtesy Thomas Jefferson University Hospital, Philadelphia, PA.

Assessment notes
  Assessment guidelines/falls risk potential
  Assessment guidelines/pressure sore potential
  Nursing assessment
  Daily assessment
Medication administration record
Nursing Kardex
Nursing care record
Critical care flow sheet
Flow sheet
Neurologic assessment sheet
Neurologic checklist
Diabetes control chart
Intake-output chart
Graphic record

OB CHART*
Diagnosis worksheet
Admission form
Consent forms
Obstetric discharge summary
Prenatal
  Initial pregnancy profile
  Health history summary
  Prenatal flow record
Perinatal data base
Patient care plan
Progress notes
Discharge instruction sheet
Operative notes
Delivery room count record
Labor unit prep room assessment
Holister forms
  Obstetric admitting record
  Labor progress chart
  Labor and delivery summary
  Postpartum progress notes
Labs
Radiology
EKG
Obstetric ultrasound
Antenatal evaluation center form
Physician's treatment sheets
Medication sheets
Nursing Kardex
Nursing care record
(Antenatal unit) pad count
Intake-output chart
Graphic record

BABY CHART*
Diagnosis worksheet
Admission form

---

*Newborn identification/footprints to be kept with birth certificate on mother's chart.

Birth certificate
Consent forms
Newborn discharge summary
Pediatric admission nursing assessment and discharge planning
Patient care plan
Progress notes
Discharge instructions
Holister forms
  Obstetric admitting record
  Labor and delivery summary
  Labor progress chart
  Initial newborn profile
  Newborn flow record
Footprints
MicroBase
Labs
Newborn maturity rating and class
Growth record for infants
Audiologic record
Impedance measurement
Neonatal neurosonography
Pulmonary evaluation and diagnostic system neonatal test report
Physician's treatment sheets
Nursing Kardex
Flow sheets
IV therapy record
Apnea and bradycardia record

REHAB CHART
Same order as medical chart except for the following forms:
  1. Patient discharge/readmission form: before discharge summary
  2. Assessment/treatment/plan/goals form: before progress notes
Department of Rehabilitation Medicine progress note sheet: behind progress notes
  3. Interdisciplinary conference summary and discharge plan form: after progress notes
The following forms are placed in the miscellaneous section of the chart in the order listed:
  4. Neurologic examination
  5. Record of patient visits
  6. Occupational therapy section form
  7. Physical therapy section, general rehabilitation in patient summary form

PSYCHIATRY ASSEMBLY ORDER
  1. Application for involuntary emergency examination and treatment forms are placed behind consent forms
  2. Psychiatric data base form: after ER sheets
  3. 12-Hour treatment plan: after psychiatric data base

4. Creative arts therapies form: after 72-hour treatment plan
5. Psychiatric data base, corresponds to admissions
6. Crisis medication sheet: before medication administration sheets

7. Seclusion/restraint observation record: behind flow sheets
8. Observation checklist for patients in seclusion or on suicide precautions form: behind seclusion/restraint observation record

■ APPENDIX V

Universal Precautions

KATHRYN A. GILL

Increased concern for healthcare workers becoming infected with bloodborne diseases through accidental needle sticks and spills was the impetus for the Occupational Safety and Health Administration (OSHA) to issue a standard designed to protect healthcare workers. The major bloodborne diseases that healthcare providers may be exposed to on the job include the various forms of hepatitis, such as hepatitis B (HBV), and syphilis, malaria, and human immunodeficiency virus (HIV). Of these, HBV and HIV are the two most significant. These diseases can be transmitted in body fluids such as blood, saliva, semen, vaginal secretions, amniotic fluid, cerebrospinal fluid, synovial fluid, and pericardial fluid. Other sources of transmission could include dental procedures, handling unfixed tissues or organs from living or dead humans, handling cell or tissue cultures contaminated with HIV/HBV as well as organ cultures and culture mediums or similar solutions. Research workers must also be careful when handling blood, organs, or tissues from HIV/HBV-contaminated experimental animals.

There are many ways these diseases can be transmitted. Accidental injuries from contaminated sharp objects, such as needles, scalpels, broken glass, and exposed dental wires are among the most common. Exposure can occur from open cuts and skin abrasions, including dermatitis and acne and by way of the mucous membranes of the mouth, nose, and eyes. Touching contaminated surfaces and transferring the infectious material to the mouth, nose, or eyes is a more indirect means of transmission. Healthcare workers must be aware that work surfaces can be heavily contaminated without visible evidence. Surface contamination is a major mode of transmission for HBV, especially in hemodialysis units. It is known that HBV can survive dried on surfaces at room temperature for at least 1 week.

Since we cannot know, with certainty, every patient carrying or infected with a bloodborne disease, univer-

sal precautions require us to treat all patients as if they were known to be infected with HIV, HBV, or other bloodborne diseases. OSHA guidelines provide us with five major tactics to reduce our risks of exposure. They include establishing engineering controls, employee work practices, housekeeping protocols, providing personal protective equipment, and offering vaccination against hepatitis B.

Engineering controls involve things such as the utilization of autoclaves and sterilization methods, self-sheathing needles, and the use of biosafety cabinets and disposal methods. Work practice protocols include wearing protective gear such as gloves, and concentration on personal hygiene, such as frequent hand washing. Housekeeping controls include keeping equipment clean and contaminant free as well as disposing of sharps and laundry into the appropriate containers. Last, vaccination against hepatitis B is optional and is provided at no cost to the healthcare employees if their jobs put them at risk for exposure. The vaccine is administered over a 6-month period and in three injections and is 85% to 97% effective for 9 years or longer. Those who should not be vaccinated include individuals whose antibody test indicates they are immune, those who have already received the complete vaccination series, or those with a specific medical reason.

Medical facilities are now required to offer an inservice to employees regarding the OSHA requirements and guidelines. Please check with the Human Resource or Infection Control Departments for a schedule of inservices at your facility.

BIBLIOGRAPHY

American Medical Association: *Bloodborne pathogens*, Chicago, The Association.

Occupational Safety and Health Administration: *OSHA standard for bloodborne pathogens*, Washington, DC, 1991, U.S. Department of Labor.

Illustration Credit Page

Chapter 1

Figures 1-1, 1-2, 1-3, 1-6, 1-7, 1-8, 1-9, 1-10, 1-11, 1-12, and 1-13: Modified from Pinkney N: *A review of concepts of ultrasound physics and instrumentation,* ed 4, Copiague, NY, 1992, Sonicor, Inc.

Chapter 2

Figures 2-1, 2-5, 2-6, 2-9, 2-14, 2-20, 2-26, 2-27, and 2-29: Modified from Pinkney N: *A review of concepts of ultrasound physics and instrumentation,* ed 6, Copiague, NY, 1997, Sonicor, Inc.

Figure 2-12: From Pinkney N: *A review of concepts of ultrasound physics and instrumentation,* ed 4, Copiague, NY, 1992, Sonicor, Inc.

Figures 2-10, 2-15, 2-18, 2-19, 2-21, 2-22, 2-23, 2-24, 2-25, 2-26, 2-27, 2-28, 2-30, 2-31, 2-32: Modified from Pinkney N: *Ultrasound physics, imaging, instrumentation, and Doppler,* Copiague, NY, 2001, Sonicor, Inc.

Chapter 3

Figure 3-2, *A:* From Thibodeau G: *Anatomy and physiology,* ed 4, St. Louis, 1999, Mosby, pp 280-281.

Figures 3-5 and 3-6: From Herlihy B: *The human body in health and illness,* ed 1, Philadelphia, 2000, WB Saunders, p 309.

Chapter 4

Figures 4-6, 4-10, 4-11, 4-12, 4-13, and 4-14, *D:* From Tempkin BB: *Ultrasound scanning: principles and protocols,* Philadelphia, 1993, WB Saunders.

Unnumbered Figure 4-1 and Figure 4-14, *A* and *C:* From Lane A, Sharfaei H: *Modern section anatomy,* Philadelphia, 1992, WB Saunders.

Chapter 13

Figure 13-6, *A:* From Copenhaver WM: *Bailey's textbook of histology,* ed 16, Baltimore, 1971, Williams & Wilkins, p 361.

Chapter 22

Opening Figure and Figures 22-1, 22-2, 22-7, 22-8, 22-9, 22-10, 22-11, 22-12, 22-13, 22-14, 22-15, 22-16, 22-17, 22-18, and 22-20: Redrawn from Tempkin BB: *Ultrasound scanning: principles and protocols,* Philadelphia, 1993, WB Saunders.

Chapter 23

Figures 23-17, 23-24, and 23-30: From Park MK: *Pediatric cardiology for practitioners,* ed 2, Chicago, 1988, Year Book.

Figure 23-27: Modified from Park MK: *Pediatric cardiology for practitioners,* ed 2, Chicago, 1988, Year Book.

Chapter 25

Figure 25-18: From Neumeyer MM, Thiele BL: Evaluation of lower extremity occlusive disease with Doppler ultrasound. In Taylor KJW, Burns PN, Wells PNT, editors: *Clinical applications of Doppler ultrasound,* New York, 1988, Raven Press.

Index

Page references followed by "f" indicate figures and by "t" indicate tables.